Sports Injury Management

Sports Injury Management

Marcia K. Anderson, Ph. D., L.A.T.,C.

Professor and Director, Athletic Training Program

Department of Movement Arts, Health Promotion, and Leisure Studies

Bridgewater State College

Bridgewater, Massachusetts

Susan J. Hall, Ph. D.

Professor and Director of Graduate Studies

Department of Kinesiology and Physical Education

California State University, Northridge

Northridge, California

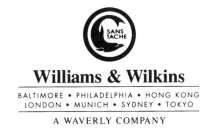

Williams & Wilkins

BALTIMORE • PHILADELPHIA • HONG KONG
LONDON • MUNICH • SYDNEY • TOKYO

A WAVERLY COMPANY

Williams & Wilkins

Executive Editor: Donna Balado
Developmental Editor: Lisa Stead
Production Coordinator: Mary Clare Beaulieu
Manuscript Editor: Raymond Lukens

Copyright© 1995
Williams & Wilkins
Rose Tree Corporate Center
1400 North Providence Rd., Suite 5025
Media, PA 19063–2043 USA

Accurate indications, adverse reactions, and dosage schedules for drugs are provided in this book, but it is possible they may change. The reader is urged to review the package information data of the manufacturers of the medications mentioned.

Printed in the United States of America

Library of Congress Cataloging in Publication Data
Anderson, Marcia K.
    Sports injury management / Marcia K. Anderson, Susan J. Hall.
      p. cm.
    Includes index.
    ISBN 0-683-00175-2
    1. Sports injuries. I. Hall, Susan J. (Susan Jean). 1953– .
  II. Title
  RD97.A53 1995
  617.1'027—dc20   94-22447

94 95 96 97 98
1   2   3   4   5   6   7   8   9   10

Our primary goal for *Sports Injury Management* is to integrate basic medical concepts and related scientific information to provide a foundation in the prevention, recognition, assessment, management, disposition, and rehabilitation of sports-related injuries and illnesses. Any individual responsible for providing health care to sports participants should be able to recognize life-threatening injuries, determine if a possible fracture or major ligament damage is present, manage the immediate injury, and determine whether immediate referral to a physician is necessary.

Written as an introductory text for a one-term athletic training class, this book is suitable for students interested in athletic training, coaching, exercise physiology, health education, health fitness, physical therapy, recreation, physical education, and youth sports. Its unique format introduces the student to new topics through a problem-solving approach using pertinent case studies. The text is easy to read and is supplemented with detailed line art, photographs, and tables to further promote understanding and retention of material introduced in the text.

CONTENT AND ORGANIZATION

The text is divided into six parts. Each part opens with a special feature highlighting a noted professional in the athletic training field. Among those featured are:

Earlene Durrant, Ph.D., A.T.,C.
Director Athletic Training Curriculum
Brigham Young University
Provo, Utah

Kathy Fox, M.A., L.A.T.,C., P.T., S.C.S.
Director of the Sports Medicine Program
Braintree Hospital Rehabilitation Network
Braintree, Massachusetts

Ron O'Neil, L.A.T.,C.
Head Athletic Trainer
New England Patriots Professional Football Team
Foxboro, Massachusetts

Yoshitaka Ando, B.S., L.A.T.,C.
Head Athletic Trainer
Lincoln-Sudbury Regional High School
Sudbury, Massachusetts

Maria Hutsick, M.S., L.A.T.,C.
Head Athletic Trainer
Boston University
Boston, Massachusetts

Marsha Grant, M.Ed., A.T.,C.
Head Athletic Trainer
Sterling High School
Somerdale, New Jersey

These interviews are designed to introduce the student to individuals who work in traditional and nontraditional athletic training settings. These individuals provide a unique look at the field of athletic training, and discuss how they got interested in athletic training as a career option. Each NATA-Certified Athletic Trainer speaks frankly about the ups and downs of the job, and many share personal stories about why athletic training is so important to the overall health care of sports participants.

Section I: Foundations of Sports Injury Management (Chapters 1–2). Chapter 1 opens with an introduction to sports injury management and outlines the key role athletic trainers play as part of the primary sports medicine team. In addition, standards of professional practice, legal liability, record keeping, and career opportunities in athletic training are discussed. Chapter 2 provides the student with information on the mechanics of injury to soft tissues, bones, and nerves. The healing process for specific tissues, the basis of pain, and factors that mediate pain are also explained.

Section II: Sports Injury Management (Chapters 3 to 6). Chapter 3 introduces the HOPS format (**H**istory, **O**bservation and inspection, **P**alpation, and **S**pecial Tests) used in basic injury assessment, and relates this process to emergency procedures. The process is further expanded upon in Chapter 4 as it relates specifically to sports injury assessment. Chapter 5 discusses therapeutic exercise and therapeutic modalities used to facilitate healing and introduces the student to the SOAP format (**S**ubjective, **O**bjective, **A**ssessment, and **P**lan) used in advanced injury assessment. Chapter 6 provides information on protective equipment used to prevent injury to specific body regions.

Section III: Injuries to the Lower Extremity (Chapters 7 to 9), Part IV: Injuries to the Upper Extremity (Chapters 10 to 12), Part V: Injuries to the Axial Region (Chapters 13 to 15). Each chapter begins with a general review of anatomy and biomechanical overview of the joint or body region. Next, prevention of injury is discussed, followed by information on specific sports injuries and their management. Finally, a step-by-step injury assessment of the region is presented using the HOPS format, and examples of rehabilitation exercises are provided for the treatment plan.

Section VI: Special Conditions Related to Sports (Chapters 16 and 17). Chapter 16 discusses injuries and conditions related to the reproductive system, including injuries to the genitalia, sexually transmitted diseases, and menstrual irregularities. Chapter 17 concludes with other health conditions that can affect sport performance, such as respiratory tract infections, gastrointestinal problems, viral diseases, diabetes, anemia, epilepsy, hypertension, substance abuse, and eating disorders.

PEDAGOGICAL FEATURES

As educators, we have highlighted information in the text by incorporating several pedagogical features to enhance the text's usefulness as a teaching tool. This is designed to increase readability and retention of pertinent and necessary information. These in-text features include:

Learning Objectives

Each chapter opens with a set of learning objectives. These objectives list the most important concepts in the chapter that the student should focus on during reading.

Thought Questions

Thought questions, identified by a question mark, are found at the beginning of each major section within each chapter. These questions encourage the student to analyze information critically and to solve problems in the scenario presented. The answer to each thought question is provided at the end of that section within the text, and is identified by a light bulb.

Marginal Definitions and Tips

New or unfamiliar words are in bold print within the text, and their definition is provided in the margin. This allows the student easy access to and better retention of new vocabulary terms. Important sentences or facts are also summarized in the margins to assist the learning process.

Tables

Several chapters have tables that expand upon pertinent information discussed in the text. This allows a large amount of didactic knowledge to be organized in an easy-to-read summary of information.

Field Strategies

A unique feature of this book is the use of Field Strategies to clinically apply cognitive knowledge. In Parts III, IV, and V, for example, the charts move step by step through the signs and symptoms of a specific injury, list immediate management, and provide several rehabilitation exercises for the condition. This careful integration of cognitive knowledge and the practical application of that knowledge is designed to assist the learning process.

Art and Photography Program

Art plays a major role in facilitating the learning process. The editor and authors have worked hard to incorporate appropriate illustrations and photographs to supplement material presented in the text. A graphic artist with extensive experience as a medical illustrator has provided realistic and accurate figures to depict anatomical structures, and has devised innovative approaches to illustrate injury mechanisms. Each illustration was carefully reviewed to assess detail and accuracy.

Summary

Each chapter has a summary of the key concepts discussed in the text. Several chapter summaries also contain a list of injuries or conditions that necessitate immediate referral to a physician for further care.

References

Any valuable teaching tool must include a listing of cited references used to gather information for the text. This provides the instructor and student with an accurate bibliography that can be referred to if additional information on the topic is needed.

Glossary and Index

At the end of the book, the student will find an extensive glossary of terms, many of which have appeared as marginal definitions. Furthermore, the comprehensive index contains cross-referencing information to locate specific information within the text.

Supplements

To facilitate the classroom experience, we have developed several teaching tools to assist the instructor in presenting information and in assessing student retention. In addition, material is also available for the student to add further reinforcement of material presented in the text. These features include:

Instructor's Manual

Written by Dr. Malissa Martin, Director of the Undergraduate Athletic Training Curriculum Program at the University of South Carolina, the Instructor's Manual provides suggestions and exercises to supplement material presented in each chapter. The modules include chapter objectives, vocabulary terms, and laboratory exercises including injury scenarios to facilitate the learning process. These injury scenarios parallel those presented in the Student Manual. At the end of the Instructor's Manual are over 1,000 sample test questions that cover pertinent information in each of the chapters.

Computerized Testbank

For your convenience, this computerized test bank offers a flexible, time-saving method to create original, challenging tests using over 700 test questions in the testbank. With this program, you will be able to create, format, edit, and print exams to fit your specific needs. This testbank is available to adopters of the text on both Macintosh and IBM-compatible computers.

Student Manual

Also developed by Dr. Malissa Martin, Director of the Undergraduate Athletic Training Curriculum Program at the University of South Carolina, the Student Manual uses a problem-solving approach to challenge the student in the clinical application of cognitive knowledge presented in the text. The injury scenarios parallel those presented in the Instructor's Manual, and are designed to move the student step by step through the HOPS format, emphasizing proper vocabulary skills, and techniques to thoroughly assess and manage each injury. In addition, short answers to questions are provided for students to review the basic concepts presented in each chapter.

Bridgewater, Massachusetts   Marcia K. Anderson

Northridge, California   Susan J. Hall

Acknowledgments

The authors would like to express sincere appreciation for the support and guidance provided by friends and colleagues, many of whom assisted in the development of the text through critical analysis and review of the initial drafts. These colleagues include: Kim Barrett, University of Florida; John Cottone, SUNY Cortland; Bill Holcomb, San Jose State University; Malissa Martin, University of South Carolina; John Miller, University of New Hampshire; and Charles J. Redmond, Springfield College.

In addition to the reviewers, several colleagues and friends assisted in the preparation of the manuscript. Special thanks are extended to Marjorie A. King, M.S., A.T.C., R.P.T., who did the initial draft of Chapters 4 and 5, and Therese Joseph, R.P.T., who assisted in the development of the rehabilitation exercises listed in the individual joint chapters. Frank Forney of BioGraphics did a superb job on the line art illustrations, and Denise Passaretti of Passaretti Photography did an outstanding job on many of the set shots used in the text. A special thanks to my good friend and colleague Professor Cheryl Hitchings for her valued input and patience in assuming additional tasks within the department so that I could successfully complete this important contribution to the profession.

We would like to acknowledge all the help, direction, and guidance provided by our good friends Pat Coryell and Grace Wong, who assisted us through the first draft, and continue to provide valued support. Finally, a special thanks to the many dedicated and talented people at Williams & Wilkins, publishers, who took on the ominous task of polishing the manuscript and pulling the loose ends together. We are indebted to Lisa Stead, Developmental Editor, and Tina D'Antonio, Editorial Assistant, whose quick responses to our many phone calls and continual feedback was most helpful in maintaining our sanity. Thank you!

Marcia K. Anderson
Susan J. Hall

Contents

Field Strategies

Sports Injury Management

Foundations of Sports Injury Management

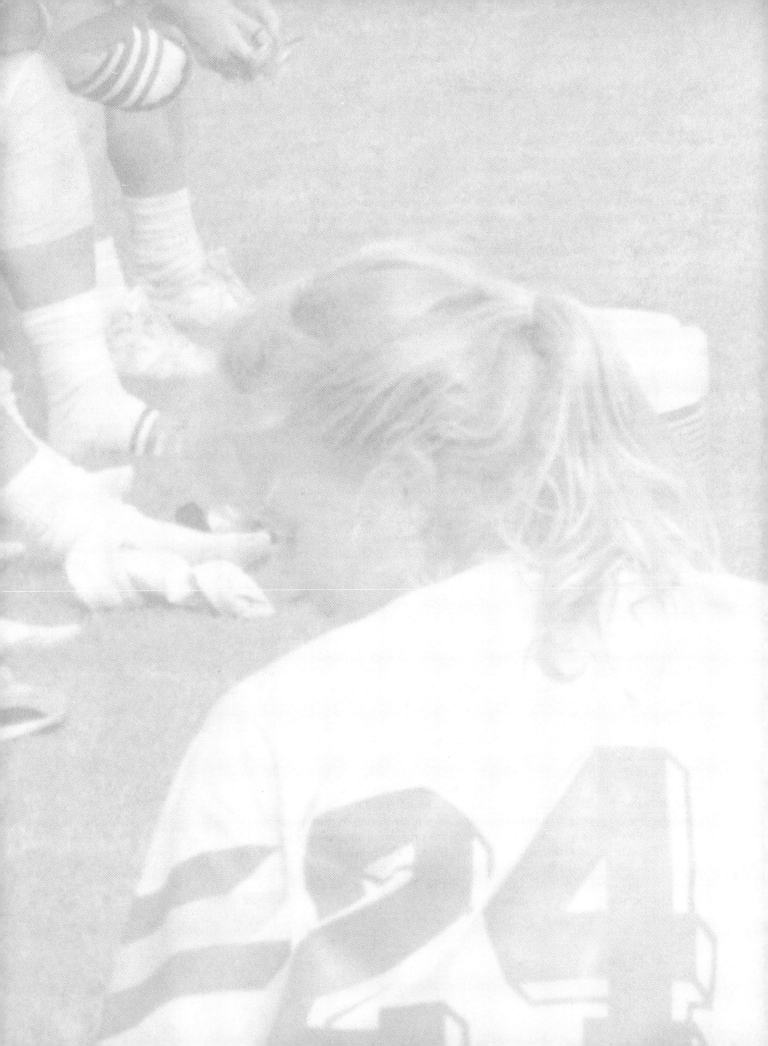

Earlene Durrant, Ph.D., A.T.,C.

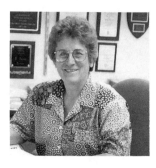

Dr. Earlene Durrant is a Professor and Director of the Athletic Training Curriculum Program at Brigham Young University in Provo, Utah. As one of the first athletic trainers ever to receive a Ph.D., she was the first woman elected President of the Utah Athletic Trainer's Association, and the first woman ever appointed to chair a national NATA committee.

I came to BYU in 1973 to complete my Ph.D. in Physical Education. Title IX had just been passed, and the university realized they needed a women's athletic trainer. Because I was the only female on the staff who had ever taped an ankle, I was elected. My clinical hours were completed under the direction of the certified staff trainers at BYU, and I became certified in 1975, when there were fewer than a dozen certified women in the United States.

I started out as the Women's Athletic Trainer for ten Division I teams and six extramural teams. In 1980, when the athletic curriculum was approved by the NATA, my workload tripled when I became the primary educator and administrator of the curriculum program. Despite this, I love the job and would not trade it for the world.

As a curriculum coordinator, I am responsible for the day-to-day functional running of the academic program, including recruiting students, interviewing and testing students for admission into the program, academic advising, scheduling, working with the clinical instructors, doing annual reports for the NATA and NATA Board of Certification, and developing the curriculum to keep our students abreast of the information and research they need to compete in this profession.

The best thing about teaching in a curriculum program is working with dynamic students who are not afraid of a challenge. Teaching athletic training gives me the opportunity to inspire these students to grow both professionally and personally. It is personally gratifying to know that I had a major role in making them better professionals, who may some day shape the direction of our profession. It's exhilarating to see the excitement in their eyes when they finally grasp the concepts in the classroom and translate them into the practical application of providing quality health care to their patients. To see them take personal interest in the welfare of their athletes and to unselfishly give of themselves is inspiring to me as a teacher. Many of my students continue to write me or call just to say hello and thank me for introducing them into this challenging profession.

That is not to say that my assignment does not have its down side. Being a Professor at a large university carries with it an obligation to do active research and publish. In addition, I raise funds to supplement the clinical program. I recruit donations from area physicians, physical therapists, schools, and clinics to provide stipends for the students to complete clinical hours at off-site locations. All of this takes time away from the personal interaction with my students.

For students considering a career in athletic training, I would recommend broadening your academic background with another program, such as teaching or health promotion, to make you more marketable. A master's degree with a focus on research is also highly recommended. Realize that competition in the field is keen, and today you have to be better at your job than your clinical instructor is. Commitment is the key. Athletic training is a people-oriented service profession, and you have to be willing to give of yourself 12 to 15 hours a day, 7 days a week. Get involved in the profession as a student by attending your state, district, and national conferences. Get to know those in the field and begin to develop your own networking system. Always remember that you are a professional. You have to act like a professional, and dress like one. That is how you succeed. Welcome to the athletic training profession.

Sports Injury Management and the Athletic Trainer

After you have completed this chapter, you should be able to:

■ Identify the health care services in sports medicine that enhance health fitness and sport performance

■ Identify members of the primary sports medicine team, their role, and their responsibility in sport injury management

■ Explain basic parameters of ethical conduct and standards of professional practice for athletic trainers

■ Specify academic and clinical requirements necessary to become a NATA certified athletic trainer, and continuing education requirements needed to maintain certification

■ Explain standard of care and what factors must be proven to show breach of that duty of care

■ Describe preventive measures to reduce potential risk of litigation

■ Discuss potential job opportunities for an individual interested in athletic training as a career

Sport, with its inherent risks, leads to injury at one time or another for nearly all participants. Physicians and athletic trainers responsible for the health and safety of sport participants are called "sports medicine specialists." These individuals are essential in the prevention, recognition, assessment, management, and rehabilitation of sport injuries. Furthermore, these individuals serve as a valuable resource to educate and counsel sport participants to prevent chronic degenerative injuries and diseases through life-long activity-related fitness and health education.

This chapter examines the roles of the physician and athletic trainer as parts of the primary sports medicine team. In the absence of an athletic trainer, the coach or designated supervisor of the sport-related activity must assume the role of health care provider. Standards of professional practice and criteria for national certification as an athletic trainer are presented in detail. Legal liability surrounding sports injury care will be presented relative to reducing the risk of litigation. Finally, potential job opportunities for individuals interested in athletic training as a career are discussed.

SPORTS MEDICINE

? *Many medical and health care professionals refer to themselves as sports medicine specialists. Think for a minute about what this term implies. Where do sport supervisors, coaches and athletic trainers fit into the scheme of providing health care to sport participants?*

Sports medicine is a broad and complex branch of health care encompassing several disciplines. Essentially it is an area of health care and special services that applies medical and scientific knowledge to prevent, recognize, assess, manage, and rehabilitate injuries or illnesses related to sport, exercise, or recreational activity, and in doing so, enhances health fitness and performance of the participant (1). Sport performance is enhanced through several mediums including:

1. Provision of a clean, safe, and accessible participation environment
2. Prevention of injury through preparticipation screening; development and supervision of physical conditioning and exercise

Sports medicine
Area of health and special services that apply medical and scientific knowledge to prevent, recognize, manage, and rehabilitate injuries related to sport, exercise, or recreational activity

programs; design, use, and fitting of protective equipment; and proper skill instruction
3. Recognition and assessment of a sport injury or illness
4. Management and disposition of an injury or illness
5. Injury rehabilitation through therapeutic exercise, reconditioning, and analysis of skill technique
6. Education and counseling to maintain life-long fitness and good health

Health care involves a variety of medical, paramedical, and professional personnel working together to provide a safe environment to permit maximal sport performance. The primary sports medicine team provides on-site supervision to prevent injury and deliver immediate health care. This team includes the team physician or primary care physician, athletic trainer, coach or sport supervisor in the absence of an athletic trainer, and the sport participant (2). Other professionals, not necessarily on-site but readily accessible to the primary sports medicine team, contribute their knowledge and expertise and may include orthopedic physi-

cians, physical therapists, emergency medical technicians (EMTs), podiatrists, radiologists, nutritionists, exercise physiologists, and sport psychologists. In addition, the primary sports medicine team may consult other professionals periodically to further complement the total health care provided to a sport participant. Professionals who may be included on the sports medicine team are listed in **Table 1-1**.

Providing a safe, healthy, and accessible environment coupled with proper supervision will prevent many injuries. Due to inherent risks in some sports, and the forces involved in contact and collision activities, some injuries will still occur. The National Athletic Trainers' Association (NATA) has projected that nearly 25 percent of all interscholastic athletes are injured each year. During a single high school football season, over 37 percent of all players were sidelined with injuries that required at least one week away from sport participation. Of these injuries, over 60 percent occurred during practice sessions (3). Despite the report that direct deaths due to injuries sustained in high school football have greatly diminished, the National Center for Catastrophic Sports Injury Research confirm that serious injuries continue (4). It is imper-

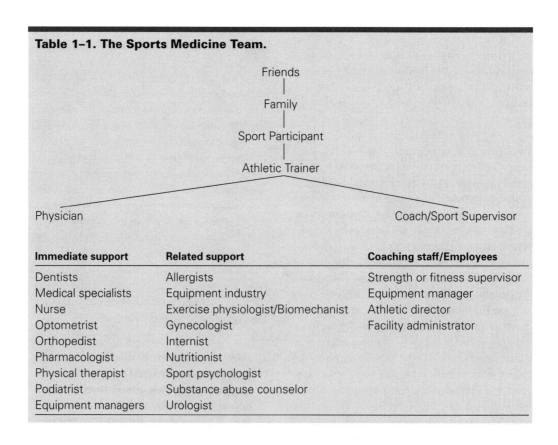

Table 1–1. The Sports Medicine Team.

Friends
|
Family
|
Sport Participant
|
Athletic Trainer

Physician   Coach/Sport Supervisor

Immediate support	Related support	Coaching staff/Employees
Dentists	Allergists	Strength or fitness supervisor
Medical specialists	Equipment industry	Equipment manager
Nurse	Exercise physiologist/Biomechanist	Athletic director
Optometrist	Gynecologist	Facility administrator
Orthopedist	Internist	
Pharmacologist	Nutritionist	
Physical therapist	Sport psychologist	
Podiatrist	Substance abuse counselor	
Equipment managers	Urologist	

ative the primary sports medicine team work together to provide quality comprehensive health care to all sport participants.

Sports medicine is the combination of health care and special services that applies medical and scientific knowledge to prevent, recognize, assess, manage, and rehabilitate injuries or illnesses related to sport, exercise, or recreation, and in doing so, enhances health fitness and performance of the participants. The athletic trainer, coach, and sport supervisors are the individuals responsible for daily on-site health care.

RESPONSIBILITIES OF THE PRIMARY SPORTS MEDICINE TEAM

Think for a minute or two about the individuals who make up the primary sports medicine team. What duties do you think each should be responsible for?

Total health care encompasses the prevention, recognition, assessment, management, and rehabilitation of sport injuries and illnesses, the organization and administration of health care, and education and counseling of the sport participant. No single profession can provide the expertise to carry out this enormous responsibility. As such, the team approach has proven to be the most successful method of addressing health care for sport participants (5). The primary sports medicine team is the pivotal group of individuals with specialized training and expertise in their chosen fields that provides on-site immediate health care. Each has responsibilities toward the prevention and care of sport injuries.

Team Physician

In organized sport, such as interscholastic, intercollegiate, or professional athletic programs, a team physician may be hired, or may volunteer their services to direct the primary sports medicine team in providing on-site medical care for sport participants. This individual supervises the various aspects of health care and is the final authority to determine the mental and physical fitness of athletes in organized programs (1,5).

In an athletic program, the team physician should administer and review preseason physical exams; review preseason conditioning programs; assess the quality, effectiveness, and maintenance of protective equipment; dispense medications; educate the athletic staff on emergency policies, proce-

dures, health care insurance coverage, and legal liability; and review all medical forms, policies and procedures to ensure compliance with school and athletic association guidelines (1,5). This individual may also serve as a valuable resource on current therapeutic techniques, facilitate referrals to other medical specialists, and provide educational counseling to sport participants, parents, athletic trainers, coaches, and sport supervisors.

In many high school and collegiate settings, financial constraints may prevent hiring a full-time team physician. Instead, several physicians rotate the responsibility of being present at competitions and are paid a per-game stipend. Primary care physicians, orthopedists, and other specialists, such as osteopaths, internists, general surgeons, and pediatricians who have a broad and thorough understanding of sport injuries may also serve as team physician.

The team physician should be present at competitions, particularly with high risk sports, such as football, hockey, or lacrosse to conduct emergency injury assessment, manage, and treat any injury and illness. Team physicians should be sensitive not only to the observable injuries, but also address the emotional and psychological needs of an injured participant. Preserving the health and safety of the participant is the team physician's top priority.

Primary Care Physician

In the absence of a team physician, the primary care physician or family physician assumes the duties of the team physician. This individual can be an important resource providing information on the growth and development of an adolescent, immunization records, and medical history. In addition, they may administer preparticipation exams, provide initial clearance for sport participation, diagnose sport injuries, prescribe medication, and clear individuals for sport participation after an injury (5).

Athletic Trainer

Athletic trainers are the critical link between the sport program and medical community, and are certified by the National Athletic Trainers' Association (NATA). Although athletic trainers work under the direction of a physician, they provide a much broader range of direct services to the sport participant on a

The team approach has proven to be the most successful method to provide health care to sport participants

A team physician directs the primary sports medicine team and is the final authority to determine the mental and physical fitness of athletes in school programs

Athletic trainers are the critical links between the sport program and medical community, and are certified by the NATA

daily basis. Athletic trainers have a strong background in human anatomy and physiology, kinesiology/biomechanics, psychology, health and nutrition, exercise physiology, organization and administration, first aid and emergency care, injury prevention, assessment, therapeutic rehabilitation, and use of modalities. Because of this broad background, the athletic trainer serves as the facilitator and liaison between the physician and athlete, and physician and coach. Their primary duties and responsibilities are summarized in **Table 1-2** and include (6):

1. Injury prevention
2. Recognition and evaluation of injuries/illnesses
3. Injury management/treatment and disposition
4. Injury rehabilitation
5. Organization and administration
6. Education and counseling

Injury Prevention

Injury prevention is a goal in any fitness related activity, and can be accomplished through preparticipation physical exams; regular safety checks of equipment, facilities and field areas; designing and implementing year-round conditioning programs to develop strength, flexibility, agility, and endurance; promoting proper lifting technique and safety in the weight room; and following universal safety precautions to prevent the spread of infectious diseases. With a working knowledge of joint mechanics and injury mechanisms, the athletic trainer can prevent injuries by designing and applying appropriate taping, wrappings, protective devices, or braces to prevent injury or reinjury from occurring. Monitoring environmental conditions, such as temperature, humidity, or lightning during thunderstorms can help the athletic trainer adhere to guidelines for safe participation in adverse weather, thus reducing the potential for injury (6).

Recognition and Evaluation of Injuries and Illnesses

The athletic trainer is responsible for recognizing and evaluating injuries that occur during sport participation. To do so, this individual needs a strong background in human anatomy and physiology, joint biomechanics, neuroanatomy, and tissue healing and repair. With this knowledge, the athletic trainer can recognize the body's normal physiologic

response to trauma, evaluate common soft tissue injuries, such as sprains, strains, contusions, dislocations, and fractures, and determine the extent or seriousness of injury. The process of injury evaluation and assessment follows a consistent, systematic format including the history, observation and inspection of the injury site, palpation of soft tissue and bony structures, and special tests (i.e., range-of-motion testing, muscle strength, sensory and motor neurologic testing, ligamentous/capsular stress testing, and functional testing) (6).

Injury Management, Treatment and Disposition

After injury evaluation, the athletic trainer must determine what steps are appropriate to prevent additional pain or discomfort for the individual. Appropriate referral may include summoning local emergency medical services (EMS) to immobilize the individual with emergency care equipment (i.e., cervical collars, special splints, or backboards) for transportation to the nearest medical facility. In less serious cases, appropriate management may involve applying ice to control inflammation, strapping the area for support, or removing the individual from participation **(Figure 1-1)** (6).

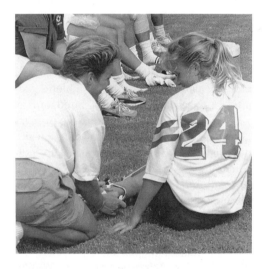

Fig. 1.1: Injury management. After evaluating an injury, the athletic trainer can determine what action is appropriate to manage the situation. This may include sideline treatment to control inflammation or immediate referral to a physician.

After injury evaluation, the athletic trainer must determine what steps are appropriate to prevent additional pain and discomfort

Modalities
Therapeutic agents that enhance tissue healing while reducing pain and disability

Documentation and record keeping are two of the most important duties an athletic trainer performs

Table 1–2. Duties of the Athletic Trainer.

Injury Prevention

Develop, implement, and assess preseason, inseason, and offseason conditioning programs
Educate the athlete to prevent use of dangerous skills and techniques
Assist the team physician in preparticipation physical exams
Design, fabricate, fit, and apply appropriate taping, wrapping, and protective devices to prevent injury or reinjury
Select and use protective devices and equipment to protect the athlete
Maintain and repair athletic apparatus and activity areas
Monitor environmental conditions

Recognition and Evaluation of Injuries/Illnesses

Obtain a medical history of the athlete including mechanism of injury, type and extent of pain, location of pain, predisposing factors and obvious signs and symptoms
Inspect the injured area for deformity, discoloration, bleeding, edema
Palpate anatomic sites for pain, effusion, deformity and obvious pathologic signs
Perform specific tests to determine decreased range of motion, muscle weakness, joint laxity, circulatory impairment, and nerve dysfunction
Recognize severity of trauma and functional status of athlete

Injury Management/Treatment and Disposition

Select and administer appropriate first aid using proper emergency care equipment
Refer the athlete to appropriate medical personnel and facility
Administer appropriate procedures to the injured or ill athlete to provide optimal opportunity for recovery

Rehabilitation

Develop criteria for the return of the athlete to full functional participation to minimize reinjury
Restore the injured or ill athlete to normal functional status by using therapeutic modalities and exercise
Evaluate the use of rehabilitation equipment, manual techniques, and therapeutic modalities to determine their appropriate use and application

Organization and Administration

Establish a standardized written procedure for planning, organizing, and implementing health care services
Establish with emergency support services, an emergency triage plan
Document all athletic training treatments and services provided by health care professionals
Purchase equipment and supplies
Inspect all athletic training facilities, equipment, therapeutic modalities, and maintain records to comply with mandated safety and sanitation standards

Education and counseling

Review previous injuries and counsel athletes to assess personal status for safe participation
Provide information on health topics, and refer the athlete to specialists for consultation on social or personal problems
Continue education by reading, attending educational programs, workshops, or through research
Counsel and advise athletic staffs and teams on potentially hazardous situations to ensure safe participation
Instruct student athletic trainers within the athletic training environment to develop entry level proficiency for athletic trainers
Instruct student athletic trainers in clinical and interpersonal communication skills to facilitate professionalism
Counsel and advise the public of the roles and responsibilities of the athletic training professional

Injury Rehabilitation

After acute inflammation has subsided, usually within 24 to 72 hours, the athletic trainer can begin a rehabilitation program to help the individual return to their preinjury status (**Figure 1-2**). In consultation with a physician, a comprehensive rehabilitation program is developed including therapeutic goals and objectives, selection of therapeutic **modalities** and exercise, use of prescription and nonprescription pharmacologic agents to aid in recovery, methods to assess and document progress, and criteria for return to participation. Information documented and gathered during rehabilitation will assist the physician in determining if the individual can be cleared for participation (6).

Organization and Administration

The athletic trainer is responsible for documenting and recording all administrative components of an athletic training program including those pertaining to health services (i.e., preparticipation exams and screening, injury evaluations, first aid treatment and emergency care, follow-up care and rehabilitation, and medical clearance to participate); other services rendered to an injured party (counseling, educational programs, referrals to other specialists); financial management; training room management; personnel management; and public relations. Regular inspection records of athletic training facilities, therapeutic modalities and equipment, gymnasiums, pools, and fields verify compliance with mandated safety and sanitation standards. The purchase of equipment and supplies, equipment reconditioning records, policies and procedures for drug testing and screening programs can verify compliance with safety standards established by national governing athletic associations. Written policies and procedures, such as supervision of student athletic trainers, emergency care protocols, confidentiality of medical records, and normal operating procedures should also be documented (6).

Education and Counseling

Athletic trainers educate sport participants about injury prevention and safety through educational materials and programs on specific safety and health topics. Many athletic trainers work closely with physicians, sport supervisors, coaches, and parents to counsel participants on important social and personal health areas, such as alcohol or other chemical substance abuse, weight control and eating disorders, proper nutrition, infectious diseases, personal hygiene, depression, family problems, or school-related stress. Because of the athletic trainer's unique working relationship, they can serve as an important resource to refer an individual to an appropriate specialist for further care or counseling (6).

The Coach or Sport Supervisor

A coach is responsible for teaching skills and strategies of a sport. A sport supervisor may not necessarily be a coach, but instead may be responsible for administering and supervising recreational sport activities or activity areas within health club facilities. Both individuals are responsible for encouraging good sportsmanship and developing an overall awareness of safety and injury prevention. To increase brevity, coaches and sport supervisors will henceforth be jointly referred to as sport supervisors.

If a sport supervisor has access to an athletic trainer, the athletic trainer assumes a more pivotal role on the primary sports medicine team to provide health care to an injured individual. Although nearly all professional and intercollegiate athletic programs have at least one athletic trainer on staff, it is estimated that less than 20 percent of all high schools in the United States have an athletic trainer (3). In the absence of an athletic trainer, the sport supervisor must assume a more active role in providing health care to sport participants.

> In the absence of an athletic trainer, the coach or sport supervisor must assume a more active role in providing health care to sport participants

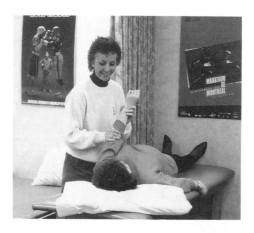

Fig. 1.2: Injury rehabilitation. The athletic trainer can do range of motion and strengthening exercises to help the individual return safely to sport participation.

Sport supervisors do not typically have the background in human anatomy and physiology, health and nutrition, injury prevention, assessment, management, and rehabilitation, or first aid and emergency care as do athletic trainers. Because of this, all sport supervisors should maintain current certification in cardiopulmonary resuscitation (CPR) and emergency first aid care. In the absence of an athletic trainer, sport supervisors, with the assistance of a physician, are expected to evaluate the physical condition of all sport participants prior to any activity, properly fit and use quality safety equipment, teach proper skill development and technique, and constantly reinforce the importance of safety and injury prevention throughout the year (5). Concern for safety and injury prevention must be communicated during the preseason team meeting with players and parents. Each player and parent should be informed of the risk of injury, how to prevent injuries, and what to do if an injury occurs. Conditioning programs should be based on sound physiologic principles and training techniques, and be properly supervised. Activities should be planned so as not to predispose the participants to excessive fatigue or heat injury. Sport supervisors should meet with their respective staff to develop and practice emergency procedures, skills, techniques, and use of emergency equipment. If possible, at least one staff person should have advanced training in emergency care.

Sport Participant

Sport participants play an essential role in working with the athletic trainer and sport supervisor to maximize injury prevention. Participants are responsible for maintaining a high level of fitness, eating nutritional foods, and playing within the rules of the sport. All sport participants should refrain from ingesting alcohol and other chemical substances, such as anabolic steroids, human growth hormones, and amphetamines to enhance performance. Each can impair judgment, alter coordination, and place the individual at risk for injury. The participant should be responsible for maintaining and wearing safety equipment at all times during activity. In the event of an injury, the individual should know where to seek immediate health care and follow medical advice from the physician or athletic trainer. If sport participants understand

and practice safety and preventive measures, the number of injuries or illnesses associated with sport participation can be reduced.

Student Athletic Trainer

Student athletic trainers provide the work force in organized sport programs to implement the policies and procedures of daily health care at team practices and games (**Figure 1-3**). Many students gain practical experience on the high school level, and enroll in a college to pursue a degree program in athletic training, human performance, physical education, or a health related area. On the college level, NATA certified athletic trainers supervise and guide the student athletic trainer through the clinical application of sports injury care. Initially the student athletic trainer may only observe the staff athletic trainers and assist when needed. As the student's skills and knowledge improve, the athletic trainers will help the student learn NATA competencies in athletic training and prepare the college student to meet the NATA Board of Certification standards. Student athletic trainers can view first hand the contributions athletic trainers provide in the total health care of sport participants.

Each player and parent should be informed of the risk of injury, how to prevent injuries, and of what to do should an injury occur

Student athletic trainers provide the work force to implement the policies and procedures of daily health care at team practices and games

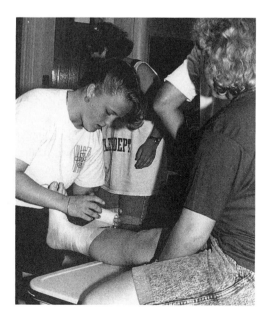

Fig. 1.3: Student athletic trainers provide the work force to implement the policies and procedures of daily health care to sport participants.

Physical Therapist

Physical therapists are not a part of the on-site primary sports medicine team, yet they provide a unique and valuable resource in the overall rehabilitation of a sport participant. While the athletic trainer typically works with healthy athletes, the physical therapist has a broader background in treating patients of all ages and with a wider variety of physical problems. Physical therapists often supervise the rehabilitation of an injured sport participant in an industrial medical clinic, hospital, or sports medicine clinic. In many cases, athletic trainers are also registered physical therapists. Likewise, many physical therapists are also working toward certification as an athletic trainer. Dual certification is a strong asset in the job market.

Athletic and Clinical Administrators

Administrators do not provide health care, however, they are ultimately responsible for directing, managing, administering the facility and personnel. Duties may include the development, administration, and assessment of programs; fiscal management; ensuring compliance with safety and sanitation standards; facility maintenance; personnel management, and professional development of employees. Each of these areas can influence the risk of injury for sport participants, employees, and visitors to the facility. Administrators should work with the primary sports medicine team to develop standard operating procedures to handle emergency care procedures and on-site health care. These procedures may include establishing an emergency care plan, developing uniform reporting and documentation of injuries, standards for inspection and maintenance of the facility and safety equipment, and criteria for hiring and retaining employees.

Administrators set an example of safety awareness through sound fiscal management in providing safe field areas and facilities, hiring qualified personnel to implement the health care plan, purchasing high quality equipment and supplies, and supporting decisions made by the primary sports medicine team. In addition, administrators are responsible for providing regular inservice educational workshops to keep staff informed of current trends in the profession, and facilitating meetings to discuss work load, standard of care, safety measures, and professional development.

After reading about the responsibilities of the primary sports medicine team, what role will you play in providing health care to sport participants?

STANDARDS OF PROFESSIONAL PRACTICE

If you were injured, what standards of care and professional conduct would you expect to receive from the immediate health care provider?

Standards of professional practice are ethical responsibilities that guide one's actions and promote high standards of conduct and integrity to assure high quality health care (7). These standards reflect what the profession believes is right and wrong. The role of a health care provider should never compromise the health of any sport participant. Decisions concerning whether or not a sport participant should be allowed to participate in an activity must be based on sound medical consideration. Individuals should be informed of the risks for injury, protected from injury whenever possible, and receive expedient health care and rehabilitation if injury occurs. In addition, all participants have a right to confidentiality about their health status. Litigation due to breach of confidentiality relative to medical records has occurred. Athletic trainers, sport supervisors, and physicians should be sensitive about dissemination of health information and should honor the wishes of an individual to make the information public or not. The National Athletic Trainers' Association (NATA) has established 5 basic ethical principles for athletic trainers to abide by. These include (8):

1. Members shall respect the rights, welfare, and dignity of all individuals
2. Members shall comply with the laws and regulations governing the practice of athletic training
3. Members shall accept responsibility for the exercise of sound judgment
4. Members shall maintain and promote high standards in the provision of services
5. Members shall not engage in any form of conduct that constitutes a conflict of interest or that adversely reflects on the profession

---

Administrators have a major responsibility to direct, manage, and administer the facility and personnel

Administrators set an example of safety awareness by providing a safe environment, hiring qualified personnel, purchasing quality safety equipment, and supporting decisions made by the primary sports medicine team

Standards of professional practice are ethical ideals that guide your actions and promote high standards of conduct and integrity

Sport participants have a right to confidentiality about their health status

NATA Certification for the Athletic Trainer

Individuals seeking to become NATA certified athletic trainers must complete the following core requirements (8,9):

1. Clinical athletic training hours may not begin to accumulate until after the high school degree has been completed
2. Proof of graduation at the baccalaureate level at an accredited college or university
3. Proof of current American National Red Cross Standard First Aid Certification and current Basic CPR (American Red Cross or American Heart Association), or EMT equivalent
4. At least 25% of all clinical athletic training experience hours must be attained in actual (on location) practice and/or game coverage with one or more of the following sports: football, soccer, hockey, wrestling, basketball, gymnastics, lacrosse, volleyball, and rugby
5. Endorsement of certification application by a NATA certified athletic trainer

An individual may qualify for application through two options: (1) by graduating from an undergraduate or graduate college that has an educational program accredited through the Commission on Accreditation of Allied Health Educational Programs (CAAHEP), and passing the national certification examination, or (2) by completing an internship and passing the national certification examination. Students in CAAHEP-accredited entry-level programs must complete formal instruction in the following core curriculum subject matter (9):

Human anatomy
Human physiology
Psychology
Kinesiology/biomechanics
Exercise physiology
Prevention of athletic injuries/illnesses
Evaluation of athletic injuries/illnesses
First aid and emergency care
Therapeutic modalities
Therapeutic exercise
Personal/community health
Nutrition
Administration of athletic training programs

In addition to core subject matter, additional coursework is highly recommended in chemistry, physics, pharmacology, statistics and research design. Students are also required to complete 800 clinical hours under the supervision of a NATA certified athletic trainer at the college or affiliated site (i.e., an area high school or local college) (9).

Students who do not attend a college with a CAAHEP-accredited entry-level program may complete requirements for certification through internship. Requirements for this option are established by the NATA Board of Certification (NATABOC) and include the following subject areas (9):

Health (i.e., nutrition, drugs/substance abuse, health education)
Human anatomy
Human physiology
Kinesiology/biomechanics
Physiology of exercise
Basic athletic training; and
Advanced athletic training (one course in therapeutic modalities and rehabilitative exercise are acceptable alternatives to satisfy the advanced athletic training requirement).

If seeking certification via the internship route, the NATABOC requires 1500 hours of athletic training experience under the supervision of a NATA certified athletic trainer. Of these, at least 1000 hours must be attained in a traditional athletic training facility at the interscholastic, intercollegiate, or professional sports level. The remaining 500 hours may be completed at an allied clinical setting, such as in a sports medicine clinic, campus health center, industrial health facility, other health care facility, and/or sport camp setting under the supervision of a NATA certified athletic trainer. These hours must be accumulated in no less than two, nor more than five years (9).

Continuing Education Requirements

Continuing education programs provide an opportunity for athletic trainers to acquire new innovative skills and techniques, and learn about current research within the profession. Once certified as a NATA athletic trainer, the NATABOC requires eight continuing education units over a three-year period. Currently there are several methods to accumulate continuing education units, which include attendance at workshops, seminars, conferences, and conventions; being a speaker or panelist at a clinical symposium; professional publications; enrolling in a related correspondence or post graduate education course; reading professional journals and completing Continuing Education Unit (CEUs) quizzes; and becoming involved in the NATA certification exam testing program. In addition, current proof of CPR certification is required at least once during the CEU requirement period (10). For current standards of certification and continuing education requirements write to: NATA, 2952 Stemmons Freeway, Dallas, Texas 75247 or to NATABOC, 3725 National Drive, Suite 213, Raleigh, NC 27612.

Registration and Licensure

As of April 1994, thirty-one states now require athletic trainers to meet specific standards of practice within the individual state, referred to as state licensure, certification, or registration **(Table 1-3)** (11,12). These laws define the role of the athletic trainer and set the legal parameters under which the athletic trainer can operate within that state. These laws may delineate the specific clientele and services that can be provided in the various work settings. Although standards vary, in most states athletic trainers provide services to athletes under the direct supervision of a physician licensed in that state. Nearly all states accept the successful completion of the NATA examination as a basis for obtaining licensure (11). In nontraditional settings or in states that do not have licensure laws, athletic trainers may be restricted in the services they provide. Being properly licensed and practicing within the established standards of prac-

tice are two of the strongest safeguards against litigation.

💡 *Did you determine what standard of care and professional conduct you should expect to receive if injured during an organized sport activity? If you determined the individual should be a NATA certified athletic trainer, you are correct.*

LEGAL LIABILITY

❓ *You have learned that several high school athletes are using the weight room when a supervisor is not present. Although the individuals have been instructed in proper lifting technique and safety, you are concerned about legal liability. What implications exist concerning your legal responsibility to these athletes? What action(s) can be taken to ensure a safe weight training facility?*

Prevention of injuries, and reducing further injury or harm is a major responsibility for all athletic trainers and sport supervisors. Legal action involving the practice of athletic training is typically tried under tort law. A **tort** is a wrong done to an individual whereby the injured party seeks a remedy for damages suffered. In lawsuits, actions are measured against a standard of care provided to those individuals for whom you are directly responsible. **Standard of care**, or liability, is defined as what another minimally competent individual educated and practicing in that profession would have done in the same or similar circumstance to protect an individual from harm or further harm (13). For example, an individual responsible for providing ath-

---

State licensure laws define the role of the athletic trainer and set legal parameters under which the athletic trainer can operate within that state

Tort
A wrong done to an individual whereby the injured party seeks a remedy for damages suffered

Standard of Care
What another minimally competent professional educated and practicing in the same profession would have done in the same or similar circumstance to protect an individual from harm

---

Table 1–3. States that Require Certification, Licensure or Registration for Athletic Trainers.

Alabama	Louisiana	North Dakota
*Arizona	Massachusetts	Ohio
*Connecticut	Minnesota	Oklahoma
Delaware	Mississippi	*Oregon
Georgia	Missouri	Pennsylvania
*Hawaii	Nebraska	Rhode Island
Idaho	*New Hampshire	South Carolina
Illinois	New Jersey	South Dakota
Indiana	New Mexico	Tennessee
Kentucky	New York	Texas

*States that are exempt from existing licensure standards that limit other related professions.
Note: For information on individual state licensure laws or an up-date on states regulating the practice of athletic training contact: Government Affairs Committee, The National Athletic Trainers Association, 2952 Stemmons, Dallas, TX 75247

letic training services would be held to a standard of care expected of a NATA certified athletic trainer. Therefore, in states with specific registration, certification, or licensure laws, valid NATA certification and registration or licensure for individuals providing athletic training services would be minimal protection against litigation.

In the absence of an athletic trainer, the sport supervisor indirectly assumes the duty of care, and will also be held to a certain standard of care. Duty of care is measured by what is learned, or should have been learned in the professional preparation of that individual. For example, sport supervisors should be able to assess and recognize potentially severe injuries, provide emergency first aid, and initiate appropriate referral for advanced medical care if necessary. Completing a basic athletic training class, and having current certification in basic first aid and CPR would be minimal protection against litigation.

The question may arise as to who is the final authority to clear an individual for play. The final authority in measuring an individual's status for participation rests with the supervising team physician, regardless of the age of the participant. In the absence of a team physician, the final authority rests with the family physician. Parents of minors can not assume the risk involved in sport for their child (1).

Negligence

Athletic trainers and sport supervisors are expected to teach, supervise, inspect and provide quality equipment, ensure a safe environment, and provide a duty of care to all sport participants (14). Failure to provide this care can result in liability, or **negligence**.

Negligent torts may occur as a result of **malfeasance**, **misfeasance**, **nonfeasance**, **malpractice**, or **gross negligence (Table 1-4)**.

To find an individual liable, the injured person must prove that (1) there was a duty of care, (2) there was a breach of that duty, (3) there was harm (e.g., pain and suffering, permanent disability, or loss of wages), and (4) that the resulting harm was a direct cause from that breach of duty (14). If a spectator notices a large hole in the field prior to a game, and a player steps into the hole and breaks an ankle, the spectator is not liable because that individual has no duty of care for the player. However, an athletic trainer or supervisor does have a duty of care to check the field for hazards prior to competition. As such, the athletic trainer or sport supervisor could be held liable for the injury sustained by the participant.

Although a sport participant does assume some risk inherent in any activity, the individual does not assume the risk that the professional will breach their duty of care. Fortunately, the number of lawsuits brought against athletic trainers in the performance of their duties is rare. Since 1973, an athletic trainer was a named defendant in only nine lawsuits (15). Negligence may occur as a result of an action, or lack of action. Situations that may result in litigation can be seen in **Table 1-5**.

Failure to Warn

A legal duty of care for athletic trainers and sport supervisors is to inform individuals of the risks for injury during sport participation. Participants and parents of minor children must be informed that risk for injury exists,

Negligence
Breach of one's duty of care that causes harm to another individual

Participants and parents of minor children must be informed that risk for injury exists, and understand the nature of that risk so informed judgments can be made concerning participation

To find an individual liable, the injured must prove that:
- there was a legal duty of care
- there was a breach of that duty
- there was harm caused by that breach
- the harm was a direct cause of the breach of duty

Table 1–4. Negligent Torts.

Malfeasance occurs when an individual commits an act that is not their responsibility to perform. If you suspect a neck injury and remove the football helmet, you could be liable

Misfeasance occurs when an individual commits an act that is their responsibility to perform, but uses the wrong procedure, or does the right procedure in an improper manner. If you suspect a neck injury and improperly secure the head and neck region to the rigid spine board, you could be held liable

Nonfeasance occurs when an individual fails to perform their legal duty of care. If you suspect, or should have suspected, a neck injury and failed to use a rigid back board to stabilize the individual, you could be held liable

Malpractice occurs when an individual commits a negligent act while providing care

Gross negligence occurs when an individual has total disregard for the safety of others

Table 1–5. Actions that May Result in Litigation

Failing to warn an individual about the risks involved in sport participation

Treating an injured party without their consent

Failing to provide medical information concerning alternative treatments or the risks involved with the treatment to an athlete

Failing to provide safe facilities, fields, and equipment

Being aware of a potentially dangerous situation and failing to do anything about it

Failing to provide an adequate injury prevention program

Allowing an injured or unfit player to participate resulting in further injury or harm

Failing to provide quality training, instruction, and supervision

Using unsafe equipment

Negligently moving an injured athlete before properly immobilizing the injured area

Failing to employ qualified medical personnel

Failing to have a written emergency care plan

Failing to properly recognize an injury or illness, both as immediate acute care and as long-term treatment

Failing to immediately refer an injured party to the proper physician

Failing to keep adequate records

Treating an injury that did not occur within the school athletic environment

---

Informed consent
Condition whereby an injured adult, or parents of minor children are reasonably informed of needed treatment, possible alternative treatments, and the advantages and disadvantages of each course of action, and give written consent to receive the treatment

Consent can only be obtained from one who is competent to grant it; that is, an adult who is physically and mentally competent, or in the case of children under 18, the parent

Battery
Unpermitted or intentional contact with another individual without consent

Foreseeability of harm
Condition whereby danger is apparent, or should have been apparent, resulting in an unreasonably unsafe condition

Unsafe conditions should be identified, reported in writing to appropriate personnel, restricted from use, and repaired or replaced as soon as possible

---

and must understand the nature of that risk so informed judgments can be made about participation. Understanding and comprehending the nature of the risk is determined by the participant's age, experience, and knowledge of pertinent information about the risk. An advanced gymnast, for example, would know of and appreciate the risk of injury much more than a novice gymnast. Therefore, it is crucial to warn the novice of all inherent dangers in the activity and continually reinforce that information throughout the entire sport season.

Warning of the risks can be done in a variety of ways, such as at a preseason or organizational meeting with parents and participants, posting visible warning signs around equipment, requiring protective equipment, playing by the rules, and discouraging dangerous techniques. Other methods warning of risks are listed in **Table 1-6.**

Informed Consent

In providing health care, **informed consent** implies that an injured party has been reasonably informed of needed treatment, possible alternative treatment, and advantages and disadvantages of each course of action. To be valid, consent can only be obtained from one who is competent to grant it; that is, an adult who is physically and mentally competent, or in the case of children under 18, only the parent can grant consent on behalf of the minor.

For minors, exceptions may exist in emergency situations when parents are unavailable. Authorization to treat in the absence of the parent, or in the event the individual is physically unable to consent to treatment, should be obtained in writing prior to the start of sport participation. This consent may be obtained during preparticipation meetings as part of the documentation depicting consent to participate in that activity. An example of a consent form can be seen in **Field Strategy 1-1**.

Failure to receive informed consent may constitute battery. **Battery** is any unpermitted or intentional contact with another individual without their consent. Although many courts require that intent to harm be present in an allegation of battery, written documentation of informed consent should be obtained from an individual, or parents of minor children to avoid litigation.

Foreseeability of Harm

To recognize the potential for injury first, then remove that danger before an injury occurs, is another duty of care for athletic trainers and sport supervisors. **Foreseeability of harm** exists when danger is apparent, or should have been apparent, resulting in an unreasonably unsafe condition (**Figure 1-4**). This potential for injury can be identified during regular inspections of gymnasiums, field areas, swimming pools, safety equipment, and

Table 1-6. Strategies to Avoid Litigation.

Ensure that all personnel are properly licensed for practicing within the laws of the state, particularly in providing athletic training services

Hire qualified coaches, sport supervisors, athletic trainers, and fitness instructors, and establish strict rules for supervision and use of the facility

Have an established preparticipation plan including:
  Annual preparticipation health examination
  Insurance verification
  Medical data information cards
  Physician's clearance to participate

Hold a preseason/preparticipation meeting to:
  Inform participants and parents of the risks involved in sport participation
  Obtain written informed consent from the parents of minor children before participation
  Document what was said at the preseason or preparticipation meeting

Have a well-established primary sports medicine team to:
  Develop a total health care plan including staff responsibilities during emergency situations
  Obtain adequate health insurance for participants and liability insurance for the staff
  Establish a communication system at each field or gymnasium station
  Maintain appropriate standard injury documentation and referral forms
  Develop criteria to return an injured player to participation
  Select and purchase quality safety equipment from a reputable dealer
  Inspect safety equipment and supervise proper fitting, adjustment, and repair of equipment
  Inspect equipment, facilities and fields for hazards and prohibit their use if found to be dangerous
  Establish policies for documentation, confidentiality, and storage of medical records
  Keep accurate records of equipment purchases, reconditioning, and repairs

Post warning signs in plain sight on and around equipment to inform of the risks involved in abuse of equipment, and to describe proper use of the equipment

Post visible signs in the swimming pool area giving the depth of the pool and prohibiting diving in the shallow area

Post warning signs in the whirlpool area to inform individuals not to touch the turbine device while standing or sitting in water

Require participants to wear protective equipment regularly, including protective eyewear in appropriate racquet sports

Issue only those helmets that meet standards established by the National Operating Commission on Standards for Athletic Equipment (NOCSAE). Inform players the helmet cannot prevent all injuries and the possibility exists that serious head and neck injuries may occur in the sport

Develop appropriate skill instruction and provide positive feedback on proper execution of skills and techniques

Place ropes or signs along the sidelines of fields to keep spectators off the playing field

Provide continuing education for coaches, sport supervisors, and athletic trainers through inservice workshops and programs

Act as a reasonably prudent professional in caring for all sport participants

---

athletic training facilities. For example, unpadded walls under the basketball hoops, glass or potholes on playing fields, slippery floors near a whirlpool, exposed wiring, and failure to follow universal safety precautions against the spread of infectious diseases all pose a threat to safety. Unsafe conditions should be identified, reported in writing to appropriate personnel, restricted from use, and repaired or replaced as soon as possible.

Product Liability

Athletes, parents, coaches, and athletic trainers place a high degree of faith in the quality and safety of equipment used in sport participation. Manufacturers have a duty of care to

Manufacturers have a duty of care to design, manufacture, and package safe equipment that will not cause injury when used as intended

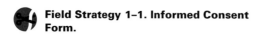

Field Strategy 1–1. Informed Consent Form.

ATHLETIC CLUB REGISTRATION

Athlete's Full Name:_____
Address:_____
Age:____Weight: _____Phone No.:_____
School: _____Grade Next Sept.:_____
Father's Full Name: _____
Address:_____
City: _____State: ___Zip:_____
Mother's Full Name: _____
Address:_____
City: _____State: ___Zip:_____
Do Parents Carry Hospitalization?YES NO

THIS CLUB DOES NOT CARRY MEDICAL INSURANCE FOR PARTICIPANTS. THE PARTICIPANT'S PARENTS AND/OR LEGAL GUARDIAN ASSUME ALL RESPONSIBILITY FOR SAID INSURANCE

CONSENT TO PARTICIPATE, RELEASE, WAIVER OF LIABILITY AND INDEMNITY AGREEMENT

In consideration of your acceptance of the undersigned athlete into the athletic program, we the undersigned, with the intent to be legally bound, do for ourselves, our heirs, executors, administrators and all others claiming by or through us, or as a result of any claim related to the athlete's participation in the club's activities or programs, do hereby state that we the undersigned consent to the participant's participation in the activities and that we are aware of all risks, hazards and uncertainties connected with participation in the programs and activities of the Club, and do hereby waive, release and discharge the Club, and all of its officers, directors, officials, coaches, employees, volunteers, umpires and any other individuals acting for or on behalf of the Club, from any and all claims while participating in, traveling to, or from or competing in any of the activities or functions of the Club or those it attends. It is the undersigned's specific intent to release, acquit and forever discharge the Club all of its officers, directors, officials, coaches, employees, volunteers, umpires and any other individuals acting for or on behalf of the Club, from all claims, demands, actions, causes of action, and for all liability for injury, damage or loss of whatsoever, kind, nature or description that may arise or be sustained by the participant which is due in any way or connected in any way with the participants participation in the Club or any of its functions or activities. It is further our specific intent that this release apply to any injury, damage or claims arising from any act or omission of the Club or any of the individuals released hereby including any injury, damage or claim arising from any negligent act or negligent omission of such organization or individuals.

The participant and the undersigned hereby assume full responsibility for all risk of bodily injury, death or property damage due to the negligent or other conduct of those parties released hereby or otherwise, as a result of any activities connected in any way with the Club. The undersigned on behalf of the participant and for themselves, and all of their heirs, executors and administrators and all others, do hereby further covenant not to sue the Club or any of the individuals released hereby in the event of any injury or damage of any kind or description whatsoever and should any such suit or claim be instituted at any time, including any claim, demand or suit by the minor participant either before he reaches the age of majority or thereafter, the undersigned do hereby further agree to indemnity and hold the Club, and all of those individuals released hereby, completely and absolutely harmless from all expenses, demands, claims, fees, and costs of whatever description or nature which may arise as the result of any such claims being instituted at any time including all costs, fees and expenses involved in defending or investigating any and all claims, demands or causes of action whatsoever that may hereafter be asserted or brought by the participant or anyone on his or her behalf for the purpose of enforcing any claim for damages on account of any injuries or damages sustained during participation in any of the activities of the Club.

EMERGENCY MEDICAL AUTHORIZATION

We, the undersigned, do hereby consent and authorize any duly authorized doctor, emergency medical technician, hospital or other medical facility to treat or attempt to treat the participant for any injuries received by said participant while he participates in any activity of the Club, or while traveling to or from or competing in any Club activity. We further authorize any licensed physician to perform any procedure which he or she deems advisable in attempting to treat or relieve any injuries or any related unhealthy conditions in said participant that may be encountered during any necessary procedure or operation. We further consent to the administration of any anesthesia as deemed advisable by any licensed physician, and do hereby further authorize any x-ray examination, medical or surgical diagnosis or treatment, and hospital care to be rendered to the participant in our absence under the general or special supervision and on the advice of a licensed physician, surgeon, anesthesiologist, dentist or other qualified personnel acting under their supervision.

We, the undersigned, realize and appreciate that there is a possibility of complication and unforeseen consequence in any medical treatment, and we assume any such risk on behalf of ourselves and the participant as stated herein. We acknowledge that there has been no warranty made as to the results of any such treatment or diagnostic procedure.

Each of the undersigned expressly acknowledge and agree that they have read and understood the terms of this form, including the CONSENT TO PARTICIPATE, RELEASE, WAIVER OF LIABILITY AND INDEMNITY AGREEMENT coupled with the EMERGENCY MEDICAL AUTHORIZATION and further state that no oral representations, statements or inducements apart from the foregoing written provisions have been made.

WE HAVE READ, UNDERSTOOD AND VOLUNTARILY SIGNED THIS RELEASE

_____   _____
Parent or Guardian   Parent or Guardian

_____   _____
Athlete-Participant   Date

Implied warranty
Unwritten guarantee that the product is reasonably safe when used for its intended purpose

Expressed warranty
Written guarantee that states the product is safe for consumer use

design, manufacture, and package safe equipment that will not cause injury to an individual when the equipment is used as it was intended (14,16) This is called an **implied warranty**. An **expressed warranty** is a written guarantee that the product is safe for use. In football there is an implied warranty that if fitted and used properly, the helmet can pro-

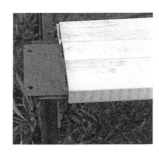

Fig. 1.4: Regular safety checks of equipment can foresee the possibility of injury. Dangerous or hazardous bleachers should be repaired or replaced immediately.

tect the head and brain from certain injuries. The National Operating Committee on Standards for Athletic Equipment (NOCSAE) has established minimum standards for football helmets to tolerate certain forces when applied to different areas of the helmet. Manufacturers and reconditioners of helmets place a visible expressed warranty on all helmets that meet NOCSAE standards. This statement informs players that the helmet is not intended to be used to butt, ram or spear an opposing player, and that use in this manner could result in serious head, brain, or neck injuries, paralysis, or death for the player or opposing player. Strict liability makes the manufacturer liable for any and all defective or hazardous equipment that unduly threatens an individual's personal safety (14,16).

Teachers, coaches, athletic trainers, fitness specialists, and supervisors should know the dangers involved in using sport equipment, and have a duty to properly supervise its fitting and intended use. Supervisors also have a duty to warn participants of the dangers inherent in using the equipment.

Preventing Litigation

All members of the sports medicine team should be aware of their duty of care consistent with existing state law, and complete that duty of care within established policies and standards of practice. Several steps can be taken to reduce the risk of subsequent litigation and include: safety checks of equipment and facilities, hiring qualified personnel, proper supervision and instruction, purchasing quality equipment, posting appropriate warning signs, maintaining accurate and complete health care records, and having a well organized emergency care plan. Other steps are listed in **Table 1-6**.

After reading this section, have you determined what your duty of care is relative to the individuals lifting weights in an

unsupervised room? You should have foreseen the possibility of injury, warned the individuals to leave, and taken immediate steps to close the room until competent personnel could supervise the area. Failure to do so could make you liable through an act of nonfeasance. You might also want to place visible signs on the walls depicting proper lifting technique for each station, and post signs warning that no one should use the equipment without proper supervision.

MEDICAL RECORDS AND RECORD KEEPING

A individual received a severe blow to the anterior part of the right leg, which resulted in rapid swelling. The sport supervisor applied ice to limit swelling and told the individual to see a physician that day. The individual decided not to see the physician and returned home to ice the leg. Three days later the swelling was still present and the individual was unable to move the foot. If litigation occurred as a result of this incident, what should the supervisor have done to protect against possible legal action?

One of the most important responsibilities athletic trainers and sport supervisors can do is develop and implement a comprehensive record-keeping system. Accurate records are critical in litigation and serve to improve communication between all members of the primary sports medicine team. Although the specific nature of record keeping will vary with the needs and function of the facility, several records should always be maintained. Direct communication concerning preparticipation exams, insurance forms, personal data information cards, accident reports and injury management, daily treatment or status reports, rehabilitation programs and progress charts, clearance for participation, supply and equipment inventory, and annual reports will document that personnel are providing their duty of care.

Preparticipation Exams

Preparticipation screening can determine the general health, maturity, and fitness level of an individual; detect those at risk for injury or those who may have conditions that may limit participation; identify individuals who may need counseling on health-related issues; and can meet insurance requirements (17,18). This screening is usually done at least six

Strict liability makes the seller liable for any or all defective or dangerous equipment that unduly threatens an individual's personal safety

All members of the sports medicine team should be aware of their duty of care and complete that duty within established policies and standards of practice

Accurate records are a major defense in litigation and serve to improve communication among all members of the primary sports medicine team

weeks prior to participation in the activity. Muscular weakness or abnormalities can then be detected and treated prior to beginning the sport program. Ideally, exams should be performed in the physician's office where a more thorough and comprehensive exam can be completed. The initial screening examination should focus on the individual's medical history and physical examination of the musculoskeletal and cardiovascular systems. Annual reevaluations should focus on medical history and a limited physical examination including maturity assessment, height and weight measurement, cardiovascular assessment, skin examination, and assessment of new problems occurring since the initial screening (18).

Medical history information should be confirmed by the parents of minor children to ensure accuracy (**Field Strategy 1-2**). Information gathered may include: immunization records; past episodes of infectious diseases, loss of consciousness, recurrent headaches, musculoskeletal injuries, heat stroke, chest pains during or after exercise, seizures, breathing difficulties, eating disorders, and chronic medical problems; medication and drug use; allergies; heart murmurs or unusual heart palpitation; use of contact lenses, corrective lenses, dentures, prosthetic devices, or special equipment (pads, braces, neck rolls, or eye guards); and family history of cardiac, vascular, or neurologic problems, such as sickle cell anemia, diabetes, high blood pressure, or sudden death. A supplemental health history questionnaire can be provided for female participants to gather information on menstrual or vaginal irregularities, eating habits, urinary tract disorders, and use of birth control pills or hormones (**Field Strategy 1-3**) (19).

The physical examination includes a general assessment of the body, and an orthopedic assessment for the individual's specific sport including assessment of muscle strength, joint laxity, posture, and cardiovascular fitness. Examples of suggested forms can be seen in **Field Strategies 1-4** and **1-5**. An example of a large station-type mass screening format can be seen in **Field Strategy 1-6**.

After the prescreening exam, the physician must determine the individual's eligibility to participate in sport. Although there are no universal standards regarding sport participation, several guidelines do exist. Conditions that may exclude an individual from participation include atlantoaxial instability, severe hypertension, aortic disorders, tuberculosis, severe pulmonary insufficiency, uncontrolled diabetes or convulsive disorders, serious bleeding tendencies, acute infections, enlarged liver or spleen, hernias, symptomatic abnormalities or inflammations, functional instability, previous serious head trauma or surgery, renal disease, or absence of one kidney (20). **Table 1-7** provides a more complete list of disqualifying conditions for sport participation.

Insurance Forms

Every sport participant should have health insurance coverage. Documentation of the insurance carrier and policy number for each individual should be available to the athletic trainer or sport supervisor in case the individual must seek medical care in an emergency. This information can be written on file cards and carried with the supervisor at all practices and games.

Medical Data Information Cards

In school programs personal data information cards can document the individual's address and phone number, parent's address and phone number, who to contact in case of an emergency, and may also list pertinent health information, such as past injuries, medic alert conditions, and the health insurance carrier and policy number (**Figure 1-5**). These cards should be easily accessible to the athletic trainer or sport supervisor, and should be carried when competitions are held at a site away from home.

Accident Reports

Accident reports document an injury, the immediate care, and instructions for follow-up care. Sport injuries or illnesses should be documented if the individual has to be removed from sport participation to be treated, or if the injury or illness affects participation. For example, if an individual injures an ankle during participation and is removed for the rest of practice to ice the region, this should be documented. If the individual injures the ankle in an unrelated sport accident and cannot participate in an activity the next day, the circumstance of injury should also be documented. This pro-

Field Strategy 1-2. Medical History Form.

This evaluation is only to determine readiness for sports participation. It should not be used as a substitute for regular health maintenance examinations.

Name _____ Age (Yrs) _____ Grade _____ Date _____
Address _____ Phone_____
Sports _____

The Health History (Part A) and Physical Examination (Part C [table 3]) must both be completed, at least every 24 months, before sports participation. The Interim Health History (Part B) must be completed at least annually.

Part A: Health History
To be completed by athlete and parent.

		Yes	No
1.	Have you ever had an illness that:		
	a. required you to stay in the hospital?	☐	☐
	b. lasted longer than a week?	☐	☐
	c. caused you to miss 3 days of practice or competition?	☐	☐
	d. is related to allergies (e.g., hay fever, hives, asthma, insect sting reactions)?	☐	☐
	e. required an operation	☐	☐
	f. is chronic (e.g., asthma, diabetes)?	☐	☐
2.	Have you ever had an injury that:		
	a. required you to go to an emergency room or see a doctor?	☐	☐
	b. required you to stay in the hospital?	☐	☐
	c. required x-rays?	☐	☐
	d. caused you to miss 3 days of practice or a competition?	☐	☐
	e. required an operation?	☐	☐
3.	Do you take any medication or pills?	☐	☐
4.	Have any members of your family under age 50 had a heart attack, had a heart problem, or died unexpectedly?	☐	☐
5.	Have you ever:		
	a. been dizzy or passed out during or after exercise?	☐	☐
	b. been unconscious or had a concussion?	☐	☐
6.	Are you able to run ½ mile (2 times around the track) without stopping?	☐	☐
7.	Do you:		
	a. wear glasses or contacts?	☐	☐
	b. wear dental bridges, plates, or braces?	☐	☐
8.	Have you ever had a heart murmur, high blood pressure, or a heart abnormality?	☐	☐
9.	Do you have any allergies to any medicine?	☐	☐
10.	Are you missing a kidney?	☐	☐
11.	When was your last tetanus booster? _____	☐	☐
12.	For women.		
	a. At what age did you experience your first menstrual period? _____		
	b. In the last year, what is the longest time you have gone between periods? _____		

Explain any "yes" answers. _____
_____
_____
_____

I hereby state that, to the best of my knowledge, my answers to the above questions are correct.

Date _____
Signature of athlete _____
Signature of parent _____

Part B: Interim Health History
This form should be used during the interval between preparticipation evaluations. Positive responses should prompt a medical evaluation.

1. Over the next 12 months, I wish to participate in the following sports:
   a. _____
   b. _____
   c. _____
   d. _____

                                                                          Yes   **No**
2. Have you missed more than 3 consecutive days of participation in
   usual activities because of any injury this past year?   ☐   ☐
   If yes, please indicate:
   a. Site of injury _____
   b. Type of injury_____

3. Have you missed more than 5 consecutive days of participation in
   usual activities because of an illness, or have you had a medical illness
   diagnosed that has not been resolved in the past year?   ☐   ☐
   If yes, please indicate:
   a. Type of illness _____

4. Have you had a seizure or a concussion or been unconscious for
   any reason in the last year?   ☐   ☐

5. Have you had surgery or been hospitalized in this past year?   ☐   ☐
   If yes, please indicate:
   a. Reason for hospitalization _____
   b. Type of surgery_____

6. List all medications you are currently taking and what condition the medication is for.
   a. _____
   b. _____
   c. _____

7. Are you worried about any problem or condition at this time?   ☐   ☐
   If yes, please explain: _____
   _____

I hereby state that, to the best of my knowledge, my answers to the above questions are correct.

Date _____
Signature of athlete _____
Signature of parent _____

vides a record of the initial injury and lays the foundation for follow-up care. The accident report should include information such as that found in **Table 1-8**.

In litigation, these reports can document that duty of care was provided in a responsible manner. **Field Strategy 1-7** provides an example of an accident reporting form. Litigation may be brought years after an injury. A statute of limitations can vary from 3 to 7 years depending on state law. Check statutes in your state and keep all medical records in a safe secure location for the designated time.

Name _____ Age _____

Directions: Please answer the following questions to the best of your ability.

1. How old were you when you had your first menstrual period? _____
2. How often do you have a period? _____
3. How long do your periods last? _____
4. How many periods have you had in the last 12 months? _____
5. When was your last period? _____
6. Do you ever have trouble with heavy bleeding? _____
7. Do you have questions about tampon use?_____
8. Do you ever experience cramps during your period? _____
   If so, how do you treat them? _____
9. Do you take birth control pills or hormones? _____
10. Do you have any unusual discharge from your vagina? _____
11. When was your last pelvic exam? _____
12. Have you ever had an abnormal PAP smear? _____
13. How many urinary tract infections (bladder or kidney) have you had?
14. Have you ever been treated for anemia? _____
15. How many meals do you eat each day? How many snacks? _____
16. What have you eaten in the last 24 hours? _____
17. Are there certain food groups you refuse to eat (e.g., meats, breads)? _____
18. Have you ever been on a diet?_____
19. What is your present weight? _____
20. Are you happy with this weight? If not, what would you like to weigh?_____
21. Have you ever tried to control your weight by vomiting? _____
    Using laxatives? _____Diuretics? _____Diet pills?_____
22. Have you ever been diagnosed as having an eating disorder? _____
23. Do you have questions about healthy ways to control weight? _____

Injury Management, Rehabilitation and Progress Charts

The physician and athletic trainer should work together to develop goals and objectives to return the injured individual to full activity. Documentation of records may include day-to-day treatment logs (**Figure 1-6**) that record strapping or taping; therapeutic exercise logs; education, or counseling provided to the individual; rehabilitation charts that detail the therapeutic exercise program; and progress notes to record the individual's movement toward attaining the goals. These documents and a final functional evaluation can help the physician determine when the individual is ready to return to full competition. All records and the physician's clearance for full participation may also be used to document duty of care, and should be stored in a safe, secure location.

Supply and Equipment Inventory

Having supplies and equipment available when needed can make the job easier. At the end of the year a full inventory and inspection of supplies, equipment, and storage areas in the athletic training room or clinic should be conducted. Doing so will determine which supplies need replenishing, and if equipment needs to be repaired or replaced. A running inventory done throughout the year can identify anything in short supply so adequate time is available to replenish it.

Annual Reports

Nearly all employers require an annual report to assess the status of the facility and program. The annual report evaluates strengths and weaknesses of the health care program and provides recommendations for

All treatment and rehabilitation records, including the physician's clearance for participation, should be kept on file in a safe secure location

A running inventory can identify what supplies are running low so new supplies can be ordered before they are exhausted

⊕ Field Strategy 1-4. Physical Examination Record.

Name _____ Date _____ Age _____ Birth date _____

Height _____ Vision: R ____/_____ corrected _____uncorrected _____
Weight _____   L ____/_____ corrected _____uncorrected _____
Pulse_____ Blood Pressure _____Percent body fat (optional)_____

	Normal	Abnormal Findings	Initials
1. Eyes			
2. Ears, nose, throat			
3. Mouth, teeth			
4. Neck			
5. Cardiovascular			
6. Chest, lungs			
7. Abdomen			
8. Skin			
9. Genitalia: hernia (male)			
10. Musculoskeletal: ROM, strength, etc.			
a. neck			
b. spine			
c. shoulders			
d. arms, hands			
e. hips			
f. thighs			
g. knees			
h. ankles			
i. feet			
11. Neuromuscular			

12. Physical maturity (Tanner stage)   1   2   3   4   5

Comments re abnormal findings:_____
_____
_____
_____
_____
_____
_____

Participation Recommendations
1. No participation in: _____
_____

2. Limited participation in: _____
_____

3. Requires:_____
_____

4. Full participation in:_____
_____

Physician Signature _____
Telephone number_____Address_____

Field Strategy 1–5. The Two-minute Orthopedic Exam.

Instructions	Points of Observation
Stand facing examiner	Acromioclavicular joints, general posture
Look at ceiling, floor, over both shoulders; touch ears to shoulders	Cervical spine motion
Shrug shoulders (examiner resists)	Trapezius strength
Abduct arms 90° (examiner resists at 90°)	Deltoid strength
Fully rotate arms externally	Shoulder motion
Flex and extend elbows	Elbow motion
Pronate and supinate wrists with arms at sides, elbows flexed 90°	Elbow and wrist motion
Spread fingers; make fist	Hand or finger motion and deformities
Contract and relax quadriceps	Symmetry and knee effusion; ankle effusion
"Duck walk" four steps away from examiner with buttocks on heels	Hip, knee, and ankle motion
Stand with back to examiner	Shoulder symmetry, scoliosis
Straighten knees, touch toes	Scoliosis, hip motion, hamstring tightness
Raise up on toes	Calf symmetry, leg strength

 Field Strategy 1–6. Mass Station Screening Exam.

Station	Additional points	Personnel
1. Sign in, height, weight, vital signs, vision, body fat analysis	Blood pressure, pulse (radial, femoral), heart (rhythm, rate, size, murmurs) visual acuity, paired eyes, equal size of pupils, protective eyewear	Trainer, nurse, or physician
2. Medical history	Personal, orthopedic, and family medical history	Trainer or nurse
3. Medical examination	Skin analysis, abdominal masses, genitalia (undescended testicle, testicular mass, hernia), single organs, cardiovascular, urine analysis	Physician
4. Orthopedic examination	Postural assessment, range of motion and strength measurements (see specific orthopedic assessment)	Trainer or physician
5. Anaerobic assessment	Shuttle run, sit-ups, 40-yard dash, vertical jump	Trainer or coach
6. Aerobic assessment	Step test, timed mile run	Trainer or coach
7. Check out	Review records to determine: Full clearance for participation Clearance with limitations after certain conditions have been met Limited participation No participation	Physician

Table 1–7. Disqualifying Conditions for Sport Participation.

Recommendations for Participation in Competitive Sports

Physical condition	Contact/ collision	Limited contact/ impact	Noncontact— strenuous	Noncontact— moderately strenuous	Noncontact— nonstrenuous
Atlantoaxial instability	No	No	Yes; in swimming, no butterfly, breast stroke or diving starts	Yes	Yes
Acute illness	Requires individual assessment (e.g., contagiousness, exacerbation of illness)				
Cardiovascular					
Carditis	No	No	No	No	No
Hypertension					
Mild	Yes	Yes	Yes	Yes	Yes
Moderate	Requires individual assessment				
Severe	Requires individual assessment				
Congenital heart disease	Patients with mild forms can be allowed a full range of physical activities; patients with moderate or severe forms or those who are postoperative should be evaluated by a cardiologist before athletic participation				
Absence or loss of function in one eye	Eye guards may allow the athlete to participant in most sports, but this must be judged on an individual basis				
Detached retina	Consult an ophthalmologist				
Inguinal hernia	Yes	Yes	Yes	Yes	Yes
Absence of one kidney	No	Yes	Yes	Yes	Yes
Enlarged liver	No	No	Yes	Yes	Yes
Musculoskeletal disorders	Requires individual assessment				
History of serious head or spine trauma, repeated concussions or craniotomy	Requires individual assessment		Yes	Yes	Yes
Convulsion disorder					
Poorly controlled	Yes	Yes	Yes	Yes	Yes
Well controlled	No	No	Yes; no swimming or weight lifting	Yes	Yes; no archery or riflery
Absence of one ovary	Yes	Yes	Yes	Yes	Yes
Pulmonary insufficiency	May be allowed to compete if oxygenation remains satisfactory during a graded stress test				Yes
Asthma	Yes	Yes	Yes	Yes	Yes
Sickle cell trait	Yes	Yes	Yes	Yes	Yes
Skin: boils, herpes, impetigo, scabies	While contagious, no contact sports or gymnastics using mats		Yes	Yes	Yes
Enlarged spleen	No	No	No	Yes	Yes
Absent or undescended testicle	Yes; certain sports may require a protective cup		Yes	Yes	Yes

improvement. These reports may include the number of individuals cared for by the health care staff, the number and types of injuries treated, professional involvement or community service done by the staff, identification of equipment or facilities that need to be replaced or repaired, and recommendations for further improvement in the program. This report is then forwarded to the facility administrator.

💡 *In administering immediate care to the individual who received a direct blow to the anterior leg, did you determine that an injury report should be completed document-*

Medical Data Information Card

Name _____ Age _____ Gender _____ ID# _____
Activity _____ Sport _____

Home Address _____ Phone _____
City _____ State _____ Zip _____

Parents/Guardian _____
Home Address _____ Phone _____
City _____ State _____ Zip _____

In case of emergency contact: [if different than above.]
Name _____ Relationship _____
Home Address _____ Phone _____
City _____ State _____ Zip _____

Insurance carrier_____ Policy number _____

Past injuries/illnesses that affected participation & dates: _____
_____

Special medic alerts or health concerns: _____
_____

Fig. 1.5: Medical data information cards document pertinent personal and medical information on the individual, the contact in case of an emergency, and the current health insurance carrier and policy number.

Table 1–8. Information Needed on an Accident Report.

Who was injured?
When did the injury occur and what activity was the individual participating in?
Where did the injury occur?
What body part was injured?
Was the individual wearing any protective equipment at the time of injury?
How did the injury occur (mechanism)?
What did you do to assess and manage the injury, including:
   History of the injury
   Injury assessment and severity
   Immediate first aid care provided
What recommendation for referral to a physician was made?
Was determination of eligibility for continued participation made?
If referred to a physician, this determination should be completed by the physician and
   documented on the report

---

ing the injury and the need to see a physician? The individual should have been instructed to have the physician complete and return the form to the supervisor to document the physician's orders for further care and eligibility for participation.

CAREER OPPORTUNITIES IN ATHLETIC TRAINING

Career opportunities for athletic trainers are becoming increasingly available in both the public and private sectors. Envi-

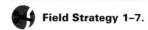 **Field Strategy 1–7.**

FALL RIVER PUBLIC SCHOOLS
STANDARD STUDENT ACCIDENT REPORT FORM
Part A. Information on ALL Accidents

No.
Date Rec'd
Office Use Only

1. Name: .... Home Address: ....
2. School: .... Sex: M ☐; F ☐. Age: .... Grade or classification ....
3. Time accident occured: Hour .... A.M.; .... P.M. Date: ....
4. Place of Accident: School Building ☐   School Grounds ☐   To or from School ☐   Home ☐   Elsewhere ☐

5. **NATURE OF INJURY**	Abrasion	Fracture	DESCRIPTION OF THE ACCIDENT
	Amputation	Laceration	How did accident happen? What was student doing? Where was student? List specifically unsafe acts and unsafe conditions existing. Specify any tool, machine or equipment involved. ....
	Asphyxiation	Poisoning	
	Bite	Puncture	
	Bruise	Scalds	
	Burn	Scratches	
	Concussion	Shock (el.)	
	Cut	Sprain	
	Dislocation		
	Other (specify)		
PART OF BODY INJURED	Abdomen		
	Ankle	Foot	
	Arm	Hand	
	Back	Knee	
	Chest	Leg	
	Ear	Mouth	
	Elbow	Nose	
	Eye	Scalp	
	Face	Tooth	
	Finger	Wrist	
	Other (specify)		

6. Degree of Injury: Death ☐   Permanent Impairment ☐   Temporary Disability ☐   Nondisabling ☐
7. Total number of days lost from school: .... (To be filled in when student returns to school)

Part B. Additional Information on School Jurisdiction Accidents

8. Teacher in charge when accident occurred (Enter name): ....
    Present at scene of accident: No: .... Yes: .... Does student have school insurance No: .... Yes: ....

9. **IMMEDIATE ACTION TAKEN**	First-aid treatment ...... By (Name): ....
	Sent to school nurse ...... By (Name): ....
	Sent home ...... By (Name): ....
	Sent to physician ...... By (Name): ....
	Physician's Name: ....
	Sent to hospital ...... By (Name): ....
	Name of Hospital: ....

10. Was a parent or other individual notified, No: .... Yes: .... When .... How: ....
    Name of Individual notified: ....
    By whom? (Enter name): ....
11. Witness: 1. Name: .... Address: ....
    2. Name: .... Address: ....

12. **LOCATION**		Specify Activity		Specify Activity		Remarks
	Athletic field	...................Locker	....			What recommendations do you have for preventing other accidents of this type, ...
	Auditorium	...................Pool	....			
	Cafeteria	...................Sch. grounds	....			
	Classroom	.... shop	....			
	Corridor	...................Showers	....			
	Dressing room	...................Stairs	....			
	Gymnasium	...................Toilets and				
	Home Econ.	.... washrooms				
	Laboratories	...................Other (specify)				

Signed: Principal: .... Teacher: ....

sion yourself 5 years from now as an athletic trainer. Where would you like to be working at that time?

Today, athletic training is an excellent career choice for many women and men who want to work with children, interscholastic, intercollegiate, recreational, and professional athletes in a health care environment. This allied health profession provides a challenging and valuable service needed at all levels of

State College
Sports Medicine
Daily Treatments

Date _____

Name	Injury Area	Sport	Ice	Ice Massage	Ice Soak	Cold Pack	Cold Whirlpool	Contrast	Warm Whirlpool	Hydroculator	Ultrasound	Sound-Stim Come	EMS	FITRON/BIKE	BAPS Board	Multi-Axial	Cybex-Orthotron	Proprioception	Flexibility EX	Achilles Slant	Rehabilitation	Wound Cleansing	Padding	Wrap	Tape	Other	Trainer Initials

Fig. 1.6: Daily treatment logs record strapping and taping, therapeutic exercise, use of modalities, and education or counseling of the individual.

sport participation. Athletic trainers are generally employed in secondary school, intercollegiate, or professional athletic programs, sports medicine clinics, clinical and industrial health care programs, health and fitness clubs, or a combination of any of the above.

In a 1992 NATA Professional Education Committee report, 92% of the graduates from NATA-approved graduate athletic training educational programs found employment at either sports medicine and related clinics (51%), in high schools (10%), colleges (29%), or professional athletic programs (1%). Of the remaining 8%, 2% went directly into post-graduate study, 4% found employment in other occupations, and 2% were unknown. In the NATA-approved undergraduate athletic training educational programs, 39% went directly into graduate education programs, while 43% found employment in sports medicine or related clinics (27%), in high schools (9%), in colleges (2%), or professional athletic programs (1%). Nine percent found other employment in non-related fields and nine percent were unemployed or of unknown status (21). Entry-level salaries for a bachelor's degree (BS) average $23,065 (±4,635) and $25,368 (±5,826) for a master's degree (MS) (22). The more common employment sites will be discussed.

High School and Collegiate Settings

High school and collegiate settings are often referred to as traditional athletic training settings. Because of the number and seriousness of injuries in competitive sport programs, the need exists for an athletic trainer on every school staff. However, less than 20% of high schools have access to an athletic trainer.

In high schools, the athletic trainer is often hired as a faculty member and given a reduced teaching load, or paid additional monies for athletic training duties. The individual begins work 2 to 3 weeks prior to the start of school with preseason practice sessions, and provides health care coverage to athletes throughout the school year.

At the college level, athletic training responsibilities vary. At most colleges the athletic trainer is hired to provide services only to intercollegiate athletes. The individual is placed on a 10 or 12 month work schedule depending on the demands of the job. In smaller schools the athletic trainer may teach part-time in the physical education or health department, and provide athletic training services to athletes. The athletic trainers may also be asked to work in the campus health center assessing general health, supervising rehabilitation programs, or educating students on health issues.

An advantage to working at a school site is the opportunity to see a variety of injuries and illnesses, and the general satisfaction in helping competitive athletes stay healthy. Many individuals enjoy the prestige of working in a highly visible high school or college program. Depending on the number of athletic trainers working at the school, disadvantages may involve long work hours and excessive travel responsibilities in providing coverage to the various teams.

Sports Medicine Clinics

Privately owned sports medicine clinics and related clinics provide a variety of job opportunities for athletic trainers (**Figure 1-7**). The patients vary in age, level of perfor-

High school and collegiate settings are often referred to as traditional athletic training sites

An advantage to working at a school site is seeing a variety of injuries, and having the satisfaction in helping competitive athletes stay healthy

Athletic trainers working in a sports medicine clinic can expect to work a standardized work day, and see a variety of patients and conditions

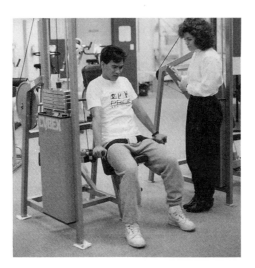

Fig. 1.7: Patients at a sports medicine clinic vary in age, level of performance, and have a wider variety of conditions needing treatment.

mance, and have a wider variety of conditions needing treatment. Under the direction of a physician, the athletic trainer provides activity related health care services. Some clinics may specialize in only sport related injuries, while others may deal in cardiac rehabilitation, exercise physiology, biomechanical analysis, workman's compensation injuries, or may serve the general population. Athletic trainers working in a sports medicine clinic can expect to work a standardized work day during which they see a variety of patients and conditions. In some states direct billing or licensure standards may restrict the athletic trainer from providing certain services, such as initial patient evaluation or using electrical modalities.

Dual High School/Clinic Trainer

Many sports medicine clinics are subcontracting athletic training services to area high schools. The clinic hires the athletic trainer full-time but splits the trainer's time between the clinic in the mornings and high school in the afternoon or evening. As mentioned earlier, direct billing or licensure laws may restrict some services provided by the athletic trainer in a clinic setting. This arrangement is growing in popularity throughout the United States, as evidenced in recent NATA studies (21). As licensure laws begin to adapt to the changing athletic training profession, the clinical setting may provide an excellent career option.

Industrial Health Care Programs

Many companies hire athletic trainers to provide employees with in-house athletic training services. Working under the direction of a physician, the athletic trainer can perform injury assessment, management, rehabilitation, develop wellness and fitness programs, and provide education and counseling for employees. Not only is this cost effective, it is also time efficient as employees do not need to leave work for these services.

Professional Sport Teams

Athletic trainers for professional sport teams are usually hired by a single sport team to perform athletic training services throughout the year. During the competitive season the athletic trainer will concentrate on traditional duties, but during the remainder of the year the trainer may be asked to develop and supervise general conditioning programs, rehabilitate injured athletes, or recruit players, do scouting, manage equipment, or make travel arrangements for the team. Salaries vary considerably depending on the length of the playing season, revenues from television, and potential monies from playoffs and championships.

Have you determined what setting you would like to be working in as an athletic trainer? What advantages and disadvantages exist in each setting?

SUMMARY

Sports medicine is a branch of medicine that applies medical and scientific knowledge to improve sport performance. The primary sports medicine team provides on-site supervision to prevent injury and deliver immediate health care. The athletic trainer, coach, sport supervisor, team physician, primary care physician, and sport participant are all members of this team. Athletic trainers serve as the essential link between the sport program and medical community. Working under the direction of a physician, athletic trainers are responsible for the prevention, recognition and evaluation, management and treatment, and rehabilitation of injuries; organization and administration of the athletic training program; and education and counseling of sport participants.

Standards of professional practice are ethical judgments that guide your actions and

Many sports medicine clinics hire athletic trainers to work in the clinic in the mornings and in local high schools in the afternoon

Industries hire athletic trainers to provide employees with cost effective in-house athletic training services

promote high standards of conduct and integrity. For an athletic trainer, NATA certification and state licensure can help meet one's duty of care in providing health care to sport participants. Decisions concerning whether or not an individual should participate in an activity should be made by the physician based on sound medical consideration, and should never compromise the health of the individual.

Prevention of accidents and injuries is a major task for all athletic trainers and sport supervisors. To find an individual liable, the injured person must prove that there was a duty of care, there was a breach of that duty, and there was harm caused by that breach. Steps to reduce the risk of injury and subsequent litigation should include obtaining informed consent; recognizing the potential for injury and correcting it; warning participants of the risk of injury; hiring qualified personnel; proper supervision and instruction; purchasing, fitting, and maintaining quality equipment; posting appropriate warning signs; maintaining accurate and complete health care records; and having a well-organized emergency care system.

Accurate records are a major defense in litigation and serve to improve communication among all members of the primary sports medicine team. Direct communication concerning preparticipation exams, insurance forms, personal data information cards, accident reports and injury management forms, daily treatment or status reports, rehabilitation programs and progress charts, clearance for participation, supply and equipment inventory, and annual reports will document that personnel are providing their duty of care.

Athletic trainers are generally employed in secondary school, intercollegiate, or professional athletic programs, sports medicine clinics, clinical and industrial health care programs, at research facilities, health clubs, or a combination of any of the above. Each setting provides positive attributes for the athletic trainer who wants to work with children, with interscholastic, intercollegiate, recreational, or professional athletes in a health care environment.

REFERENCES

1. Herbert, DL. *Legal Aspects of Sports Medicine*. Canton, OH: Professional Reports Corporation, 1990.

2. Mellion, MB. *Office Management of Sports Injuries and Athletic Problems*. Philadelphia: Hanley & Belfus, 1988.

3. Powell, J. 1989. Injury toll in prep sports estimated at 1.3 million, Ath Train (JNATA), 24(4):360-373.

4. Ramotar, JE. 1990. No direct deaths in high school football. Phys and Sportsmed, 19(9):48-49.

5. Mellion, MB, and Walsh, WM. "The team physician." In *The Team Physician's Handbook*, edited by MB Mellion, WM Walsh, and GL Shelton. Philadelphia: Hanley & Belfus, 1990.

6. Magnus, BC, and Ingersoll, CD. 1990. Approaches to ethical decision making in athletic training. Ath Train (JNATA), 25(4):340-343.

7. National Athletic Trainers' Association. 1992. New NATA code of ethics approved. NATA News, 4(7): 15-16.

8. National Athletic Trainers' Association. 1993. NATA Code of Ethics. Approved at the annual meeting of the National Athletic Trainers' Association, Kansas City, June, 1993.

9. Committee on Allied Health Education and Accreditation. *Essentials and Guidelines for an Accredited Educational Program for the Athletic Trainer*. Chicago: American Medical Association, 1992.

10. NATA Board of Certification Continuing Education Office. Continuing Education File 1994-1996. NATA Board of Certification, Inc., 1994.

11. National Athletic Trainers' Association. 1992. Governmental Affairs. NATA News, 4(3):25.

12. Governmental Affairs Committee, National Athletic Trainer's Association, Inc.. Personal communication with author, 15 April, 1994.

13. Clement, A. *Law in sport and physical activity*. Indianapolis: Benchmark Press, 1988.

14. Leverenz, LJ, and Helms, LB. 1990. Suing athletic trainers: Part I, A review of the case law involving athletic trainers. Ath Train (JNATA), 25(3):212-216.

15. Bailey, JA, and Matthews, DL. *Law and liability in athletics, physical education, and recreation*. Dubuque: Wm C Brown Publishing, 1989.

16. Leverenz, LJ, and Helms, LB. 1990. Suing athletic trainers: Part II, Implications for the NATA competencies. Ath Train (JNATA), 25(3):219-226.

17. Smith, DM, Lombardo, JA, and Robinson, JB. "The preparticipation evaluation." In *Primary Care*, edited by MB Mellion, vol. 18, no. 4. Philadelphia: WB Saunders Company, 1991.

18. Tanji, JL. 1990. The preparticipation physical examination for sports. Amer Fam Phys, 42(2):397-405.

19. Johnson, MD. 1992. Tailoring the preparticipation exam to female athletes. Phys and Sportsmed, 20(7):61-72.

20. Magnes, SA, Henderson, JM, and Hunter, SC. 1992. What conditions limit sports participation? Experience with 10,540 athletes. Phys and Sportsmed, 20(5):143-158.

21. Professional Education Committee. Athletic Training Education Newsletter. National Athletic Trainers' Association, Inc. November, 1993:12-15.

22. Moss, CL. 1993. 1992 Entry-level Salaries for Athletic Trainers. J of Ath Train (JNATA), 28(2):151.

Chapter 2

The Mechanics of Tissue Injury and Healing

After you have completed this chapter, you should be able to:

- Define compression, tension, shear, stress, strain, bending, and torsion, and explain how each can play a role in injury to biological tissues

- Explain how the material constituents and structural organization of skin, tendon, ligament, muscle, and bone affect the ability of these structures to withstand the mechanical loads to which each is subjected

- List and describe common injuries of skin, tendons, ligaments, muscles, and bone

- Describe the processes by which tissue healing occurs in skin, tendons, ligaments, muscles, and bone

- Explain the mechanisms by which nerves are injured and the processes by which nerves can heal

- Discuss the types of altered sensation that can result from nerve injury

Human movement during sport and exercise is typically faster and produces greater force than is normally the case during activities of daily living. As a result, the potential for injury is also heightened. Understanding the different ways in which forces act upon the body is necessary for understanding how to best prevent injuries. Likewise, understanding the material and structural properties of skin, tendon, ligament, muscle, bone, and nerve is essential for understanding how these tissues respond to applied forces.

This chapter begins with a general discussion of injury mechanisms, including descriptions of force and torque and their effects. Next are sections on soft tissues, bone, and nerve that address the mechanical characteristics of these tissues, the types of sport injury to which each can be subjected, and the processes by which the tissues heal.

INJURY MECHANISMS

Athletes routinely sustain larger than usual forces during both training and competition. What factors determine whether a given force results in injury?

Analyzing the mechanics of injuries to the human body is complicated by several factors. First, potentially injurious forces applied to the body act at different angles, over different surface areas, and over different periods of time. Second, the human body is composed of many different types of tissue, which respond differently to applied forces. Finally, injury to the human body is not an all or none phenomenon. That is, injuries range in severity. This section introduces the types of mechanical loading that can cause injury, and describes the basic mechanical responses of biological tissues to these forms of loading.

Force and Its Effects

Force may be thought of as a push or a pull acting on a body. A multitude of forces act on our bodies routinely during the course of daily activities. The forces of gravity and friction enable us to move about in predictable ways when internal forces are produced by muscles. During sport participation we apply forces to balls, bats, racquets, and clubs and we absorb forces from impacts with the ball used in the sport, the ground or floor, and our opponents in contact sports.

When a force acts there are two potential effects on the target object. The first is acceleration, or change in velocity, and the second is deformation, or change in shape. For example, when a racquetball is struck with a

Force produces acceleration and/or deformation of the object acted upon

racquet, the ball is both accelerated (put in motion in the direction of the racquet swing) and deformed (flattened on the side struck). The greater the stiffness of the material to which a force is applied, the greater the likelihood that the deformation will be too small to be easily seen. The more elastic the material to which a force is applied, the greater the likelihood that the deformation will be temporary, with the body springing back to regain its original shape.

When a force is sustained by the tissues of the human body, two primary factors help to determine whether injury results. The first is the size, or magnitude of the force, and the second is the material properties of the involved tissues. **Figure 2-1** is a load-deformation curve, which shows the deformation of a structure in response to progressive loading, or force application. With relatively small loads, the response of the structure is elastic, meaning that when the load is removed, the material will return to its original size and shape. Within the elastic region of the load-deformation curve, the greater the stiffness of the material, the steeper the slope of the line. Greater stiffness, therefore, translates to less deformation in response to a given load. With loads exceeding the material's **yield point**, or **elastic limit**, however, the response of the structure is plastic, meaning that when the load is removed, some amount of deformation will remain. Loads exceeding the ultimate failure point on the load-deformation curve result in mechanical **failure** of the structure, which translates to fracturing of bone or rupturing of soft tissues.

The direction in which force is applied to biological materials also has important implications for injury potential. Many tissues are **anisotropic**, meaning that the structure is stronger in resisting force from some directions than from others. The anatomical makeup of many of the joints of the human body also make them more susceptible to injury from a given direction. For example, lateral ankle sprains are much more common than medial ankle sprains because ligamentous support of the ankle is much stronger on the medial side. Consequently, in discussing injury mechanisms, force is commonly categorized according to the direction from which the force acts on the affected structure.

Force acting along the long axis of a structure is termed axial force. When the opponent in fencing is touched with the foil, the foil is loaded axially. When the human body is in an upright standing position, body weight creates axial loads on the femur and the tibia, the major weight bearing bones of the lower extremity.

Axial loading that produces a squeezing or crushing effect is termed compressive force or compression (**Figure 2-2**). The weight of the human body constantly produces compression on the bones that support it. The 5th lumbar vertebra must support the weight of the head, trunk, and arms when the body is erect, producing compression on the intervertebral disc below it. When a football player is sandwiched between two opposing players, the force acting on the player is compressive. In the absence of sufficient padding, compressive forces sustained during contact sports often result in bruises, or contusions.

Axial loading in the direction opposite that of compression is called tensile force or tension (**Figure 2-2**). Tension is a pulling force that tends to stretch the object to which it is applied. Muscle contraction produces tensile force on the attached bone, enabling movement of that bone. When the foot and ankle

Yield point (elastic limit)
The maximum load that a material can sustain without permanent deformation

Failure
Loss of continuity; rupturing of soft tissue or fracture of bone

Anisotropic
Having different strengths in response to loads from different directions

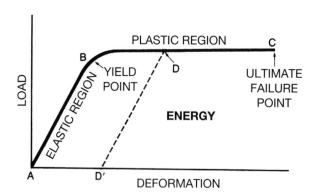

Fig. 2.1: Load-deformation curve for a structure composed of pliable material.

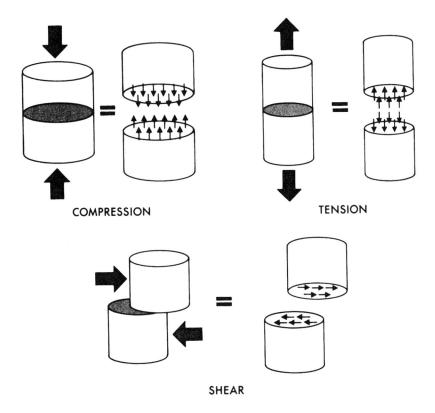

Fig. 2.2: Compression and tension are directed along the longitudinal axis of a structure, whereas shear acts parallel to a surface.

are inverted or rotated excessively, the tensile forces applied to the ligaments may result in an ankle sprain.

Whereas compressive and tensile forces are directed toward and away from an object, a third category of force, termed shear, acts parallel or tangent to a plane passing through the object **(Figure 2-2)**. Shear force tends to cause one part of the object to slide or dis-place with respect to another part of the object. Shear forces acting on the spine can cause spondylolisthesis, a condition involving anterior slippage of a vertebra with respect to the vertebra below it.

When force is sustained by the human body, another important factor related to the likelihood of injury is the magnitude of the **stress** produced by that force. Mechanical

Stress
The distribution of force within a body; quantified as force divided by the area over which the force acts

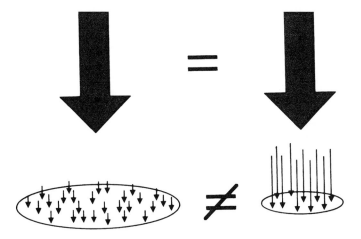

Fig. 2.3: The stress produced by a force depends on the area over which the force is spread.

stress is defined as force divided by the surface area over which the force is applied (**Figure 2-3**). When a given force is distributed over a large area, the resulting stress is less than if the force were distributed over a smaller area. Alternatively, if a force is concentrated over a small area, the mechanical stress is relatively high. It is a high magnitude of stress, rather than a high magnitude of force, that tends to result in injury to biological tissues. One of the reasons that football and ice hockey players wear pads is that a pad distributes any force sustained across the entire pad, thereby reducing the stress acting on the player.

Strain may be thought of as the amount of deformation an object undergoes in response to an applied force. Application of compressive force to an object produces shortening and widening of the structure, whereas tensile force produces lengthening and narrowing of the structure. Shear results in internal changes in the structure acted upon. The ultimate strength of biological tissues determines the amount of strain that a structure can withstand without fracturing or rupturing.

Injury to biological tissues can result from a single traumatic force of relatively large magnitude, or from repeated forces of relatively smaller magnitude. When a single force produces an injury, the injury is called an acute injury and the causative force is termed macrotrauma. An acute injury, such as a ruptured anterior cruciate ligament or a fractured humerus, is characterized by a definitive moment of onset followed by a relatively predictable process of healing. When repeated or chronic loading over a period of time produces an injury, the injury is called a chronic injury or a stress injury, and the causative mechanism is termed microtrauma. A chronic injury, such as glenohumeral bursitis or a metatarsal stress fracture, develops and worsens gradually over time, typically culminating in a threshold episode in which pain and inflammation become evident. Chronic injuries may persist for months or years.

Many biological tissues, including tendon, ligament, muscle, and bone, tend to respond to gradually increased mechanical stress by becoming larger and stronger. When a runner's training protocol incorporates progressively increasing mileage, it is important that this occur in a gradual fashion so the body can adapt to the increased mechanical stress to prevent a stress injury. Overuse syndromes and

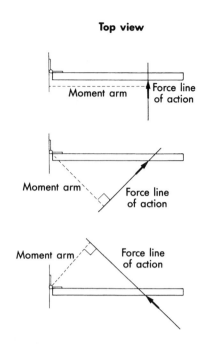

Top view

Fig. 2.4: Torque created at the hinges of a door is the product of force and the force's moment arm.

stress fractures result from the body's inability to adapt to an increased training regimen.

Torque and Its Effects

Consider what happens when a swinging door is opened. A hand applies force to the door, causing it to rotate about its hinges (**Figure 2-4**). Two factors influence whether the door will swing in response to the force. One factor is the force's magnitude. Equally important, however, is the force's moment arm. The moment arm is the perpendicular distance from the force's line of action to the axis of rotation. The product of a force and its moment arm is called torque, or moment. Torque may be thought of as rotary force. It is the amount of torque acting that determines whether a rotating body such as a door will move.

In the human body, it is torque that produces rotation of a body segment about a joint. When a muscle develops tension it produces torque at the joint that it crosses. The amount of torque produced is the product of muscle force and the muscle's moment arm with respect to the joint center (**Figure 2-5**). For example, the torque produced by the biceps brachii is the product of the tension developed by the muscle and the distance between its attachment on the radius and the center of rotation at the elbow.

It is a high magnitude of stress rather than a high magnitude of force which causes injury

Strain
Amount of deformation with respect to the original dimensions of the structure

Acute injuries are caused by a single force called macrotrauma

Stress injuries are caused by repeated loading called microtrauma

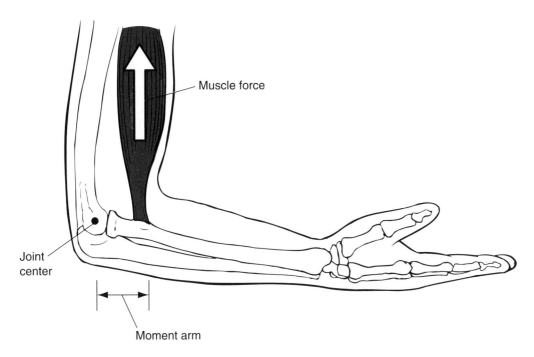

Muscle force

Joint center

Moment arm

Fig. 2.5: The torque produced at a joint is the product of the magnitude of muscle force and the muscle's moment arm (perpendicular distance of the muscle's line of action to the axis of rotation at the joint center).

Excessive torque can produce injury. Such torque is usually generated by forces external to the body rather than by the muscles. The simultaneous application of forces from opposite directions at different points along a structure such as a long bone generate a torque known as a bending moment, which can cause **bending** and ultimately fracture of the bone (**Figure 2-6**). If a football player's leg is anchored to the ground and he is tackled on that leg from the front while being pushed into the tackle from behind, a bending moment is created on the leg. When bending is present the structure is loaded in tension on one side and in compression on the opposite side (**Figure 2-6**). Because bone is stronger in resisting compression than tension, the side of the bone loaded in tension will fracture if the bending moment is sufficiently large.

The application of torque about the long axis of a structure such as a long bone can cause **torsion**, or twisting of the structure (**Figure 2-6**). Torsion results in the creation of shear stress throughout the structure. In skiing accidents where one boot and ski are firmly planted and the skier rotates during a fall, torsional loads can cause a spiral fracture of the tibia.

Factors that influence the likelihood of injury when a force is sustained include force magnitude and direction, the area over which the force acts, the force's moment arm (which determines the amount of torque generated), and the type(s) of tissue affected.

SOFT TISSUE INJURIES

Tendon and ligament are both collagenous connective tissues, yet they are somewhat different in both structure and function. Based on these differences, what are the implications for injury?

Skin, tendon, ligament, and muscle are soft (non-bony) tissues that behave in characteristic ways when subjected to different forms of loading. Anatomic structure and material composition influence the mechanical behavior of each tissue.

Anatomical Properties of Soft Tissue

Skin, tendon, and ligament are known as collagenous tissues after their major building block: collagen. Collagen is a protein that is strong in resisting tension. Collagen fibers have a wavy configuration in a tissue that is not in tension (**Figure 2-7**). This enables collagenous tissues to stretch slightly under tensile loading as these fibers straighten. Thus, collagen fibers provide strength and flexibility to tissues, but are relatively inelastic. Elastin, another protein, provides added elas-

Bending
Loading that produces tension on one side of an object and compression on the other side

As a bone bends, the side loaded in tension tends to fracture first

Torsion
Twisting around an object's longitudinal axis in response to an applied torque

Collagen resists tension and provides strength and flexibility to tissues but is relatively inelastic

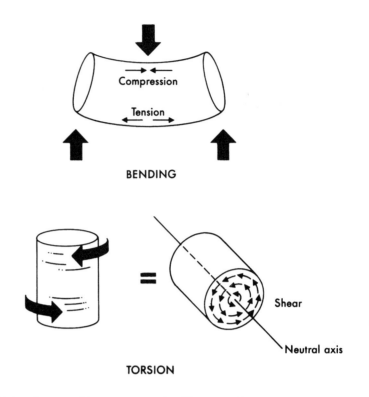

BENDING

TORSION

Shear

Neutral axis

Fig. 2.6: Bones loaded in bending are subject to compression (C) on one side and to tension (T) on the other. Bones loaded in torsion develop internal shear stress, with maximal stress at the periphery and no stress at the neutral axis, as shown above.

ticity to some connective tissue structures, such as the ligamentum flavum of the spine.

Skin

The skin is composed of two major regions. The outer region, known as the epidermis, has multiple layers containing the pigment melanin, along with the hair, nails, sebaceous glands, and sweat glands (**Figure 2-8**). Beneath the epidermis is the dermis, contain-

ing blood vessels, nerve endings, hair follicles, sebaceous glands, and sweat glands.

The dermis is composed of dense irregular connective tissue, characterized by a loose, multidirectional arrangement of collagen fibers. This fiber arrangement enables the resistance of multidirectional loads, including compression, tension, and shear. This type of tissue also forms the fascia, fibrous sheets of connective tissue that surround muscles.

The epidermis and dermis are the major outer and inner layers of skin

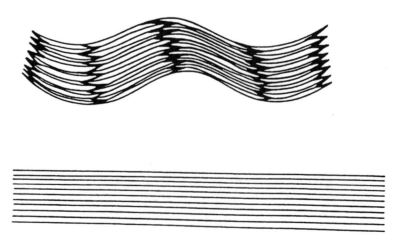

Fig. 2.7: Collagen fibers are wavy in configuration when unloaded, and straightened when loaded in tension.

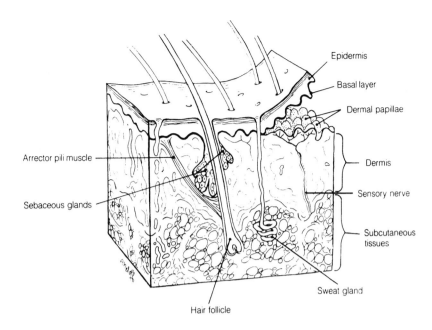

Fig. 2.8: Skin. The structures contained in the epidermis and dermis.

Dense irregular connective tissue also covers internal structures such as the liver, lymph nodes, and testes, as well as the bones, cartilages, and nerves.

Other components of the skin are elastic fibers and reticular fibers. Elastic fibers provide the skin with some elasticity. Reticular fibers are composed of a type of collagen known as reticulin. These fibers function like collagen fibers, but are much thinner. Reticular fibers also form a meshed network that provides support for internal structures such as the lymph nodes, spleen, bone marrow, and liver.

Tendons, Ligaments, and Aponeuroses

Tendons connect muscle to bone, whereas ligaments connect bone to bone. Both structures are composed of dense regular connective tissue, consisting of tightly packed bundles of unidirectional collagen fibers. In tendons, the collagen fibers are arranged in a parallel pattern, enabling resistance of high, unidirectional tensile loads when the attached muscle contracts (**Figure 2-9**). In ligaments, the collagen fibers are largely parallel, but are also interwoven among each other (**Figure 2-9**). This arrangement is well-suited to ligament function, enabling

The arrangements of collagen fibers in tendon and ligament provide strength against the loads to which the tissues are subjected

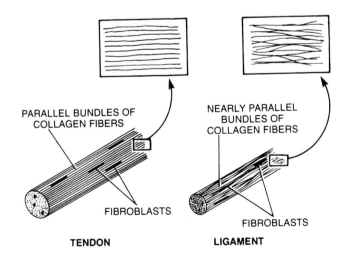

Fig. 2.9: Collagen arrangements in tendon and ligament.

resistance of large tensile loads along the long axis of the ligament, but also providing resistance to smaller tensile loads from other directions.

Ligaments contain more elastin than tendons, and so are somewhat more elastic than tendons. From a functional standpoint this is appropriate, because ligaments are connected at both ends to bones, while tendons attach on one end to muscle, a tissue with some elasticity. Although most ligaments contain only small amounts of elastin, the ligamentum flavum of the spine is composed of approximately two-thirds elastic fibers and one-third collagen fibers (1). This ligament has a specialized role in providing stability to the multisegmented spine; it stretches to allow spinal flexion, but remains taut when the spine is in a neutral position.

The aponeuroses are another set of structures formed by dense, regular, connective tissue. These are strong, flat, sheet-like tissues that attach muscles to other muscles or to bones.

Muscle

Muscle is a highly organized structure. Each muscle cell, or fiber, is surrounded by a sheath known as the endomysium. Small numbers of fibers are bound up into fascicles by a dense connective tissue sheath called the perimysium. A muscle is composed of several

fascicles surrounded by the epimysium (**Figure 2-10**).

The structure and composition of muscle enable it to function in a **viscoelastic** fashion —that is, muscle is characterized by both time-dependent extensibility and elasticity. Extensibility is the ability to be stretched or to increase in length, whereas elasticity is the ability to return to normal length after either lengthening or shortening has taken place. The viscoelastic aspect of muscle extensibility enables muscle to stretch to greater lengths over time in response to a sustained tensile force. This means that a static stretch maintained for 30 seconds is more effective in increasing muscle length than a series of short ballistic stretches.

Another of muscle's characteristic properties, irritability, is the ability to respond to a stimulus. Stimuli affecting muscles can be either electrochemical, such as an action potential from the attaching nerve, or mechanical, as with an external blow to the muscle. If the stimulus is of sufficient magnitude, muscle responds by developing tension.

The ability to develop tension is a property unique to muscle. Although some sources refer to this ability as *contractility*, a muscle may or may not contract (shorten) when tension is developed. For example, isometric "contraction" involves no joint movement and no change in muscle length, and eccentric "contraction" actually involves lengthening of

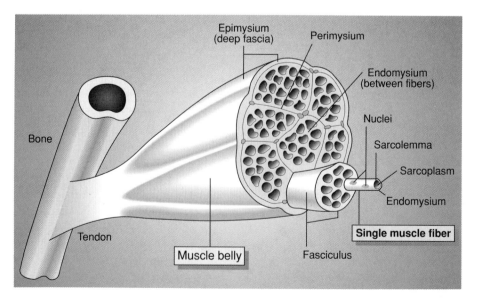

Fig. 2.10: Muscle tissue.

the muscle developing tension. Only when a muscle develops tension concentrically does it also shorten. When a stimulated muscle develops tension, the amount of tension present is the same throughout the muscle and tendon and at the site of the tendon attachment to bone.

Skin Injury Classifications

Forces applied to the body in different ways and from different directions result in different types of injury. Because the skin is the body's first layer of defense against injury it is the most frequently injured body tissue.

Abrasions are common minor skin injuries caused by shear when the skin is scraped with sufficient force, usually in one direction, against a rough surface. The greater the applied force, the more layers of skin that are scraped away.

Blisters are minor skin injuries caused by repeated application of shear in one or more directions, as happens when a shoe rubs back and forth against the foot. The result is the formation of a pocket of fluid between the epidermis and dermis as fluid migrates to the site of injury.

Skin bruises are injuries resulting from compression sustained during a blow. Damage to the underlying capillaries causes the accumulation of blood within the skin.

Incisions, lacerations, avulsions, and punctures are breaks in the skin resulting from injury. An incision is a clean cut, produced by the application of a tensile force to the skin as it is stretched along a sharp edge. A laceration is an irregular tear in the skin that typically results from a combination of tension and shear. An avulsion is a severe laceration that results in complete separation of the skin from the underlying tissues. A puncture wound results when a sharp, cylindrical object penetrates the skin and underlying tissues with tensile loading. The care of skin wounds with bleeding present is discussed in Chapter 3.

Other Soft Tissue Injury Classifications

Injuries to the soft tissues below the skin are also dependent upon the nature of the causative force. Other factors of relevance are the location (superficial vs. deep) and the material properties of the involved tissues.

Muscle **contusions** or bruises result from compression sustained from heavier blows.

Such injuries vary in severity in accordance with the area and depth over which blood vessels are ruptured. **Ecchymosis**, or tissue discoloration, may be present if the hemorrhage is superficial. As blood and lymph flow into the damaged area swelling occurs, often resulting in the formation of a hard mass composed of blood and dead tissue called a **hematoma**. This mass may restrict joint motion. Nerve compression usually accompanies such injuries, leading to pain and sometimes temporary paralysis.

Muscle contusions are rated in accordance with the extent to which associated joint range of motion is impaired. A first degree contusion causes little to no range of movement restriction, a second degree contusion causes a noticeable reduction in range of motion, and a third degree contusion causes severe restriction of motion. With a third degree contusion the fascia surrounding the muscle may also be ruptured, causing swollen muscle tissues to protrude.

Muscle and tendon strains and ligament sprains are caused by abnormally high tensile force that produces rupturing of the tissue and subsequent hemorrhage and swelling. The likelihood of strains and sprains depends on the magnitude of the force acting and the structure's cross-sectional area. The greater the cross-sectional area of a muscle, the greater its strength, meaning the more force it can produce and the more force that is translated to the attached tendon. The larger the cross-sectional area of the tendon, however, the greater the force that it can withstand, because increased cross-sectional area translates to reduced stress. It is almost always the muscle portion of the musculotendinous unit that ruptures first, because tendons, by virtue of their collagenous composition, are about twice as strong as the muscles to which they attach (2). Tendon begins to develop tears when it is stretched to approximately 5 to 8% beyond normal length (3).

Strains and sprains are categorized as first, second, and third degree. First degree strains or sprains are accompanied by some pain, but may involve only microtearing of the collagen fibers, with no readily observable symptoms. There may be mild discomfort, local tenderness, mild swelling, and ecchymosis, but no loss of function. Second degree tensile injuries of these tissues are characterized by more severe pain, more extensive rupturing of the tissue, detectable joint instability, and/or

Contusion
Compression injury involving accumulation of blood and lymph within a muscle

Ecchymosis
Superficial tissue discoloration

Hematoma
A localized mass of blood and lymph confined within a space or tissue

Strains and sprains are tension injuries to tendons and ligaments, respectively

Tendons are about twice as strong as the muscles to which they are attached

Cramp
Painful involuntary muscle contraction, either clonic or tonic

Spasm
Transitory muscle contractions

Myositis
Inflammation of connective tissues within a muscle

Fascitis
Inflammation of the fascia surrounding portions of a muscle

Tendinitis
Inflammation of a tendon

Tenosynovitis
Inflammation of a tendon sheath

Myositis ossificans
Accumulation of mineral deposits in muscle

Calcific tendinitis
Accumulation of mineral deposits in tendon

Bursitis
Inflammation of a bursa

Stages of healing and repair are a) acute response (reaction phase), b) repair and regeneration, and c) remodeling.

The acute phase of inflammation begins with local vasoconstriction

Hypoxia
Having a reduced concentration of oxygen

Necrosis
Death of a tissue

Zone of primary injury
Region of injured tissue prior to vasodilation

Edema
Swelling resulting from collection of exuded lymph fluid in the interstitial tissues

muscle weakness. Third degree injuries of this nature produce severe pain, a major loss of tissue continuity, loss of range of motion, and complete instability of the joint (4).

Although typically not associated with injury, muscle **cramps** and **spasms** are painful involuntary muscle contractions common to the sport setting. A cramp is a painful involuntary contraction that may be clonic, with alternating contraction and relaxation, or tonic, with continued contraction over a period of time. Cramps appear to be brought on by a biochemical imbalance, sometimes associated with muscle fatigue. A muscle spasm is an involuntary contraction of short duration caused by reflex action that can be biochemically derived or initiated by a mechanical blow to a nerve or muscle.

Myositis and **fasciitis** refer respectively to inflammation of a muscle's connective tissues and inflammation of the sheaths of fascia surrounding portions of muscle. These are chronic conditions that develop over time as the result of repeated body movements that irritate these tissues.

Tendinitis and **tenosynovitis** involve inflammation of a tendon or the tendon sheath. Tendinitis is a chronic condition characterized by pain and swelling with tendon movement. Tenosynovitis may be either acute or chronic. Acute tenosynovitis is characterized by a snapping sound with movement, inflammation, and local swelling. Chronic tenosynovitis has the additional symptom of nodule formation in the tendon sheath.

Prolonged chronic inflammation of muscle or tendon can result in the accumulation of mineral deposits resembling bone in the affected tissues known as ectopic calcification. Accumulation of mineral deposits in muscle is known as **myositis ossificans**. A common site is the quadriceps region. In tendons the condition is called **calcific tendinitis** .

Bursitis involves irritation of one or more bursae, the fluid-filled sacs that serve to reduce friction in the tissues surrounding joints. Bursitis may also be either acute or chronic, brought on by either a single traumatic compression, or by repeated compressions associated with overuse of the joint.

Soft Tissue Healing

After an athletic injury has occurred, proper care involves immediate treatment and rehabilitation. Because the normal healing process

takes place in a regular and predictable fashion, the knowledgeable athletic trainer or sport supervisor can follow the various signs and symptoms exhibited at the injury site to monitor how healing is progressing. Healing of soft tissues is a three phase process involving acute response, repair and regeneration, and remodeling. Knowing when it is appropriate to begin rehabilitation and when it is acceptable to return an athlete to practice and competition require knowledge and understanding of the healing process.

The immediate response to injury is the acute inflammatory phase, also known as the reaction phase, which occurs for the first several days following an injury. The characteristics of inflammation include redness (rubor), local heat (calor), swelling (tumor), pain (dolor), and in severe cases, loss of function (functio laesa). The beginning of the acute phase involves local vasoconstriction lasting from a few seconds to as long as 10 minutes. This vasoconstriction curtails loss of blood and enables the initiation of clotting. However, the same vasoconstriction can also result in **hypoxia** and tissue **necrosis**, or death, due to lack of oxygen to the area. Following vasoconstriction, vasodilation is brought on by heparin, an anticoagulant, and other chemical mediators. In conjunction with this, increased blood flow to the region causes swelling. Blood from the broken vessels and damaged local tissues form a hematoma, which, in conjunction with necrotic tissue, forms the **zone of primary injury**.

Swelling, or **edema**, occurs as the vascular walls become more permeable and increased pressure within the vessels forces plasma out into the interstitial tissues (**Figure 2-11**). These processes act to speed the arrival of leukocytes, mast cells, platelets, and plasma proteases. Leukocytes are white blood cells that ingest dead cells, any foreign material, and infectious agents through a process known as **phagocytosis**. Mast cells are connective tissue cells carrying heparin and histamine. Platelets and basophil leukocytes also transport histamine, which serves as a vasodilator and increases blood vessel permeability. The leukocytes release enzymes that interact with phospholipids in the cell membranes to produce arachidonic acid. Arachidonic acid activates further inflammation of the affected cells through production of chemical mediators, including prostaglandins and leukotrienes. Bradykinin, a major plasma

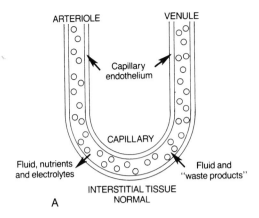

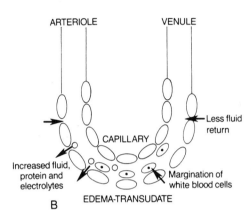

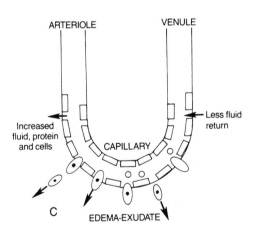

Fig. 2.11: Edema forms when histochemical agents open the pores in the vascular walls, allowing plasma to migrate into the interstitial space.

protease present during inflammation, increases vessel permeability and stimulates nerve endings to cause pain. This chain of chemical activity produces the **zone of secondary injury**, which includes all of the tissues affected by inflammation, edema, and hypoxia. After the debris and waste products from the damaged tissues are ingested through phagocytosis, the leukocytes reenter the blood stream and the acute inflammatory reaction subsides.

Repair and regeneration of injured tissue takes place from approximately two days following the injury through the next six to eight weeks, overlapping the later part of the acute inflammation phase. This stage begins when the hematoma's size is sufficiently diminished to allow room for the growth of new tissue. Although the skin has the ability to regenerate new skin tissue, the other soft tissues replace damaged cells with scar tissue.

Healing through scar formation begins with the accumulation of exuded fluid containing a large concentration of protein and damaged cellular tissues. This accumulation forms the foundation for a highly vascularized mass of immature connective tissues that include fibroblasts, which are cells capable of generating collagen. The fibroblasts begin to produce immature collagen through the process known as fibroplasia. By the fourth or fifth day following the injury, a weak, vascular connective tissue has been produced over the injury. Over the next two to four weeks this scar tissue increases in tensile strength and decreases in vascularity. As less new collagen is required, the number of fibroblasts at the site is reduced.

Because scar tissue is fibrous, inelastic, and non-vascular, it is less strong and less functional than the original tissues. Scar formation can reduce the structure's tensile strength by as much as 30% as compared to pre-injury strength. The development of the scar also typically causes the wound to shrink in size, resulting in decreased flexibility of the affected tissues following the injury.

The final phase of injury recovery is known as the remodeling phase. This period involves maturation of the newly formed tissue, decreased fibroblast activity, increased organization of the extracellular matrix, and a return to normal histochemical activity. In soft tissue the process begins about three weeks post-injury, overlapping the repair and regeneration phase. It continues for a year or more as collagen fibers become oriented along the lines of mechanical stress to which the tissue is usually subjected.

Muscle fibers are permanent cells that do not reproduce in response to injury or training. There are, however, reserve cells in the basement membrane of each muscle fiber

Phagocytosis
Process by which white blood cells surround and digest foreign particles

Histamine is a vasodilator and increases blood vessel permeability

Bradykinin increases vessel permeability and stimulates nerve endings to cause pain

Zone of secondary injury
Region of damaged tissue following vasodilation

Repair and regeneration overlap the acute phase and last 2 days through the next 6 to 8 weeks

By the 4th or 5th day following injury, a weak, vascular connective tissue has been produced over the injury

Scar tissue is fibrous, inelastic, and nonvascular, making it less strong and less functional than the original tissues

Adhesions
Tissues that bind healing tissue to adjacent structures, such as other ligaments or bone

---

High tensile stress before scar formation is complete can cause elongation of the new, formative tissues

---

Complete immobilization of an injury leads to atrophy, loss of strength, and decreased rate of healing

---

Collagen provides bone with some degree of flexibility and strength in resisting tension

---

Most epiphyses close around age 18, although some may be present until about age 25

---

that are able to regenerate muscle fiber following injury (3). Severe muscle injury can result in scarring or the formation of **adhesions** within the muscle, which inhibits muscle fiber regeneration. Following severe injury, muscle may regain only about 50% of its pre-injury strength (3).

Because tendons and ligaments have few reparative cells, healing of these structures can take more than a year. If these tissues undergo abnormally high tensile stress before scar formation is complete, the newly forming tissues can be elongated. In ligaments, this can result in joint instability.

Because tendons, ligaments, and muscles hypertrophy and atrophy in response to levels of mechanical stress, complete immobilization of the injury leads to atrophy, loss of strength, and decreased rate of healing in these tissues. The amount of atrophy is generally proportional to the time of immobilization. Thus, although immobilization may be necessary to protect the injured tissues during the early stages of recovery, strengthening exercises should be implemented as soon as appropriate during rehabilitation of the injury. The sport participant is at increased risk for reinjury as long as the affected tissues are below pre-injury strength.

Because tendons are stronger than the muscles to which they attach, the muscle typically ruptures rather than the tendon when the musculotendinous unit is overloaded. Although ligaments have more elasticity than tendons because they attach at both ends to bone, they tend to rupture and/or become permanently stretched when bones displace at a joint.

BONE INJURIES

A distance runner complains of localized pain around the head of the second metatarsal in the right foot that increases after training sessions. The pain has been present for three weeks and is getting worse. What injury might you suspect? What are the implications for the athlete's continued training?

Bone behaves predictably in response to stress in keeping with its material constituents and structural organization. The composition and structure of bone make it strong for its relatively light weight.

Anatomical Properties of Bone

The primary constituents of bone are calcium carbonate, calcium phosphate, collagen, and water. The minerals, making up 60 to 70% of bone weight, provide stiffness and strength in resisting compression. Collagen provides bone with some degree of flexibility and strength in resisting tension. Aging causes a progressive loss of collagen and increase in bone brittleness. Thus, children's bones are more pliable than adults' bones.

As bones develop, longitudinal bone growth continues only as long as the bone's epiphyseal plates, or growth plates, continue to exist **(Figure 2-12)**. Epiphyseal plates are cartilaginous discs found near the ends of the long bones. These are the sites where longitudinal bone growth takes place on the diaphysis (central) side of the plates. During or shortly after adolescence, the plate disappears and the bone fuses, terminating longitudinal growth. Most epiphyses close around age 18, although some may be present until about age 25.

Although the most rapid bone growth occurs prior to adulthood, bones continue to grow in diameter throughout most of the lifespan. The internal layer of the periosteum builds new concentric layers of bone tissue on top of the existing ones. At the same time, bone is resorbed or eliminated around the sides of the medullary cavity, so that the diameter of the cavity is continually enlarged. The bone cells that form new bone tissue are called osteoblasts, and those that resorb bone are known as osteoclasts. In healthy adult

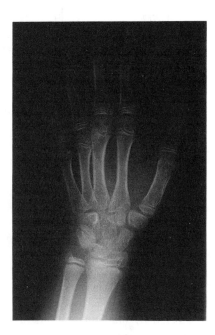

Fig. 2.12: Epiphyseal growth plate.

bone the activity of osteoblasts and osteo-clasts, referred to as bone turn-over, is largely balanced. The total amount of bone remains approximately constant until women reach their forties and men reach their sixties, when a gradual decline in bone mass begins. Sport participants past these ages may be at increased risk for bone fractures. However, regular participation in weight-bearing exer-cise has been shown to be effective in reduc-ing age-related bone loss.

No matter what the athlete's age, some bones are also more susceptible to fracture as a result of their internal composition. Bone tissue is categorized as either **cortical** , if the porosity is low—with 5 to 30% nonmineral-ized tissue, or as **cancellous**, if the porosity is high—with 30 to over 90% of nonmineralized tissue **(Figure 2-13)**. Most human bones have outer shells of cortical bone, with can-cellous bone underneath. Cortical bone is stiffer, which means that it can withstand greater stress but less strain than cancellous bone. Cancellous bone, however, has the advantage of being spongier than cortical bone, which means that it can undergo more strain before fracturing. The mineralization of cancellous bone varies with the individual's age and with the location of the bone in the body. Both cortical and cancellous bone are anisotropic, which means that they exhibit different strengths and stiffnesses in response to forces applied from different directions. Bone is strongest in resisting compressive stress, and weakest in resisting shear stress.

Bone size and shape also influence the likelihood of fracture. The shapes and sizes of bones are largely determined by the direc-tions and magnitudes of the forces to which they are habitually subjected. The direction in which new bone tissue is formed has been found to be adapted to best resist the loads encountered, particularly in regions of high stress such as the femoral neck. The mineral-ization and girth of bone increase in response to increased stress levels. For example, the bones of the dominant arm of professional tennis players and professional baseball players have been found to be larger

Osteoblasts form new bone tissue, whereas osteoclasts resorb bone

Regular participation in weight-bearing exercise has been shown to be effective to some extent in mediating age-related bone loss

Cortical
Compact bone tissue of higher density

Cancellous
Bone tissue of lower density

Bone is strongest in resisting compression and weakest in resisting shear

The mineralization and girth of bone increase in response to increased stress levels

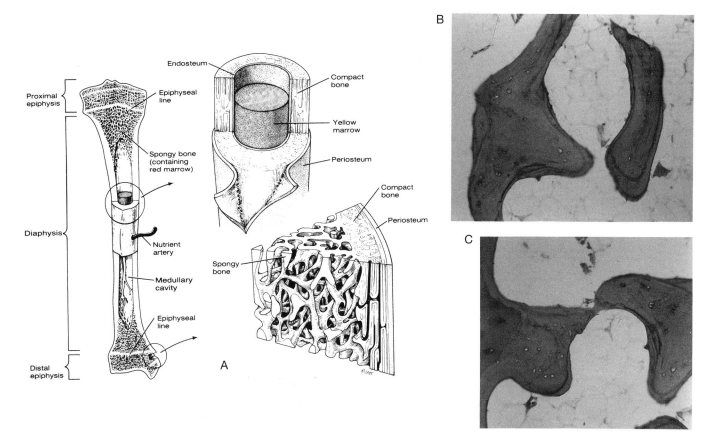

Fig. 2.13: Bone macrostructure. Note the epiphyseal growth lines at either end of the bone (A). The cortical bone surrounds the cancellous bone and medullary cavity. Cancellous bone is more porous than cortical bone, as can be seen in the electron micrograph photo above (B,C).

Fracture Type		Description
Simple (closed)		Bone breaks cleanly, but ends do not break the skin.
Compound (open)		Bone ends penetrate through soft tisssues and the skin.
Greenstick		Bones break incompletely, as a green stick breaks.
Transverse		Break occurs in a straight line across the bone.
Oblique		Break ocurs diagonally when torsion occurs on one end while the other is fixed.
Spiral		Jagged bone ends are S-shaped because excessive torsion is applied to a fixed bone.
Avulsion		Bone fragment is pulled off by an attached tendon or ligament.

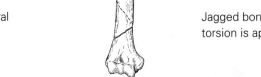

Fracture Type		Description
Comminuted	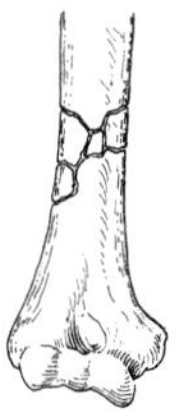	Bone fragments into several pieces.
Epiphyseal	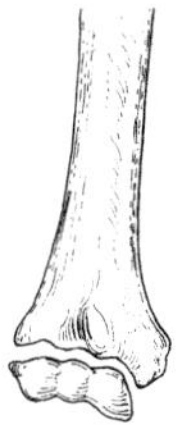	Separation involves the epiphysis of the bone.
Impacted	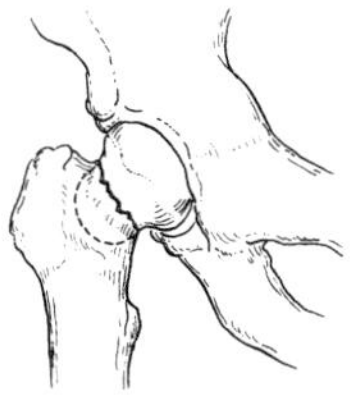	Another bone is impacted, or driven into, another piece of bone.
Depressed	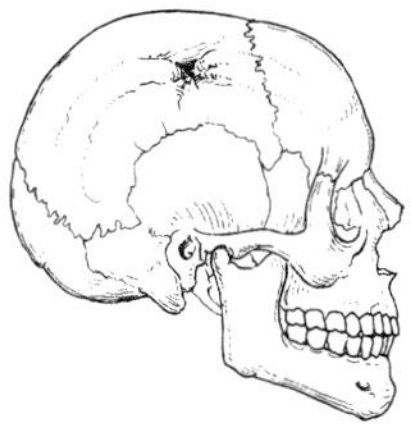	Occurs more frequently on flat bones when the broken bone portion is driven inward.

Fig. 2.14: Types of fractures.

and stronger than the bones of their nondominant arms (5,6).

Bone Injury Classifications

A **fracture** is a disruption in the continuity of a bone **(Figure 2-14)**. The type of fracture sustained depends on the type of mechanical loading that caused it, as well as the health and maturity of the bone at the time of injury. Fractures are considered to be simple when the bone ends remain intact within the surrounding soft tissues and compound when one or both bone ends protrude from the skin.

Spiral fractures of the long bones are often produced by excessive torsional and bending loads, as exemplified by tibial fractures resulting from skiing accidents. Such fractures are the result of a combined loading pattern of shear and tension, producing failure at an oblique orientation to the longitudinal axis of the bone (7).

Because bone is stronger in resisting compression than both tension and shear, acute compression fractures of bone are rare. Under combined loading, however, a fracture resulting from a torsional load may be affected by the presence of a compressive load. An impacted fracture is one in which the opposite sides of the fracture are compressed together. Fractures that result in depression of bone fragments into the underlying tissues are termed depressed.

Because the bones of children contain relatively larger amounts of collagen than adult bones, they are more flexible and more resistant to fracture under day-to-day loading than adult bones. Consequently, greenstick fractures, or incomplete fractures, are more common in children than in adults. A greenstick fracture is an incomplete fracture typically caused by bending or torsional loads.

Avulsions are another type of fracture caused by tensile loading that involve a ten-

Fracture
A disruption in the continuity of a bone

Fractures are simple when the bone ends remain intact within the surrounding soft tissues and compound when one or both bone ends protrude from the skin

Greenstick fractures are more common in children than adults

don or ligament pulling a small chip of bone away from the rest of the bone. Explosive throwing and jumping movements may result in avulsion fractures. When loading is very rapid, a fracture is more likely to be comminuted, meaning it contains multiple fragments.

Stress fractures, also known as fatigue fractures, result from repeated low magnitude forces. Stress fractures differ from acute fractures in that they can worsen over time, beginning as a small disruption in the continuity of the outer layers of cortical bone and ending as complete cortical fracture with possible displacement of the bone ends. Stress fractures of the metatarsals, the femoral neck, and the pubis have been reported among runners who have apparently over-trained. Stress fractures of the pars interarticularis region of the lumbar vertebrae have also been reported to occur in higher than normal frequencies among female gymnasts and football linemen (8).

Osteopenia, a condition of reduced bone mineral density, predisposes the athlete to fractures of all kinds, but particularly to stress fractures. The condition is primarily found among adolescent female athletes, especially distance runners, who are **amenorrheic**. Although amenorrhea among this group is not well understood, it appears to be related to a low percentage of body fat and/or high training mileage. The link between cessation of menses and osteopenia is also not well understood. Possible contributing factors include hyperactivity of osteoclasts, hypoactivity of osteoblasts, hormonal factors, and insufficiencies of dietary calcium or other minerals or nutrients.

Epiphyseal Injury Classifications

The bones of children and adolescents are vulnerable to epiphyseal injuries, including injuries to the cartilaginous epiphyseal plate, articular cartilage, and apophysis. The apophyses are sites of tendon attachments to bone, where bone shape is influenced by the tensile loads to which these sites are subjected. The epiphyses of long bones are termed pressure epiphyses and the apophyses are termed traction epiphyses after the types of physiological loading present at these sites. Both acute and repetitive loading can injure the growth plate, potentially resulting in premature closure of the epiphyseal junction and termination of bone growth. "Little League elbow," for example, is a stress injury to the medial epicondylar epiphysis of the humerus.

Salter (9) has categorized acute epiphyseal injuries into five distinct types (**Figure 2-15**).

Type I   Complete separation of the epiphysis from the metaphysis with no fracture to the bone

Type II   Separation of the epiphysis and a small portion of the metaphysis

Type III Fracture of the epiphysis

Type IV Fracture of a part of the epiphysis and metaphysis

Type V   Compression of the epiphysis without fracture, resulting in compromised epiphyseal function

Another category of epiphyseal injuries is referred to collectively as osteochondrosis. Osteochondrosis results from disruption of blood supply to an epiphysis, with associated tissue necrosis and potential deformation of the epiphysis. Because the cause of the condition is poorly understood, it is typically termed idiopathic osteochondrosis. The osteochondroses occur most commonly between the ages of three and ten and are more prevalent among boys than girls (9). Specific disease names have been given to osteochondrosis at the sites of most common occurrence. For example, Legg-Calvé-Perthes disease is osteochondrosis of the femoral head, as discussed in Chapter 9.

The apophyses are also subject to osteochondrosis, particularly among children and adolescents. These conditions, referred to as apophysitis, may be idiopathic. They are also often associated with traumatic avulsion type fractures. Common sites for apophysitis are the calcaneus and the tibial tubercle at the site of the patellar tendon attachment. Osteochondrosis at these sites is referred to respectively as Sever's disease and Osgood-Schlatter disease, discussed in Chapters 7 and 8.

Bony Tissue Healing

Healing of acute bone fractures is a three phase process, as is soft tissue healing. The acute inflammatory phase lasts approximately four days. Damage to the periosteum and surrounding soft tissues results in the formation of a hematoma in the medullary canal and surrounding tissues. The ensuing inflammatory response involves vasodilation, edema formation, and the histochemical changes associated with soft tissue inflammation.

During repair and regeneration, osteoclasts resorb damaged bone tissues, whereas osteoblasts build new bone. Between the

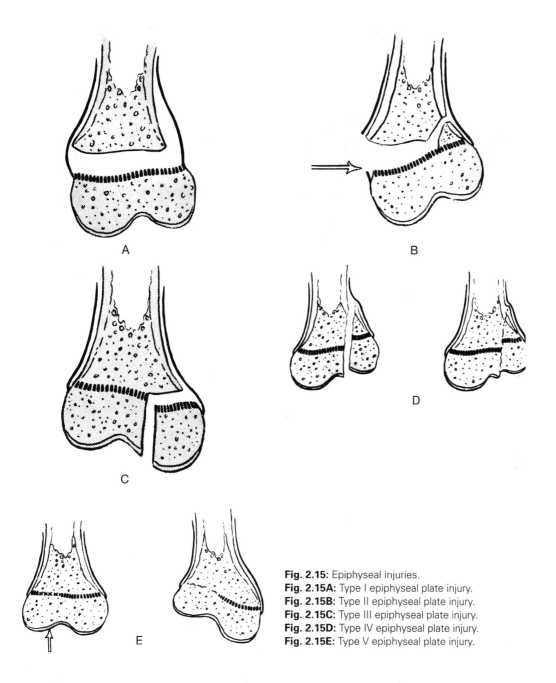

A

B

C

D

E

Fig. 2.15: Epiphyseal injuries.
Fig. 2.15A: Type I epiphyseal plate injury.
Fig. 2.15B: Type II epiphyseal plate injury.
Fig. 2.15C: Type III epiphyseal plate injury.
Fig. 2.15D: Type IV epiphyseal plate injury.
Fig. 2.15E: Type V epiphyseal plate injury.

fractured bone ends, a fibrous vascularized tissue known as a **callus** is formed **(Figure 2-16)**. The callus contains weak, immature bone tissue that strengthens with time through bone remodeling. The process of callus formation is known as enchondral bone healing. An alternative process, known as direct bone healing, can occur when the fractured bone ends are immobilized in direct contact with one another. This enables new, interwoven bone tissue to be deposited without the formation of a callus. Unless a fracture is fixed by metal plates, screen, or rods, healing normally takes place through the enchondral process (3). Because noninvasive

treatment is generally preferred, a fixation device is only implanted when it appears unlikely that the fracture will heal acceptably without one.

Remodeling of bone tissue involves osteoblast activity on the concave side of the fracture, which is loaded in compression, and osteoclast activity on the convex side of the fracture, which is loaded in tension. The process continues until normal shape is restored and bone strength is commensurate with the loads to which the bone is routinely subjected.

Because stress fractures continue to worsen as long as the site is over-loaded, it is

Callus
Fibrous tissue containing immature bone tissue that forms at fracture sites during repair and regeneration

Fracture healing normally involves callus formation

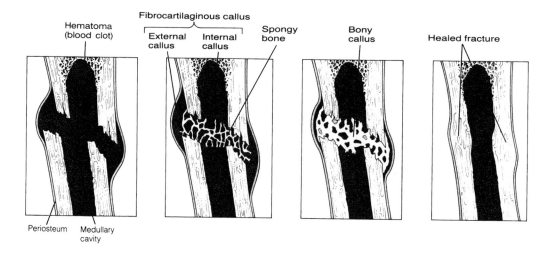

Fig. 2.16: The process of endochondral bone healing through callus formation.

Afferent nerves
Nerves carrying sensory input from receptors in the skin, muscles, tendons, and ligaments to the central nervous system

Efferent nerves
Nerves carrying stimuli from the central nervous system to the muscles

Both tensile and compressive forces can injure nerves

Neurotmesis
Complete severance of a nerve

important to recognize these injuries as early as possible. Elimination or reduction of the repetitive mechanical stress causing the fracture is the primary factor necessary for healing. This allows a gradual restoration of the proper balance of osteoblast and osteoclast activity present in the bone.

Pain localized around the second metatarsal head in a runner's foot is a classic symptom of a stress injury. The runner should be referred to a physician. If a fracture is present, activity should be curtailed until the injury has healed.

NERVE INJURIES

A weight lifter complains of pain radiating down the posterior aspect of the left leg. What condition might you suspect? Is medical referral appropriate?

The nervous system is divided into the central nervous system, consisting of the brain and spinal cord, and the peripheral nervous system, which includes 12 pairs of cranial nerves and 31 pairs of spinal nerves, along with their branches (**Figure 2-17**). Injuries to any of these nerves can be devastating to the individual, potentially resulting in temporary or permanent disability.

Anatomical Properties of Nerve

Each spinal nerve is formed from anterior and posterior roots on the spinal cord that unite at the intervertebral foramen. The posterior branches are the **afferent** (sensory) **nerves** that transmit information from sensory receptors in the skin, tendons, ligaments,

and muscles to the central nervous system. The anterior branches are the **efferent** (motor) **nerves** that transmit control signals to the muscles. The nerve fibers are heavily vascularized and are encased in a multi-layered protective sheath of connective tissue.

Nerve Injury Classifications

Nerves are most commonly injured by tensile or compressive forces. Tensile injuries of nerves typically occur during severe high-speed accidents, such as automobile accidents or impact collisions in contact sports (10). When a nerve is loaded in tension, the nerve fibers tend to rupture prior to the rupturing of the surrounding connective tissue sheath (11). Because the nerve roots on the spinal cord are not protected by connective tissue, they are particularly susceptible to tensile injury, especially to stretching of the brachial plexus or cervical nerve roots. Complete separation of a nerve is termed **neurotmesis**.

Compressive injuries of nerves are more complex because their severity depends on the magnitude and duration of loading and whether the applied pressure is direct or indirect (10). Because nerve function is highly dependent on oxygen provided by the associated blood vessels, damage to the blood supply caused by a compressive injury results in damage to the nerve.

Nerve injuries can result in a range of afferent symptoms, from complete loss of sensation through severe pain. Terms used to describe altered sensation include hypoesthesia, a reduction in sensation, hyperesthesia,

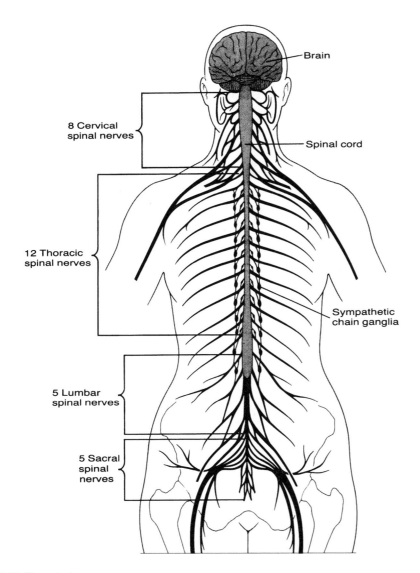

Fig. 2.17: The spinal nerves.

- 8 Cervical spinal nerves
- 12 Thoracic spinal nerves
- 5 Lumbar spinal nerves
- 5 Sacral spinal nerves
- Brain
- Spinal cord
- Sympathetic chain ganglia

heightened sensation, and paresthesia, a sense of numbness, prickling, or tingling. Pinching of a nerve can result in a sharp wave of pain that is transmitted through a body segment. Irritation or inflammation of a nerve can result in chronic pain along the nerve's course known as neuralgia.

Nerve Healing

When a nerve is completely severed, healing does not occur and loss of function is typically permanent. Unless such injuries are surgically repaired, random regrowth of the nerve occurs, resulting in the formation of a **neuroma**, or nerve tumor.

When nerve fibers are ruptured in a tensile injury, but the surrounding myelin sheath remains intact, it is sometimes possible for a nerve to regenerate along the pathway provided by the sheath during healing. Such regeneration is relatively slow, however, proceeding at a rate of less than 1 mm per day or about 2.5 cm per month (3).

Pain radiating down the posterior aspect of the legs is symptomatic of a sciatic nerve injury or impingement and may indicate a herniated disc. The athlete should be referred immediately to a physician for evaluation.

PAIN

You notice that in two individuals who are working to rehabilitate ankles that were sprained at about the same time, one shirks exercises because of excessive pain, while the other performs workouts without

Pinching of a nerve can result in a sharp wave of pain or burning sensation that is transmitted through a body segment

Neuroma
A nerve tumor

Nociceptors
Specialized nerve endings
that transduce pain

The substantia gelatinosa of the dorsal spinal cord is believed to function as a gatekeeper for pain impulses entering the central nervous system

Morphine-like chemicals called endorphins and encephalins are produced naturally by the body in response to stressors

Referred pain is perceived by the brain to emanate from a location away from the source of the pain

Radiating pain is felt both at its source and along a nerve

Dermatomes
A region of skin supplied by a single afferent neuron

complaint. What variables may be at work here?

Pain is a universal symptom common to most injuries. The individual's perception of pain is influenced by various physical, chemical, social, and psychological factors.

The Neurological Basis of Pain

Pain is brought about by stimulation of specialized afferent nerve endings called **nociceptors**. With most acute sport related injuries, pain is initiated by **mechanosensitive** nociceptors responding to the traumatic force that caused the injury. With chronic injuries and during the early stages of healing of acute injuries, pain persists due to the activation of **chemosensitive** nociceptors. Bradykinin, serotonin, histamines, and prostaglandins are all chemicals transported to the injury site during inflammation that activate the chemosensitive nociceptors.

Small diameter, slow transmission nerves carry pain impulses, whereas large diameter, fast transmission nerves carry other sensations, such as touch, temperature, and proprioception. Both types of fibers communicate with the spinal cord through the substantia gelatinosa (SG) of the cord's dorsal horn. Specialized T cells then transmit impulses from all of the afferent fibers up the spinal cord to the brain, with each T cell carrying a single impulse.

According to the gate control theory of pain, the SG acts as a gate keeper by allowing either a pain response or one of the other afferent sensations to be transported by each T cell (12). The theory is substantiated by the observation that increased sensory input can reduce the sensation of pain. For example, extreme cold can often numb pain. Because hundreds or thousands of "gates" are in operation, however, it is more common that added sensory input reduces rather than eliminates the feeling of pain because pain impulses get through to some of the T cells.

Factors that Mediate Pain

The body produces pain-killing chemicals similar to morphine called beta-endorphin and methionine enkephalin. Both work by blocking neural receptor sites that transmit pain. Several different sites in the brain produce endorphins. Stressors such as physical exercise, mental stress, and electrical stimulation provoke the release of endorphins into the cerebrospinal fluid. A phenomenon called "runner's high," a feeling of euphoria that occurs among long distance runners, has been attributed to endorphin release. The brain stem and pituitary gland produce enkephalins. Enkephalins block pain neurotransmitters in the dorsal horn of the spinal cord.

The central nervous system also imposes a set of cognitive and affective filters on both the perception of pain and the subsequent expression of perceived pain. Social and cultural factors can be powerful influences on pain tolerance level. In American society, for example, it is much more acceptable for females than for males to express feelings of pain. Individual personality and a state of mental preoccupation can also be significant mediators of pain.

Referred Pain and Radiating Pain

Referred pain is perceived at a location remote from the site of the tissues actually causing the pain. A proposed explanation for referred pain begins with the fact that neurons carrying pain impulses split into several branches within the spinal cord. Although some of these branches connect with other pain transmitting fibers, some also connect with afferent nerve pathways from the skin. This cross-branching can cause the brain to misinterpret the true location of the pain (13).

In at least some instances, referred pain behaves in a logical and predictable fashion. For example, pain from the internal organs is typically projected outward to corresponding **dermatomes** of the skin, as is the case with heart attacks and ruptured spleens and kidneys.

Referred pain should not be confused with radiating pain, which is pain that is felt both at its source and along a nerve. Pinching of the sciatic nerve at its root may cause pain that radiates along the nerve's course down the posterior aspect of the leg.

Differences in pain perception and tolerance can be caused by differences in chemical, social, and psychological influences as well as by differences in the severity of the original injury and the progression of the healing process.

SUMMARY

The nature of a sports related injury depends on the magnitude, direction, and point of application of the applied force(s) as well as on the health and strength of the affected tissues. When the force acting on a structure exceeds the structure's yield point, failure occurs. This translates to fracturing of bone and rupturing of soft tissues. Biological tissues are strongest in resisting the form of loading to which they are most commonly subjected. The material compositions of skin, tendon, ligament, and muscle make them particularly strong in resisting tension, whereas bone is strongest in resisting compression.

The body's response to injury is a well-ordered, predictable process. The initial reaction is the acute inflammatory phase, which lasts for approximately four days following injury. During this phase, subcellular agents are rushed to the site to remove the damaged tissue. From about two days through the next six weeks following the injury, the repair and regeneration phase sets in. In this phase fibroblasts produce a scar over soft tissue ruptures, and osteoblasts produce a callus across most bone fractures. The final phase, known as the remodeling or maturation phase, begins about three weeks postinjury and lasts a year or more as the tissues strengthen and become reoriented along lines of mechanical stress.

The pain associated with injuries is caused by mechanical and/or chemical insult to the nerves. Nerves can be injured through both tensile and compressive overloads. Only when the protective sheath surrounding the nerve remains intact can nerve regeneration occur following an injury.

REFERENCES

1. Nachemson AL, and Evans JH. 1968. Some mechanical properties of the third human lumbar interlaminar ligament (ligamentum flavum). J Biomech, 1(1):211–215.
2. Elliott, DH. 1967. The biomechanical properties of tendon in relation to muscular strength. Ann Phys Med, 9:1.
3. American Academy of Orthopaedic Surgeons. *Athletic Training and Sports Medicine*. Park Ridge, IL: American Academy of Orthopaedic Surgeons, 1991.
4. Carlstedt, CA, and Nordin, M. Biomechanics of tendons and ligaments. In *Basic Biomechanics of the Musculoskeletal System*, edited by M Nordin and VH Frankel. Philadelphia: Lea & Febiger, 1989.
5. Jones, HH, et al. 1977. Humeral hypertrophy in response to exercise, J Bone Joint Surg Am, 59:204–208.
6. Watson, RC. Bone growth and physical activity. In *International Conference on Bone Measurements*, edited by RB Mazess. DHEW Pub No NIH 75–683, Washington, DC, 1973.
7. Nordin, M, and Frankel, VH. Biomechanics of bone. In *Basic Biomechanics of the Musculoskeletal System*, edited by M Nordin and VH Frankel. Philadelphia: Lea & Febiger, 1989.
8. Jackson, DW, Wiltse, LL, and Cirincione, RJ. 1976. Spondylolysis in the female gymnast. Clin Orthop, 117:68–73.
9. Salter, RB. *Textbook of Disorders and Injuries of the Musculoskeletal System*. Baltimore: Williams & Wilkins, 1983.
10. Rydevik, B, Lundborg, G, and Skalak, R. Biomechanics of peripheral nerves. In *Basic Biomechanics of the Musculoskeletal System*, edited by M Nordin and VH Frankel. Philadelphia: Lea & Febiger, 1989.
11. Sunderland, S. *Nerves and Nerve Injuries*. Edinburgh: Churchill Livingstone, 1978.
12. Newton, RA. Contemporary views on pain and the role played by thermal agents in managing pain symptoms. In *Thermal Agents in Rehabilitation*, edited by S Michlovitz. Philadelphia: FA Davis, 1990.
13. Ottoson, D, and Lundberg, T. *Pain Treatment by Transcutaneous Electrical Nerve Stimulation: A Practical Manual*. New York: Springer-Verlag, 1988.

Sports Injury Management

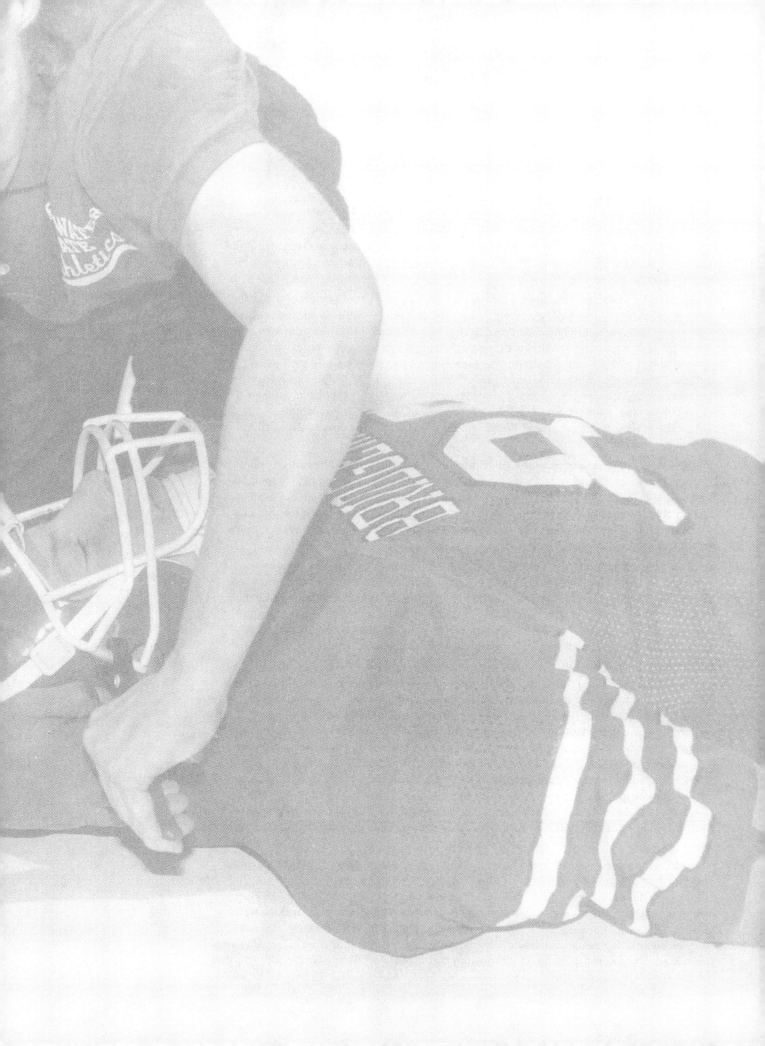

Kathy Fox, M.A., A.T., C., P.T., S.C.S.

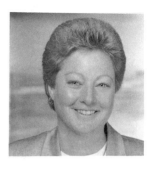

Like many people in athletic training, I got interested in the profession after an injury. As a result, I went to the State University of New York at Cortland for an undergraduate degree in education with emphasis in athletic training, then went right into graduate school at Miami University in Ohio. Although I currently work at Braintree Hospital in the outpatient physical therapy clinic, I administer the entire sports medicine program for the hospital and its 35 satellite clinics

As an administrator, I am responsible for the budget, hiring, and evaluation of the athletic trainers, procuring high school contracts, marketing and public relations for the program, and serving as a sounding board and ombudsman for the staff. I love the administrative part of this job, especially working with the public to advance the visibility of the athletic training profession. As an advocate for the profession, I require my entire staff to do community service presentations three to four times each year. At first, some were reluctant to do public speaking; however, many now present regularly at the state athletic training meetings, annual physical education, recreation, and dance conventions, and participate in regular workshops and seminars for C.E.U. credit for area NATA certified athletic trainers.

The athletic trainers who work in the clinic really have a limited role. They serve mainly as clinical aides and perform tasks such as applying superficial heat and cold, supervising an established strengthening program, assisting in setting up the treatment area, and making sure the facility is clean and neat. Unfortunately, in our state, these trainers are not being utilized to their fullest potential because of the current licensure law and third-party billing policies.

All of the trainers split their time between the clinic and an area high school or college. The workload averages about 40 hours per week, and as such, there is less burnout among our employees. We provide a full-time salary and health benefits, and pay the trainers for their travel time to the school and mileage. A dual position provides a unique opportunity to maintain skills in two separate environments, treat a more diverse clientele over a wider age range, and see a broader array of orthopedic injuries and conditions.

Although area schools could benefit more from a full-time trainer on staff to supervise on-site rehabilitation and follow the athlete through the entire injury healing process, we provide a community service that is unequaled in the area. We provide on-site health care for the athletic program, immediate access to any medical specialist in the field, a comprehensive rehabilitation team, and an array of professional consultants who work with area communities to provide a holistic health care system for their children. From a business perspective, the hospital loses out in that the athletic trainers are locked into a morning schedule in the clinic to accommodate the schools in the afternoon, evenings, and weekends. In the summer, however, the athletic trainers are in the clinic 40 hours a week. While there, they cannot practice to the full potential of their license in the non-traditional setting. This is really unfortunate. To my knowledge, only one state, Missouri, has taken a leadership role in changing this dilemma.

If you are interested in working in a clinic in a dual role, I would suggest getting dual certification as a physical therapy assistant or physical therapist, just because of the third-party billing situation. I also think it's imperative that people in athletic training be committed to teaching athletic training in one way or another. This doesn't necessarily have to be in a classroom setting, but it means being an advocate for the profession by taking your knowledge and respecting it enough to share it with others. It implies that you are committed to your profession and to improving that profession. That's what really identifies great athletic trainers.

Kathy Fox is a vocal advocate for the athletic training profession. In her dual role as an athletic trainer and physical therapist, she has worked extensively in sports medicine clinics and in area high schools. She is now the Director of the Sports Medicine Program for the Braintree Hospital Rehabilitation Network in Braintree, Massachusetts.

Chapter 3

Emergency Procedures

After you have completed this chapter, you should be able to:

- Describe the signs, symptoms, and management of potentially life-threatening conditions.
- Identify preventive measures to reduce the risk of life-threatening conditions
- Describe the procedures and techniques used in primary and secondary injury assessment
- Identify emergency conditions that warrant immediate action by emergency medical services (EMS)
- Describe proper procedures to transport a seriously injured individual.

Serious injuries can be frightening, particularly if breathing or circulation is impaired. As the first person on the scene, you are expected to evaluate the situation, assess the extent and seriousness of injury, recognize life-threatening conditions, provide immediate emergency care, and initiate any emergency procedures to provide follow-up medical care. Although few sport related injuries are serious enough to impair breathing or circulation, these injuries do occur. Furthermore, assessment and recognition of some serious injuries can be significantly hampered if the individual is unconscious and unable to respond to verbal questions about the condition.

In this chapter you will first learn which conditions can pose a threat to an individual's life. Next, the importance of developing an emergency care plan to speed action by facility personnel and local emergency medical services (EMS) in providing emergency health care will be discussed. You will then move step-by-step through a primary and secondary survey to determine if an emergency situation exists and EMS should be summoned. Finally, after summoning EMS, you will learn how to assist the emergency medical team to secure a seriously injured individual to a stretcher to transport the individual to a medical facility.

EMERGENCY SITUATIONS

❓ *Think for a minute or two about what injuries or conditions might be life-threatening to an individual. Although these injuries or conditions may occur during sport participation, they may not be directly related to the actual participation. As such, an understanding of these conditions can aid in early recognition and treatment.*

Injuries or conditions that impair, or have the potential to impair, vital function of the central nervous system and cardiorespiratory system are considered emergency situations. Many serious injuries are clearly evident and recognizable, such as lack of breathing or absence of a pulse. The presence of these conditions is identified in checking the **ABCs: A**irway, **B**reathing, **C**irculation, and severe arterial bleeding. This immediate assessment, called a **primary survey**, determines unresponsiveness, recognizes and identifies immediate life threatening situations, and dictates what action is needed to care for the individual. However, conditions such as internal bleeding, shock, or heat stress may slowly cause the individual's condition to deteriorate. A **secondary survey** involves a more detailed hands-on, head-to-toe assessment to detect conditions that may not in themselves pose an immediate threat to life, but if left unrecognized and untreated, could lead to serious complications.

In recognizing any injury or condition, symptoms and diagnostic signs are gathered to determine the seriousness of injury. A **symptom** is information provided by the injured individual regarding their perception of the problem. These conditions, or subjective feelings, include blurred vision, ringing

Always check the ABCs: *A*irway, *B*reathing, *C*irculation, and *s*evere arterial bleeding.

Primary survey
Immediate assessment to determine unresponsiveness and status of the ABCs

Secondary survey
Detailed head-to-toe assessment to detect medical and injury-related problems that if unrecognized and untreated could become life-threatening

Symptom
Subjective information provided by an individual regarding their perception of the problem

in the ears, fatigue, dizziness, nausea, headache, pain, weakness, or an inability to move a particular body part. A diagnostic **sign** is a measurable physical finding regarding the individual's condition. A sign is what you hear, feel, see, or smell when assessing the individual (1). Interpreting the symptoms and signs is the foundation used to recognize and identify the injury or condition. In sport injuries, the secondary survey comprises the largest portion of the total injury assessment process. Emergency conditions that will be discussed include:

1. Obstructed airway emergencies
2. Cardiopulmonary emergencies
3. Unconscious athlete
4. External hemorrhage
5. Internal hemorrhage
6. Shock
7. Fractures
8. Hyperthermia (heat stress)
9. Hypothermia (cold stress)

Where appropriate, the mechanism of injury, signs and symptoms, prevention, and treatment of the conditions will be discussed. Assessment is presented in the primary and secondary survey sections.

OBSTRUCTED AIRWAY

You are watching a field hockey game when a player stops running and suddenly grabs the throat with both hands and appears to be choking. Think for a minute or two about what has occurred and what you need to do to handle this situation.

The airway can become partially or totally blocked by a solid foreign object (mouth guard, bridgework, chewing gum, chaw of tobacco, or mud), fluids (blood clots from head injuries or vomitus), swelling in the throat caused by allergic reactions, or more commonly, the back of the tongue (due to unconsciousness). An obstructed airway prevents adequate oxygen from being exchanged in the lungs and can lead to **cyanosis** and death.

Partial Airway Obstruction

When a person has a **partial airway obstruction,** there is still some air exchange in the lungs. The individual will typically grasp the throat in the universal distress signal for choking (**Figure 3-1**). If there is adequate air exchange, the individual will be able to cough forcefully. Listen for other unusual breathing sounds between breaths, such as

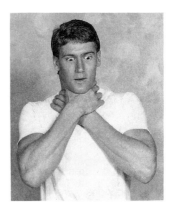

Fig. 3.1: Universal distress sign for choking.

gurgling that may indicate a foreign object, blood, or other fluids in the throat; snoring, caused by the tongue obstructing the airway; crowing, caused by spasm in the larynx; or wheezing, due to serious edema or spasm in the airway (2,3). If the individual is able to cough forcefully, do not interfere. Stand beside the individual and encourage them to continue coughing in an attempt to dislodge the obstruction. The individual may have an ineffective cough and emit a high-pitched noise while breathing. This sign indicates poor air exchange and should be treated as a total airway obstruction.

Total Airway Obstruction

In a **total airway obstruction**, no air is passing through the vocal cords, so the individual will be unable to speak, breathe, or cough. The universal distress signal is almost always apparent. You must react quickly to clear the airway and stimulate the breathing process. Protocols for clearing the airway and restoring respirations are explained in the primary survey section.

The field hockey player is giving the universal distress sign but is coughing, indicating only a partial airway obstruction. Did you determine that you should not interfere, but instead should encourage the individual to cough in an attempt to dislodge the mouthguard? If so, you are correct.

CARDIOPULMONARY EMERGENCIES

You are on the sideline watching a soccer game when suddenly a spectator grabs the chest, staggers, then collapses. Think for a minute or two about what might have occurred and what you may need to do to provide emergency care in this situation.

Sudden death from cardiac arrest is one of the most prominent medical emergencies today. When an ineffective heart fails to pump oxygenated blood to the brain, the brain becomes seriously impaired within a matter of four to six minutes. If not immediately corrected, death is imminent. Heart attacks and cardiac arrest may result from strenuous physical activity, direct trauma, electrical shock, excessive alcohol or other chemical substance abuse, suffocation, drowning, or heart anomalies (3,4,5). Cardiopulmonary resuscitation (CPR) combines ventilation and heart compression to artificially pump oxygenated blood to the brain, heart, and other vital organs of the body to sustain life until advanced medical care can be obtained.

The National Athletic Trainers' Association requires all athletic trainers to be certified in CPR. The American College of Sports Medicine (ACSM) has also recognized the need to maintain minimal standards and guidelines for providing health care services to individuals utilizing health/fitness facilities. The standard requires that the facility manager, fitness/athletic director, instructor/leader, and all support staff be certified in cardiopulmonary resuscitation (CPR) before working with participants. Furthermore if the need arises, the facility and employees must respond with current CPR protocols and/or emergency first aid (6).

Cardiopulmonary emergencies frequently follow physical exertion or stress. Signs and symptoms of acute disorders indicating a possible heart attack include pain originating behind the sternum and radiating into either or both arms (usually the left), into the neck, jaws, teeth, upper back, or superior middle abdomen. Shortness of breath, nausea, and a feeling of impending doom are also present (4). CPR protocol is explained in the primary survey.

The individual clutched the chest and collapsed. If you determined a possible heart attack, you are correct. Tell someone to call an ambulance while you initiate the primary survey to determine if breathing and circulation are impaired.

UNCONSCIOUS ATHLETE

A basketball player goes up for a shot, gets tangled with another player, and falls onto the back striking the head on the floor. It does not appear the individual is moving. As you approach the player, think for a minute or two about how you will handle this situation.

Consciousness is defined on a continuum that grades levels of behavior in response to stimuli. These levels include (1) alertness, (2) drowsiness or lethargy (which proceeds to sleep), (3) stupor, (4) unconsciousness, and (5) coma (2). *Alertness* is the highest level of consciousness and cortical activity whereby the individual is fully alert, aware of the surroundings, and can respond to questions. *Lethargy* is the state in which the individual seems less alert and somewhat unaware of the surroundings, but can be aroused with a nudge or sound to respond to questions. *Stupor* is the level when the individual is nearly unconscious and unable to stay alert for any appreciable length of time. When prodded, the individual may initially respond to questions, but repeatedly lapses into unconsciousness and must be constantly aroused. **Unconsciousness**, on the other hand, is defined as an impairment of brain function whereby the individual lacks conscious awareness and is unable to respond to superficial sensory stimuli, such as pinching in the armpit or rapping knuckles on the sternum. *Coma* is the most depressed state of consciousness in which the individual is not aroused even by stimuli as powerful as pin pricks (3). The eyes are closed and the individual has no recognizable speech.

Head injuries are the leading cause of loss of consciousness in sport activity and are discussed in detail in Chapter 13. A transient lapse of consciousness, as in fainting, is called **syncope**. Other conditions that may alter consciousness include respiratory distress; tumors, hemorrhage, edema, or infections that invade the brain stem structures; seizures or epilepsy; heatstroke; metabolic disturbances such as hypoglycemia (abnormally low blood sugar); drug overdose (from opiates, barbiturates, aspirin, Tylenol, or alcohol); poisoning; liver and kidney failure; or cerebrovascular or cardiac malfunctions (2,7).

In emergency situations consciousness is determined through verbal and sensory stimuli. Try to communicate by calling the individual's name. You may need to shout loudly to get a response. Pinch the soft tissue in the armpit or rap your knuckles on the sternum and observe any painful withdrawal. If the individual does not respond, immediately

The NATA and ACSM recommend that all facility personnel be certified in CPR before working with participants

Levels of consciousness include:
  alertness
  drowsiness or lethargy
  stupor
  unconsciousness
  coma

Unconsciousness
Impairment of brain function wherein the individual lacks conscious awareness and is unable to respond to superficial sensory stimuli

Syncope
Fainting or lightheadedness

Determine consciousness through verbal and sensory stimuli

check the ABCs. If the individual is unconscious but breathing, proceed to the secondary survey for a more thorough head-to-toe assessment. A more detailed discussion of consciousness can be found in Chapter 13 in the section on assessment of cranial injuries.

💡 *Did you call the individual's name and try to arouse the person through sensory stimulation? Make sure breathing and circulation are not impaired before moving to the secondary survey.*

HEMORRHAGE

❓ *A second baseman collided with a runner and was cleated across the front of the shin. The area is bleeding profusely. Think for a minute or two about how you will control hemorrhage to limit blood loss and risk of infection.*

Severe hemorrhage causes a decrease in blood volume and blood pressure. To compensate for this factor, the heart's pumping action must increase. However, because there is less blood in the system, the strength of the pumping action is weakened resulting in a characteristic rapid, weak pulse. The human body can tolerate the loss of one pint of blood. The loss of two to three pints of blood, particularly in a short amount of time, however, such as one or two hours, can be fatal (4,5). Severity of bleeding is dependent upon age, weight, general physical condition, whether the bleeding is arterial or venous, speed of flow, where bleeding originated, if the blood is flowing freely or into a body cavity, and whether the bleeding is a threat to respiration.

Arterial bleeding from an oxygen rich vessel is characterized by a spurting, bright red color. Major arteries when completely severed often constrict and seal themselves for a short period. However, if the artery is only punctured or partially severed, bleeding can be severe. The spurting action of arterial bleeding can lead to a delay in clotting. Venous bleeding from an oxygen depleted vessel appears as a dark, bluish-red, almost maroon color. The continuous steady loss of blood can be heavy. Most veins collapse if they are cut. However, bleeding from deep veins can be as profuse and as difficult to control as arterial bleeding (5). If the large veins in the neck are cut, an air bubble or air embolism can be sucked into the vein and then travel to the heart. Capillary bleeding is usually very slow and often described as ooz-

ing. The blood is red but a duller shade than arterial blood. This type of bleeding clots easily. **Hemophilia** is an inability of blood to clot leading to excessive blood loss. Hospitalization is often required to control hemorrhage in these individuals.

External Bleeding

External bleeding is the result of an exposed skin wound. Large exposed wounds carry a higher threat of infection than smaller ones. The most common methods used to control external bleeding include direct pressure and elevation (**Figure 3-2**). Universal safety precautions should always be followed when dealing with external hemorrhage and body fluids (**Table 3-1**).

Pressure is applied directly over the wound with a sterile gauze pad compressing the region against the underlying bone. Elevation utilizes gravity to reduce blood pressure, and thus, aids blood clotting. In more severe bleeding, indirect pressure points can also help control hemorrhage but should not be used if a fracture is suspected distal to the pressure point because of possible movement of the fractured bone ends. **Field Strategy 3-1** explains the immediate control of hemorrhage and proper disposal of blood-soaked materials.

Internal Hemorrhage

Internal bleeding can result from blunt trauma or certain fractures (such as those of the pelvis, rib, or skull). Because internal hemorrhage is not visible it can be overlooked leading to shock. The history of injury (i.e., a fall, a deceleration injury, or severe blunt trauma), coupled with signs and symptoms of shock should indicate possible internal bleeding exists. Immediate action is necessary to manage the situation. **Field Strategy 3-2** lists signs and symptoms that may indicate internal bleeding, and explains emergency management of the condition.

External devices can be used to decrease external and internal hemorrhage, and reduce the risk of shock from excessive blood loss. Inflatable air splints and vacuum splints can apply direct compression on damaged vessels to limit the amount of blood loss after a fracture. Pneumatic counter-pressure, or anti-shock garments are placed around the

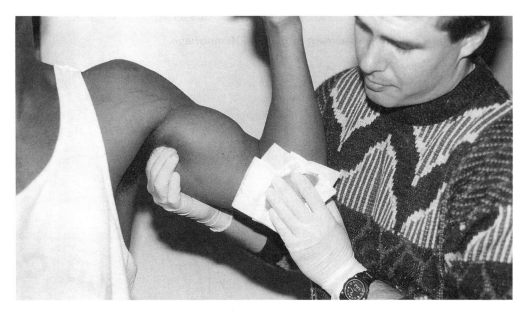

Fig. 3.2: Direct pressure over the wound and elevation above the heart are the best methods to control hemorrhage. Make sure latex gloves are always worn when handling blood or body fluids.

Table 3–1. Universal Safety Precautions in Treating Wounds.

Whenever an individual suffers a laceration or wound in which oozing or bleeding occurs, the activity should be stopped as soon as possible. The individual should be removed for treatment, and should not be returned to participation until cleared by appropriate medical personnel

Wash hands with germicidal soap before and after using latex gloves

Wear gloves for all routine procedures such as:

Caring for wounds including abrasions, lacerations, avulsions, blisters, pustules or boils, and aspiration of a bursa or hematoma

Being in contact with contaminated material containing blood or bodily fluids (such as bandages, ace wraps, urine samples, towels)

On-the-field evaluations where bleeding must be controlled (lacerations, bloody nose, open fracture)

Change gloves after each treatment. Discard gloves that are torn, cut, or punctured

Wear a protective facemask and eyewear if a procedure could generate droplets of fluid that may spray into the practitioner's mouth, nose, or eyes

Sterilize instruments thoroughly and handle them with care. Dispose of needles, scalpels and other "sharp" sticks in a biohazard container. Needles, once used, should never be recapped nor removed from disposable syringes by hand. Any needle pricks or cuts should be reported to the supervising physician so appropriate supportive therapy may be instituted

Clean all tables and counters regularly with a 10:1 bleach solution

Wash all blood-stained towels and linens in hot water and bleach

Have a well-marked designated biohazard container for soiled materials easily accessible in the training room. A specific policy should be established for disposal of materials

Use an approved mouth shield when giving artificial respiration

Health care workers with open lesions should refrain from direct contact with individuals until the lesions have healed

Inoculations for hepatitis should be required for all staff and student athletic trainers

Education of staff, coaches, athletes, and student athletic trainers about the risks for contracting and spreading contagious diseases should be a priority

For confidential information, referrals, and educational materials on HIV, hepatitis, and other communicable diseases, call the CDC National Hotline at 1-800-342-2437

Field Strategy 3–1. Management of External Hemorrhage.

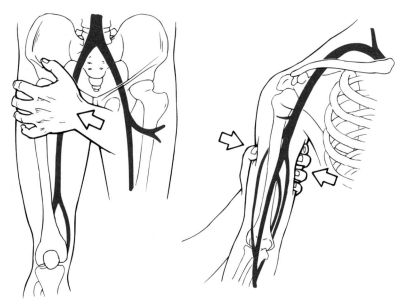

A. Femoral artery. B. Brachial artery

Put on latex or rubber gloves before you attempt to control hemorrhage
Apply direct pressure

Place a sterile gauze dressing directly over the wound, compressing the tissues and blood
vessels against the underlying bone
If bleeding stops, cleanse the wound with a normal saline solution
If bleeding is extensive, secure the dressing in place. *Never* remove a dressing that becomes
blood soaked
Place another dressing on top of the previous one and hold both in place

Elevate the injured area

Placing the limb above the heart slows the flow of blood and speeds clotting
Elevation is contraindicated in cervical injuries, internal injuries, impaled objects, fractures or
dislocations of the involved site because movement may cause further damage or intensify
the bleeding

Apply indirect digital pressure

Pressure points are places where an artery is close to a bony surface, and can be compressed
against the underlying bone to reduce blood flow to the distal injury site
Hold the pressure point only as long as necessary to stop the bleeding. Reapply pressure if
bleeding recurs
There are twenty-two pressure point sites in the body, eleven on each side. The two most
common are the brachial artery in the upper arm, and femoral artery in the anterior hip.
Discard all blood-soaked gauze pads in a properly labeled red biohazard bag. Do *not* throw them
into a wastebasket. To remove soiled gloves, use the dominant hand to reach to the opposite
hand and grasp the wrist band of the soiled glove. Pull the wrist band away from the wrist and
distal to the palm of the hand so the soiled portion of the glove is enveloped by the glove
itself. Once removed, that glove is now placed in the palm of the remaining gloved hand. The
process is repeated. Both gloves are then discarded in a biohazard receptacle. The hands
should then be washed with soap and water. If you are away from the training room or clinic
area, discard the pads and soiled gloves in a plastic bag, and discard that bag in the red
biohazard bag when you return to the room. The biohazard bag is then disposed of according
to the facility's procedures for disposal of biohazard waste. [*For information on proper disposal
of biohazard waste contact your local hospital*]

abdomen, pelvis, and lower extremities. Air is then pumped into the garment to apply steady compression to push fluids from the lower extremities into the body core. In doing so, the vascular compartment size is reduced and the heart does not have to work as hard to pump blood to the vital organs. As a result, blood pressure is increased and shock is limited. Pneumatic anti-shock devices are used by emergency medical technicians (EMTs) and paramedics to stabilize the patient's condition while traveling to the trauma center.

 After applying latex gloves, you should control hemorrhage on the baseball player by using direct compression and elevation. After bleeding has stopped, cleanse the wound with a saline solution and cover with a sterile dressing. Discard the gloves and any gauze pads containing blood or bodily fluids in a properly identified biohazard bag. Refer the individual to a physician if suturing is needed. Check the wound daily for signs of infection.

SHOCK

A football player was tackled resulting in a lower leg fracture. You have immobilized the leg and are awaiting the arrival of the ambulance. Think for a minute or two about what possible complications might occur as a result of this traumatic injury.

If the heart is unable to exert adequate pressure to circulate enough oxygenated blood to the vital organs, shock occurs. This condition may be due to a damaged heart that fails to pump properly, low blood volume from blood loss or dehydration, or because blood

---

Field Strategy 3–2. Management of Internal Bleeding.

Signs and symptoms may include:

Bleeding from the mouth, rectum, or other body openings; bloody fluid from the nose or ears
Low blood pressure, usually 90/60 mm Hg or lower
Rapid, weak pulse
Severe respiratory distress; rapid breathing, possibly becoming shallow
Pale, cold and clammy skin with profuse sweating
Feeling of impending doom, restlessness, or anxiety
Dull eyes, dilated pupils that are slow to respond to light
Pain, tenderness, swelling, or discoloration at the injury site
Dizziness in the absence of other symptoms
Nausea and vomiting blood; the blood may look like used coffee grounds
Blood in the urine or decreased urinary output
Rigidity or spasms of the abdominal wall muscles
Altered levels of consciousness

Emergency management

Activate EMS as quickly as possible
Maintain an open airway
Monitor vital signs
Check for fractures. Splint if appropriate
Treat for shock
Loosen any restrictive equipment or padding at the neck and waist
Anticipate vomiting; place the individual on their side with the head pointing downward to allow for drainage, provided you have ruled out a spinal injury
Keep the individual quiet
Continue to monitor vital signs until the ambulance arrives

vessels dilate, leading to blood pooling in larger vessels away from vital areas **(Figure 3-3)** (4,5). This results in a lack of oxygen and nutrition at the cellular level. The heart pumps faster, but due to reduced volume, pulse rate is weakened and blood pressure drops (hypotension). This rapid, weak pulse is the most prominent sign of shock. As the individual's condition deteriorates, breathing becomes rapid and shallow. Sweating is profuse. Vital body fluids pass through the weakened capillaries thereby causing further circulatory distress. If not corrected, circulatory collapse can lead to unconsciousness and death.

Shock occurs in injuries involving severe pain, bleeding, spinal injuries, fractures, or intra-abdominal or intrathoracic injuries, but may also occur to some degree in minor injuries. The severity of shock depends on age, physical condition, pain tolerance, fatigue, dehydration, presence of any disease, extreme cold or heat exposure, or improper handling or movement of an injured area (5). Types of shock include hypovolemic, respiratory, neurogenic, psychogenic, cardiogenic, metabolic, septic, and anaphylactic.

> Shock occurs in injuries with severe pain, bleeding, spinal injuries, fractures, or abdominal or thoracic injuries, but may also occur in minor injuries

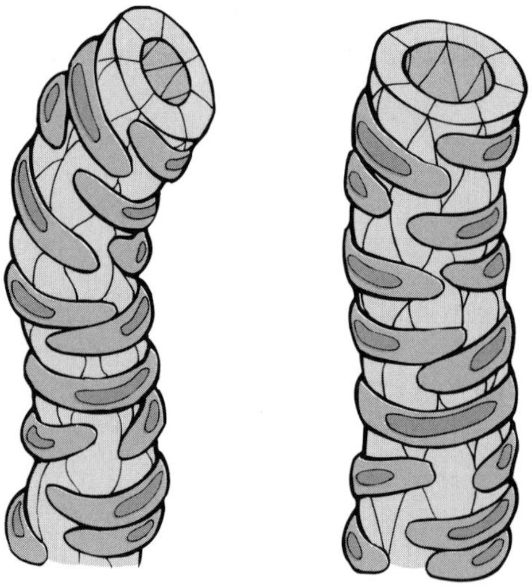

Hypovolemic shock results from excessive blood or fluid loss leading to an inadequate circulation and oxygen supply to all body organs. Possible causes include hemorrhage, dehydration, multiple trauma, and severe burns.

Respiratory shock results from insufficient oxygen in the blood from inadequate breathing. Possible causes are spinal injury to the respiratory controlled nerves, airway obstruction, or chest trauma, such as from pneumothorax, hemothorax, or a punctured lung.

Neurogenic shock occurs when peripheral blood vessels dilate and an insufficient blood volume cannot supply oxygen to the vital organs. This may occur in a spinal or head injury when nerves that control the vascular system are impaired, thereby altering the integrity of blood vessels.

Psychogenic shock refers to a temporary dilation of blood vessels resulting in the draining of blood from the head with pooling of blood in the abdomen. This is commonly seen in fainting from the sight of blood.

Cardiogenic shock occurs when the heart muscle is no longer able to sustain enough pressure to pump blood through the system. Possible causes are injury to the heart or previous heart attack.

Metabolic shock results from a severe loss of body fluids due to an untreated illness that alters the biochemical equilibrium. Possible causes are insulin shock, diabetic coma, vomiting, or diarrhea.

Septic shock derives from severe, usually bacterial, infection whereby toxins attack the walls of small blood vessels causing them to dilate, therefore decreasing blood pressure.

Anaphylactic shock refers to a severe allergic reaction of the body to a foreign protein that is ingested, inhaled, or injected from foods, drugs, or insect stings. This type of shock can occur in minutes or even seconds following contact with the substance to which the person is allergic, and thus may not exhibit typical signs and symptoms seen in other types of shock.

Signs and symptoms of shock develop over time. In most cases shock begins with a feeling of uneasiness or restlessness, increased respirations, and increased weakened heart rate. The individual's skin turns pale, clammy, and profuse sweating is usually present. The lips, nail beds, and membranes in the mouth show cyanosis. Thirst, weakness, nausea, and vomiting may then become apparent. In later

Fig. 3.3: (A) The diameter of an arteriole blood vessel is controlled by circular layers of smooth muscles that either constrict or relax to regulate peripheral blood flow. (B) During shock, blood vessels vasodilate. This action increases the size of the vascular bed and decreases resistance to blood flow resulting in blood pooling in larger vessels, depriving the brain and vital organs of needed oxygen. As a result, heart rate increases giving the characteristic rapid, weak pulse that is often the first sign of shock.

stages, a rapid, weak pulse and labored, weakened respirations may lead to decreased blood pressure and possible unconsciousness. Immediate management involves activating local Emergency Medical Services (EMS), maintaining an open airway, controlling bleeding, splinting any fractures, and maintaining body temperature. If you do not suspect a head or neck injury, elevate the feet and legs eight to twelve inches. Vital signs should be taken and recorded every five minutes, and given to the ambulance attendants when they arrive. **Field Strategy 3-3** summarizes immediate care.

 A fracture can lead to shock. With a lower leg fracture, elevate the limb after the leg is immobilized and keep the individual warm to maintain body heat to minimize the risk of shock.

FRACTURES

 In the previous example, the football player was tackled and fractured the lower leg. What immediate care is necessary to handle this situation and prevent possible shock from setting in?

A fracture is a break in the continuity of a bone and may be classified as simple or compound. Because of the risk of infection, compound or open fractures are more serious than simple or closed fractures. Signs of fracture include swelling and bruising (discoloration), deformity and/or shortening of the limb, point tenderness, grating or **crepitus**, guarding or disability, or exposed bone ends. Assessment and recognition is confirmed through the use of palpation, percussion, compression, and distraction. These techniques will be discussed in the secondary survey.

A suspected fracture should be splinted before the individual is moved to avoid damage to surrounding ligaments, tendons, blood vessels, or nerves. If nerves are damaged, sensation or muscle movement may become impaired. Damaged blood vessels may impair circulation to distal body parts. Fractures of the femur and fractures resulting in no distal

> Signs of fracture include swelling, discoloration, deformity and/or shortening, point tenderness, grating or crepitus, guarding, disability, or exposed bone ends

Crepitus
Cracking or grating sound heard during palpation that indicates a possible fracture

---

Field Strategy 3–3. Management of Shock.

Signs and symptoms may include:

Restlessness, anxiety, fear, or disorientation	Nausea and/or vomiting
Cold, clammy moist skin	Shallow, irregular breathing, but may also be
Profuse sweating	labored, rapid or grasping
Extreme thirst	Dizziness
Eyes are dull, sunken, with pupils dilated	Pulse is rapid and weak
Skin is initially chalky, but later may appear cyanotic	

Management of shock

Activate EMS immediately. Secure and maintain an open airway. Control any major bleeding and monitor vital signs.

If you do not suspect a head or neck injury, or leg fracture, elevate the feet and legs 8 to 12 inches. If there are breathing difficulties, the individual might be more comfortable with the head and shoulders raised in a semi-reclining position. With a head injury, elevate the head and shoulders to reduce pressure on the brain. The feet may also be slightly elevated. In a suspected neck injury, keep the individual lying flat.

If the individual vomits or is unconscious, place them on their side to avoid blocking the airway with any fluids. This allows the fluids to drain from the mouth.

Splint any fractures. This will reduce shock by slowing bleeding and will help ease pain. If the individual has a leg fracture, keep the leg level while splinting the fracture. Raise the leg only after it has been properly immobilized.

Move the individual to a warm environment. Maintain body heat by keeping the individual warm, but do not overheat. Remove any wet clothing if possible and cover the individual with a blanket. Keep the individual quiet and still. Avoid any rough or excessive handling.

Do not give the individual anything by mouth, in case surgery is indicated.

Monitor vital signs every two to five minutes until the ambulance arrives.

pulse are considered to be priority emergencies requiring immediate transportation to the nearest medical facility. Open fractures or injuries involving multiple fractures are considered to be second priority injuries (See Determination of Findings).

Splints are used to support, immobilize, and protect possible fracture sites. *If in doubt, always immobilize the joint above and below the suspected fracture site.* There are four major types of splints (**Figure 3-4**). The more common rigid splints are made of wood, wires, aluminum, or cardboard. Soft splints may include pneumatic (air) splints which are easy to apply and can be left on for x-rays. Air splints, however, should not be used in a compound fracture, or in a simple fracture with deformity as the bone ends may move during application. Other soft splints include pillows, blankets, towels, and dressings, such as the sling and swathe. Traction splints are used for long bone fractures. Vacuum splints use a pump to remove air from the splint encircling the fractured limb. This allows the limb to remain in the exact position in which it was found.

The choice of splint depends on the bone(s) involved and equipment available. Because fingers and toes may be covered in any splint, be sure to check them regularly for circulatory impairment by observing bilateral skin color, temperature, and capillary refill. Capillary refill is checked by blanching the nails and watching for a rapid return of the normal pink color under the nail. **Field Strategy 3-4** summarizes general principles used to splint fractures (2).

Did you determine the individual with the fractured lower leg should have the leg immobilized from above the knee to the foot? It may be best to use a traction splint. The leg should then be elevated to prevent the onset of shock. What else might you do to reduce the risk of shock?

HYPERTHERMIA

A runner has just completed a half-marathon on a warm sunny day. Think for a minute or two about how the body dissipates internal heat generated during exercise. Under what circumstances would the immediate environment alter thermal regulation in the body?

Hyperthermia, or elevated body temperature, occurs when internal heat production is no longer in balance with external heat loss

(**Figure 3-5**). The hypothalamus maintains **homeostasis** by initiating cooling or heat retention mechanisms as needed to maintain a relatively constant body core (skull, thoracic, and abdominal region) temperature between 36.1° and 37.8°C (97° to 100°F). Heat-regulating mechanisms, such as sweating or shivering are activated by two means: (a) when peripheral thermal receptors in the skin are stimulated, and (b) when changes in blood temperature are noted as blood flows through the hypothalamus.

Internal Heat Regulation

Internal heat is generated during muscular activity through energy metabolism. During exercise, the circulatory system must deliver oxygen to the working muscles and deliver heated blood from deep tissues to the periphery for dissipation. The increased blood flow to the muscles and skin is made possible by increasing cardiac output and redistributing regional blood flow (i.e., blood flow is reduced to the visceral organs). As exercise begins, heart rate and cardiac output increase while superficial venous and arterial blood vessels dilate to divert warm blood to the skin surface. Heat is dissipated when the warm blood flushes into skin capillaries (2). This is evident when the face becomes flushed and reddened on a hot day or after exercise.

At rest with air temperature below 30.6°C (87°F), about two thirds of the body's normal heat loss occurs as a result of conduction, convection, and radiation. As air temperature approaches skin temperature and exceeds 30.6°C (87°F), evaporation becomes the predominant means of heat dissipation (**Figure 3-6**) (8).

Radiation

Radiation is the loss of heat from a warmer object to a cooler object in the form of infrared waves (thermal energy) without physical contact. Usually body heat is warmer than the environment and radiant heat energy is dissipated through the air to surrounding solid, cooler objects. When the temperature of surrounding objects in the environment exceed skin temperature, such as the sun or hot artificial turf, radiant heat is absorbed.

Conduction

Conduction is the direct transfer of heat through a liquid, solid, or gas from a warm

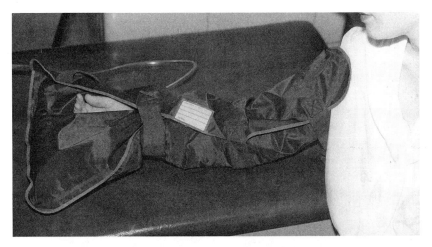

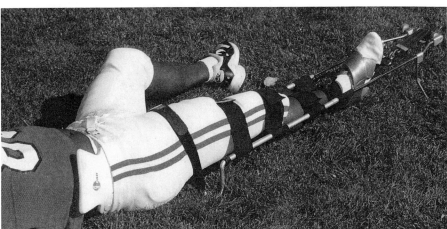

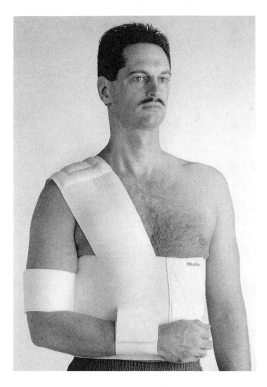

Fig. 3.4: Splints used to immobilize fractures come in a variety of styles. (A) Vacuum splint. (B) Traction splint. (C) Sling and swathe.

Field Strategy 3–4. Principles of Emergency Splinting for Suspected Fractures

Establish an open airway and complete the primary survey.

Remove any clothing and jewelry around the injury site. Clothing should be cut away with scissors to avoid unnecessarily moving the injured area.

Check the distal pulse beyond the fracture site. If pulse is weak, check for internal hemorrhage.

Cover all wounds, including open fractures with sterile dressings and secure them. Do not attempt to push the bone ends back underneath the skin.

Apply minimal in-line traction, and maintain it until the splint is in place and secured. Immobilize the joint above and below the fracture site. Severely angulated fractures should not be straightened. With such injuries, immobilize in the position you find the limb in.

Splint firmly, but not too tightly to impair circulation. Recheck distal pulse. Check vital signs and arrange for transportation to the nearest medical facility.

object to a cooler object. For example, a football player can absorb heat through the feet simply by standing on hot artificial turf.

Convection

The effectiveness of heat loss by conduction depends on convection, or how fast the air (or water) next to the body is exchanged once it becomes warmed. If air movement is slow, air molecules next to the skin are warmed and act as an insulation. In contrast, if warmer air molecules are continually replaced by cooler air molecules, such as on a breezy day or in a room with a fan, heat loss increases as the air currents carry heat away.

Evaporation

At rest, sweat glands assist thermoregulation by secreting unnoticeable amounts of sweat (about 500 ml/day). Sweat is a weak saline

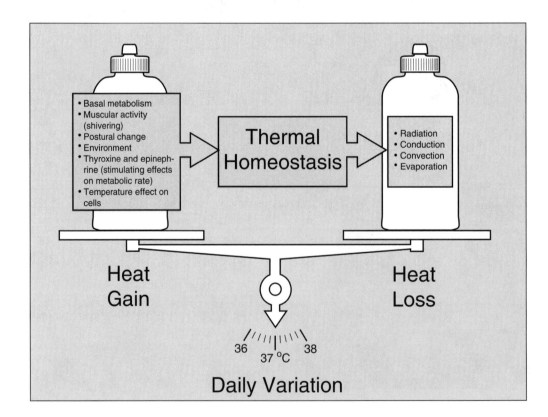

Fig. 3.5: Thermal homeostasis is achieved when internal heat production and heat loss are properly balanced to maintain a relatively constant body core temperature.

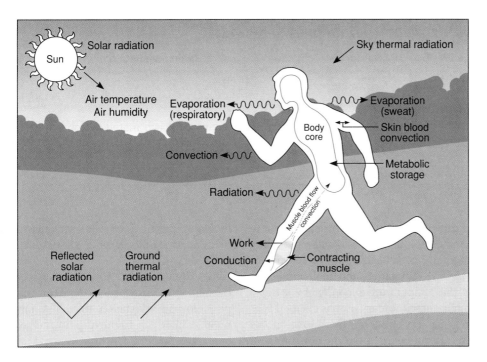

Fig. 3.6: Heat production from within working muscles is transferred to the body core and skin. During exercise, body heat is dissipated into the surrounding environment by radiation, conduction, convection, and evaporation.

solution, largely (99%) water, that evaporates when molecules in the water absorb heat from the environment and become energetic enough (that is, vibrate fast enough) to escape as a gas. As body temperature rises during exercise or illness, peripheral blood vessels dilate and sweat glands are stimulated to produce noticeable sweat, which can amount to a loss of one to two L of body water in one hour (2). Sweating itself does not cool the body; evaporation of the sweat cools the body.

In addition to heat loss through sweating, about 350 ml of water seeps through the skin every day, and another 300 ml of water is vaporized from mucous membranes in the respiratory passages (9). This is illustrated when you "see your breath" in very cold weather. Furthermore, it is not uncommon for sport participants to lose 1.5 to 2.5 L/hr of water during exercise. Although an individual may continually drink water (**ad libitum**) throughout an exercise bout, less than 50% of fluid lost will be replenished (9).

Measuring the Heat Stress Index

The heat stress index is a measure of ambient air temperature, humidity, and solar radiant energy. Relative humidity is the most impor-

tant factor that determines the effectiveness of evaporative heat loss. Relative humidity is the ratio of water in the ambient air to the total quantity of moisture that can be carried in air at a particular ambient temperature, and is expressed as a percentage. For example, 65% relative humidity means that ambient air contains 65% of the air's moisture carrying capabilities at the specific temperature. When air is completely saturated with water vapor (100% relative humidity), and ambient temperature is higher than skin temperature, no heat dissipation occurs (10).

The most commonly used heat-stress index is the Wet Bulb-Globe Temperature Index (WBGT) illustrated in **Table 3-2**. This index is calculated as follows:

$$WB - GT = (0.1 \times DBT) + (0.7 \times WBT) + (0.2 \times GT)$$

Ambient temperature is measured by a dry-bulb thermometer (DBT), but does not take into account vapor pressure, which has a direct impact on the ability to evaporate sweat. Wet-bulb temperature (WBT) is the temperature recorded by a thermometer with the mercury bulb surrounded by a wet wick, commonly called a sling psychrometer **(Figure 3-7)**. A sling psychrometer measures heat stress by exposing dry-bulb and wet-bulb thermometers to rapid air flow.

Ad libitum
At pleasure or at will

Relative humidity is the most important factor that determines the effectiveness of evaporative heat loss

Table 3–2. WBGT Index for Outdoor Activities

Range (°F)	Signal Flag	Recommendations
Below 64	None	Unlimited activity
64 to 76	Green	Stay alert for increases in the index and look for symptoms of heat stress
73 to 82	Yellow	Curtail active exercise for unacclimated persons
82 to 85.9	Red	Curtail active exercise for all persons, except well-acclimated individuals
86+	Black	Curtail all active exercise

Great differences in the recorded temperatures indicate a high rate of evaporation and low humidity. Smaller differences indicate a low rate of evaporation and high humidity. GT is the temperature recorded by a thermometer whose mercury bulb is encased in a sphere painted black. The black globe absorbs radiant energy from the environment to measure this important factor that dry- or wet-bulb thermometers cannot (10). **Table 3-2** lists recommendations for activities when temperature, humidity, and radiation are measured using the WB-GT index. Guidelines for safe participation in hot, humid environments using only a sling psychrometer for measurement are listed in **Table 3-3**.

Recent studies comparing females and males exercising at the same relative intensity found little difference in heat tolerance between genders (11,12,13,14). Although women possess more heat-activated sweat glands per unit skin area than men, women sweat less than men. Women begin to sweat at higher skin and core temperatures, produce less sweat than men for a comparable heat-exercise load, yet show a heat tolerance equivalent to men (9,15). This suggests that women rely on circulatory mechanisms for heat dissipation, whereas men depend more on evaporation for cooling (9). The production of less sweat to maintain thermal balance can provide significant protection from dehydration during work at high ambient temperatures.

Preventing Heat Emergencies

Several steps can be taken to reduce the risk of heat injury and include:

Identify individuals at risk. Healthy individuals at risk for heat injuries include those poorly acclimatized or conditioned, individuals inexperienced with heat injuries, individuals with a large muscle mass, children, and the elderly. Others at risk are listed in **Table 3-4**.

Acclimatization. Exercising moderately during repeated heat exposure can result in physiological adaptation to a new environment, which can improve performance and heat tolerance. This process is called

> Women rely on circulatory mechanisms for heat dissipation, whereas men depend more heavily on evaporation for cooling

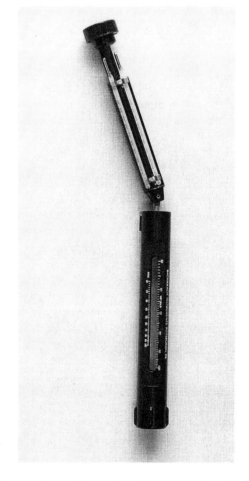

Fig. 3.7: A sling psychrometer measures heat by exposing a dry-bulb and wet-bulb thermometer to rapid air flow, which can help determine safe participation levels on hot humid days.

Table 3–3. Participation Guidelines using WBT Range.

°F	°C	Recommendations
60	15.5	No prevention necessary
61 to 65	16.2 to 18.4	Alert persons to symptoms of heat stress and the importance of adequate hydration
66 to 70	18.8 to 21.1	Insist that adequate water be ingested
71 to 75	21.6 to 23.8	Rest periods and water breaks every 20 to 30 minutes; place limits on intense activity
76 to 79	24.5 to 26.1	Modify practice considerably and curtail activity for unacclimated individuals
80	26.5	Cancel practice

acclimatization, and is one of the most effective measures to prevent heat stress. In general, a minimum of eight daily exposures for 1.5 to 2 hours/day is sufficient to acclimate the body to the environment. Intensity of each exercise bout should produce a target core temperature of 38° to 38.5°C (100.4° to 101.3°F) in the first half hour of the exercise bout (10). Gradual acclimatization decreases heart rate, body temperature, salt concentration in sweat; increases peripheral blood flow, plasma volume, sweat capacity; and more evenly distributes sweat over the skin and sustains the increased sweat rate over a longer period (10). The NCAA recommends gradual participation over 7 to 10 days to provide an adequate acclimatization to the environment. In addition, exercise intensity and duration should increase over days to weeks until exercise intensity and duration is comparable to competitive levels (16).

Heat acclimatization is lost rapidly. As a general rule, one day of heat acclimatization is lost over 2 to 3 days without heat exposure. Therefore, after about 3 weeks, most of the beneficial effects of acclimatization are lost (10).

Clothing. Light-colored, lightweight, porous clothing is preferred to dark-colored, heavyweight, nonporous clothing. Evapora-

Acclimatization
Physiologic adaptations of an individual to a different environment, especially climate or altitude

Exercise intensity should produce a target core temperature of 38° to 38.5°C (100.4° to 101.3°F) in the first half hour of the exercise bout

Table 3–4. Individuals at Risk for Heat Illness.

Healthy individuals who are:

Poorly acclimatized or poorly conditioned
Inexperienced individuals with limited knowledge about heat
Using some oil-based or gel-based sunscreens that block evaporative cooling
Elderly
Individuals with excessive muscle mass

Individuals with:

Pre-existing dehydrated state or pre-existing heat injury
Sleep deprivation due to decreased heart rate and decreased skin blood flow response to heat load
Chronic illnesses including cardiac disease, uncontrolled diabetes, eating disorders, hypertension, or malignant hyperthermia
Acute illnesses including fever or gastrointestinal illnesses
Alcohol and substance abuse involving amphetamines, cocaine, hallucinogens, laxatives, or narcotics
Medications including anticholinergics, diuretics, antihistamines, and beta blockers

Overweight or large athletes

Children

Heavy sweat suits and rubberized plastic suits produce high relative humidity close to the skin and retard evaporation

The rate of gastric emptying can be retarded when ingested fluids contain even the smallest amount of salt or simple sugars

Diuretics
Drugs that promote the excretion of urine

Substances used to induce vomiting and diarrhea lead to dehydration and cause excessive potassium loss and muscle weakness

On hot, humid days reschedule activities during the morning or evening to avoid the worst heat of the day

tive heat loss occurs only when clothing is thoroughly wet and sweat can vaporize. Therefore, changing into a dry shirt hinders heat dissipation (9). Heavy sweat suits or rubberized plastic suits produce high relative humidity close to the skin and retard evaporation, increasing the risk of heat illness (8,9).

Even with loose-fitting porous jerseys, wrappings or protective pads, and football helmets can seal off 50% of the body surface of football players and severely limit evaporative cooling. Increased metabolic rate needed to carry the weight of the equipment and increased temperatures on artificial surfaces also increase the risk for heat related illnesses (9). To counter this, football players should initially practice in short sleeved tee shirts, shorts, and low cut socks. On hot humid days uniforms should not be worn, and if possible, shoulder pads and helmets should be removed often to allow for radiation and evaporative cooling. Rubberized suits should never be worn (9,16).

Fluid hydration and electrolyte replacement. Thirst is not indicative of the need for water. Ten to twenty minutes prior to exercise, participants should consume 13 to 20 oz. of cold water (5°C; 41°F) and should have unlimited access to water at all times during exercise. Cold liquids, especially water, empty from the stomach and small intestines into the blood stream significantly faster than warm liquids (9,17). The rate of gastric emptying can be retarded when ingested fluids contain even the smallest trace of salt or simple sugars, whether glucose, fructose, or sucrose.

The minerals sodium, chloride, magnesium, and potassium are called electrolytes because they are dissolved in the body as electrically charged particles called ions. Electrolytes regulate fluid balance, nerve conduction, and muscle contraction. Ionic concentration within sweat is greatly influenced by the rate of sweating and an individual's state of heat acclimatization. Four liters of sweat equals approximately a 5.8 percent loss of body weight and contains high levels of sodium and chloride, but little potassium, calcium, or magnesium. These losses lower the body's sodium and chloride content by 5 to 7 percent; potassium by less than 1.2 percent. Because the body loses more water than electrolytes, the ionic concentration of these minerals rises in the body fluids. This illustrates that during periods of heavy sweating, the need to replace body water is greater than replacing electrolytes.

Electrolyte solutions are unnecessary for individuals with a normal diet. Evidence suggests that electrolyte intake during exercise does not improve performance or reduce physiological strain including muscle cramps, unless the individual is involved in continuous or repeatedly prolonged activity for over two to three hours in the heat (8,9,17). Commercial drinks should be diluted with twice as much water than suggested to produce a solution that is no more than 8 percent glucose polymer (16,17). While maintaining hydration, the participant should avoid excessive amounts of protein, caffeine, alcoholic beverages, and foods that increase urine production.

If individuals are taking **diuretics**, they should be carefully watched for dehydration, because these drugs reduce plasma volume and may adversely affect thermoregulation and cardiovascular function (9). Substances used to induce vomiting and diarrhea also lead to dehydration and may cause excessive electrolyte loss with an accompanying muscle weakness.

Weight charts. Losing 2 percent of body weight can affect sport performance. A weight loss of 3 to 5 percent can affect the thermoregulatory mechanisms (9). A rule of thumb is for every pound of water lost, 1 pint of water must be consumed. Recommended fluid intake to compensate for water loss can be seen in **Table 3-5**.

Temperature/humidity. A sling psychrometer should be used on questionable days to determine safe participation before activity begins. On days when the WBT reading ranges below 21.1°C (70°F), sport participants should have a 10-minute rest period every hour. When the WBT reading is between 21.6° to 23.8°C (71° to 75°F), water breaks should be every twenty to thirty minutes, and limits should be placed on intense activity. Practice should be seriously modified when readings exceed 24.5° to 26.1°C (76° to 79°F), and cancelled over 26.5°C (80°F) (9).

Practice schedules. On hot, humid days reschedule workouts, practices, and competitions in the morning or evening to avoid the worst heat of the day. Allow frequent water breaks (i.e. 10 minutes every half hour), shorten the practice, and lessen the intensity. Whenever possible get the players out of the sun and remove any restrictive equipment, pads, and helmets.

Table 3–5. Recommended Fluid Intake[a] for a Strenuous 90-minute Exercise Bout.

Weight loss/lbs.	Minutes between waterbreak	Fluid/break/oz.
8	No practice recommended	—
7½	No practice recommended	—
7	10	8 to 10
6½	10	8 to 9
6	10	8 to 9
5½	15	10 to 12
5	15	10 to 11
4½	15	9 to 10
4	15	8 to 9
3½	20	10 to 11
3	20	9 to 10
2½	20	7 to 8
2	30	8
1½	30	6
1	30	6
½	30	6

Based on 80% replacement of weight loss.

Heat Cramps

Heat cramps are painful, involuntary muscle spasms caused by excessive water and electrolyte loss during and after intense exercise in heat. Paradoxically, the condition more frequently occurs in a well conditioned acclimated athlete who has overexerted in hot weather and rehydrated with only water (8). Cramps commonly occur in the calf and abdominal muscles, but may involve the upper extremity muscles. Predisposing factors include lack of acclimatization, use of diuretics, and sodium depletion in the normal diet.

With heat cramps, body temperature is not usually elevated, and the skin remains moist and cool (8,10). Pulse and respiration may be normal or slightly elevated, and dizziness may be present.

Heat Exhaustion

Heat exhaustion usually occurs in unacclimatized people early in the summer or during the first hard training sessions. Individuals who wear protective equipment or heavy uniforms are also at risk, as evaporation through the material may be retarded.

Symptoms develop due to increased metabolic heat load from physical activity and reduced blood volume from dehydration and/or salt depletion secondary to fluid loss.

The individual may appear ashen and gray. Other symptoms include fatigue, weakness, uncoordinated gait, dizziness, nausea or vomiting, small urine output, headache, low blood pressure in the upright position, rapid and shallow respirations, and a rapid, weak pulse (**Figure 3-8**). Sweating mechanisms are generally working profusely making the skin wet, cool, and clammy, however, sweating may be reduced if the person is dehydrated. An elevated core temperature generally does not exceed 39.5°C (103°F) (10).

Heat Stroke

Heat stroke is the least common but most serious heat related illness. In football, heat stroke is second only to head injuries as the most frequent cause of death. The condition is also seen in distance runners, and wrestlers dehydrated through weight loss. Heat stroke is almost always preceded by prolonged, strenuous physical exercise in individuals who are poorly acclimatized, or in situations where evaporation of sweat is inhibited. During exercise, metabolic heat continues to rise. Decreased blood plasma volume causes the heart to beat faster and work harder to pump blood through the circulatory system. The thermoregulatory system is overloaded and the body's cooling mechanisms fail to dissipate the rising core temperature. The hypo-

Heat cramps
Painful involuntary muscle spasms caused by excessive water and electrolyte loss

Factors that place individuals at risk for heat cramps include lack of acclimatization, use of diuretics, and dietary sodium depletion

Heat exhaustion can lead to fatigue, dizziness, confusion, rapid and shallow respirations, and a rapid, weak pulse

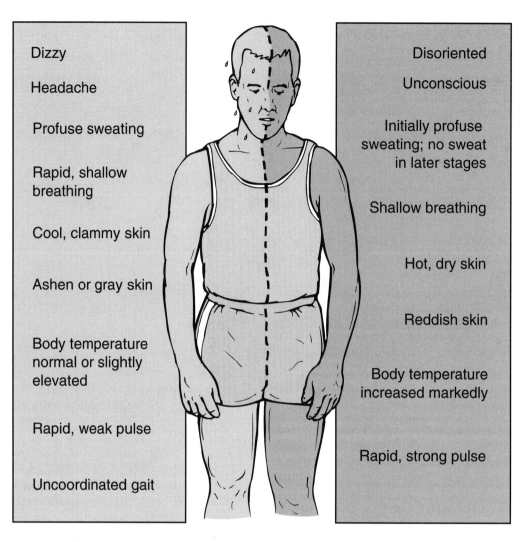

Dizzy		Disoriented
Headache		Unconscious
Profuse sweating		Initially profuse sweating; no sweat in later stages
Rapid, shallow breathing		Shallow breathing
Cool, clammy skin		Hot, dry skin
Ashen or gray skin		Reddish skin
Body temperature normal or slightly elevated		Body temperature increased markedly
Rapid, weak pulse		Rapid, strong pulse
Uncoordinated gait		

Fig. 3.8: Comparison of the signs and symptoms associated with heat exhaustion and heat stroke.

thalamus shuts down all heat-control mechanisms, including the sweat glands, to conserve water loss. As a result, a vicious circle is created: as temperature increases the metabolic rate increases, which in turn, increases heat production. The skin becomes hot and dry. As temperature continues to elevate, permanent brain damage may occur. Core temperature can rise to 105°F and has been known to reach 107° to 108°F (18). If untreated, death is imminent.

Initial symptoms include a feeling of burning up. Deep breaths, irritability, disorientation, profuse sweating, and an unsteady gait may be present. As the condition deteriorates, sweating ceases. The skin is hot and dry, and appears reddened or flushed (**Figure 3-8**). The individual will have dilated pupils giving the appearance of a glassy stare. As core temperature rises, the pulse becomes rapid and strong, as high as 150 to 170 beats per minute. Tissue damage by excessive body heat leads to vasomotor collapse, shallow breathing, decreased blood pressure, and a rapid and weak pulse. Muscle twitching or seizures may occur just before the individual lapses into coma (8,18).

Emergency Care for Heat Stress

Treatment for all heat conditions involves immediately moving the person to a cool place, removing all equipment and unnecessary clothing, and cooling the body. Place the individual supine with the feet elevated above the heart to maintain blood pressure and circulation to the brain. Cool fluids with a diluted electrolyte solution may be administered unless the individual is stuporous or unconscious.

With heat cramps, passive stretching and ice massage over the affected area is helpful. The individual should be watched carefully as this condition may precipitate heat exhaustion or heatstroke.

In suspected heat exhaustion and heat stroke, activate EMS. Rapid cooling of the body and fluid replacement is a priority. Cooling can be enhanced by sponging or toweling the individual with cool water or place them in front of a fan. Particular attention should be directed to cooling the major blood vessels in the armpit, groin, and neck regions. Core temperature should be taken every 10 minutes and should not fall below 38°C (100°F) to avoid hypothermia (8,18). Heat stroke victims usually require airway management, intravenous fluids, and in severe cases, circulatory support. Continue body cooling during transport to the nearest trauma center. **Field Strategy 3-5** lists the signs, symptoms, and immediate care for heat related conditions. Physical activity should not be resumed until the individual has returned to the predehydrated state and has been cleared by a physician.

 During the half marathon, the runner's body heat was dissipated through radiation, conduction, convection, and evaporation. Environmental stresses including high temperature, relative humidity, radiation, and wind velocity can overload these heat dissipating mechanisms leading to hyperthermia.

HYPOTHERMIA

? *Think for a minute or two about how the body maintains heat in cold weather. How can you prevent heat loss during adverse weather conditions?*

Hypothermia, or reduced body temperature, occurs when the body is unable to maintain a constant core temperature. With cold weather, or decreased circulating blood temperature, heat promoting mechanisms attempt to maintain or increase core temperature. Vasoconstrictor fibers in surface blood vessels prevent blood from shunting to the skin. Because skin is insulated with a layer of subcutaneous fat, heat loss is reduced. Cold also stimulates the release of certain chemicals that increase metabolic activity and heat production in the heart, liver, brain, and endocrine organs. If vasoconstriction and increasing metabolic rate are insufficient to maintain core temperature, shivering begins, thus producing heat through involuntary contractions in skeletal muscles as long as energy supplies last (2). During gradual seasonal changes, the hormone thyroxine is released by the thyroid gland and serves as another avenue to increase metabolic rate. During

Particular attention should be directed to cooling the major blood vessels in the armpits, groin, and neck

Hypothermia
Decreased body temperature

Shivering can produce heat through involuntary muscle contractions only as long as energy supplies last

Field Strategy 3–5. Management of Heat Related Conditions.

Condition	Signs and symptoms	Treatment
Heat cramps	Involuntary muscle spasms or cramps; normal pulse and respirations; profuse sweating and dizziness	Rest in cool place; massage cramp with ice and do passive stretching; drink cool water with diluted electrolyte solution
Heat exhaustion	Weakness; confusion; headache; profuse sweating; skin is wet, cool, clammy, and may appear ashen; breathing is rapid and shallow; pulse is weak, discontinue activity until thoroughly recovered	Rest in cool room; remove equipment and clothing; execute rapid cooling of body; sponge or towel the individual with cool water or use fan; individual may need IV fluids
Heat stroke	Irritability progresses to apathy; unsteady gait and disorientation; pulse is rapid and strong; skin is hot and dry and appears red or flushed; blood pressure falls; may have convulsions, seizures, or slip into coma	ACTIVATE EMS! Rest in cool room; rapidly cool the body with ice on the major blood vessels, or use wet compresses in path of an electric fan; treat for shock and transport to trauma center immediately

Active skeletal muscles produce 30 to 40 times the amount of heat produced at rest	

Clothing should be light, porous enough to allow free exchange of perspiration, and should not restrict movement

The insulating ability of clothing can be decreased by as much as 90% when saturated through either external moisture or condensation from sweating

Cold urticaria
Condition characterized by redness, itching, and large blister-like wheals on skin that is exposed to cold

Raynaud's phenomenon
Condition characterized by intermittent bilateral attacks of ischemia of the fingers or toes, marked by severe pallor, numbness, and pain

vigorous exercise, skeletal muscles produce 30 to 40 times the amount of heat produced at rest and as such, are important in regulating body temperature (2).

Cold emergencies happen in two ways. In one, the core temperature remains relatively constant but the shell temperature decreases. This leads to localized injuries from frostbite. The other occurs when both core temperature and shell temperature decrease leading to general body cooling. All body processes slow down and systemic hypothermia occurs. If left unabated, death is imminent.

Women are less able to produce heat through exercise or shivering because of less lean body mass, although the additional subcutaneous fat does provide more tissue insulation (19,20). In cold, men tend to maintain a lower heart rate, higher stroke volume, and higher mean arterial blood pressure than women, but there are no distinct differences in cold tolerance when genders are matched for aerobic fitness at the same relative work load (21).

Preventing Cold Related Injuries

During cold weather, body heat is lost through respiration, radiation, conduction, convection, and evaporation. Although the body will attempt to generate heat through heat producing mechanisms, this may be inadequate to maintain a constant core temperature. **Table 3-6** lists factors that contribute to cold injuries.

Several steps can be taken to prevent heat loss and are summarized in **Field Strategy 3-6**. The "layer principle" of clothing allows for several thin layers of insulation rather than a thick one. Fabrics should be light, yet porous enough to allow free exchange of per-

spiration, and should not restrict movement. Fabrics may include wool, wool/synthetic blends, polypropylene, or treated polyesters such as Capilene (18). Cotton has poor insulating ability that is markedly decreased when saturated with sweat. Pile garments containing down, Dacron, Hollofil, or Quallofil are more useful when worn during warm-up, time-outs, or during the cooldown period following exercise (19). Jackets with a hood and drawstring, and pants made of wind resistant material, such as Gore-Tex, Nylon, or 60/40 cloth, can protect against the wind.

A ski cap, face mask, and neck warmer can protect the face and ears from frostbite. Ski goggles can protect the eyes but they must be well ventilated to prevent fogging, and can be treated with anti-fog preparations. Polypropylene gloves, or in extreme temperatures, woolen mittens can be worn with windproof outer mittens of Gore-Tex or Nylon. Athletic shoes should be large enough to accommodate an inner layer of polypropylene socks and an outer pair of heavy wool socks. Avoid getting wet because heat loss can be increased by evaporation. The insulating ability of clothing can be decreased as much as 90% when saturated through either external moisture or condensation from sweating (3). If conditions are bad enough, it is better to cancel the practice or event for the day.

Frostbite Injuries

Frostbite is caused by freezing soft tissue. Individuals who have **cold urticaria** or **Raynaud's phenomenon** are at a higher risk for frostbite. These conditions are discussed in more detail in Chapter 17 with environmental considerations. Superficial frostbite involves the skin and underlying tissue. Deep frostbite involves the

---

Table 3–6. Predisposing Factors to Cold Related Injuries.

Inadequate insulation from the cold or wind
Restrictive clothing or arterial disease that prevents peripheral circulation, especially in the feet
Poor diet lacking adequate glycogen and fat
Presence of chronic metabolic disorders
Pre-existing fatigue or general weakness
Use of alcohol or other substance abuse
Use of tobacco products, especially smoking
Age (very young or old)
Decreased circulation
Enhanced effect by the body's normal effort to maintain its core temperature by shunting blood flow away from the shell to the core to prevent hypothermia

Field Strategy 3–6. Reducing the Risk for Cold Injuries.

Check weather conditions and consider possible deterioration.
Identify individuals who may be susceptible to cold and keep a watchful eye on them.
Dress in several light layers instead of one heavy layer.
Wear windproof, dry, well-insulated garments that allow water vapor to escape. Wool is excellent.
Carry windproof pants and jacket if conditions warrant. Keep your back to the wind.
Have well-insulated, wind-proof mittens, gloves, hats, and scarves. Wear them!
Wear foot wear that will keep your feet dry and insulated from the cold.
Avoid dehydration by drinking water. Do not drink alcoholic beverages or snow because this will worsen hypothermia.
Carry nutritious snacks that contain carbohydrates and sugars for quick energy during exercise.
Eat small amounts of food often.
Do not stand in one position for an extended period. Keep wriggling your toes to bring warm blood to the area.
Stay dry by wearing appropriate rain gear or protective clothing. If you get wet, change as soon as you can into dry clothing.
Breathe through the nose, rather than the mouth, to minimize heat and fluid loss.
Do not touch any metal with bare skin.
Watch the faces of those around you for signs of frostbite.

---

tissues deep to the skin and subcutaneous layers, and may result in complete destruction of the injured tissue (**Figure 3-9**). Damage depends on the depth and penetration of the cold resulting from varying duration, temperature, and wind velocity (22).

Areas commonly affected are the fingertips, toes (especially in constricting footwear), earlobes, and tip of the nose. The skin initially appears red and swollen, and the individual complains of diffuse numbness that may or may not be preceded by a itchy or prickly sensation. The area then turns white with a yellow or blue tint that looks "waxy" (18,22).

In superficial frostbite the area may feel firm to the touch, but the tissue beneath is soft and resilient. If the frostbite extends into deep tissues, the skin feels hard because it is actually frozen tissue (see **Table 3-7**). The person should be taken indoors, protected from any further refreezing, and subjected to careful, rapid rewarming of the area. Do not rub the skin with snow. Remove any clothing, jewelry or rings, and immerse the injured area in water heated 40° to 42°C (104° to 108°F) for 30 to 45 minutes (18). A whirlpool is ideal, but if unavailable, use a basin large enough so skin does not touch the sides of the container. Avoid hot water as this may burn the person. In deep frostbite, as the area thaws it will feel numb and appear mottled blue or purple (22). Capillary damage and plasma may leak into surrounding tissues causing swelling.

When the part is completely rewarmed, gently dry the affected area and apply a sterile dressing. If fingers or toes are being rewarmed, place sterile dressings between the digits before covering (22). Cover the entire area carefully with towels or a blanket to keep it warm, and transport the individual to the nearest trauma center with the limb slightly elevated. If severe, blisters may form in the tissues beneath the outer layers of skin and gangrene may develop within two to three weeks (22). Throbbing, aching, and burning sensations may last for weeks. The skin may remain permanently red, tender, and sensitive to re-exposure to cold.

Systemic Body Cooling

Normal skin temperature in cool weather ranges between 32° to 34°C (90° to 93°F) and can drop as low as 21° to 23°C (70° to 73°F) before the body core begins to cool. Exposed surfaces on the hands, face, head, and neck lose most of the body heat through radiation. At 4.4°C (40°F) over half the body's generated heat can be lost from an uncovered head. At 15°C (5°F) up to 75 percent of the body's heat is lost through the head (22). Air movement coupled with cold produces a wind chill factor that causes heat loss from the body faster than in still air. The faster the wind, the higher the wind chill factor.

Tissue damage is dependent on the depth and penetration of the cold resulting from varying degrees of duration, temperature of exposure, and wind velocity

In frostbite the skin initially appears red and swollen, and the individual will complain of diffuse numbness that may or may not be preceded by a itchy or prickly sensation

At 4.4°C (40°F) over 50% of the body's heat can be lost from an uncovered head

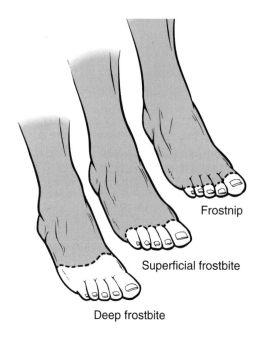

Frostnip

Superficial frostbite

Deep frostbite

Fig. 3.9: The stages of frostbite.

When core temperature falls below 34.4°C (94°F), essential biochemical processes begin to slow (18). Heart and respirations slow down, cardiac output and blood pressure fall, and as the skin and muscles cool, shivering increases violently. Numbness sets in and even the simplest task becomes difficult to perform. If core temperature continues to drop below 32°C (90°F), shivering ceases and muscles become cold and stiff. **Cold diuresis** occurs as blood is shunted away from the shell to the core in an effort to maintain vascular volume. If intervention is not initiated, death is imminent. **Table 3-8** further highlights the stages of systemic hypothermia, or general body cooling.

Treatment involves maintenance of the ABC's and rapid rewarming of the entire body. Activate EMS because advanced life support is often necessary. If the individual is conscious, warm fluids may be given, however, alcohol and caffeine should be avoided.

The body maintains heat through vaso-constriction of blood vessels, stimulation of metabolic activity, and shivering. Localized and systemic cold injuries can be prevented by covering exposed skin, wearing a hat, and dressing in layers to conserve body heat.

THE EMERGENCY PLAN

A gymnast slipped off the springboard on an approach to a vault and collided full force into the vaulting horse. The individual is now lying on the floor and does not appear to be moving. Think for a minute or two about what you should do to provide immediate care to this person and how additional help can be summoned.

An **emergency plan** is a well developed process that activates the emergency health care services of the facility and community to provide immediate health care to an injured individual. In serious injuries, prompt medical care is vital to maintain the cardiorespiratory system to sustain central nervous system function. Any delay may increase the severity of injury. As discussed in Chapter 1, health care is dependent on procedures developed and implemented by the primary sports medicine team. The facility manager, physician, athletic trainer, and sport supervisor have a legal duty of care to develop and implement an emergency plan to provide health care to sport participants. The ACSM has developed recommendations for health/fitness facilities relative to standards of health care. Along with CPR certification for all employees working with participants, the ACSM recommends that every health/fitness facility develop an emergency procedures plan to address staff skills, supplies and equipment, support personnel, practice, risk management, documentation of emergency situations, and any follow-up actions taken. Furthermore, at least one staff person should be identified as a medical liaison and have

---

Table 3–7. Signs and Symptoms of Frostbite.

1° Skin appears initially red, then white, and is usually painless. The condition is typically noticed by friends first. Skin is soft to the touch.

2° Skin appears initially red and swollen. Diffuse numbness may be preceded by an itchy or prickly sensation. White or waxy skin color appears later. Skin is firm, but tissue beneath is soft.

3° Skin appears blotchy white to yellow-gray or blue-gray. Skin is hard the entire depth and totally numb.

Table 3–8. Stages of Systemic Hypothermia.

Core temperature °F	Symptoms
96 to 99	Intense, uncontrollable shivering is present.
91 to 95	Violent shivering persists. If conscious, it may be difficult to speak.
86 to 90	Shivering decreases and is replaced by strong muscular rigidity. Muscle coordination deteriorates to jerky erratic movements. Thinking is clouded and the person may have total amnesia.
81 to 85	Person becomes irrational, loses awareness of the surroundings and drifts into a stuporous state. Muscular rigidity continues, and heart rate and respirations slow. Cardiac arrhythmias may be present.
78 to 80	Person becomes unconscious and cannot respond to spoken word. Reflexes cease to function and the heartbeat becomes erratic.
Below 78	Cardiac and respiratory centers in the brain fail. Edema and hemorrhage occur in the lungs leading to death.

advanced first aid training (6). Likewise, the NATA also requires certification in first aid for all athletic trainers, and the establishment of emergency procedures protocol in athletic training rooms.

At least once each year the primary sports medicine team and related individuals should meet with representatives from the local Emergency Medical System (EMS) to discuss, develop, and evaluate the emergency procedures plan. A written emergency plan should be developed for each activity site, and may include information such as, who will render emergency care and control the situation, what type of care will be initiated, who will call the ambulance, what care will be provided while the ambulance is coming to the facility, who will supervise the other activity areas if supervisors must leave those areas to go to the accident scene, and proper use and disposal of items and equipment exposed to blood or bodily fluids. It is critical during emergencies that everyone work together to ensure medical attention is not delayed. **Field Strategy 3-7** lists several important issues and questions to address in developing an emergency care plan.

All employees, along with local EMTs or paramedics, should practice the emergency plan through regular educational workshops and training sessions. These workshops can provide continuing education in emergency care management and recertification in first aid and cardiopulmonary resuscitation protocols. This will help prepare each individual to assume their role in rendering emergency care to an injured participant.

As the first person on the scene, you should initiate the facility's emergency procedures plan, do a primary survey, and summon help from your colleagues, one of whom should call the local EMS.

PRIMARY INJURY ASSESSMENT

You witnessed the gymnast lying motionless after colliding with the vaulting horse. In initiating the facility's emergency procedures plan, what priorities do you need to assess to determine if breathing or circulation is impaired.

The primary injury assessment, or primary survey, should establish the level of unresponsiveness, initiate, or maintain adequate breathing and circulation to sustain cardiorespiratory function until help arrives. Assessment of all injuries, no matter how minor, should always include a primary assessment. In most cases, this is completed quickly as you approach the injured individual and observe the person moving or talking. As such, you can proceed immediately to the secondary injury assessment. If the person is not moving or is unresponsive, however, initiate the primary survey before moving to the secondary survey.

Occasionally collisions occur in sport activities where more than one player is injured. **Triage** refers to assessing all injured individuals quickly, then returning to the most seriously injured and giving immediate treatment to that person. **Table 3-9** indicates a category system commonly used to determine priority of care with multiple injuries (4).

As you approach an individual, check the surrounding area to see if any equipment or apparatus may have contributed to the injury. Scan the individual and note any noticeable

Triage
Assessing all injured individuals to determine priority of care

Field Strategy 3–7. Developing an Emergency Care Plan.

Are all supervisors working with participants currently certified in emergency first aid and CPR? Is one individual identified as the medical liaison, or "captain"? Does this person have advanced first aid training?

When an emergency occurs, who will activate EMS? If the medical liaison must summon additional staff to help control the situation, who will supervise the other activity areas and do crowd control? Who has access to locked gates or doors? Who will direct the ambulance to the accident scene?

Do all supervisors understand their roles during an emergency and nonemergency situation? Has the facility invited representatives from EMS to become familiar with the floor plan of the facility? Does the facility regularly have announced and unannounced mock emergency drills to practice the procedures? Is EMS involved in these drills?

Have all sport participants been medically cleared to participate? Are appropriate documents completed (i.e., physical examination, permission to participate, informed consent, and emergency information)? Have the athletic trainers and sport supervisors been informed of any orthopedic or health problems that might affect participants?

Do you have emergency cards for each participant with family phone numbers, physician's names and numbers, special instructions/considerations, and who to contact when parents/guardians are unavailable?

Is the facility checked regularly for safety hazards? Does everyone know the location and have easy access to first-aid kits, splints, stretchers, and a phone? Are emergency numbers posted near each phone (i.e., EMS, hospital, training room, school nurse, facility medical liaison, fire and police departments)?

What information will be provided over the telephone, such as:
    Type of emergency situation
    Possible injury/condition
    Current status of the injured party
    Type of assistance being given to the injured party
    Exact location of the facility or injured individual (give cross streets to assist EMS) and specific point of entry to the facility
    Telephone number of phone being used

Do you have different emergency procedures for the various facilities (pool, gymnasia, weight room, training room, and fields)?

Who will be responsible for informing the individual's parents/guardians that an emergency has occurred?

Are proper injury records completed after the injury and kept on file in a central, secure location?

As you approach an individual, check the surrounding area to see if any equipment or apparatus may have contributed to the injury

Decerebrate rigidity
Extension of all four extremities

Decorticate rigidity
Extension of the legs with flexion of the elbows, wrists, and fingers

deformities and body position. In severe brain injuries, a neurological sign called posturing of the extremities, may occur. **Decerebrate rigidity** is a postural attitude characterized by extension in all four extremities **(Figure 3-10)**. **Decorticate rigidity** is a postural attitude characterized by extension of the legs and marked flexion in the elbows, wrist, and fingers. When posturing is evident, an emergency exists and medical assistance should be summoned immediately. Unless you have ruled out a possible spinal injury, always assume one is present and stabilize the head and neck before proceeding.

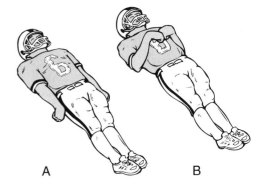

Fig. 3.10: Body posturing. (A) Decerebrate rigidity is characterized by extension in all four extremities. (B) Decorticate rigidity is characterized by extension of the legs and flexion of the elbows, wrist and fingers. Both conditions indicate a severe brain injury.

Table 3–9. Triage for Priority Care.

Highest priority	Second priority	Lowest priority
Respiratory arrest or airway obstruction	Blood loss of less than two pints Severe burns	Minor lacerations or soft tissue injury
Cardiac arrest	Open or multiple fractures	Minor or simple fractures
Severed artery	Stable abdominal injuries	Sprains
Spinal injury	Eye injuries	Strains
Head injuries with unconsciousness Severe shock		Those, who because of extensive injuries, have little chance of survival
Joint fractures with no distal pulse		No pulse for more than 20 minutes
Fractured femur		

Assess Unresponsiveness

Without moving the individual, tap the shoulder or arm while calling the individual's name. You may have to shout to get a response. Look at the facial expression and any eye movement. Does the individual respond to your voice by opening the eyes, moving a body part, or answering a question? Do they withdraw from painful stimuli (i.e., knuckle to the sternum or being pinched)? Are they totally unresponsive? If the individual cannot open the eyes on verbal command, or does not demonstrate withdrawal from painful stimulus, activate EMS and proceed to check the ABCs. This step should take 5 to 10 seconds.

Open the Airway

The tongue is attached directly to the lower jaw. In a supine position the tongue may slide posterior to close the epiglottis over the windpipe. By moving the jaw forward the tongue is lifted away from the epiglottis to open the airway. This may be all that is necessary for spontaneous breathing to return. If breathing does not spontaneously recur, a foreign object may be obstructing the airway. Remove the face mask of a football player. *Under no circumstances should the helmet be removed unless special circumstances are present (i.e., the screws securing the face mask are stripped and the individual is in respiratory distress, or you are unable to assess the airway)* (16). In either case, helmet removal should be performed only be personnel trained in the procedure. To remove the face mask, have a colleague stabilize the head and neck by placing the index fingers or thumbs in the helmet earholes and holding tightly (**Figure 3-11**). With the head and neck stabilized, use a screwdriver, wire cutters, or specialized tool to remove the plastic clips (23). In older helmets, bolt cutters may need to be used to remove the facemask. Remove the entire facemask and mouthguard to allow easy access to the mouth and nose. There are two methods to open the airway when no obstruction is present: head tilt/chin lift method and jaw thrust method. If the airway is obstructed by a foreign object, the Heimlich maneuver, abdominal thrusts, and a finger sweep can be used to clear the airway.

Head Tilt/Chin Lift Method

Open the airway by placing the tips of your fingers under the jaw. Lift forward while simultaneously pushing down on the individual's head. Avoid any excessive force (**Figure 3-12-A**). Keep the mouth slightly open. This method is recommended except where head or neck injury is suspected.

Jaw Thrust Method

If you suspect a head or neck injury, maintain the head in a fixed position. Rest your elbows on either side of the individual's head. Grasp the individual's lower jaw and lift forward

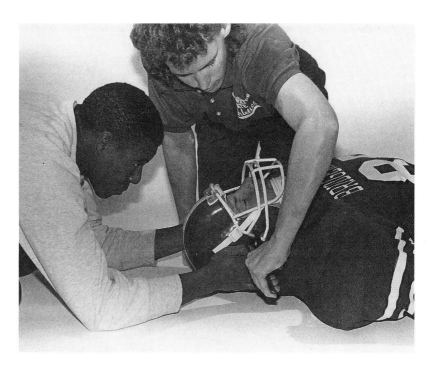

Fig. 3.11: To remove the face mask, have one assistant stabilize the helmet by grasping the ear holes with the middle fingers. Cut the side supports with a "Trainer's Angel," wire cutter, bolt cutter, or use a screwdriver to remove the screws. Do not remove the helmet unless special circumstances are present.

with both hands, keeping the mouth slightly open **(Figure 3-12-B)**.

Heimlich Maneuver

Stand behind the individual and wrap your arms around their waist. Make a fist with one of your hands and place the thumb side of the fist half way between the navel and lower tip of the sternum (xiphoid process) **(Figure 3-13-A)** . Grasp the fist with your other hand.

Keeping the elbows out, press the fist into the individual's abdomen with quick upward thrusts. Each thrust should be a separate, distinct movement. The action of the thrust pushes up on the diaphragm, compressing air in the lungs and creating a forceful pressure against the blockage, thus expelling or exploding the object from the airway. Repeat the thrusts until the obstruction is cleared or the individual becomes unconscious.

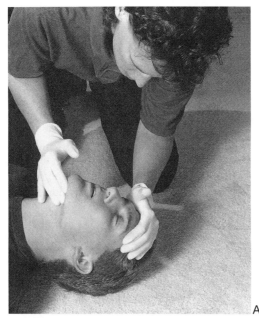

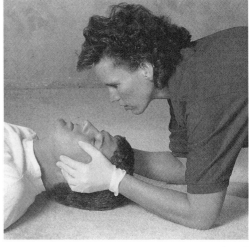

B

A

Fig. 3.12: Head tilt/chin lift method (A). Jaw thrust method (B).

Abdominal Thrusts

When unconscious, position the individual's head and open the airway to check for breathlessness. Straddle the thighs keeping your weight centered over your knees. Place the heel of one hand midway between the individual's navel and lower tip of the sternum (**Figure 3-13-B**). Place the other hand directly on top of the first hand. Press into the abdomen 6 to 10 times with quick upward thrusts.

Finger Sweep

If a foreign object is lodged in the back of the throat, and is visible, you may be able to remove the object. Be careful not to push the object further into the throat. With the hand closest to the victim's feet, open the mouth by grasping both the tongue and lower jaw between your thumb and fingers. Insert the index finger from the other hand into the mouth along the far cheek, extending deep into the throat to the base of the tongue (**Figure 3-14**). Using a hooking motion, dislodge the object and move it into the mouth for removal. **Field Strategy 3-8** lists protocol used to clear an obstructed airway.

Establish Breathing

Breathing is assessed with the look, listen, feel principle: *look* to see if the chest is rising or falling; *listen* for air exchange through the mouth or nose, or both; *feel* with your cheek to determine if there is air exchange (**Figure 3-15**). The depth of respirations indicates the volume of air being exchanged. **Dyspnea** refers to labored or difficult breathing and is a sign of respiratory distress. If the respiratory control center is depressed, **apnea**, or temporary cessation of breathing, can occur. Unless this condition is altered, respiratory arrest will lead to death. Take 3 to 5 seconds to assess the presence of breathing. If breathing is absent, send someone to activate EMS while you perform the following steps.

1. Using the hand placed on the forehead, pinch the nostrils closed. Take a deep breath. Place your mouth over the individual's mouth to establish an airtight seal and give two successive breaths. The chest should rise.
2. Remove your mouth to allow air to escape from the injured person's mouth and do the look, listen, feel technique to note air exchange.
3. Check the pulse at the carotid artery. Locate the Adam's apple with the index and middle finger. Slide the fingers to the side of the neck closest to you between the large neck muscle and windpipe (**Figure 3-16**). Do not use the thumb, as it has its own pulse. Very little pressure is needed to detect the pulse. Take 5 to 10 seconds to establish the presence of a pulse.

> Methods to open the airway:
> Head tilt/chin lift method
> Jaw thrust method
> Abdominal thrusts
> Finger sweep

Dyspnea
Labored or difficult breathing

Apnea
Temporary cessation of breathing

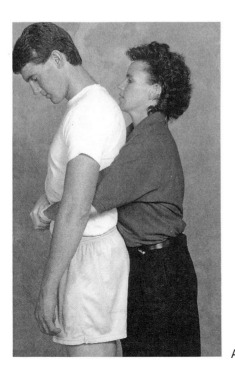

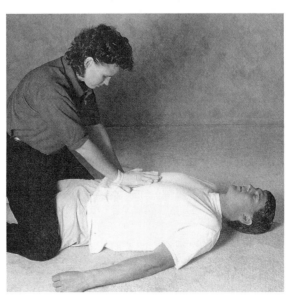

B

A

Fig. 3.13: Abdominal thrusts in a conscious individual (A). Abdominal thrusts in an unconscious individual (B).

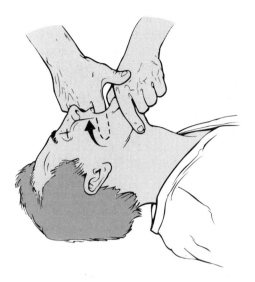

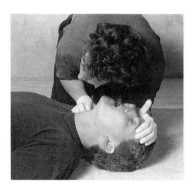

Fig. 3.15: To assess respirations: Look to see if the chest is rising, listen for air exchange through the mouth or nose, and feel on your cheek if there is air exchanged.

Fig. 3.14: Use the index finger to sweep away any visible foreign matter that may be obstructing the airway.

Establish Circulation

Each heart beat circulates blood to the vital organs. Combined with oxygen, minimal life support is sustained until advanced emergency care can be provided by trained emergency personnel. Circulation is maintained through chest compressions.

4. If a pulse is present but the individual does not resume breathing, continue giving a breath every five seconds (12 breaths per minute) for an adult; every four seconds (15 breaths per minute) for a child; and every three seconds (20 breaths per minute) for an infant.

5. If no pulse is present, proceed with cardiopulmonary resuscitation (CPR).

1. Locate the substernal notch with the hand closest to the individual's feet. Place the middle finger in the notch and index finger on the sternum.

2. Place the other hand on the midline of the sternum with the thumb against the index finger of the distal hand.

 Field Strategy 3–8. Management of an Obstructed Airway.

Ask, "Are you choking? Can you speak?"

Look for the universal distress sign or nodding of the head. Reassure the individual you are there to help.

Perform several Heimlich maneuver thrusts. Ask, "Are you still choking?" Repeat abdominal thrusts until the object is dislodged or the individual collapses. *If* the person collapses, then—

Position the head. Give two full breaths, each breath lasting from one to one and a half seconds. If your breath is unable to enter into the individual's mouth, then—

Reposition the individual's head and give two more breaths. If you are still unable to breathe into the individual, then—

Tell someone to call for an ambulance; say, "Airway is obstructed, call 911 (or your local emergency number or the telephone operator)"

Perform 6 to 10 abdominal thrusts

Do a finger sweep. If the object is visible, attempt to remove it

Give two full breaths again. If you are unable to breathe air into the individual, then repeat the full sequence until the airway is cleared or the ambulance arrives. The total sequence for an unconscious individual is: 6 to 10 abdominal thrusts, finger sweep, and 2 breaths.

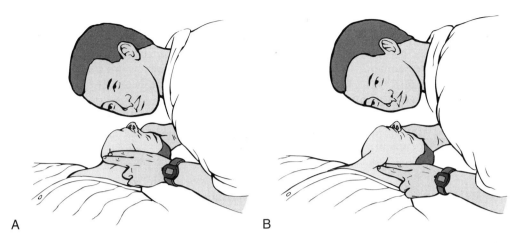

A   B

Fig. 3.16: To take a carotid pulse, place two on the larynx (Adam's apple), then gently slide the fingers into the groove between the larynx and sternocleidomastoid muscle on the side closest to you.

3. Place the distal hand on top of the proximal base hand and bring your shoulders directly over the individual's sternum. Interlace the fingers to hold them off the chest wall and begin a cycle of 15 chest compressions and 2 breaths for an adult **(Figure 3-17)**. The sternum should be compressed 1 ½ to 2 inches at a rate of 80 to 100 times per minute. In a child the ratio is 5 chest compressions to 1 breath. The heel of one hand is used to compress the midsternum 1 to 1 ½ inches (3,4).

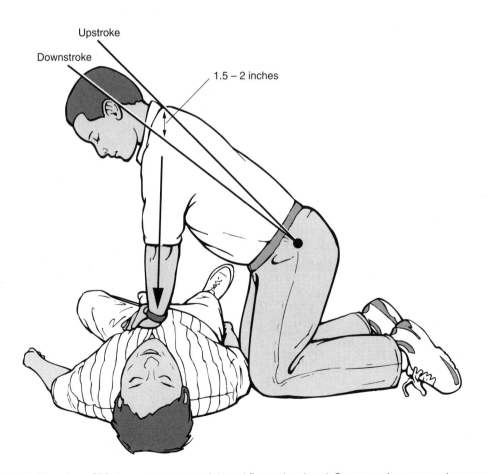

Upstroke

Downstroke

1.5 – 2 inches

Fig. 3.17: To perform CPR, keep your arms straight and fingers interlaced. Compress the sternum downward 1½ to 2 inches.

4. After one minute of CPR take another pulse for 5 to 10 seconds.
5. If the individual's pulse does return, check and maintain breathing. If breathing does not return, begin rescue breathing and continue to monitor the pulse.
6. If breathing returns, monitor the ABCs and proceed with a secondary assessment.
7. If the pulse does not return, continue CPR until the ambulance arrives.

Never interrupt CPR for more than 5 seconds, because blood flow will drop to zero. If you are alone and no one has responded to your shouts for help by the end of the first minute, however, you must summon an ambulance yourself (3). Then, quickly return to the individual and continue giving CPR. **Field Strategy 3-9** demonstrates a full primary survey without an obstructed airway. **Table 3-10** is a flow chart that outlines the various action steps taken during a primary survey.

 The gymnast was not moving as you approached. However, as you arrived at the scene and spoke to the person, the individual groaned and moved an arm. You have determined that breathing and circulation are present. Proceed to the secondary survey but continue to monitor the ABCs in case shock occurs.

Field Strategy 3–9. Primary Survey.

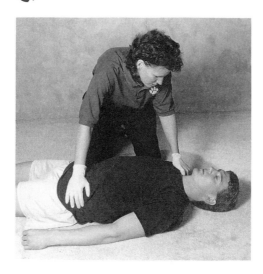

Establish unresponsiveness

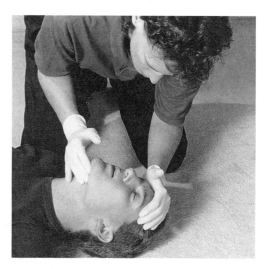

Open airway

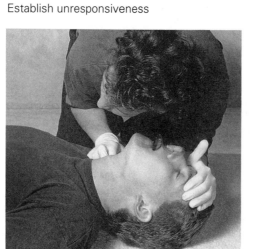

Breathing: look, listen, feel
Note breathing rate and depth

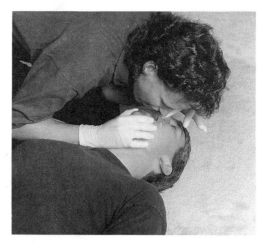

Give two breaths

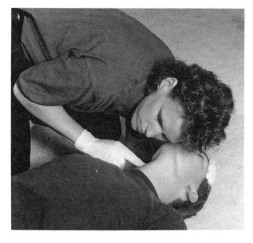

Check the carotid pulse
Note pulse rate and strength

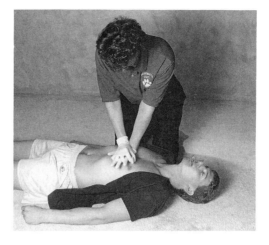

Locate proper hand position. Do chest
compressions
15 compressions; 2 ventilations

Table 3–10. Flow Chart for the Primary Survey.

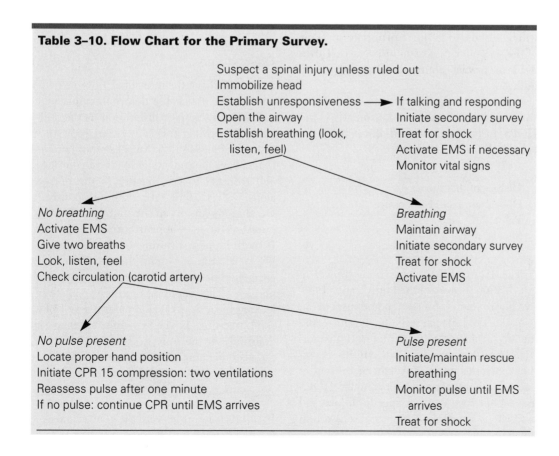

Suspect a spinal injury unless ruled out
Immobilize head
Establish unresponsiveness ⟶ If talking and responding
Open the airway   Initiate secondary survey
Establish breathing (look,   Treat for shock
    listen, feel)   Activate EMS if necessary
                                   Monitor vital signs

No breathing   *Breathing*
Activate EMS   Maintain airway
Give two breaths   Initiate secondary survey
Look, listen, feel   Treat for shock
Check circulation (carotid artery) Activate EMS

No pulse present   *Pulse present*
Locate proper hand position   Initiate/maintain rescue
Initiate CPR 15 compression: two ventilations   breathing
Reassess pulse after one minute   Monitor pulse until EMS
If no pulse: continue CPR until EMS arrives   arrives
                                   Treat for shock

HOPS sports injury assessment:
History of the injury
Observation and inspection
Palpation
Special tests

Vital signs
Objective measurements of pulse, respiration, blood pressure and skin temperature indicating normal body function

Observe body position and any deformities, bleeding, discoloration, swelling, respirations, pupillary response to light, and the general attitude of the individual

SECONDARY INJURY ASSESSMENT

❓ *You have assessed the gymnast and determined the individual is somewhat lethargic but does respond to verbal commands. Breathing is shallow but pulse is normal. Think for a minute or two about how you will proceed to determine the seriousness of injury.*

A secondary injury assessment involves a detailed hands-on, head-to-toe assessment to detect conditions that may not in themselves pose an immediate threat to life, but if left unrecognized and untreated, could lead to serious complications. If the individual is moving and speaking, or if the individual is unconscious and ABCs are adequate, begin the secondary injury assessment. In nearly all cases, an individual will regain consciousness in a short period and can then respond to your questions.

Many athletic trainers and other medical personnel begin the secondary survey with an assessment of vital signs to establish a baseline of information about the health status of the individual. **Vital signs** include pulse, respiration, blood pressure, and skin temperature. Although not specifically cited as a vital sign, skin color, pupillary response to light, and eye movement should also be documented. Each of these factors will be discussed in the appropriate sections of the secondary assessment process. **Table 3-11** lists what abnormal vital signs may indicate.

A popular methodical process used extensively in sports injury assessment is the HOPS format and is used throughout the text. HOPS is an acronym for:

History of the injury
Observation and inspection
Palpation
Special tests

The HOPS format uses both subjective information (history of the injury), and objective information (observation and inspection, palpation, and special tests) to recognize and identify problems contributing to the condition. In emergency situations, HOPS assessment includes an overall scan of the entire body. In a nonemergency sport injury, HOPS assessment focuses on a specific injury and associated structures, and is discussed in detail in Chapter 4.

History of the Injury

An accurate history of the injury can help determine the extent and seriousness of injury. The individual's response, or lack of response, to verbal commands can also determine the level of consciousness. In a semiconscious or unconscious individual, information can be gathered by other players, officials, or bystanders. Remember, however, that an individual who is not fully responsive may have a head or neck injury. As such, you must maintain stabilization of the head and neck throughout the entire secondary survey. Ask the conscious individual to describe their perception of the problem including the primary complaint, mechanism of injury, site and severity of pain, and any weakness or disability resulting from the injury.

Position yourself close to the individual and speak in a calm confident manner. Tell the individual not to move the head or neck for any reason. Reassure the individual you are there to help. Questions should be open-ended to allow the person to provide as much information as possible about their perception of the problem. Listen attentively for clues that may indicate the nature of the injury. **Field Strategy 3-10** lists several questions to determine a history of the injury and assess the level of consciousness.

Observation

As you approach the individual, observe body position for noticeable deformities that may indicate a fracture or dislocation. Is the individual breathing normally or in respiratory distress? Take steps to control serious hemorrhage. Can the individual focus on your face and respond to commands? Is the person alert, restless, lethargic, or nonresponsive? Do they moan, groan, or mumble? Do the pupils of the eyes appear normal or dilated? Is there redness, bruising, or discoloration in the facial area or behind the ears. Note any clear fluid or bloody discharge from the ears or nose. This could be cerebrospinal fluid leaking from the cranial area as a result of a skull fracture. Is there visible swelling or deformity in the muscle(s) or joint? Always do bilateral comparison whenever possible.

Respiration

Breathing rate varies with the gender and age of an individual but averages between 12 and

Table 3–11. Abnormal Vital Signs and What They May Indicate.

Pulse

Rapid, weak	Shock, internal hemorrhage, diabetic coma, or heat exhaustion
Rapid, bounding	Heat stroke, fright, fever, hypertension, apprehension, or normal exertion
Slow, bounding	Skull fracture, stroke, drug use (barbiturates and narcotics), certain cardiac problems or some poisons
No pulse	Blocked artery, low blood pressure, or heart in cardiac arrest with death imminent

Respiration

Shallow breathing	Shock, heat exhaustion, insulin shock, chest injury, or cardiac problems
Irregular breathing	Airway obstruction, chest injury, diabetic coma, asthma, or cardiac problems
Rapid, deep	Diabetic coma, hyperventilation, some lung diseases
Frothy blood	Lung damage, such as a puncture wound to the lung from a fractured rib or other penetrating object
Slowed breathing	Stroke, head injury, chest injury, or use of certain drugs
Wheezing	Asthma
Crowing	Spasms of the larynx
Apnea	Hypoxia (lack of oxygen), congestive heart failure, head injuries
No breathing	Cardiac arrest, poisoning, drug abuse, drowning, head injury, or intrathoracic injuries with death imminent if action is not taken to correct condition

Blood Pressure

Systolic is <100 mm	Hypotension caused by shock, hemorrhage, heart attack, internal injury, or poor nutrition
Systolic is >135 mm	Hypertension

Skin Temperature

Dry, cool	Exposure to cold or cervical, thoracic, or lumbar spine injuries
Cool, clammy	Shock, internal hemorrhage, trauma, anxiety, or heat exhaustion
Hot, dry	Disease, infection, high fever, heat stroke, or overexposure to environmental heat
Hot moist	High fever
Isolated hot spot	Localized infection
Cold appendage	Circulatory problem
"Goose pimples"	Chills, communicable disease, exposure to cold, pain, or fear

Skin color

Red	Embarrassment, fever, hypertension, heat stroke, carbon monoxide poisoning, diabetic coma, alcohol abuse, infectious disease, inflammation, or allergy
White or ashen	Emotional stress (fright, anger, etc.), anemia, shock, heart attack, hypotension, heat exhaustion, insulin shock, or insufficient circulation
Blue or cyanotic	Heart failure, some severe respiratory disorders, and some poisoning. In dark skinned individuals, a bluish cast can be seen in the mucous membranes (mouth, tongue, and inner eyelids), the lips, and nail beds
Yellow	Liver disease or jaundice

Pupils

Constricted	Individual is using opiate-based drug, or has ingested a poison
Unequal	Head injury or stroke
Dilated	Shock, hemorrhage, heat stroke, use of a stimulant drug, coma, cardiac arrest, or death

Field Strategy 3–10. Determining the History of Injury and Level of Consciousness.

Stabilize the head and neck. Do not move individual unnecessarily until a spinal injury is ruled out.

If unconscious:

Call the person's name loudly and gently tap the sternum or touch the arm. If no response, rap the sternum more forcibly with a knuckle or pinch the soft tissue in the armpit (axillary fold) and note if there is a withdrawal from the painful stimulus. If no response, immediately initiate the primary survey.

If ABCs are adequate, proceed with the secondary survey. If you did not see what happened, question other players, supervisors, officials, and bystanders. Ask:

What happened?

Did you see the individual get hit or did the individual just collapse?

How long has the individual been unconscious?

Did the individual lapse into total unconsciousness or deteriorate gradually?

If it was gradual, did anyone talk to the individual before you arrived?

What did the person say? Was it coherent? Did the person moan, groan, or mumble?

Has this ever happened before to this individual?

If conscious, ask:

What happened? If the individual is lying down, find out if they were knocked down, fell, or rolled voluntarily into that position.

Did you hear any sounds or any unusual sensations when the injury occurred? Note if the individual is alert and aware of their surroundings, or has any short term or long term memory loss.

Do you have a headache? Where is the pain? Can you point to the area? On a scale of one to ten, with ten being the most painful, how would you rate the pain? Is the pain getting worse or better? If there is more than one painful area, ask which area hurts the most.

Can you describe the pain? Is it localized or does it radiate into other areas?

Have you ever injured this body part before, or experienced a similar injury? When did this previous injury happen?

How are you feeling now? Are you nauseated or sick to your stomach? Are you dizzy? Can you see clearly?

Are you taking any medication (prescription, over-the-counter, vitamins, birth control, etc.)? Are you allergic to anything?

Do not prompt the individual. Let them describe what happened, and *listen attentively* for clues that will indicate the nature of the injury. Be professional and reassuring.

Rubor
Reddish skin

Pallor
Ashen or pale skin

20 breaths per minute in an adult and between 20 to 28 breaths per minute in a child. Breathing rate is assessed by doubling the number of respirations in a 30 second period. Shallow breathing may indicate shock, heat exhaustion, chest injury, or a cardiac condition. Frothy blood during respirations may indicate lung damage due to a fractured rib.

Skin Color

Skin color can indicate abnormal blood flow and low blood oxygen concentration in a particular body part or area. Three colors are commonly used in light skinned individuals: red, white or ashen, and blue. A reddish skin, or **rubor**, may indicate dilated capillary vessels resulting from an increased blood flow indicating fever, hypertension, or heat stroke. A **pallor**, ashen, or white colored skin is caused by vasoconstriction of the capillaries resulting in a decreased blood flow. This may indicate shock, heart attack, or hypotension. Skin that is bluish indicates low oxygen concentration, or cyanosis, indicating possible heart failure, or a respiratory disorder, such as an airway obstructed by chewing tobacco or gum. In dark skinned individuals, skin pigments mask cyanosis. However, a bluish cast can be seen in mucous membranes (mouth, tongue, and inner eyelids), the lips, and nail beds. Fever in these individuals can be seen by a red flush at the tips of the ears.

Pupils

Rapid constriction of pupils when the eyes are exposed to intense light is called the **pupillary light reflex**. Upon examination with a small bright light source, such as a pen light, the eyes may appear normal, constricted, unequal, or dilated (**Figure 3-18**). Unequal pupils indicate a possible head injury or stroke. Dilated pupils indicate shock, hemorrhage, cardiac arrest, coma, or death.

Eye movement is tested by asking the individual to focus on a single object. If the individual sees two images instead of one, it is called **diplopia**, or double vision. This condition occurs when the external eye muscles fail to work in a coordinated manner. Ask the individual to watch your fingers move through the six cardinal fields of vision (**Figure 3-19**). Test the individual's depth perception by placing a finger several inches in front of the individual and ask the person to reach out and touch the finger. Move the finger to several different locations.

Palpation

Palpation involves using the pads of the fingers in small circular or side-to-side motions to detect anomalies in bony and soft tissue structures. Palpations can detect eight different physical findings: temperature, swelling, point tenderness, crepitus, deformity, muscle spasm, cutaneous sensation, and pulse. Palpations begin at the head and move methodically down the trunk of the body to the feet. **Field Strategy 3-11** lists the process commonly used in a head-to-toe assessment.

Pupillary light reflex
Rapid constriction of pupils when exposed to intense light

Diplopia
Double vision

Palpate for temperature, swelling, point tenderness, crepitus, deformity, muscle spasm, cutaneous sensation, and pulse

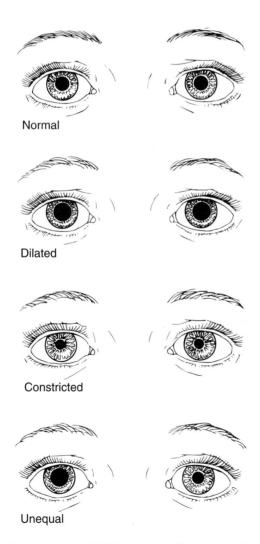

Normal

Dilated

Constricted

Unequal

Fig. 3.18: Pupil size. (A) Normal pupil size. (B) Dilated pupils. (C) Constricted pupils. (D) Unequal pupils.

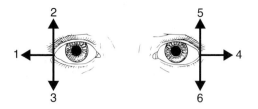

Fig. 3.19: Six cardinal fields of vision.

perature in the body's core (skull, thoracic and abdominal regions) (1,8). Body temperature can also be reflected in the skin. Normally the skin is dry but certain conditions, such as cold, shock, or fever, can alter surface blood vessels indicating a serious problem. Skin temperature is assessed by placing the back of the hand against the individual's forehead or by palpating appendages bilaterally **(Figure 3-20)**.

Temperature

Core temperature is measured by a thermometer placed under the tongue, in the armpit, or in case of unconsciousness, in the rectum. Rectal temperatures, usually .5° higher than oral temperatures, are considered to be a more accurate measurement of tem-

Bony Palpations

Possible fractures can be detected with palpation, percussion, use of a tuning fork, compression, and distraction. Palpation can detect deformity, crepitus, swelling, or increased pain at the fracture site. Percussion utilizes a tap-

---

 Field Strategy 3–11. Protocol for Head-to-Toe Palpations.

Continue to stabilize the head and neck until a spinal injury is ruled out.

Palpate the scalp and facial area for lacerations, deformities, or depressions. Discoloration over the mastoid process behind the ear (*Battle's sign*) or around the eyes (*raccoon eyes*), or presence of blood or cerebrospinal fluid from the ears or nose may indicate a skull fracture.

Check the eyes for any injury, presence of contact lenses, pupil size, equality and pupillary response to light. Both pupils may appear slightly dilated in an unconscious athlete. If the individual is conscious, check eye movement and tracking.

Check the mouth for a mouthguard, dentures, broken teeth, or blood that may have caused or could cause a possible airway obstruction. Sniff for any odd breath odor, such as a fruity smell (diabetic coma) or alcohol.

Palpate the cervical spine for any point tenderness or obvious deformity. Check the anterior neck for indications of impact, or bruising.

Inspect and palpate the chest for possible wounds, discoloration, deformities, and chest expansion upon breathing. If the patient is unconscious, rap the sternum to see if the individual withdraws from the touch. With conscious patients, use sternal or lateral rib compression to determine the possibility of a fracture.

Inspect and palpate the abdomen for tenderness, rigidity, distention, spasms or pulsations. Palpate the lower back for deformity and point tenderness. Be careful not to move the individual.

Inspect and palpate the upper extremities for deformity, point tenderness, swelling, muscle spasm, and discoloration. Pinch in the axillary area (armpit). Touch the fingers and ask if the individual can feel it? Does it feel the same on both hands? Can the individual move the fingers and squeeze your hand? Is there bilateral grip strength? Take a radial pulse and feel for skin temperature. Do not move the limbs or change body position.

Inspect and palpate the pelvis and lower extremities for deformity, point tenderness, swelling, muscle spasms, and discoloration. Take a distal pulse at both the medial ankle (posterior tibial artery) and dorsum of the foot (dosalis pedis). Feel for skin temperature. Squeeze the gastrocnemius and pinch the top of the foot. Touch the toes and ask if the individual can feel it? Does it feel the same on both feet? Have the individual wiggle the toes and move the feet. Do not move the limbs or change body position.

Recheck vital signs every two to five minutes until the ambulance arrives.

Remember: *Do not harm the individual.* If in doubt, assume the worst and treat accordingly.

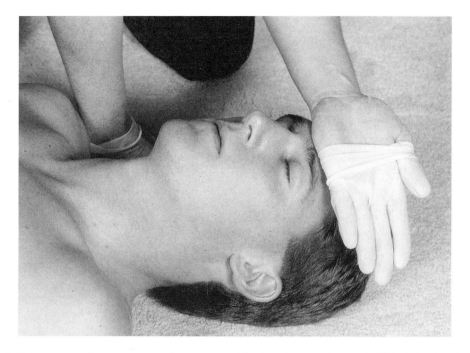

Fig. 3.20: To assess skin temperature, place the back side of the hand against the individual's forehead, or compare appendages bilaterally by palpation and blanching of the nails.

ping motion of the finger over a bony structure. A tuning fork works in the same manner. Vibrations travel through the bone and typically cause increased pain at a fracture site **(Figure 3-21)**. For example, if you suspect a fracture in the arm (humerus) tap lightly on the inside bony prominence at the elbow (medial epicondyle of the humerus). If the individual complains of pain in the midarm region you should suspect a possible fracture. Compression is performed by gently compressing the distal end of the bone toward the proximal end, or by encircling the body part, such as a foot or hand and gently squeezing, thereby compressing the heads of the bones together. Again, if a fracture is present pain will increase at the fracture site. Distraction employs a tensile force, whereby the application of traction to both ends of the fractured bone will help relieve pain.

Soft Tissue Palpation

Deformity, such as an indentation, may indicate a rupture in a musculotendinous unit. A protruding firm bulge may indicate a joint dislocation, ruptured bursa, or hematoma. Swelling may indicate diffuse hemorrhage or inflammation in a muscle, ligament, bursa, or joint capsule. Note where the point tenderness is elicited. This may indicate the injured structure.

Cutaneous Sensation

Run your fingernails along both sides of the arms and legs, and ask the individual if it feels the same on both sides of the body part. Pain perception can also be tested by applying a sharp and dull point to the skin. Note whether the individual can distinguish the difference.

Pulse

Factors such as age, gender, aerobic physical condition, degree of physical exertion, medications or chemical substances being taken, blood loss, and stress all influence pulse rate and strength (4). Pulse is usually taken at the carotid artery because it is not normally obstructed by clothing, equipment, or strappings. Normal adult resting rates range between 60 and 80 beats a minute; children from 80 to 150 beats. Aerobically conditioned athletes may have a pulse rate as low as 44 to 50 beats a minute. Pulse is assessed during the secondary survey by doubling the pulse rate during a 30 second period. A rapid, weak pulse indicates shock. A slow, bounding pulse may indicate possible skull fracture, stroke, or a cardiac problem.

Distraction employs a tensile force, whereby pain should be relieved if a fracture is present

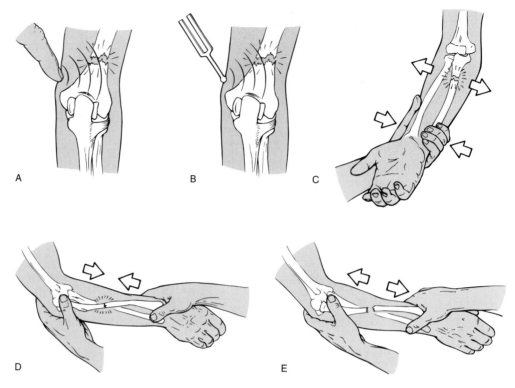

Fig. 3.21: Ruling out fracture. (A) Percussion. (B) Use of a tuning fork. (C and D) Compression. (E) Distraction. If the bone is fractured, pain will increase with percussion, use of a tuning fork, and compression, but will decrease with distraction.

Special Tests

In an emergency, special tests are usually limited to determining whether a spinal injury is present. This can be assessed by the individual's response to verbal and motor commands. Although initial assessment of unresponsiveness will be completed in the primary survey, further assessment of muscular movement should be completed before moving the individual. In a semiconscious or conscious individual, the inability to move a body part may indicate serious nerve damage to the central nervous system.

Muscular Movement

In evaluating muscle movement avoid any unnecessary movement of the individual. Ask the individual to wiggle the fingers and toes on both hands and feet. If this task is completed, place your fingers in both of their hands and ask the person to squeeze the fingers. Compare grip strength in both hands. Then, have the individual dorsiflex and plantarflex both feet and compare bilateral strength.

In an unconscious individual, a verbal or motor response is obviously not possible. Painful stimulation may produce a reaction movement, however. For example, pinching the soft tissue in the injured person's armpit, striking the sternum with your knuckle, or pinching the nipple may produce an eyelid flutter or involuntary movement away from the stimulus. If there is no reaction, this indicates a serious head or neck injury, or that the individual is in a coma. This individual should not be moved until emergency personnel arrive. Monitor the ABCs, recheck the vital signs, and treat for shock.

Blood Pressure

Blood pressure is the force per unit area exerted on the walls of a blood vessel, generally considered to be the aorta (2). As one of the most important vital signs, blood pressure reflects the effectiveness of the circulatory system. Changes in blood pressure are very significant. **Systolic blood pressure** is measured when the left ventricle contracts and expels blood into the aorta. It is approximately 120 mm Hg for a healthy adult. **Diastolic blood pressure** is the residual pressure present in the aorta between heart beats and averages 70 to 80 mm Hg in healthy adults. Blood pressure may be affected by gender,

Systole
Pressure in aorta when left ventricle contracts

Diastole
Residual pressure in aorta between heart beats

weight, race, lifestyle, and diet. Blood pressure is measured in the brachial artery with a sphygmomanometer and stethoscope, and is illustrated in **Figure 3-22**. Low blood pressure may indicate shock, hemorrhage, or heart attack.

💡 *The gymnast reported pain on the left side of the chest that increased during deep inhalations. Discoloration is present on the lower left side of the anterior chest wall. Palpation elicited pain in the region of the 9th and 10th ribs on the lateral side and increased with compression on the sternum. Muscle strength and sensation in the hands and feet appear normal.*

DETERMINATION OF FINDINGS

❓ *You have completed your emergency assessment of the gymnast. Pain is present in the thoracic region and deep respirations are inhibited and painful. Should you activate EMS and have this individual transported to the nearest trauma center?*

After completing the secondary assessment, a decision must be made on how best to handle the situation. If EMS has already been activated, control hemorrhage, splint suspected fractures, treat for shock, reassess vital signs every 2 to 5 minutes, and wait for the ambulance to arrive before moving the individual. As a general rule, an individual should be referred to the nearest trauma center or clinic if any life threatening situation is present, or if any loss of normal function occurs. Conditions that warrant activation of EMS and referral to a physician are listed in **Table 3-12**. If in doubt, always refer.

💡 *This individual has painful, limited respirations, palpable pain, and discoloration in the thoracic region over the 9th and 10th ribs. EMS should be activated to transport this individual to the nearest trauma center for further assessment and treatment.*

MOVING THE INJURED PARTICIPANT

❓ *How should this individual be transported to avoid additional pain or to keep the condition from getting worse?*

The safest way to move an individual is with a stretcher. Ideally, five trained individuals should roll, lift, and carry an injured person. The captain (the most medical trained individual) will stabilize the head and give commands for each person to slowly lift the injured individual onto the stretcher. The individual is then secured onto the stretcher.

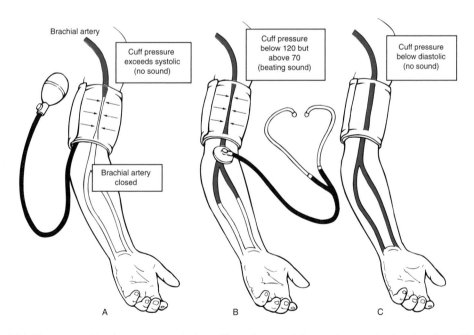

Fig. 3.22: To measure blood pressure, apply the cuff snugly around the arm just proximal to the elbow (A). Inflate until the pressure gauge registers about 200 mm Hg. Blood flow is occluded and the brachial artery can no longer be palpated in the cubital fossa. Place the stethoscope over the brachial artery in the cubital fossa (B). Slowly deflate the cuff and listen for the first soft beating sounds (systolic pressure). As pressure is reduced still further, the sound will become louder and more distinct, but will gradually disappear as blood no longer becomes constructed. The pressure at which the sound disappears is the diastolic pressure (C).

Table 3–12. Emergency Conditions to Be Referred to the Nearest Trauma Center or Physician

Medical emergencies that require activations of EMS (911)

Respiratory arrest or any irregularity in breathing

Severe chest or abdominal pains that may indicate heart attack, cardiac arrest, or internal hemorrhage

Excessive bleeding from a major artery or loss of a significant amount of blood

Suspected spinal injury resulting in back pain, paralysis, or inability to move any body part

Head injury with loss of consciousness

Open or multiple fractures, and fractures involving the femur, pelvis, or several ribs

Joint fracture or dislocation with no distal pulse

Severe signs of shock or possible internal hemorrhage

Injuries that require immediate referral to a physician

Eye injuries

Dental injuries where a tooth has been knocked loose or knocked out

Minor or simple fractures

Lacerations that may require suturing

Injuries where a functional deficit is noticeable

Loss of normal sensation, diminished or absent reflexes that may indicate a nerve root injury

Noticeable muscular weakness in the extremities that may indicate peripheral nerve injury

Any injury if you may have doubts about its severity or nature

---

An individual should be referred to the nearest trauma center if there is a loss of function or a life-threatening situation present

On command the stretcher is raised to waist level. The individual should be carried feet first so the captain can constantly monitor the individual's condition. **Field Strategy 3-12** describes how to secure and move an individual on a stretcher. **Field Strategy 3-13** describes how to move and secure an individual in the water onto a stretcher.

When referring an individual to a trauma facility, document information including the mechanism of injury, symptoms and vital signs, and any weakness, change of sensation, or disability as a result of the injury. Relay this information and what actions were taken to the appropriate individual (EMT, paramedic, or physician). A competitive school athlete seen by a physician should provide the school athletic trainer or coach with a written report stating the diagnosis and status of the athlete relative to return to sport participation. The athlete should not be allowed to return to competition until clearance is provided in writing by the supervising physician.

💡 *This injured individual should be transported on a stretcher by EMTs. Provide the EMTs with information on the history of the injury, symptoms, vital signs, and any weakness, change of sensation, or disability as a result of the injury. Indicate how you managed the situation and the results.*

SUMMARY

Athletic trainers and sport supervisors must have a thorough knowledge of emergency procedures to recognize and assess life threatening conditions. These emergencies may involve obstructed airway, cardiopulmonary emergencies, unconscious athlete, serious hemorrhage, shock, fractures, hyperthermia, and hypothermia. The NATA and ACSM require that all athletic trainers and employees in health/fitness facilities be certified in CPR and kept current on emergency first aid protocols. Furthermore, the facility should develop and implement an emergency procedures plan in consultation with local emergency medical services to address emergency situations.

Unless you have ruled out a possible spinal injury, always assume one is present and stabilize the head and neck before proceeding. Assessment of all injuries, no matter how minor, should always include a primary injury assessment. Primary injury assessment determines unresponsiveness and assesses the ABCs: Airway, Breathing, Circulation,

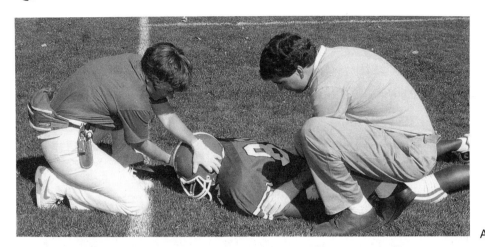

A

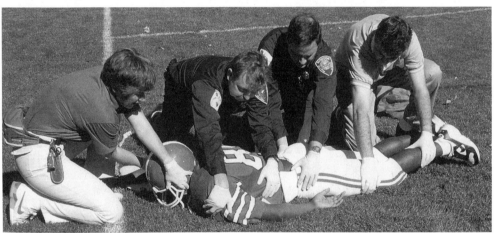

B

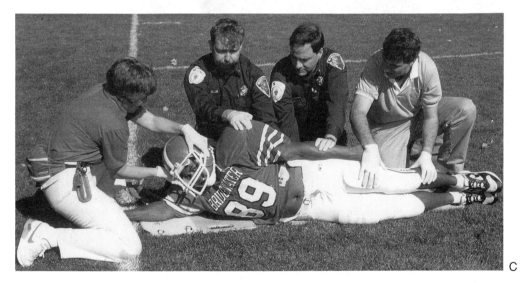

C

A.   *Unless ruled out, assume the presence of a spinal injury.* Place all extremities in an axial alignment. If the individual is lying face down, roll the individual supine. Four or five people are required to "log roll" the individual. The "captain" of the team (the most medically-trained individual) stabilizes the head and neck in the position as they were found, regardless

(*continued*)

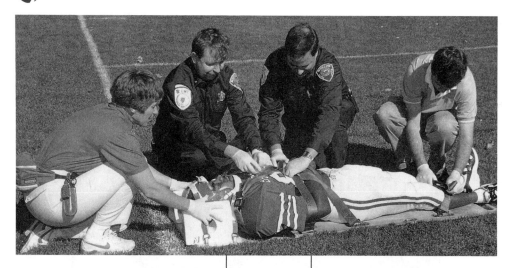

D

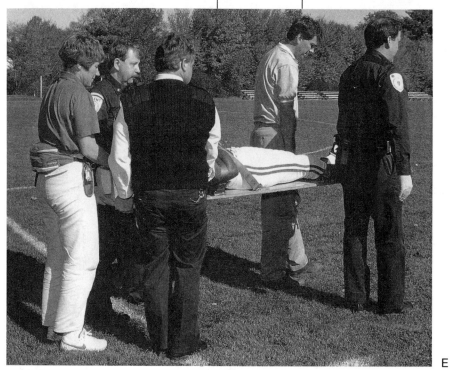

E

of the angle. The captain should position the arms in the cross arm technique so that during the log roll the arms will end in the proper position.

B. Place the spine board as closely as possible beside the individual. When possible, padding can be placed at the levels of the neck, waist, knees, and ankles to help fill voids between the body and the board. Each person is responsible for one body segment: one at the shoulder, one at the hip, one at the knees, and if needed, one at the feet.

C. The captain will give the command to roll the individual on the board in a single motion.

D. Once the patient is on the board, the captain continues to stabilize the head and neck, and if not done previously, another person applies support around the cervical region. The chest is secured to the board first, then the feet. With a football player, *do not* remove the helmet unless special circumstances exist, but the face mask should be completely removed.

E. With the head and neck securely supported, four people lift the stretcher while the captain continues to monitor the individual's condition. Transport the individual feet first.

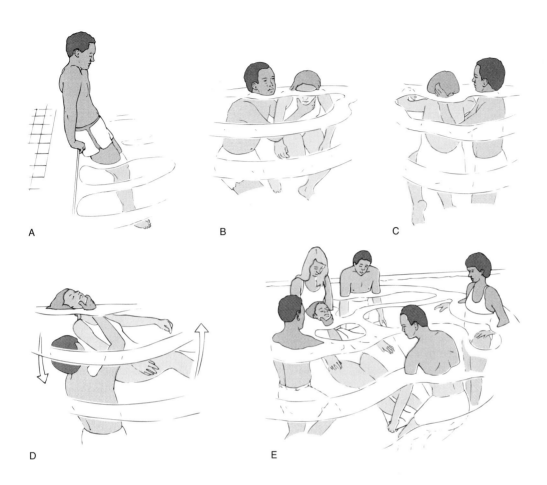

A. Ease yourself into the water near the individual and avoid any additional wave movement
B. Face the individual's side, and presume a spinal injury is present. Place one forearm along the length of the individual's sternum. Support the chin by placing the thumb on one side of the chin and the fingers on the other
C. Place the other forearm along the length of the individual's back and cradle the head near the base of the skull. Lock both wrists. Press the forearms inward and upward to provide mild traction and stabilization of the neck.
D. Turn the individual supine by slowly rotating the person toward you as you submerge and go under the individual. Avoid any unnecessary movement of the individual's trunk or legs. Slowly tow the individual to the shallow end of the pool. [*Note: In diving pools without a shallow end, move the individual to the side of the tank. The "captain" lies prone on the deck with arms in the water and takes over the in-line stabilization of the neck.*]
E. Approach the individual from the side with the backboard. Glide the foot of the board diagonally under the individual making sure the board extends beyond the head. Allow the board to rise under the individual.

(continued)

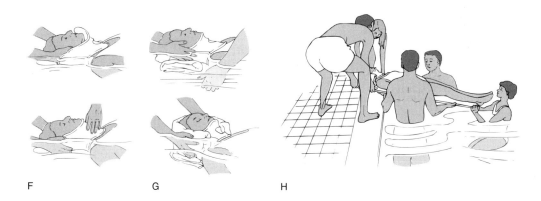

F   G   H

F. Maintain in-line stabilization while a rigid cervical collar is applied. Secure the individual to the backboard beginning at the chest, then move to the hips, thighs, and shins.

G. Before securing the head, it may be necessary to place padding under the head to fill the space between the board and head to maintain stabilization. Place a towel or blanket roll in a horseshoe configuration around the head and neck, and secure to the board.

H. Place the board perpendicular to the pool side and maintain the board in a horizontal position. Remove the board, head first. Tip the board at the head to break the initial suction holding it in the water. Two people should be on the deck to lift and slide the board onto the pool deck. Once on the deck, check vital signs and assess the individual's condition. Treat for shock and transport.

and serious bleeding. The secondary survey includes a hands-on, head-to-toe assessment to detect medical and injury related problems that do not pose an immediate life threatening situation, but may do so if left untreated. The HOPS format uses both subjective information (history of the injury), and objective information (observation and inspection, palpation, and special tests) to recognize and identify problems contributing to the condition.

As a general rule an individual should always be referred to the nearest trauma center or emergency clinic if any life-threatening situation is present, or if the injury results in loss of normal function. In moving a seriously injured or unconscious athlete, always assume the possibility of a head, neck, or spinal injury exists, and *never* move that individual unless qualified emergency medical personnel are present. If in doubt, suspect the worst and activate EMS for assistance.

REFERENCES

1. Saunders, HD. "Evaluation of a musculoskeletal disorder." In *Orthopaedic and sports physical therapy*, edited by JA Gould and GJ Davies. St. Louis: Mosby, 1989.
2. Marieb, EN. *Human anatomy and physiology*. Redwood City, CA: Benjamin/Cummings, 1992.
3. American Red Cross. *Standard first aid*. Washington, D.C.: The American National Red Cross, 1988.
4. Grant, HD, Murray, RH, and Bergeron, D. *Brady emergency care*. Englewood Cliffs, NJ: Prentice Hall, 1990.
5. Hafen BQ, and Karren, J. *First aid and emergency care workbook*. Englewood, CO: Morton, 1990.
6. American College of Sports Medicine. *Health fitness facility standards and guidelines*. Champaign, IL: Human Kinetics, 1992.
7. Parcel, GS, and Rinear, CE. *Basic emergency care of the sick and injured*. St. Louis: Times Mirror/Mosby College Publishing, 1990.
8. Ryan, AJ. "Heat stress." In *Prevention of athletic injuries: The role of the sports medicine team*, edited by FO Mueller and AJ Ryan. Philadelphia: F.A. Davis, 1991.
9. McArdle, WD, Katch, FI, and Katch, VL. *Exercise physiology: Energy, nutrition and human performance*. Philadelphia: Lea & Febiger, 1991.
10. Vogel, JA, Rock, PA, Jones, BH, and Havenith, G. "Environmental considerations in exercise testing and training." In *ACSM's resource manual for guidelines for exercise testing and prescription*, American College of Sports Medicine. Philadelphia: Lea & Febiger, 1993.
11. Avellini, BA, Kamon, E, and Krajewski, JT. 1980. Physiological responses of physically fit men and

women to acclimation to humid heat. J Appl Physiol, 49(2):254–261.

12. Frye, AJ, and Kamon, E. 1981. Responses to dry heat of men and women with similar aerobic capacities. J Appl Physiol, 50(1):65–70.

13. Horstman, DH, and Christensen, E. 1982. Acclimatization to dry heat: Active men vs active women. J Appl Physiol, 52(4):825–831.

14. Frye, AJ, and Kamon, E. 1983. Sweating efficiency in acclimated men and women exercising in humid and dry heat. J Appl Physiol, 54(4):972–977.

15. Haymes, EM. "Temperature and exercise." In *Sport science perspectives for women*, edited by J Puhl, CH Brown, & RO Voy. Champaign, IL: Human Kinetics, 1988.

16. The National Collegiate Athletic Association. *1992–1993 NCAA sports medicine handbook*. Overland Park, KS: NCAA Sport Sciences, 1992.

17. Harrelson, GL. 1986. Factors affecting the gastric emptying of athletic drinks, J of Ath Tr, 21(1):20–21.

18. Mellion, MB, and Shelton, GL. "Safe exercise in the heat and heat injuries." In *The team physician's handbook* edited by MB Mellion, WM Walsh, and GL Shelton. Philadelphia: Hanley & Belfus, 1990.

19. Burskirk, ER, Rhompson, RH, and Whedon, GD. 1963. Metabolic response to cold air in men and women in relation to total body fat content, J Appl Physiol, 18(3):603–612.

20. Wyndham, CH, and others. 1964. Physiological reactions to cold of Caucasian females, J Appl Physiol, 19(5):877–880.

21. Wells, CL. *Women, sport, & performance: A physiological perspective*. Champaign, IL: Human Kinetics, 1991.

22. Fritz, RL, and Perrin, DH. "Cold exposure injuries: Prevention and treatment." In *Clinics in sports medicine*, edited by RL Ray, Vol. 8, no. 1. Philadelphia: W.B. Saunders, 1989.

23. Putnam, L. 1992. Alternative methods for football helmet face mask removal, J of Ath Tr, 27(2):170–172.

24. Vegso, JJ, and Torg, JS. "Field evaluation and management of cervical spine injuries." In *Athletic injuries to the head, neck and face*, edited by JS Torg. St. Louis: Mosby Year Book, Inc., 1991.

Chapter 4

Sports Injury Assessment

After you have completed this chapter, you should be able to:

- Identify the two main body segments and demonstrate the anatomical position.
- Define terms relative to direction, regions, and joint motion
- Describe the HOPS injury assessment process
- Define common assessment terms
- Identify specific components in a history of an injury
- Describe what is involved in observation and inspection of an injury site
- Identify principles and techniques used in palpation, range of motion testing, neurological testing and special tests
- Differentiate between injury recognition and diagnosis
- Describe the components of SOAP notes and identify information recorded in each section.

Sports injury management involves injury prevention, assessment, recognition, treatment, disposition, and rehabilitation. As the first person on the scene, the athletic trainer, coach, or sport supervisor is expected to evaluate the situation, assess the extent and seriousness of injury, and determine if referral to a physician is necessary (**Figure 4-1**).

This vital component in sports injury management is called injury assessment. Injury assessment allows for accurate recognition of the problem, determines appropriate and

> Injury assessment allows for accurate recognition of the problem, determines an appropriate and immediate treatment, and serves as a foundation to develop a comprehensive rehabilitative program

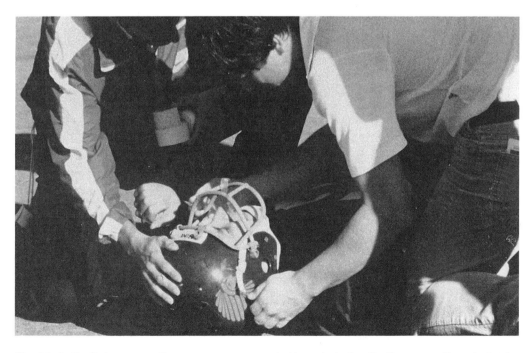

Fig. 4.1: As the first person on the scene, you are expected to evaluate the situation, assess the extent and seriousness of injury, manage the injury, and determine if referral to the physician is necessary.

immediate treatment, and provides a foundation to develop a comprehensive rehabilitation program.

Without an accurate assessment, an injury may be neglected, possibly leading to permanent deformity or disability. The role of the athletic trainer, coach, and sport supervisor is essential in providing immediate health care.

This chapter focuses on key components in injury assessment using the HOPS format.

First, you review body regions, anatomical directions, and terms used to describe injuries or illnesses. Then, beginning with an actual injury scenario, each section of the chapter will move step-by-step through the injury assessment process describing terms and general techniques used to recognize and identify the injury. An alternative assessment process, commonly called SOAP notes, is also discussed.

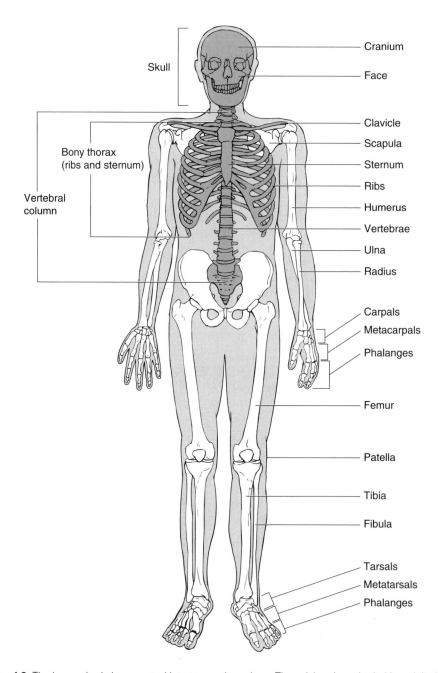

Fig. 4.2: The human body is separated into two main regions. The axial region, shaded in red, includes the head and trunk. The appendicular region, shown in black and white, includes the extremities. Direction or position on the body is based on anatomical position.

ANATOMICAL FOUNDATIONS

❓ *A soccer player fell on an outstretched arm. You suspect a fracture above the elbow. You have called the school nurse who wants to know the exact location of pain. How will you present this information so the nurse can visualize the location of injury in order to assist you in taking appropriate action?*

Using correct terminology is crucial when communicating with members of the medical community. Anatomical terms, such as superior and inferior, medial and lateral, or thoracic and abdominal help pinpoint the exact location on which to focus. Medical terms are used to describe the site, severity, and level of disability resulting from an injury. A brief overview of body segments and anatomical position, and terms related to directions, regions, and joint movements will be discussed.

Body Segments and Anatomical Position

The human body is separated into two main segments: the axial and the appendicular (**Figure 4-2**). The **axial segment** relates to the head and trunk, and includes the chest and abdomen. The abdomen is further delineated into four quadrants (**Figure 4-3**). The **appendicular segment** relates to the extremities. Direction or position on the body is based on a standardized position known as the **anatomical position**. In this position the body is erect, facing forward, with the arms at the side of the body, palms facing forward.

Directional Terms

Directional terms are used to locate one body part relative to another. For example, the elbow is superior to the wrist; the chest is on the anterior thorax; the big toe is on the medial side of the foot. These terms are always used relative to anatomical position regardless of the body's actual position. In speaking with the nurse you might report that pain is on the distal humerus, or just superior to the elbow. This way, the nurse can better visualize where the pain is located. Common directional terms used in injury assessment are defined and illustrated in **Table 4-1**.

Regional Terms

Regional terms are used to specify a general area of the body, such as the nasal, thoracic, abdominal, axillary, or popliteal regions. Regional terms are illustrated in **Figure 4-4**.

Joint Movement Terms

Injury assessment typically focuses on freely moveable joints. Although a specific joint can perform an isolated single motion, many activities, such as throwing or kicking a ball, require several simultaneous movements. In injury assessment a single movement, such as abduction or flexion, is used to assess range of motion and muscle weakness at a specific joint. The various individual motions are defined and illustrated in **Figure 4-5**. Specific joint motions are discussed in the appropriate chapters.

💡 *The soccer player fell on an outstretched arm and you suspect a fracture. In explaining the site of pain, you might report that extreme pain is present two inches proximal to the elbow joint particularly on the medial aspect of the humerus.*

ASSESSING AN INJURY

❓ *A middle-aged tennis player is complaining of a dull aching pain on the lateral side of the elbow. It is particularly bothersome after activity has stopped. Think for a minute or two about what information should be gathered from this individual to help identify factors that may have caused the injury.*

Emergency situations are evaluated using a primary and secondary survey to determine injuries or conditions that might pose a threat to life. In a specific sport related injury, the HOPS format, introduced in Chapter 3, is used extensively to assess an injury in a consistent, systematic process. HOPS is an acronym for:

History of the injury
Observation and inspection
Palpation
Special tests

The HOPS format uses both subjective information (history of the injury), and objective information (observation and inspection, palpation, and special tests) to recognize and identify the condition. These steps are followed in all injury assessments.

On-the-Field vs. Off-the-Field Assessment

Ideally, injury assessment should be conducted in a physician's office or training room where some privacy exists. In addition, pressure to complete a thorough exam is not usually a factor in these locations. Realistically, however, this may not be possible.

Axial segment
Central part of the body including the head and trunk

Appendicular segment
Relates to the extremities of the body including the arms and legs

Anatomical position
Standardized position with the body erect, facing forward, with the arms at the sides, palms facing forward

Directional terms locate one body part relative to another

Regional terms specify a general area of the body

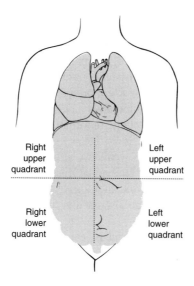

Right upper quadrant

Left upper quadrant

Right lower quadrant

Left lower quadrant

Fig. 4.3: The abdomen and pelvic cavity is divided into four quadrants.

Many injury assessments occur on the field during competition where environmental conditions, such as rain, mud, or snow may complicate the process. Officials, coaches, or parents may pressure you to assess the injury quickly, and to determine the playing status of the injured individual. After the primary survey is completed, the "on-the-field" assessment ascertains whether a moderate or serious injury is present (i.e., fracture, dislocation, unstable joint, severe bleeding, rupture of the musculotendinous unit, or nerve damage). If so, appropriate immobilization and transportation should be utilized in removing the individual from the field or court. Once off the field or court, a more thorough exam can be conducted. Decisions on the extent of injury, treatment, and playing status must be based on sound medical assessment despite external influencing

Table 4–1. Directional Terms.

Term	Definition	Illustration	Example
Superior (cranial)	Toward the head or cranium		The heart is superior to the abdomen
Inferior (caudal)	Toward the lower part of the body		The pelvic cavity is inferior to the thoracic cavity
Anterior	Toward the front of the body		The quadriceps muscles lie anterior to the femur
Posterior	Toward the back of the body		The buttock muscles lie posterior to the pelvis
Proximal	Closest to a reference point		The shoulder is proximal to the elbow
Distal	Farthest from a reference point		The wrist is distal to the elbow

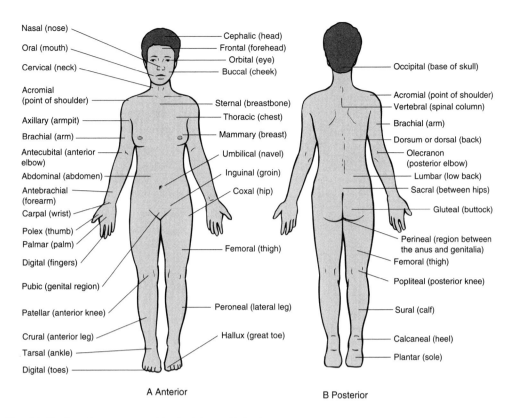

Nasal (nose)
Oral (mouth)
Cervical (neck)
Acromial (point of shoulder)
Axillary (armpit)
Brachial (arm)
Antecubital (anterior elbow)
Abdominal (abdomen)
Antebrachial (forearm)
Carpal (wrist)
Polex (thumb)
Palmar (palm)
Digital (fingers)
Pubic (genital region)
Patellar (anterior knee)
Crural (anterior leg)
Tarsal (ankle)
Digital (toes)

Cephalic (head)
Frontal (forehead)
Orbital (eye)
Buccal (cheek)
Sternal (breastbone)
Thoracic (chest)
Mammary (breast)
Umbilical (navel)
Inguinal (groin)
Coxal (hip)
Femoral (thigh)
Peroneal (lateral leg)
Hallux (great toe)

Occipital (base of skull)
Acromial (point of shoulder)
Vertebral (spinal column)
Brachial (arm)
Dorsum or dorsal (back)
Olecranon (posterior elbow)
Lumbar (low back)
Sacral (between hips)
Gluteal (buttock)
Perineal (region between the anus and genitalia)
Femoral (thigh)
Popliteal (posterior knee)
Sural (calf)
Calcaneal (heel)
Plantar (sole)

A Anterior

B Posterior

Fig. 4.4: Regional terms are used to depict specific body areas.

Table 4–1. (*continued*)

Term	Definition	Illustration	Example
Medial	Toward or at the midline of the body		The little finger is medial to the thumb
Lateral	Away from the midline of the body		The thumb is lateral to the little finger
Bilateral	Pertaining to both sides of the outer body		The ears are bilateral on the skull
Superficial	Toward or at the body surface		The skin is superficial to the muscles
Deep	Away from the body surface		The femur is deep to the skin

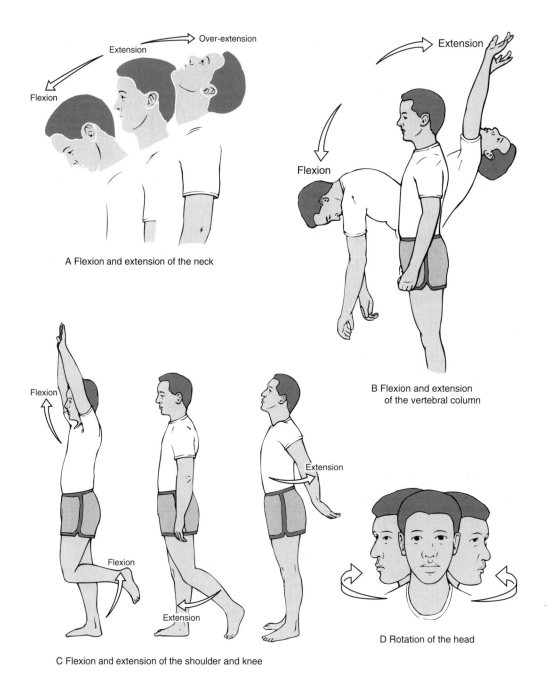

A Flexion and extension of the neck

B Flexion and extension
of the vertebral column

C Flexion and extension of the shoulder and knee

D Rotation of the head

Fig. 4.5: Movements allowed at synovial joints.

factors. Regardless of where the assessment occurs, all protocols should contain the same basic components that are relevant, accurate, and measurable.

In the interest of brevity, all sections on assessment throughout the text will explain the off-the-field assessment process. On-the-field assessment can be adapted from this information. Using the process listed above, each component of the assessment process will be described in detail. At the end of each section, symptoms and signs will be provided to help recognize and identify the injury. A

brief outline of the steps can be seen in **Field Strategy 4-1**.

Assessment Terms

Several terms are used by the medical community to describe and characterize injuries. **Etiology** is the science and study of the cause of a disease. In sport, mechanism of injury is used to describe the direct cause of an injury. Mechanisms include those forces acting on tissue which is damaged if the stress is too great for its weakest structure.

Etiology
The science and study of the cause of a disease

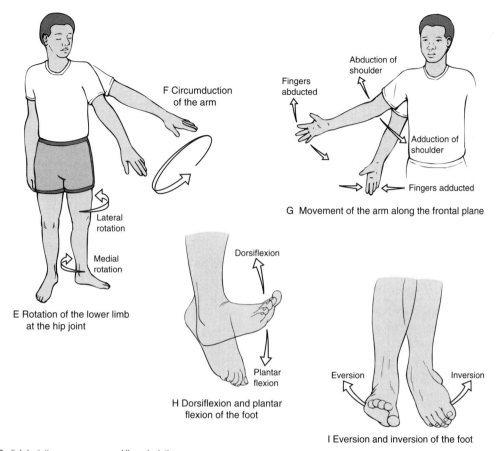

F Circumduction of the arm

Lateral rotation

Medial rotation

E Rotation of the lower limb at the hip joint

Abduction of shoulder

Fingers abducted

Adduction of shoulder

Fingers adducted

G Movement of the arm along the frontal plane

Dorsiflexion

Plantar flexion

H Dorsiflexion and plantar flexion of the foot

Eversion

Inversion

I Eversion and inversion of the foot

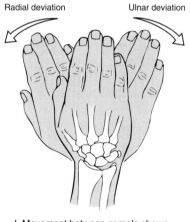

Radial deviation

Ulnar deviation

J Movement between carpals shown in dorsal view of right hand

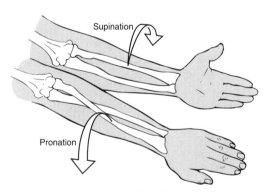

Supination

Pronation

K Supination and pronation of the forearm

Fig. 4.5: *continued.*

Examples given in Chapter 2 included compression, tension, and shear forces. **Pathology** encompasses many aspects of disease including the cause of the injury or condition, the development of abnormal conditions, and the structural and functional changes that result from the injury process. **Prognosis** is the probable course or progression of the injury and tells the individual what to expect as the injury heals. **Sequela** is a condition that may result from the injury, such as infection as the result of an open wound. **Syndrome** is an accumulation of a series of signs and symptoms associated with a particular injury or disease.

💡 *In assessing the tennis player, you want to gather both subjective (history of the injury), and objective information (observation and inspection, palpation, and special tests) to recognize and identify the condition.*

Pathology
The cause of an injury, its development, and functional changes due to the injury process

Prognosis
Probable course or progress of an injury or disease

Sequela
A condition that may follow as a consequence of an injury or disease

Syndrome
An accumulation of signs and symptoms associated with a particular injury or disease

Field Strategy 4–1. Injury Assessment Protocol.

History of the injury

Primary complaint
    Current nature, location, and onset of the condition
Mechanism of injury
    Cause of stress, position of limb, and direction of force
    Changes in running surface, shoes, equipment, techniques, or conditioning modes
Characteristics of the symptoms
    Evolution of the onset, nature, location, severity and duration of symptoms
Disability resulting from the injury
    Limitations in occupation and activities of daily living
Related medical history
    Past musculoskeletal injuries, congenital abnormalities, family history, childhood diseases,
        allergies, or cardiac, respiratory, vascular, or neurologic problems.

Observation and inspection

Observation should analyze
    Overall appearance
    Body symmetry
    General motor function
    Posture and gait
Inspection at the injury site
    Observe for deformity, swelling, discoloration, scars, and general skin condition

Palpation

Bony structures; rule out fracture first
Soft tissue structures
Palpate for skin temperature, swelling, point tenderness, crepitus, deformity, muscle spasm,
    cutaneous sensation, and pulse

Special tests

Active movement
Passive movement
    End feel
Resisted manual muscle testing
Neurologic testing
    Dermatomes
    Myotomes
    Reflexes
    Peripheral nerve testing
Stress tests
Functional testing
    Proprioception and motor coordination
    Sport specific skill performance

A complete history includes information on the:
    Primary complaint
    Cause or mechanism of injury
    Extent of pain or disability
    Previous injuries to the area
    Family history

HISTORY OF THE INJURY

The tennis player complained of a dull, aching pain on the lateral side of the elbow that increased in severity after activity had ceased. Think for a minute or two about what questions should be asked to help identify the cause and extent of the condition.

Identifying the history of the injury can be the most important step in injury assessment (1,2,3). A complete history includes information on the primary complaint, cause or mechanism of injury, extent of pain or disability due to the injury, previous injuries to the area, and family history which may have bearing on this specific condition. This information can provide possible reasons for the weakness, pain, or discomfort, and indicate possible injured structures prior to initiating the physical objective evaluation.

History taking requires patience and practice in asking the right questions. Sit with the individual in a relaxed, comfortable environment and openly discuss the condition. In an on-the-field assessment, it is imperative to focus on only vital information. Present yourself in a competent, professional manner. Listen attentively. Maintain eye contact. This establishes rapport with the injured individual and may lead that person to respond more accurately to questions and instructions (4). Standard information gathered includes the individual's name, gender, age, date of birth, occupation, and what activity the individual was participating in when the injury occurred. Comments regarding body size, body type, and general physical condition are also appropriate.

Information provided by the individual is subjective, yet should be gathered and recorded as accurately as possible. This can be accomplished by recording a number correlating with the described symptoms whenever possible. For example, when asking how bad the pain is, have the individual rate the severity of pain using a scale from 1 to 10 with 10 being severe, stabbing pain. When the pain begins, ask the individual how long it lasts. In using such measures, the progress of the injury can be determined. If the individual reports that pain begins immediately after activity and lasts for three or four hours, a baseline of information has been established. As the individual undergoes treatment and rehabilitation for the injury, a comparison with baseline information can determine if the condition is getting better, worse, or has remained the same. Documenting information during an injury assessment is important for this reason.

Although the intent of taking a history is to narrow the possibilities of conditions causing the injury, always keep an open mind. If too few factors are considered, premature conclusions may fail to adequately address the severity of injury. To avoid this, a thorough history includes determining the primary complaint, mechanism of injury, characteristics of the symptoms, disability resulting from the injury, and related medical history. These topics are summarized in **Figure 4-6**.

Primary Complaint

The primary complaint is what the injured individual believes may be the current injury. Questions should be phrased to allow the individual to describe the current nature, location, and onset of the condition (5). For example, ask: Why are you here? What is the problem? Where does it hurt? What activities or motions are weak or painful? Realize however, the individual may not wish to carry on a lengthy discussion about the injury, or may trivialize the extent of pain or disability. Be patient and keep questions simple. Pay close attention to words and gestures used to describe the condition, as they may provide clues to the quality or intensity of the symptoms.

Mechanism of Injury

After listening to the primary complaint, determine the mechanism of injury. This is probably the most important information gained in taking a history. Ask how the condition occurred. Did you fall? How did you land? Were you struck by an object or another individual? If so, in what position was the involved body part, and what direction was the force? Did you hear or feel anything? If the condition developed over time, ask when the injured person first became aware of the problem. Have there been recent changes in running surface, shoes, equipment, techniques, or conditioning modes? What motions or activities increase the pain? It is important to visualize how the injury occurred to determine possible damaged structures. This helps direct the objective evaluation.

Characteristics of the Symptoms

The primary complaint must be explored in detail from the onset to discover the evolution of symptoms including the nature, location, severity, and duration of pain or disability. The individual's pain perception, for example, can indicate what structures may be injured. There are two categories of pain; somatic and visceral. **Somatic pain** arises from the skin, ligaments, muscles, bones, or joints, and is the most common type of pain encountered in sport injuries. It is classified into two major types: deep and superficial. Deep somatic pain is described as diffuse, deep, or nagging as if intense pressure is

> Listen attentively and maintain eye contact

> Questions should be phrased to allow the individual to describe the current nature, location, and onset of the condition

> Subjective information should be gathered and recorded as accurately as possible

> The individual's pain perception can indicate what structures may be injured

> **Somatic pain**
> Pain originating in the skin, ligaments, muscles, bones, or joints

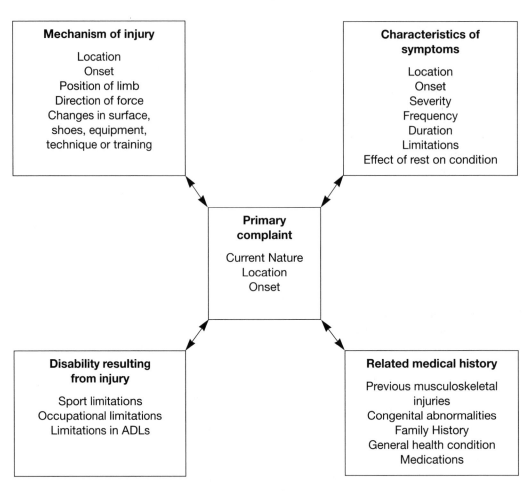

Mechanism of injury

Location
Onset
Position of limb
Direction of force
Changes in surface,
shoes, equipment,
technique or training

**Characteristics of
symptoms**

Location
Onset
Severity
Frequency
Duration
Limitations
Effect of rest on condition

**Primary
complaint**

Current Nature
Location
Onset

**Disability resulting
from injury**

Sport limitations
Occupational limitations
Limitations in ADLs

Related medical history

Previous musculoskeletal
injuries
Congenital abnormalities
Family History
General health condition
Medications

Fig. 4.6: The components to explore in taking a history of an injury.

Visceral pain
Pain resulting from injury or disease to an organ in the thoracic or abdominal cavity

Referred pain
Pain felt in a region of the body other than where the source or actual cause of the pain is located

Pain can travel up or down the length of any nerve and be referred to another region

If a nerve is injured, pain or a change in sensation, such as a numbing or burning sensation, can be felt along the length of the nerve

being exerted on the structures. It may be complicated by stabbing pain. Deep somatic pain is longer lasting and usually indicates significant tissue damage either to bone, internal joint structures, or muscles. Superficial somatic pain resulting from injury to the epidermis or dermis is usually a sharp, prickly type of pain that tends to be brief (6).

Visceral pain results from disease or injury to an organ in the thoracic or abdominal cavity, such as compression, tension, or distension of the viscera (7). Similar to deep somatic pain, it is perceived as deeply located, nagging, and pressing, and it is often accompanied by nausea and vomiting. **Referred pain** is a type of visceral pain that travels along the same nerve pathways as somatic pain. It is perceived by the brain as somatic in origin. In other words, the injury is in one region but the brain considers it in another. Referred pain, for example, occurs when an individual has a heart attack. The individual feels pain in the chest, the left arm, and sometimes the neck. **Figure 4-7** demonstrates

cutaneous areas where pain from visceral organs can be referred.

Pain can travel up or down the length of any nerve and be referred to another region. An individual who has a low back problem can feel the pain down the gluteal region into the back of the leg. If a nerve is injured, pain or a change in sensation, such as a numbing or burning sensation, can be felt along the length of the nerve. Although an individual may indicate the presence of pain or change of sensation in a specific area, it is necessary to determine if this is due to an injury at that site, or if the injury is elsewhere in the body and just perceived at that site. Keep this in mind throughout the evaluation, particularly when special tests are negative yet the individual continues to feel pain at a specific site.

To thoroughly understand the condition, ask detailed, probing questions about the location, onset, severity, frequency, and duration of the individual's symptoms. For example, to learn more about the location of pain from the tennis player, ask: Where does it

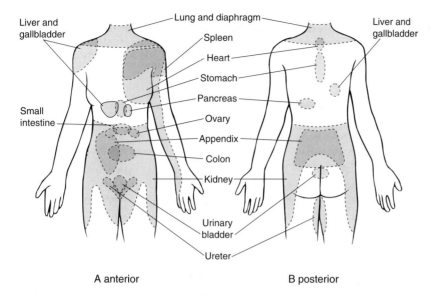

Liver and gallbladder
Lung and diaphragm
Spleen
Heart
Stomach
Pancreas
Small intestine
Ovary
Appendix
Colon
Kidney
Liver and gallbladder
Urinary bladder
Ureter

A anterior   B posterior

Fig. 4.7: Certain visceral organs can refer pain to specific cutaneous areas. Keep this in mind if all special tests are negative, yet the individual continues to feel pain at a specific site.

hurt the most? Can you point to a specific spot? Is the pain limited to that area or does it radiate into other parts of the elbow, arm, or hand? If pain is localized, limited bony or soft tissue structures are involved. Diffuse pain around the entire joint may indicate inflammation in the joint capsule, or that several structures are injured. If pain radiates into other areas of the limb or body, it may be traveling up or down the length of a nerve.

To discover the onset and severity of pain, ask: When does the pain set in (early morning, during reading, exertion, or at night)? On a scale from 1 to 10 with 10 most severe, how bad is the pain? How long does the pain last? Is the pain worse before, during, or after an activity? What activities aggravate or alleviate the symptoms? Does it wake you up at night? The onset of pain can indicate the condition. For example, morning pain and stiffness that improves with activity may indicate chronic inflammation with edema, or arthritis. Other examples of pain characteristics and what may be indicated are listed in **Table 4-2**.

To discover the nature and duration of the condition, ask: How long has the condition been present? Has the pain changed or stayed the same? What medications, treatments, or exercise programs have improved the situation in the past? These answers can determine if the individual has an acute injury resulting from a specific event leading to a sudden onset of symptoms, or a chronic injury characterized by a slow, sustained development of symptoms that culminate in a painful inflammatory condition. These answers can also determine if the condition is disabling enough to require a physician.

Disability Resulting From the Injury

Determine what the individual is unable to do because of pain, weakness, or disability from the injury. Questions should not be limited to sport participation, but should include occupational limitations, and limitations in daily activities. Activities of daily living (ADLs) are actions most people perform without thinking about, such as combing the hair, brushing the teeth, or walking up or down stairs. In questioning the tennis player, ask what activities are limited because of the injury. Has the injury affected their job, school work, or activities of daily living?

Related Medical History

Obtain information regarding other problems or conditions that might have affected this injury. Information extrapolated from the individual's preseason physical examination may verify past childhood diseases; allergies; cardiac, respiratory, vascular, musculoskeletal, or neurological problems; use of contact lenses, dentures, or prosthetic devices; and past episodes of infectious diseases, loss of consciousness, recurrent headaches, heat stroke, seizures, eating disorders, or chronic medical problems. Previous musculoskeletal

Limitation in activities should include limitations at work and daily activities

Table 4–2. Pain Characteristics and What May Be Indicated.

Morning pain with stiffness that improves with activity	Chronic inflammation with edema, or arthritis
Pain, increased aching as the day progresses	May indicate increased congestion in a joint
Sharp, stabbing pain during activity	Acute injury, such as ligament sprain or muscular strain
Dull, aching pain aggravated with muscle contraction	Chronic muscular strain
Pain that subsides during activity	Chronic condition or inflammation
Pain on activity relieved by rest	Soft tissue damage
Pain not affected by rest or activity	May indicate an injury to bone
Night pain	May indicate compression of a nerve or bursa
Muscular pain	Dull, aching, and hard to localize; is aggravated by passive stretching of the muscle and resisted muscle contractions
Bone pain	Deeply located, nagging, and very localized
Nerve pain	Sharp, burning, or numbing sensation that may run the length of the nerve
Vascular pain	Aching over a large area that may be referred to another area of the body

Observation
Visual analysis of overall appearance, symmetry, general motor function, posture, and gait

Inspection
Refers to factors seen at the actual injury site, such as redness, swelling, bruising, cuts, or scars

Note the individual's willingness and ability to move, general posture, consistency in limitations of motion, ease in motion, and general overall attitude

injuries or congenital abnormalities may place additional stress on joints predisposing the individual to certain injuries. Ask if the individual is on any medication. The type, frequency, dosage, and effect may mask some symptoms. **Field Strategy 4-2** lists useful questions for gathering a history of an injury. These are only provided as a guide and are not listed in any specific order.

The tennis player is 52 years old and a recreational player who plays two or three matches each week. His primary complaint is a dull, aching pain on the outside of the right elbow after completing a match. He rates the pain as a 7 on the 10 point scale; an 8 when he has to lift a briefcase onto a table. Pain persists for about two hours after play has ceased. This time is reduced when he uses ice over the region. He cannot recall injuring the elbow, but the aches and pains have been present for the past three months. A physician has never been consulted about this injury.

OBSERVATION AND INSPECTION

A significant amount of information has been gathered from the tennis player. The next step is to observe the individual and inspect the injury site. What observable factors might indicate the seriousness of injury?

Observation and inspection begins the objective evaluation in an injury assessment. Although explained as a separate step, obser-

vation begins the moment the injured person is seen, and continues throughout the assessment. **Observation** refers to the visual analysis of overall appearance, symmetry, general motor function, posture, and gait (**Figure 4-8**) (8). **Inspection** refers to factors seen at the actual injury site, such as redness, bruising, swelling, cuts, or scars.

Observation

Often the athletic trainer or sport supervisor sees an acute injury happen. In such a case, the severity of the condition can be somewhat determined prior to the completion of the injury assessment. However, in most instances, the individual will come to the sideline, office, training room, or clinic complaining of pain or discomfort. The individual is visually assessed from the moment they walk into the examination room. Assess the individual's state of consciousness and body language that may indicate pain, disability, fracture, dislocation, or respiratory distress. Note the individual's willingness and ability to move, general posture, consistency in limitations of motion, ease in motion, and general overall attitude (8). Using discretion in safeguarding the athlete's privacy, the injured area should be fully exposed. For example, during an assessment of the upper extremity or thoracic region, women should wear a bra, halter top, or swim suit. In a lower extremity

Field Strategy 4–2. Developing a History of the Injury.

Determine (a) primary complaint including location, onset, and current nature of the problem; (b) mechanism of injury; (c) characteristics of the symptoms including the nature, location, severity, frequency, and duration of pain or disability; (d) functional deficits relative to ADLs (Activity of Daily Living), occupation, and recreational/athletic pursuits; and (e) related medical history.

ASK:

Why are you here? What is the problem? Where is the pain or weakness located? On a scale of 1 to 10 with 10 being very severe, how would you rate your pain or weakness? Can you describe the pain (dull ache, throbbing, sharp, intermittent, red-hot or burning)?

How did the injury occur? Do you remember what position the limb was in and the direction of force? What different activities have you been doing in the last week? (Ask about changes in shoes, equipment, running surfaces, or conditioning modes, such as frequency, duration, intensity, type, or technique.)

Did the pain come on gradually (overuse problem) or suddenly (acute problem)? How long has it been a problem? Was the pain greatest when the injury first occurred or did it get worse the second or third day?

Did you hear any sounds during the incident? Any snaps, pops, or cracks? (This may indicate the tissues involved in the injury.) Did you notice any swelling or discoloration at the time of the injury? How soon did it occur? What did you do for the swelling? Have you had any muscle spasms or numbness with the injury?

What activities aggravate or alleviate the symptoms? Is the pain worse in the morning, during activity, after activity, or at night? When the pain sets in, how long does it last? Is it the same type of pain that you are experiencing now?

Have you ever injured this area before? Who evaluated the injury? What did you do for it? Have you seen a physician about this condition? What was the diagnosis? What occurred during that visit? What have you done since then to strengthen the area to prevent reinjury? Has there been any improvement in your condition?

Are there certain activities you are unable to perform because of the pain? Which ones? How old are you? (Many chronic problems are age-related). Which extremity is dominant (arm/hand; leg/foot)?

Have you had any medical problems recently? (Look for problems that may refer pain to the area from visceral organs, heart, and lungs.) Do you have any allergies? Are you on any medication?

Do you have any musculoskeletal problem elsewhere in the body? (These may result in changes in gait or technique that transfers abnormal forces to other structures.)

Has anyone in your family had a similar problem?

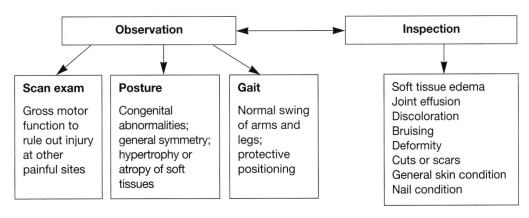

Fig. 4.8: The components of observation and inspection.

Hypertrophy
Increase in general bulk or size of an individual tissue, such as a muscle

Atrophy
Wasting-away or deterioration of tissue

Indication
A condition that could benefit from a specific action

Contraindication
A condition adversely affected by a specific action

Antalgic gait
Walking with a limp

Effusion
The escape of fluid from the blood vessels into the surrounding tissues or joint cavity

Ecchymosis
Bruise; discoloration of the skin due to subcutaneous bleeding

injury, shorts should be worn. During an on-the-field assessment, the athletic trainer must use discretion in removing equipment or clothing to assess the area.

Scan Exam

Depending on the injury, many individuals begin observation in the examination room with a scan exam to assess general motor function. The scan exam rules out injury at other joints that may be overlooked due to intense pain or discomfort at the primary injury site. In addition, pain in one area may be referred from another area. The injured person is observed doing gross motor movements in the neck, trunk and extremities. Note if there is any hesitation to move a body part, or if the individual favors one side over another. Gross motor movements may include looking up at the ceiling; rotating the head sideways in both directions; bending forward to touch the toes; rotating the trunk; bringing the palms together above the head; bringing the palms together behind the back; doing a straight leg raise forward, backward, and sideways; bending the knees; and walking on the heels and toes. This screening exam can determine if other specific areas need to be examined in more detail in addition to the primary injury site.

Posture

Posture assessment can detect congenital or functional problems that may be contributing to the injury. Specific anomalies are discussed in the separate joint chapters. Ask the individual to sit down to begin the exam. Observe any abnormalities in the spinal curves, general symmetry of the various body parts, and general attitude of the body from an anterior, side, and posterior view. For example, does the individual naturally sit with the back straight, shoulders back, and head in a straight and level position? Are the arms placed comfortably in the lap? Ask the individual to stand. Again, assess general body posture. Does the body look symmetrical? Visually scan soft tissue for **hypertrophy** or **atrophy**. Are the shoulders level? The dominant side is usually somewhat lower than the nondominant side. Is the space between the arms and body the same on both sides? Are both hands held in the same position? Do the hips look level? Are the kneecaps at the same height and pointing straight ahead? Are the

feet pointing straight ahead? From a side view, can an imaginary straight plumb line be drawn from the ear through the middle of the shoulder, hip, knee, and ankle? **Field Strategy 4-3** provides a more detailed assessment of posture in a standing position.

Gait Assessment

When not **contraindicated**, ask the individual to walk several yards while observing normal swing of the arms and legs. Stand behind, in front, and to the side of the individual to observe from all angles. A shoulder injury may be evident in a limited arm swing, or by holding the arm close to the body in a splinted position. A lower extremity injury may produce a noticeable limp, or **antalgic gait**. Running on a treadmill may show functional problems that may have contributed to a lower extremity injury.

Inspection of the Injury Site

Inspect the localized injury site for any deformity, swelling (edema or joint effusion), discoloration (redness, bruising, or ecchymosis), scars that might indicate previous surgery, and general skin condition (oily, dry, blotchy with red spots, sores, or hives) **(Figure 4-9)**. Swelling inside the joint is called localized intra-articular swelling, or joint **effusion**, and makes the joint appear enlarged, red, and puffy. **Ecchymosis** is discoloration or swelling outside the joint in the surrounding soft tissue due to a bruise or injury under the skin. Always compare the injured area to the opposite side if possible. This bilateral comparison helps to establish what is normal for this individual.

During the scan exam the tennis player was able to perform all gross motor movements, had good posture, and a normal gait. Visual inspection showed only slight redness and swelling on the lateral side of the elbow.

PALPATION

The lateral side of the elbow is red, swollen, and painful. How can the area be palpated to determine the extent and severity of injury without causing additional pain?

Bilateral palpation of paired anatomical structures can detect eight physical findings: temperature, swelling, point tenderness, crepitus, deformity, muscle spasm, cutaneous sensation, and pulse **(Figure 4-10)**. Before

Field Strategy 4–3. Postural Assessment.

touching the individual make sure your hands are clean and warm. If any injury has an opening in the skin, wear latex examination gloves as a universal precaution against disease and infection. Begin palpation with gentle circular pressure followed by gradual deeper pressure (**Figure 4-11**). Always begin proximal to the painful site. Palpate the painful area last to avoid any carry over of pain into noninjured areas.

When the fingers first touch the skin, note skin temperature. Increased temperature at the injury site could indicate inflammation or infection, whereas decreased temperature could indicate a reduction in circulation. Swelling can be localized in a small area, or diffuse. If swelling is inside the joint, motion will often be limited because of congestion caused by extra fluid. Point tenderness and crepitus indicate damage to bony or soft tissue structures and should be palpated with as little pressure as possible. Cutaneous sensation can be tested by running your fingers along both sides of the body part and asking

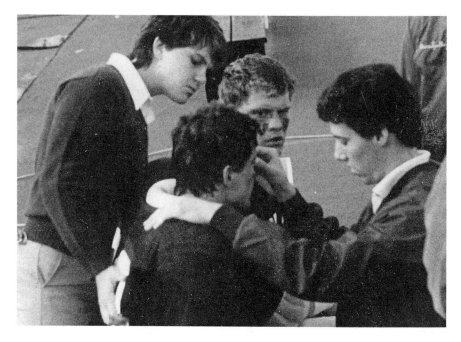

Fig. 4.9: Inspect for any deformities, swelling, discoloration, scars, and general skin condition.

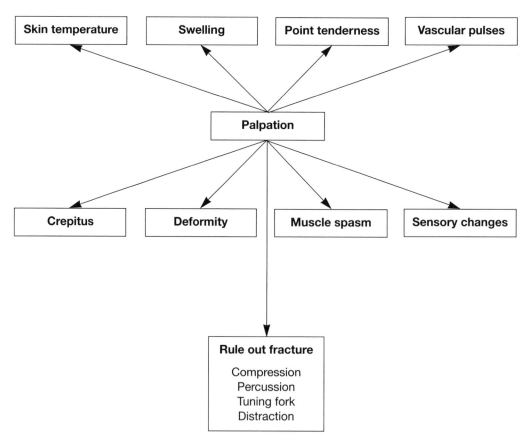

Fig. 4.10: The components of palpation.

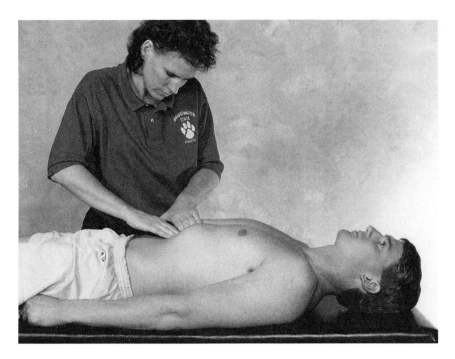

Fig. 4.11: Begin palpation with gentle circular pressure followed by gradual deeper pressure. Feel for skin temperature, swelling, point tenderness, crepitus, deformity, muscle spasm, cutaneous sensation, and pulse.

the individual if it feels the same on both sides. This technique will rule out nerve involvement, particularly if the individual has numbness or tingling in the limb. Peripheral pulses are taken distal to an injury to rule out damage to a major artery. Common sites are the radial pulse at the wrist and dorsalis pedis on the dorsum of the foot (**Figure 4-12**).

Palpation of bones determines the presence of fractures, crepitus, and loose bony or cartilaginous fragments. Possible fractures can be assessed with percussion, use of a tuning fork, compression, and distraction (See **Figure 3-21**). If test results indicate a possible fracture, assume one is present and immobilize the region.

🔦 *Palpation revealed warmth and slight swelling over the lateral elbow. Point tenderness was elicited directly over the lateral epicondyle of the humerus and in the soft muscle mass on the proximal forearm (wrist and finger extensors). All fracture tests were negative.*

SPECIAL TESTS

❓ *You have determined there is no fracture. How will you proceed to test the integrity of the soft tissue structures to determine the extent and severity of injury? What factors might limit range of motion at the joint?*

After fractures and/or dislocations have been ruled out, soft tissue structures, such as muscles, ligaments, the joint capsule, and bursae are assessed using special tests. Although a more extensive explanation will be given in the individual chapters, general principles will be discussed here. Special tests include active movement, passive movement, resisted manual muscle testing, neurological testing, stress tests for ligamentous integrity, and functional testing (**Figure 4-13**).

Active Movement

Active movement is joint motion performed voluntarily by the individual through muscular contraction. At a specific joint the amount of movement possible in a single plane is called active range of motion (AROM). Active movement determines possible damage to contractile tissue (muscle, muscle-tendon junction, tendon, and tendon-periosteal union), and measures muscle strength and movement coordination.

Although several different motions were performed during the scan exam, this testing component focuses on a specific joint. Measuring all motions, except rotation, starts with the body in anatomical position. For rotation, starting body position is midway between internal (medial) and external (lateral) rotation. Starting position is measured as zero degrees. Maximal movement away from the

Palpation of bones can determine the presence of fractures, crepitus, and loose bony or cartilaginous fragments

Special tests include active movement, passive movement, resisted manual muscle testing, neurologic testing, stress tests for ligamentous integrity, and functional testing

Active movement
Joint motion performed voluntarily by the individual through muscular contraction

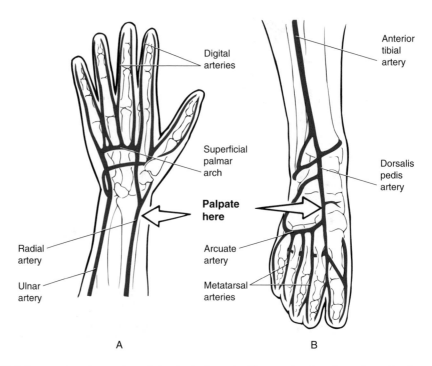

Fig. 4.12: Pulses can be taken at the radial pulse in the wrist (A), or at the dorsalis pedis on the dorsum of the foot (B).

zero degree point is the total available range of motion. For example, to subjectively measure elbow flexion, place the individual in anatomical position with the arms at the side of the body, palms facing forward. Stabilize both upper arms against the individual's body, and ask them to flex both elbows. Comparison of movement in both arms will indicate if elbow flexion is bilaterally equal.

Note the individual's willingness to perform the movement, and the fluidity and extent of movement (joint range of motion). Limitation in motion may be due to pain, swelling, muscle spasm, muscle tightness,

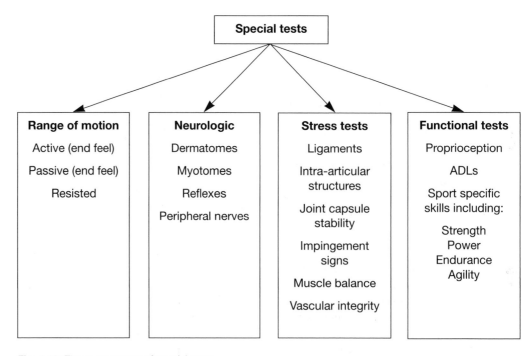

Fig. 4.13: The components of special tests.

joint contractures, nerve damage, or mechanical blocks, such as a loose body. If the individual has pain or other symptoms on motion, it is difficult to determine at this time if the joint, muscle, or both are injured. Ask if the motion causes pain and at what point in the motion does pain begin. Does the pain appear only in a limited range of motion (painful arc)? Is the pain the same type of pain associated with the primary complaint? Perform any painful movements last, because this will avoid any carryover of pain from testing one motion to the next.

Active and passive range of motion at a joint can be measured quantitatively with a **goniometer (Figure 4-14)**. The instrument is a protractor with two rigid arms that intersect at a hinge joint, and is used to measure both joint position and available joint motion (9). This measurement can determine when the individual has regained normal motion at a joint and is ready to return to participation. The arms of the goniometer measure from 0 to 180° of motion, or 0 to 360° of motion. One arm is stationary and the other arm fully moveable. Measurements are typically obtained by placing the stationary arm parallel to the proximal bone. The axis of the goniometer should coincide with the joint axis of motion. The moving arm is then placed parallel to the distal bone, utilizing specific anatomical landmarks as points of reference. **Figure 4-15** demonstrates range of motion measurement for elbow flexion. Specific range of motion and goniometry measurement techniques are listed in the individual joint chapters.

Passive Movement

If the individual is unable to perform all active movements at the injured joint because of pain or spasm, passive movement can be performed. In **passive movement** the injured limb or body part is moved through the range of motion (ROM) with no assistance from the injured individual **(Figure 4-16A & B)**. Passive range of motion (PROM) distinguishes injury to contractile tissues from noncontractile tissues (bone, ligaments, bursae, joint capsules, and neurovascular structures) (10). If pain occurs before the end of the available ROM, it may indicate an acute injury. Stretching and manipulation of the joint are contraindicated. If pain occurs simultaneously at the end of the ROM, a subacute injury may be present and a

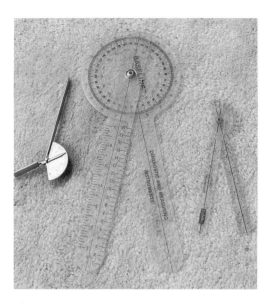

Fig. 4.14: Goniometers come in various sizes for the different body joints. Each has a protractor with two rigid arms to measure joint position and available range of motion.

mild stretching program may be started cautiously. If no pain is felt as the available ROM is stretched, a chronic injury is present. An appropriate treatment and rehabilitation program should be initiated immediately (11).

The individual should sit or lie down so the muscles are relaxed. If no pain is present during passive motion but is present during active motion, injury to contractile tissue is involved. If noncontractile tissue is injured, passive movement is painful and limitation of movement may be seen. Goniometry measurements can be taken to record available motion. Again, any painful motions should be performed last to avoid any carryover of pain from one motion to the next. At the end of the range of motion, a gentle overpressure is applied to determine **end feel** (12). Overpressure is repeated several times to see whether pain increases, which signifies damage to noncontractile joint structures. The end feel can determine the type of disorder. There are three normal end feel sensations and five abnormal end feel sensations. These end feels are summarized in **Table 4-3**.

Accessory movements are movements within the joint that accompany traditional active and passive range of motion, but cannot be voluntarily performed by the individual. Joint play motions, for example, allow the joint capsule to "give" so bones can move to absorb an external force. These movements include

Goniometer
Protractor used to measure joint position and available joint motion (ROM)

Passive movement
A limb or body part is moved through the range of motion with no assistance from the individual

If no pain is present during passive motion but pain *is* present during active motion, injury to contractile tissue is involved

If noncontractile tissue is injured, passive movement is painful and limitation of movement may be seen

End feel
The sensation felt in the joint as it reaches the end of the available range of motion

Accessory movements
Movements within a joint that cannot be voluntarily performed by the individual

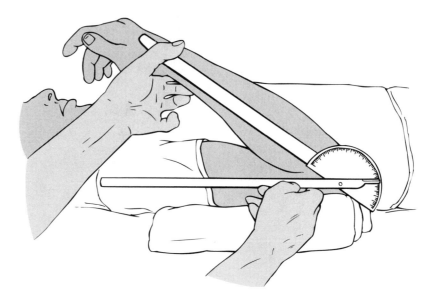

Fig. 4.15: Goniometry measurement at the elbow. In anatomical position, the elbow is flexed. The goniometer axis is placed over the lateral epicondyle of the humerus. To accommodate using a goniometer that ranges from 0° to 180°, the stationary arm is held parallel to the longitudinal axis of the radius, pointing toward the styloid process of the radius. The moving arm is held parallel to the longitudinal axis of the humerus, pointing toward the tip of the acromion process. Range of motion is measured where the pointer intersects the scale.

Loose-packed position
Resting position where the joint is under the least amount of strain

Close-packed position
Most stable joint position in which the two joint surfaces fit precisely together and supporting ligaments and capsule are maximally taut

If a bone or ligament is injured, pain will increase as the joint moves into the close packed position

Resisted manual muscle testing can assess muscle strength after an injury or surgery, and detect injury to the nervous system

Painful arc
Pain located within a limited number of degrees in the range of motion

distraction, sliding, compression, rolling, and spinning of joint surfaces. These motions occur within the joint, but only as a response to an outside force, and not as a result of any voluntary movement. The presence of accessory movement can be determined by manipulating the joint in a position of least strain, called the **loose-packed** or resting **position (Table 4-4)** (9,12). These movements are typically performed by certified athletic trainers and physical therapists to aid the healing process, relieve pain, reduce disability, and restore full normal range of motion.

In contrast to loose-packed position, **close-packed position** is the position in which two joint surfaces fit precisely together. The ligaments and joint capsule are maximally taut, joint surfaces are maximally compressed and cannot be separated by distractive forces, nor can accessory movements occur (10). Therefore, if a bone or ligament is injured, pain will increase as the joint moves into the close packed position. If swelling is present within the joint, the close packed position cannot be achieved. **Table 4-5** lists the close packed positions of the major joints of the body.

Resisted Manual Muscle Testing

Resisted manual muscle testing can assess muscle strength after an injury or surgery, and detect injury to the nervous system. Muscle weakness and pain indicates a muscular strain. Muscle weakness in the absence of pain may indicate nerve damage. Overload pressure is applied in a stationary or **static position**, or throughout the full range of motion.

In a static position, overload pressure is done with the joint in a neutral or relaxed position to relax joint structures and reduce joint stress. As such, contractile tissues (muscles) are more effectively stressed. In a fixed position the individual is asked to elicit a maximal contraction while the body part is stabilized to prevent little or no joint movement. For example, to test strength in the elbow flexors, flex the elbow at 90° and stabilize the upper arm against the body. Apply downward overpressure on the distal forearm and tell the individual not to allow the arm to move **(Figure 4-17)**. Contractions are held at least 5 seconds and repeated 5 to 6 times to indicate muscle weakening, and the presence or absence of pain (12).

Two advantages of testing throughout the full range of motion are: (1) a better overall assessment of weakness can be determined, and (2) a **painful arc** of motion can be located that might go undetected if the test is only performed in the mid-range. The body segment is placed in a specific position to isolate the muscle(s). The muscle(s) to be tested is placed on stretch in an elongated position. This position prevents other muscles in the

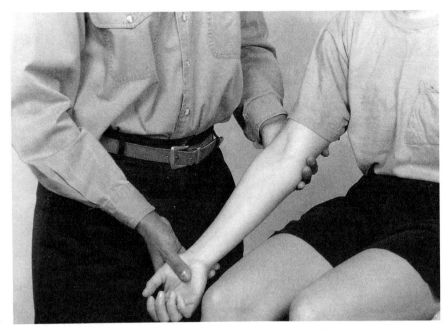

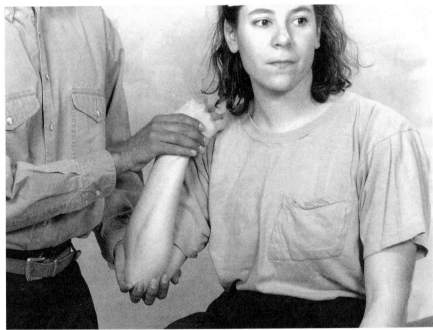

Fig. 4.16: Passive movement. The body part is moved through the range of motion with no assistance from the injured individual. Any limitation of movement or presence of pain is documented. (A) Starting position. (B) End position.

area from performing the movement. Manual pressure is exerted throughout the full range of motion, and is repeated several times to reveal weakness or pain. Ask if the motion causes pain. In this manner, both subjective information (what the individual feels) and objective information (weakness) is gathered. A standardized grading system used to measure muscle contraction is listed in **Table 4-6**.

Neurological Testing

A segmental nerve is the portion of a nerve that originates in the spinal cord, and is referred to as a **nerve root**. Each nerve root is named by its point of departure from the spinal cord. There are eight pairs of cervical nerves (C_1-C_8), twelve pairs of thoracic nerves (T_1-T_{12}), five pairs of lumbar nerves (L_1-L_5), five pairs of sacral nerves (S_1-S_5),

Advantages of testing throughout the full range of motion are:
  A better assessment of weakness is determined.
  A painful arc of motion can be detected.

Nerve root
The portion of a nerve associated with its origin in the spinal cord, such as C_6 or L_5

Table 4–3. Normal and Abnormal Joint End Feels.

Normal End Feel Sensations

Bone to bone

This is a definite, abrupt end-feel when two bony surfaces approximate, or come in contact with each other, such as when the olecranon process of the elbow contacts the posterior humerus during elbow extension

Soft tissue approximation

This indicates limited range of motion is due to normal extra-articular body tissue coming in contact with other tissue, such as when you bend your knee and the calf muscles meet the posterior thigh muscles

Tissue stretch

A springy type of movement with a slight give that comes at the end of the range of motion. It is the most common type of normal end feel. Examples include hip extension and rotation at the shoulder

Abnormal End Feel Sensations

Muscle spasm

This results in a rubber band *twang* when you reach the end of the range of motion. The muscle wants to contract to protect an acute injury. You may be able to palpate the muscle in spasm

Capsular

This has a *give to it* similar to the tissue stretch but it does not occur where you would normally expect it. This indicates an injury to the joint capsule or synovial tissue

Bone-to-bone

This is similar to the normal bone-to-bone end feel but it occurs before the normal end of the range of motion, or where you might expect it to occur

Empty end-feel

The individual may stop you before you reach the end-feel because of excessive pain in an acute condition

Springy block

This results in a rebound sensation which may be indicative of a loose bony fragment floating in the joint or damage to internal joint structures, such as a meniscus

---

Dermatome
Area of skin supplied by the cutaneous branches of each spinal nerve

Injuries to the nervous system will be reflected in both motor and sensory deficits

Myotome
A group of muscles primarily innervated by a single nerve root

An injury to a segmental nerve root will often affect more than one peripheral nerve and will not demonstrate the same motor loss or sensory deficit as an injury to a single peripheral nerve

and one pair of tiny coccygeal nerves (C_0). The first seven cervical nerve roots pass superior to the cervical vertebrae (i.e., C_7 passes superior to the 7th cervical vertebrae). In contrast, C_8, passes inferior to the 7th cervical vertebrae (between C_7 and T_1 vertebrae). Below the cervical area, all spinal nerves pass inferior to the same-numbered vertebrae (6).

In nearly all instances, each nerve root supplies nerve impulses to, or innervates, a series of muscles and an area of skin. The motor component of the nerve innervates muscle and the sensory component of the nerve innervates skin. Sensory distribution of each nerve root, called a **dermatome**, is relatively consistent, although variations may exist from individual to individual. Nerve roots leave the spinal cord to travel distally throughout the body. Several nerves may combine to form a plexus, such as the brachial plexus that innervates the upper extremity. As

the nerve roots travel distally, two or more consecutive segmental nerve roots may combine to form a peripheral nerve. The femoral nerve in the thigh has segments of L_2, L_3, and L_4 nerve roots; the axillary nerve in the shoulder has segments of C_5 and C_6 nerve roots.

Nerves are more commonly injured by tensile or compressive forces, and will be reflected in both motor and sensory deficits. The motor component of segmental nerve root function is tested using myotomes. A **myotome** is a group of muscles primarily innervated by a single nerve root. An injury to a segmental nerve root will often affect more than one peripheral nerve and not demonstrate the same motor loss or sensory deficit as an injury to a single peripheral nerve. Understanding these concepts can help assess the severity of a head or neck injury, or an individual with a suspected fracture or dislocation. Dermatomes, myotomes, and reflexes

Table 4–4. Loose Packed Position of Selected Joints.

Joint(s)	Position
Glenohumeral	55° abduction, 30° horizontal adduction
Elbow (ulnohumeral)	70° elbow flexion, 10° forearm supination
Radiohumeral	Full extension, full forearm supination
Proximal radioulnar	70° elbow flexion, 35° supination
Distal radioulnar	10° forearm supination
Wrist (radiocarpal)	Neutral with slight ulnar deviation
Carpometacarpal	Midway between abduction-adduction and flexion-extension
Metacarpophalangeal	Slight flexion
Interphalangeal	Slight flexion
Hip	30° flexion, 30° abduction slight lateral rotation
Knee	25° flexion
Ankle (talocrural)	10° plantar flexion, midway between maximum inversion and eversion
Subtalar	Midway between extremes of inversion and eversion
Tarsometatarsal	Midway between extremes of range of motion
Metatarsophalangeal	Neutral
Interphalangeal	Slight flexion

are used to assess the integrity of the central nervous system. Peripheral nerves are assessed using manual muscle testing and noting cutaneous sensory changes in peripheral nerve patterns.

Dermatomes

To assess sensitivity of a dermatome, touch the person with a cotton ball, paper clip, pads of the fingers, and fingernails. Ask the individual if each feels sharp or dull. Does the sensation feel the same on the injured body segment as it does on the uninjured body segment? Abnormal responses may be decreased tactile sensation (**hypoesthesia**), excessive tactile sensation (**hyperesthesia**), or loss of sensation (**anesthesia**). **Paresthesia** is another abnormal sensation characterized by a numbness, tingling, or burning sen-

Hypoesthesia
Decreased tactile sensation

Hyperesthesia
Excessive tactile sensation

Anesthesia
Loss of sensation

Paresthesia
Abnormal sensations, such as numbness, tingling, or burning

Table 4–5. Close Packed Positions of Selected Joints.

Joint(s)	Position
Glenohumeral	Abduction and lateral rotation
Elbow (ulnohumeral)	Extension
Radiohumeral	Elbow flexed 90°, forearm supinated 5°
Proximal radioulnar	5° forearm supination
Distal radioulnar	5° forearm supination
Wrist (radiocarpal)	Extension with ulnar deviation
Metacarpophalangeal (fingers)	Full flexion
Metacarpophalangeal (thumb)	Full opposition
Interphalangeal	Full extension
Hip	Full extension, medial rotation and abduction
Knee	Full extension, lateral rotation of tibia
Ankle (talocrural)	Maximum dorsiflexion
Subtalar	Full supination
Midtarsal	Full supination
Tarsometatarsal	Full supination
Metatarsophalangeal	Full extension
Interphalangeal	Full extension

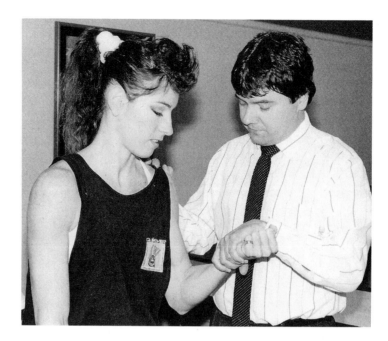

Fig. 4.17: Resisted manual muscle testing in a static position. Stabilize the arm against the body. Apply downward pressure on the distal forearm and ask the individual to prevent any movement.

sation. **Figure 4-18** illustrates dermatome patterns for the segmental nerves.

Myotomes

Nearly all muscles receive segmental innervation from 2 or more nerve roots. Selected motions may however, be innervated predominantly by a single nerve root (myotome). Resisted muscle testing of a selected motion can determine the status of the nerve root that supplies that myotome. Weakness in the myotome indicates a possible spinal cord nerve root injury. In testing a myotome, a normal response is a strong muscle contraction. A weakened muscle contraction may indicate partial paralysis (**paresis**) of the muscles innervated by the nerve root being tested. With a peripheral nerve injury, there is complete paralysis of the muscles supplied by that

nerve (12). For example, the L_3 myotome is tested with knee extension, in which the quadriceps muscle contracts. If the L_3 nerve root is damaged at its origin, there is a weak muscle contraction. This is because the quadriceps muscle also receives nerve root innervation from L_2 and L_4 segmental nerves. If however, the peripheral femoral nerve, which contains segments of L_2, L_3, and L_4 is damaged proximal to the quadriceps muscle, the muscle cannot receive any nerve impulses and therefore, will be unable to contract to execute knee extension. The most common myotomes tested are listed in **Table 4-7**.

Reflexes

Damage to the central nervous system can also be detected by stimulation of the reflexes. Exaggerated, distorted, or absent

> A weakened muscle contraction may indicate partial paralysis of the muscles innervated by the nerve root being tested

Paresis
Partial paralysis of a muscle leading to a weakened contraction

Table 4–6. Grading System used to Measure Muscle Strength.

Grade	Value	Muscle Strength
5	Normal	Complete range of motion (ROM) against gravity with maximal overload
4	Good	Complete ROM against gravity with some overload
3	Fair	Complete ROM against gravity with no overload; active range of motion (AROM)
2	Poor	Complete ROM with some assistance and gravity eliminated
1	Trace	Evidence of slight muscular contraction, no joint motion evident
0	Zero	No evidence of muscle contraction

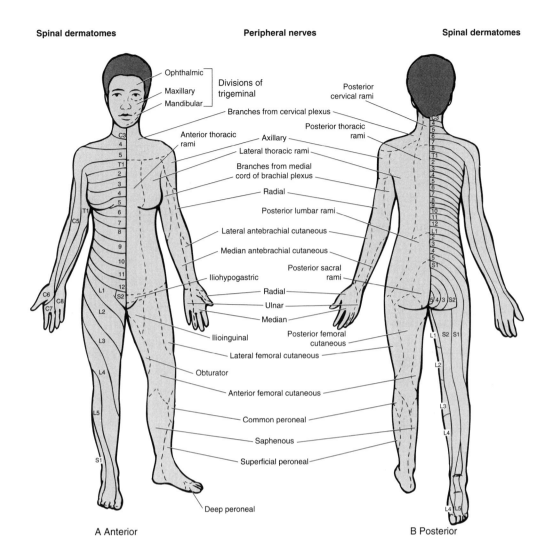

Spinal dermatomes   **Peripheral nerves**   **Spinal dermatomes**

Ophthalmic
Maxillary   Divisions of
Mandibular   trigeminal

Posterior
cervical rami

Branches from cervical plexus

Anterior thoracic
rami

Posterior thoracic
rami

Axillary

Lateral thoracic rami

Branches from medial
cord of brachial plexus

Radial

Posterior lumbar rami

Lateral antebrachial cutaneous

Median antebrachial cutaneous

Posterior sacral
rami

Iliohypogastric

Radial

Ulnar

Median

Ilioinguinal

Posterior femoral
cutaneous

Lateral femoral cutaneous

Obturator

Anterior femoral cutaneous

Common peroneal

Saphenous

Superficial peroneal

Deep peroneal

A Anterior   B Posterior

Fig. 4.18: Cutaneous sensation. Note that the cutaneous sensation patterns of the spinal nerves (*dermatomes*) differ from the patterns innervated by the peripheral nerves.

reflexes indicate degeneration or injury in specific regions of the nervous system, often before other signs are apparent (6). The most familiar deep tendon reflex is the patellar, or knee-jerk reflex, elicited by striking the patellar tendon with a reflex hammer causing a rapid contraction of the quadriceps muscle (**Figure 4-19**). Deep tendon reflexes tend to be diminished or absent if the specific nerve root being tested is damaged. **Table 4-8** lists common deep tendon reflexes and the spinal segments tested.

Peripheral Nerve Testing

Motor function in peripheral nerves is assessed with resisted manual muscle testing throughout the full range of motion. Sensory deficits are assessed in a manner identical to dermatome testing, except the cutaneous patterns differ. **Figure 4-18** demonstrates

the cutaneous patterns for peripheral nerves. Special compression tests may also be used to test peripheral nerve lesions on nerves close to the skin surface, such as the ulnar and median nerves. The "Tinel sign" test is performed by tapping the skin directly over a superficial nerve (**Figure 4-20**). A positive sign indicating irritation or compression of the nerve would result in a tingling sensation traveling into the muscles and skin supplied by the nerve.

Stress Tests

Each body segment has a series of stress tests to assess joint function and integrity of joint structures. These tests assess ligaments, intra-articular structures, joint capsule stability, impingement signs, muscle balance, and vascular integrity. For example, **Figure 4-21** demonstrates a **valgus** and **varus** stress on

Deep tendon reflexes tend to be diminished or absent when the specific nerve root being tested is damaged

Stress tests assess ligaments, intra-articular structures, joint capsule stability, impingement signs, muscle balance, and vascular integrity

Valgus
Denoting a deformity in which the distal body part angulates away from the midline of the body

Varus
Denoting a deformity in which the distal body part angulates toward the midline of the body

Table 4–7. Myotomes Used to Test Selected Nerve Root Segments

Nerve root segment	Action tested
C_1–C_2	Neck flexion*
C_3	Neck lateral flexion *
C_4	Shoulder elevation
C_5	Shoulder abduction
C_6	Elbow flexion and wrist extension
C_7	Elbow extension and wrist flexion
C_8	Thumb extension and ulnar deviation
T_1	Intrinsic muscles of the hand (finer abduction and adduction)
L_1–L_2	Hip flexion
L_3	Knee extension
L_4	Ankle dorsiflexion
L_5	Toe extension
S_1	Ankle plantar flexion, foot eversion, hip extension
S_2	Knee flexion

*These myotomes should not be performed in an individual with a suspected cervical fracture or dislocation, as they may cause serious damage or possible death.

Proprioceptors
Specialized deep sensory nerve cells in joints, ligaments, muscles, and tendons sensitive to stretch, tension, and pressure that is responsible for position and movement

the elbow joint to assess the integrity of the joint collateral ligaments. During an on-the-field assessment, tests to determine a possible fracture and major ligament damage at a joint should always be performed before moving an injured individual. Only the specific tests deemed necessary for the injury should be used. Because of the wide variety of stress tests, each will be discussed within the individual chapters.

Functional Testing

Before permitting an individual to return to sport participation after an injury, it is imperative the individual's condition be fully evaluated so risk of reinjury is minimal. Functional testing includes assessment of motor coordination or proprioception, and sport specific skill performance.

Proprioceptors are specialized deep sensory nerve cells sensitive to stretch, tension, and pressure. These cells detect minute changes in muscle dynamics and limb movement, and can instantaneously modify motor behavior consistent with changes in the environment (13). These receptors receive stimuli

Patellar ligament
Patella
Vastus lateralis
Rectus femoris (extensor)
Hamstrings (flexors)
Tibia
Fibula

Fig. 4.19: Reflexes can indicate if there is nerve root damage. The most familiar stretch reflex is the knee jerk, or patellar reflex, performed by tapping the patellar tendon with a reflex hammer causing involuntary knee extension.

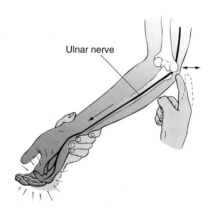

Ulnar nerve

Fig. 4.20: The "Tinel sign" test is used to detect irritation or compression of a superficial nerve. Tapping over the nerve causes a tingling sensation to travel into the muscles and skin innervated by the nerve.

Table 4–8. Commonly Tested Deep Tendon Reflexes.

Deep tendon reflexes	Segmental levels
Biceps	Cervical **5**, 6
Brachioradialis	Cervical 5, **6**
Triceps	Cervical **7**, 8
Patellar	Lumbar 2, **3**, 4
Medial hamstrings	Lumbar **5**
Lateral hamstrings	Sacral **1**
Achilles	Sacral **1**

from joints, ligaments, muscles and tendons, are responsible for position and movement, and allow us to know where the body segments are in space (6). For example, by stepping in a hole, the ankle inverts. **Muscle spindles** in the peroneal muscles respond to stretch on the muscles, and through reflex action, initiate a strong contraction to prevent excessive inversion, thus preventing damage to the supporting joint ligaments. Alterations in proprioceptive input due to injury may alter balance, reaction time, and motor control, placing the individual at a higher risk for reinjury. For an active sport participant small changes can be significant. An individual's balance can be tested by performing tasks with the eyes closed, such as walking a straight line on the toes and heels, balancing on a wobble board, or walking sideways on the hands while in a push-up position.

Sport specific tests are active movements performed by the individual during sport participation. In the rehabilitation process the individual generally performs these skills at low intensity; as the individual's condition improves, intensity is increased. With a lower leg injury the individual might begin by walking, jogging, then running forward and backward. If these skills are performed pain-free and without a limp, the individual might then be asked to run in a figure-8 pattern or a zigzag pattern. Again, each test must be performed pain-free and without a limp.

Functional tests should be sport-specific and demonstrate fluid, pain-free motion. These tests assess strength, agility, flexibility, joint stability, endurance, coordination, and proprioception. Any individual who has been discharged from rehabilitation should also pass the functional tests and be cleared by a physician for participation.

Stress tests were completed on the tennis player. Active and passive range of motion at the elbow and wrist were bilaterally normal. Resisted wrist extension on the right arm was weak and caused increased pain over the lateral epicondyle of the humerus. Joint stability tests were negative and did not increase pain. The individual has normal bilateral sensation on the hands and

Muscle spindle
Encapsulated receptor found in muscle tissue sensitive to stretch

Alterations in proprioceptive input due to injury may alter balance, reaction time, and motor control, placing the individual at a higher risk for reinjury

Functional tests assess strength, agility, flexibility, joint stability, endurance, coordination, and proprioception

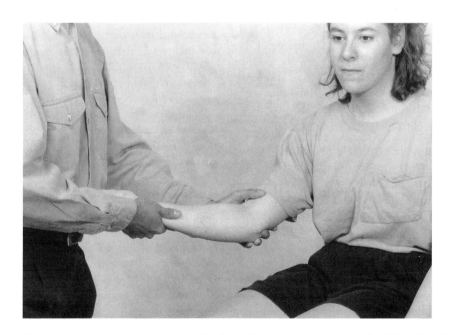

Fig. 4.21: Applying a valgus and varus stress on the elbow joint can assess the integrity of the joint collateral ligaments.

Diagnosis
Definitive determination of
the nature of the injury or illness made only by physi-
cians

An individual should always
be referred to the nearest
trauma center if any life-
threatening situation is present, or if the injury results
in loss of normal function

arms. At this point in the assessment, have
you determined what condition this individual possibly has?

INJURY RECOGNITION

The tennis player complained of dull,
aching pain on the lateral aspect of the
elbow that increased after activity stopped.
The painful site was isolated and all stress
tests were negative, except resisted wrist
extension. This muscular movement was weak
and painful. Think for a minute about what
this positive test indicates. Does the individual need to see a physician?

Injury recognition is the final step in
assessment. A fine line is drawn between
recognition of a sport related injury, and a
diagnosis. A **diagnosis** is the definitive determination of the nature of the injury or illness,
and can only be done by medical professionals trained in medical, orthopedic, and neurological factors, such as a physician, orthopedist, chiropractor, or dentist. Athletic trainers
and sport supervisors recognize a possible
injury or illness based on their assessment,
and as needed, may refer the individual for a
diagnosis. With professional preparation and
practice, your skills, as well as the ability to
recognize injuries, will improve.

A systematic and thorough assessment can
determine the extent and seriousness of injury.
The final decision in any injury assessment is
often very difficult. Subjective and objective
information gathered during the assessment
must be analyzed, and decisions made based
on what is best for the injured individual. Can
the situation be handled on-site or should the
individual be referred to a physician? A course
of action must be determined to minimize pain
and discomfort for the injured party. The athletic trainer or supervisor must decide:

1. If an ambulance should be summoned to
   transport the injured individual to the
   nearest trauma facility
2. If the individual should be referred to the
   family's primary care physician, team
   physician, or outpatient clinic for follow-
   up care
3. If the condition can be managed on-site
   with the intent to refer the individual if
   signs and symptoms fail to improve in a
   timely manner
4. What mode of transportation is best to
   move the injured individual to the sideline,

bench, training room, hospital, or physician's office

As a general rule, the individual should
always be referred to the nearest trauma center
or emergency clinic if any life-threatening situation is present, or if the injury results in loss of
normal function. For example, if the individual
is unable to walk without a limp, referral to a
physician is warranted. Conditions necessitating immediate referral to a trauma center were
listed in **Table 3-12**. In less obvious situations,
decide what is best for the health, safety, and
welfare of the individual. If in doubt, always
refer to the appropriate individual (i.e., head
athletic trainer, team physician, emergency
room, or primary care physician).

If the injured individual is referred to a
physician or trauma facility, document information gathered during the injury assessment, including the mechanism of injury, primary complaint, signs, and symptoms. Relay
this information and actions taken to the
appropriate individual (EMT, paramedic, or
physician). A competitive school athlete seen
by a physician should provide the school athletic trainer or coach with the physician's written report stating the diagnosis and if the athlete can return to sport participation, and
when. The athlete should not be allowed to
return to competition until clearance is provided by the physician in writing. Should the
injury be managed on-site, reevaluate the
injury daily to ensure satisfactory improvement. Modification in protection, treatment,
or activity level, and the need for referral to a
physician for further care will rest upon follow up assessments.

If you recognized the injury as a mild
muscle strain of the wrist extensors, you
are correct. Pain and weakness has affected
normal activities of daily living (ADLs), but
no joint instability is present. Provide medication if needed, and develop an appropriate
treatment and rehabilitation program.

SOAP NOTES

You work in a clinic with several employees. Why is it important for each
employee to be consistent and thorough in
all injury assessments and keep accurate
records?

SOAP notes provide another organized
structure for decision making and problem
solving in sports injury management. Used in
many physical therapy clinics, sports medi-

cine clinics, and athletic training rooms, these notes document patient care and serve as a vehicle of communication between the on-site clinicians and other health care professionals. The records provide information to avoid duplication of services, and state the present status and tolerance of that individual to the care being rendered by a given health care provider.

SOAP is an acronym of the components used in documentation, and includes the following sections:

Subjective evaluation
Objective evaluation
Assessment
Plan

The supervising physician determines the diagnosis of the patient and may note the results of any diagnostic testing including x-rays, magnetic resonance imaging (MRI), computed tomograms (CT) scans, laboratory testing, or personal notes. The patient is then immediately referred to an athletic trainer or physical therapist for detailed evaluation to determine an appropriate treatment and rehabilitation program. A subjective and objective evaluation, much more comprehensive than the HOPS format, is completed and correlated with short- and long-term goals in the assessment. Abbreviations are used throughout the notes for brevity. Although abbreviations vary from facility to facility, commonly used abbreviations can be seen in **Table 4-9**. There are four separate sections of SOAP notes.

Subjective Evaluation

The subjective evaluation (history of the injury) includes the primary complaint, mechanism of injury, location, onset and behavior of symptoms, functional impairments, pain perception, previous injuries to the area, and family history (14). This information is from the individual and reflects their attitude, mental condition, and perceived physical state.

Objective Evaluation

The objective evaluation (observation and inspection, palpation, and special tests) provides appropriate, measurable documentation relative to the individual's condition. This information can be repeatedly measured to track progress from the initial evaluation

through final clearance for discharge and return to sport participation. Measurable factors may include edema, ecchymosis, atrophy, range of motion, strength, joint instability, functional disability, motor and sensory function, and cardiovascular endurance. A detailed postural assessment and gait analysis may also be documented in this section.

Assessment

After the objective evaluation, the clinician will analyze and assess the individual's status and prognosis. Although a definitive diagnosis may not be known, the suspected injury site, damaged structures involved, and severity of injury should be documented.

Long-term goals are then established to accurately reflect the individual's status after rehabilitation. These long-term goals might include pain-free range of motion, bilateral strength, power, and muscular endurance, cardiovascular endurance, and return to full functional status. Short-term goals are then developed to outline the expected progress within a week or two of the initial injury. These might include immediate protection of the injured area and control of inflammation, hemorrhage, muscle spasm, or pain. Short-term goals are updated with each progress note. Progress notes may be written weekly or biweekly to document progress (**Figure 4-22**). **Table 4-10** lists several goals that may be applied to an individual with a musculoskeletal problem (15).

Plan

The final section of the note lists the **modalities**, therapeutic exercises, educational consultations, and functional activities utilized to achieve the short term goals (16). The written plan includes the following information:

1. The immediate treatment given to handle any acute problem
2. The frequency and duration of treatments, rehabilitation exercises, and evaluation standards to determine progress toward the goals
3. On-going patient education
4. Criteria for discharge

As the short-term goals are achieved and updated, periodic "in-house review" of the individual's records permit the facility and clinicians to evaluate joint range of motion, flexibility, muscular strength, power,

SOAP is an acronym for:
Subjective evaluation
Objective evaluation
Assessment
Plan

Subjective evaluation includes information on the primary complaint, mechanism of injury, location, onset and behavior of symptoms, functional impairments, pain perception, previous injuries to the area, and family history

Objective assessment measures edema, ecchymosis, atrophy, range of motion, strength, joint instability, functional disability, motor and sensory function, and cardiovascular endurance

Assessment includes long- and short-term goals

The treatment plan lists the modalities, therapeutic exercises, educational consultations, and functional activities used to achieve short term goals

Modalities
Therapeutic physical agents that promote optimal healing, such as thermotherapy, cryotherapy, electrotherapy, or manual therapy

Table 4–9. Commonly Used Abbreviations in SOAP Notes.

abnor.	abnormal	LOM	limitation of motion
AC	acute; before meals; acromioclavicular	MAEEW	moves all extremities equally well
ADL	activities of daily living	mm	muscle; millimeter; mucous membrane
ant.	anterior	MMT	manual muscle test
ante	before	MOD	moderate
AOAP	as often as possible	N	normal; never; no; not
A&O	alert & oriented	NC	neurologic check; no complaints; not completed
AP	anterior-posterior; assessment and plans	NEG	negative
AROM	active range of motion	NP	no pain; not pregnant; not present
ASAP	as soon as possible	NPT	normal pressure and temperature
B	bilateral	NSA	no significant abnormality
BID	twice daily	NSAID	nonsteroidal anti-inflammatory drug
c	with	NT	not tried
CC	chief complaint; chronic complainer	NWB	non-weight bearing
ck.	check	o	negative; without
C/O	complained of; complaints; under care of	O	objective finding; oral; open; obvious; often; other
CP	cerebral palsy; chest pain; chronic pain	OH	occupational history
		PA	posterior-anterior (x-ray); physician assistant; presents again
d/c, DC	discharged; discontinue; decrease		
DF	dorsiflexion	P&A	percussion and auscultation
DOB	date of birth	PE	physical examination
DTR	deep tendon reflexes	PF	plantar flexion
Dx	diagnosis	PH	past history; poor health
E	edema	PMH	past medical history
EENT	eyes, ears, nose, throat	PNS	peripheral nervous system
ELOP	estimated length of program	PPPBL	peripheral pulses palpable both legs
EMS	emergency medical services	prog.	prognosis
EMT	emergency medical technician	PROM	passive range of motion
EOA	examine, opinion, and advice; esophageal obturator airway	PWB	partial weight bearing
		Px	physical exam; pneumothorax
EV	eversion	rehab	rehabilitation
exam.	examination	R	right
FH	family history	R/O	rule out
FROM	full range of movement	ROM	range of motion
Fx	fracture	RTP	return to play
G1–4	grades 1 to 4	RX	therapy; drug; medication; treatment; take
GA	general appearance		
HA	headache	s	without
H/O	history of	S	subjective findings
H&P	history and physical	stat	immediately
HPI	history of present illness	STG	short-term goals
ht.	height; heart	Sx	signs, symptom
Hx	history	T	temperature
IC	individual counseling	+tive	positive
IN	inversion	UK	unknown
IPPA	inspection, percussion, palpation and auscultation	w	white; with
		WNL	within normal limits
L	left; liter	W/O	without
LAT	lateral	y.o.	year old

Physical Therapy   Daily Treatment/Progress Report _____

Patient Name: _____	Physician: _____	Diagnosis: _____
Date:	Date:	Date:
S:	S:	S:
O:	O:	O:
A:	A:	A:
STG'S:	STG'S:	STG'S:
P:	P:	P:
Initials/Treatment Time:	Initials/Treatment Time:	Initials/Treatment Time:

Signature 1 _____

Signature 2 _____

Fig. 4.22: Progress notes are added to the patient's file daily, weekly, or biweekly to document progress.

endurance, balance or proprioception, and functional status. These reviews also allow the clinicians to discuss the continuity of documentation, efficacy of treatment, average time to discharge the individuals, as well as other parameters that may reflect quality of care. As the individual progresses in the treatment plan, gradual return to activity may help motivate them to work even harder to return to full functional status. When it is determined the individual can be discharged and cleared for participation, a discharge note is written to close the file **(Figure 4-23)** (16,17). All information included within the file is confidential, and cannot be released to anyone without written approval from the patient.

In a clinical setting SOAP notes are the sole means of documenting what was done or not done for the patient. It is your ethical responsibility to keep accurate and factual records. This information verifies specific services rendered, evaluates patient progress, and efficacy of the treatment plan (15,16). Insurance companies use this information to determine if services are being appropriately rendered and therefore, qualify for reimbursement or not. More importantly, this comprehensive record-keeping system can minimize the ever-present threat of malprac-

Table 4–10. Short- and Long-Term Goals Used to Treat Musculoskeletal Problems.

Long-term Goals

Bilaterally equal:
    Musculotendinous flexibility
    Joint flexibility
    Muscular strength
    Muscular power
    Muscular speed
    Muscular endurance
Maintain or increase cardiovascular
    endurance
Restore normal biomechanical function
Restore neuromuscular re-education,
    balance, proprioception and kinesthetic
    awareness
Restore full functional abilities

Short-term Goals

Protect the injured area from further insult
Eliminate inflammation
Decrease pain
Decrease intra-articular effusion
Decrease extra-articular edema
Increase range of motion
Re-educate neuromuscular function
Educate and inform the patient

The primary error in writing SOAP notes is that of omission, whereby clinicians fail to adequately document the nature and extent of care provided to the patient

tice and litigation. In general, the primary error in writing SOAP notes is the error of omission, whereby clinicians fail to adequately document the nature and extent of care provided to the patient (17,18). Formal documentation and regular review of records can reduce this threat, and minimize the likelihood that inappropriate or inadequate care is being rendered to a patient. An illustration of an assessment as part of a SOAP note is demonstrated in **Table 4-11**.

Health care facilities should uniformly document specific services rendered, record patient evaluation, progress, and assessment particularly if several individuals are involved in the patient's rehabilitation program. SOAP notes are commonly used to keep comprehensive, concise, and accurate records.

SUMMARY

Sports injury assessment is a problem solving process that incorporates subjective and objective information about an injury that is reliable, accurate, and measurable. The HOPS format is used in injury assessment and includes history, observation and inspection, palpation, and special tests. Utilizing the HOPS format, subjective information (history) is gathered from the individual regarding their perception of the problem. This information may include:

1. The primary complaint
2. Mechanism of injury
3. Perception of pain and related symptoms
4. Disabilities resulting from the injury
5. Related medical history

To confirm information gathered in the subjective evaluation, an objective assessment is performed to discover the source of the individual's primary complaint. This segment of the assessment process includes:

1. Observation, including a scan exam to rule out referred pain from other body areas, posture and gait assessment, and inspection at the injury site
2. Bony and soft tissue palpations to determine a possible fracture or dislocation, and abnormal temperature, swelling, point tenderness, crepitus, deformity, muscle spasm, cutaneous sensation, and pulse
3. Active and passive range of motion to detect available range of motion and distinguish injuries to contractile tissue versus noncontractile tissues
4. Neurological testing through resisted manual muscle testing, dermatomes, myotomes, and reflexes
5. Stress tests for specific joints or structures

Documented information gathered during assessment establishes a baseline of information used to recognize and identify a possible cause of injury. This information can help the supervising physician accurately diagnose the problem, and provides a basis for treatment and rehabilitation programs.

SOAP notes are used in many sports medicine facilities to document the injury evaluation, assess the individual's status and prognosis, and outline the treatment plan. The treatment plan should delineate the frequency and duration of treatments, rehabilitation exercises, on-going patient education, evaluation standards to determine progress, and criteria for discharge. These notes serve as a vehicle of communication between the various health care providers and help an injured individual return safely to sport participation.

Table 4–11. Injury Assessment with SOAP Note Format.

A 52-year-old teacher complains of dull, aching pain on the lateral right elbow after playing tennis. No single episode led to the condition, but condition has now persisted for three months.

Problem:

R elbow extensor muscle strain.

Subjective:

A 52 y.o. WM in good physical condition reports dull, aching pain in lateral R elbow after playing tennis that persists for two hours. Patient reports pain started three months ago and is progressing in intensity. Discomfort is present when carrying or lifting heavy objects. Patient indicated the R elbow has never been injured before. No changes noted in racquet, grip size, or string tension.

Objective:

Visual:	R elbow shows slight erythema and swelling on lateral aspect. Patient is able to perform all gross motor movements with no limitations.
Palpation:	Patient is point tender over the lateral epicondyle and extensor muscle mass. No specific bony deviations are noted at the distal humerus or proximal radius. Percussion tap test is negative. No tenderness is noted on the ulna or medial epicondyle. Lateral aspect of the R elbow is warm to touch and slightly swollen.
ROM:	Mild restrictions and pain noted in active ROM for the R elbow, forearm, and wrist.

		AROM		Comments
		R	L	
elb	FL	140	140	PROM is WNL for R elbow;
elb	EX	0	0	NT for L; end feel for R is N
f	PR	80	85	
f	SU	85	90	
wr	FL	85	85	
wr	EX	80	85	

Neurological exam:

Motor:	MMT is 5/5 for L; 5/5 for R—all motions except 4+/5 for wr ext and supination Dynamic testing: NT Functional testing: NT
Sensory:	Dermatomes WNL to light touch C5–T1 B Biceps, Brachioradialis & Triceps reflexes WNL B Balance: NT

Special tests:

valgus stress test −R; −L
varus stress test −R; −L
common extensor tendinitis test +R; −L
pinch grip test −R; −L
Examination of Related Areas:
B shoulder, arm, and hand appear to be WNL B.

DISCHARGE SUMMARY

Patient's Name:
Physician: Dr.
Diagnosis:
Treatment & Frequency of Treatment:

Short Term Goals:

Achieved
| Yes | No |

Long-Term Goals:

Achieved
| Yes | No |

Outstanding Problems:

Home Treatment Program & Assistive Devices Needed:

Therapist: Date:

Fig. 4.23: Patients should have a discharge summary in the file signed by the supervising physician to verify completion of the rehabilitation program and final clearance to participate in sport.

REFERENCES

1. Kroenke, K. 1992. Symptoms in medical patients: An untended field. Am J of Med, 92(suppl 1A):3–6.
2. Peterson, MC, Holbrook, JH, Von-Hales, D, Smith, NL, and Staker, LV. 1992. Contributions of the history, physical examination, and laboratory investigation in making medical diagnoses. West J Med 156(2): 163–165.
3. Bates, B. *A guide to physical examination and history taking*. Philadelphia: JB Lippincott, 1991.
4. Gehring, PE. 1991. Physical assessment begins with a history. RN 54(11):27–31.
5. Urberg, MM, and Scott, NC. 1988. A self-scored medical history teaching technique. Fam Med 20(6):458–460.
6. Marieb, EN. *Human anatomy and physiology*. Redwood City, CA: Benjamin/Cummings, 1992.
7. Cailliet, R. *Pain: Mechanisms and management*. Philadelphia: FA Davis, 1993.
8. Fitzgerald, MA. 1991. Perfecting the art: the physical exam. RN 54(11):34–38.
9. Clarkson, HM, and Gilewich, GB. *Musculoskeletal assessment: Joint range of motion and manual muscle strength*. Baltimore: Williams & Wilkins, 1989.
10. Halback, JW, and Tank, RT. "The shoulder." In *Orthopaedic and sports physical therapy*, edited by JA Gould and GJ Davies. St. Louis: Mosby, 1989.
11. Barak, T, Rosen, ER, and Sofer, R. "Mobility: Passive orthopaedic manual therapy." In *Orthopaedic and sports physical therapy*, edited by JA Gould and GJ Davies. St. Louis: Mosby, 1989.
12. Magee, DJ. *Orthopedic physical assessment*. Philadelphia: WB Saunders, 1992.
13. McArdle, WD, Katch, FI, and Katch, VL. *Exercise physiology: Energy, nutrition, and human performance*. Philadelphia: Lea & Febiger, 1991.
14. Saunders, HD. "Evaluation of a musculoskeletal disorder." In *Orthopaedic and sports physical therapy*, edited by JA Gould and GJ Davies. St. Louis: Mosby, 1989.
15. Gould, JA, and Davies, GJ. "Orthopaedic and sport rehabilitation concepts." In *Orthopaedic and sports physical therapy*, edited by JA Gould and GJ Davies. St. Louis: Mosby, 1989.
16. Kettenbach, G. *Writing s.o.a.p. notes*. Philadelphia: FA Davis, 1990.
17. American Physical Therapy Association: Department of Practice. 1988. *Progress notes*. Alexandria, VA.
18. Herbert, DL. *Legal aspects of sports medicine*. Canton, OH: Professional Reports Corporation, 1990.

Chapter 5

Therapeutic Exercise and Therapeutic Modalities

After you have completed this chapter, you should be able to:

■ Identify the five theoretical emotional stages through which an individual progresses when confronted with a disabling injury

■ Identify and describe the process of designing a therapeutic exercise program

■ Explain the four phases of a therapeutic exercise programs, goals, and methodology of implementation

■ List the criteria used to clear an individual to return to full participation in sport

■ Describe the major groups of modalities, indications and contraindications for their use, and their application to manage inflammation and promote healing

■ Describe how nutrition can enhance healing

The ultimate goal of therapeutic exercise is to return the injured sport participant to full activity, pain-free, and fully functional. To do this, attention must focus on controlling inflammation and regaining normal joint range of motion, flexibility, muscular strength, muscular endurance, coordination, and power. Furthermore, cardiovascular endurance and strength in the unaffected limbs must also be maintained. Each component should be addressed within a well-organized individualized exercise program. Therapeutic modalities, medications, and proper nutrition are utilized throughout the exercise program to enhance repair and healing of damaged tissues.

In this chapter you will first learn about the emotional stages an individual may experience after injury. Second, you will learn how to develop a therapeutic exercise program following the SOAP note format introduced in Chapter 4. Next, the phases of a therapeutic exercise program will be explained, including criteria used to determine when an individual is ready to progress in the program, and ultimately return to sport activity. Finally, therapeutic modalities and medications used to control inflammation and pain, and aid the healing and repair process will be discussed. The material covered in this chap-

ter will be elaborated on in Chapters 7 to 15 for the various body segments.

PSYCHOLOGY AND THE INJURED PARTICIPANT

❓ *Think for a minute or two about how an active individual might react to the inability to participate in sport. What impact will these feelings have on their motivation to improve? How can you help this person overcome certain emotions that may hinder their progress in the therapeutic exercise program?*

To an individual who enjoys sport participation, an injury can be devastating. For many, the development and maintenance of a physically fit body provides a focal point for social and economic success important for self-esteem. A therapeutic exercise program must address not only the physical needs in returning the individual to activity, but also address the emotional and psychological needs of the injured participant.

Elizabeth Kubler-Ross identified five theoretical emotional stages that individuals progress through when confronted with grief. These stages can be adapted to an individual who has sustained an injury. The stages include denial and isolation, anger, bargaining, depression, and acceptance (1). Each

An injured individual may progress through stages of denial and isolation, anger, bargaining, depression, and finally, acceptance of the condition

individual reacts differently; some may progress rapidly through the stages in varying intensity, others may omit a phase, still others may reach a plateau and not progress.

In the denial and isolation phase, the person denies that a injury has occurred and may refuse to discuss it. The clinician should reason with the individual to convince them the condition is real and further participation could lead to more serious injury.

Once realizing they are indeed injured, many become angry with themselves, or may displace the anger toward the coach or team members. The individual may become demanding and difficult to deal with. Here, it is best to back off and allow the individual space to vent frustrations as long as the individual does not harm themselves or others with verbal or physical abuse.

As the individual's anger subsides, bargaining occurs. The individual tries to negotiate with the athletic trainer or coach to continue active participation. In return, the individual promises to do the rehabilitation program. However, if activity is limited or not allowed, depression may set in.

During the depression phase, the individual may perceive that the season is over and that there is no point in rehabilitating the injury. Motivating the person to attend regular rehabilitation sessions, or to maintain a home program of exercises can be very challenging for even the most patient and understanding athletic trainer. Realistic short-term goals can help motivate the injured individual to avoid this. Whenever possible, the rehabilitation program should mirror the individual's regular training program including the level of intensity, frequency, and duration. With activity modification, the competitive athlete may be able to do limited exercise with the team. This may reduce the feeling of isolation and being left out of daily interaction with the coach and other players. Using graphs or charts to document progress can also help the individual see improvement. This leads to stage five, acceptance of the injury.

In acceptance, the individual is resigned to the fact that hard work is necessary to rehabilitate the injury so they can return to safe participation. With a career-ending injury, final acceptance can redirect malingering or apathy toward eventual progress and near normal recovery.

💡 *An individual's emotional state will have a direct impact on success of an exercise*

program. *Charts, graphs, and activity modification that directly mirrors regular training will help motivate the individual to progress through the exercise program.*

DEVELOPING A THERAPEUTIC EXERCISE PROGRAM

❓ *In Chapter 4, you determined the problem was a mild chronic strain of the wrist extensors. What long- and short-term goals might you and the patient establish for the therapeutic exercise program? How will you measure progress?*

In designing an individualized therapeutic exercise program, several sequential steps help identify the needs and treatment goals of the patient (**Figure 5-1**) (2):

1. Assess the present level of function and dysfunction from girth measurements, goniometry assessment, strength tests, neurological assessment, stress tests, and functional activities
2. Organize and interpret the assessment to identify factors outside normal limits for the patient
3. Formulate a list of patient problems
4. Establish long-term and short-term goals
5. Develop a treatment plan to attain those goals incorporating therapeutic exercise, modalities, and medication
6. Supervise the treatment and exercise program
7. Reassess the progress of the treatment and exercise program

This process is ongoing. As continued assessment of the exercise program occurs, alterations in long- or short-term goals may result in changes in treatment or exercise progression. The process is dependent on the patient's progress and adaptation to the therapeutic exercise program.

Assess the Patient

Patient assessment initiates rehabilitation by establishing a baseline of information. This information is recorded in the **Objective**, or **O**, portion of the SOAP note, and documents the mechanism of injury, signs and symptoms, and level of dysfunction. In paired body segments, the dysfunction of the injured body part is compared to the non-injured body part to establish standards for bilateral functional status.

Patient assessment initiates the rehabilitation process by establishing a baseline of information

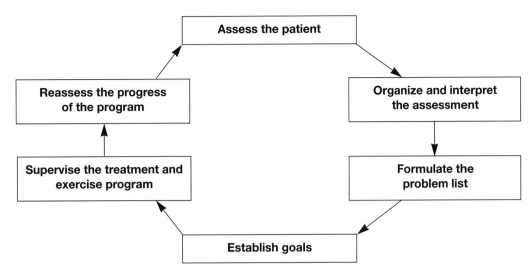

Fig. 5.1: An individualized therapeutic exercise program is developed and maintained through continual identification of the needs and treatment goals of the patient.

Organize and Interpret the Assessment

When assessment is completed, data is organized and interpreted to identify factors outside normal limits for an individual of the same age and fitness level. Primary deficits or weaknesses from injury are identified. These deficits, along with secondary problems resulting from prolonged immobilization, extended nonactivity, or lack of intervention, are organized into a priority list of concerns. Examples of major concerns might include decreased range of motion, muscle weakness or stiffness, joint contractures, sensory changes, inability to walk without a limp, or increased pain with activity. Physical assets are then identified to determine the individual's present functional status. For example, is there equal bilateral range of motion, muscle strength and endurance, and sensation? In the case of a lower extremity injury, is there normal gait? Can the individual pass functional tests?

Formulate the Problem List

From the two previous lists, analyze and interpret the information, and identify specific deficits and assets. Deficits dictate the long- and short-term goals. Activities or exercises to address the deficits should not interfere with patient progress. The assets (i.e., good cardiovascular fitness, range of motion, or muscular strength) must be maintained. The specific problems are recorded in a section called the *Problem List*, which is a part of

the **Assessment**, or **A** portion of the SOAP note.

Establish Goals

The driving forces of the exercise program are the long- and short-term goals. Long-term goals establish the individual's expected level of performance at the conclusion of the exercise program. Short-term goals develop the specific component skills needed to reach the long-term goals (3). The primary sports medicine team and patient should discuss and develop the goals. The patient must feel a part of the process, as this may educate and motivate the individual to work harder to attain the stated goals.

Many sport-specific factors, such as demands of the sport, position played, time remaining in the season, regular-season vs. post-season or tournament play, game rules and regulations regarding prosthetic braces or safety equipment, and the mental state of the athlete may affect goal development. In addition, the location, nature, and severity of injury will also impact setting goals (4).

Long-term goals typically focus on functional deficits in performing activities of daily living (ADLs). Sport participants focus on additional deficits in sport-specific skills. Long-term goals include bilateral equal range of motion; flexibility; muscular strength, endurance, and power; relaxation training; coordination; cardiovascular endurance; and performing sport-specific functional tests (i.e. throwing, running, or jumping).

Primary and secondary deficits, such as immobilization, inactivity, or lack of intervention should be listed

Long-term goals establish the individual's expected level of performance at the conclusion of the exercise program

Long-term goals typically focus on functional deficits in performing activities of daily living (ADLs)

Once long-term goals are established, short-term goals are developed in a graduated sequence to address the list of problems identified during the assessment. For example, a short-term goal with high priority is the control of inflammation, pain, and spasm. Each short-term goal should be moderately difficult, yet realistic. Specific subgoals should include an estimated time table needed to attain that goal. These subgoals are time dependent, but not fixed, as many do not take into consideration individual differences in preinjury fitness and functional status, severity of injury, motivation to complete the goals, and subsequent improvement. Constant reinforcement from the clinician to achieve the subgoals can be an incentive to continually progress toward the long-term goals. Long- and short-term goals are recorded in the **Assessment**, or **A**, portion of the note. Possible short-term goals for the injured tennis player can be seen in **Table 5-1**.

Develop the Treatment Plan

When goals are developed, determine what exercises and therapeutic modalities can be utilized to achieve those goals. The physician may also prescribe medications. This information is recorded in the **Plan**, or **P**, section of the note.

To address the problem list and return the individual to participation without risk of reinjury, four phases of rehabilitation comprise the therapeutic exercise program. The termination of one phase and initiation of the next phase may overlap. Each phase, however, has a specific role. In phase one, the inflammatory response, pain, swelling, and ecchymosis are controlled. In addition, patient education on relaxation can assist in relieving muscle spasm and pain. Phase two regains any deficits in active and passive range of motion at the affected joint. Phase three regains muscle strength, endurance, and power in the affected limb. Phase four prepares the individual for return to activity and includes analysis of motion, sport-specific skill training, regaining coordination, and improving cardiovascular conditioning. Each phase and expected outcomes are discussed in more detail later in the chapter. Throughout the program, nutritional needs and any psychological concerns of the patient should also be addressed. **Table 5-2** lists the various phases of a therapeutic exercise program.

Table 5–1. Short-Term Goals.

Week	Short-term goals
1	Control inflammation, pain, and swelling in right elbow
	Restore bilateral active range of motion (ROM) and passive range of motion (PROM), as tolerated
	Protect the involved area and decrease activity level
	Maintain strength at wrist and shoulder
	Maintain cardiovascular endurance with weight-bearing exercise
2–3	Restore full bilateral AROM and PROM at elbow
	Initiate strengthening exercises for affected elbow
	Restore bilateral strength at wrist, elbow, and shoulder
	Maintain cardiovascular endurance and general body strength
3–4	Improve strength of wrist extensors from fair to good
	Maintain full ROM at elbow, wrist, and shoulder
	Improve cardiovascular endurance
	Begin sport-specific functional patterns with no resistance
4–5	Increase muscle strength, endurance, and power in all motions at elbow
	Improve cardiovascular endurance
	Restore sport-specific functional patterns with moderate resistance
	Begin functional return to activity with necessary modification
5	Improve general body strength, endurance, and power
	Improve cardiovascular endurance
	Increase speed and resistance on sport-specific skills
	Return to full functional activity as tolerated

Supervise the Treatment and Exercise Program

Each phase of the exercise program and use of therapeutic modalities are supervised and documented. In addition, progress notes are completed on a weekly or biweekly basis. In many health care settings, these records are used for third party reimbursement of services rendered, and provide documentation of services provided to an individual should litigation occur.

Reassess the Progress of the Program

Short-term goals should be flexible enough to accommodate the progress of the individual (3). For example, if therapeutic modalities and medications are utilized, and the individual attains a short-term goal sooner than expected, a new short-term goal should be written. However, edema, hemorrhage, muscle spasm, atrophy, and infection impede the healing process and delay attaining a short-term goal. Periodic measurement of girth, range of motion, muscle strength, endurance, power, and cardiovascular fitness will determine whether progress occurs. If progress is not seen, the individual should be re-evaluated, or referred to a physician so modifications can be made in the short-term goals and treatment plan. The individual should progress through the sequential short-term goals until the long-term goals are attained, and the individual is cleared for full activity.

Long-term goals for the tennis player might include: pain-free bilateral range of motion, muscle strength, endurance, and power; maintainance of cardiovascular endurance; restoration of normal joint biomechanics; increased proprioception and kinesthetic awareness; restoration of bilateral function of ADLs; and pain-free unlimited

> Periodic measure of girth, range of motion, muscle strength, endurance, power, and cardiovascular fitness will determine if progress occurs

Table 5–2. The Therapeutic Exercise Program.

Phase One: Controlling Inflammation

Control inflammatory stage and minimize scar tissue with cryotherapy using **PRICE** principles (**P**rotect, **R**estrict activity, **I**ce, **C**ompression, and **E**levation.)
Instruct patient on relaxation techniques
Maintain range of motion, joint flexibility, strength, endurance, and power in the unaffected body parts
Maintain cardiovascular endurance

Phase Two: Restoration of Motion

Restore active and passive range of motion to within 80% of normal in the unaffected limb
Restore joint flexibility as observed in the unaffected limb
Begin pain-free isometric strengthening exercises on the affected limb
Begin unresisted pain-free functional patterns of sport-specific motion
Maintain muscular strength, endurance, and power in unaffected muscles
Maintain cardiovascular endurance

Phase Three: Developing Muscular Strength, Power, and Endurance

Restore full AROM and PROM in the affected limb
Restore muscular strength, endurance, and power using isometric, isotonic, and isokinetic exercises
Restore proprioception with closed and open kinetic chain exercises
Maintain cardiovascular endurance
Initiate minimal to moderate resistance in sport-specific functional patterns

Phase Four: Return to Sport Activity

Analyze skill performance and correct biomechanical inefficiencies in motion
Improve muscular strength, endurance, and power
Restore coordination and balance
Improve cardiovascular endurance
Increase sport specific functional patterns and return to protected activity as tolerated

The primary goal is to control inflammation by limiting hemorrhage, edema, muscle spasm, and pain

The longer the inflammatory process is allowed to progress, the more likely the resulting scar tissue will be less dense and weaker in yielding to applied stress

Analgesic effect
Condition whereby pain is not perceived, a numbing or sedative effect

Ice bags applied with a single layer of wet elastic wrap between the skin and ice pack produce a lower skin temperature than a dry elastic wrap

Increased heat may indicate inflammation and edema formation

motion in tennis specific skills with use of a tennis elbow support. Short-term goals are listed in Table 5-1.

PHASE ONE: CONTROLLING INFLAMMATION

The tennis player has pain and tenderness on the lateral side of the elbow and weakness in elbow extension. What modalities might you use to control inflammation? Would you include any exercises during this phase?

Phase one of the exercise program begins immediately after injury assessment. The primary goal is to control inflammation by limiting hemorrhage, edema, muscle spasm, and pain. The individual can move into phase two when the following criteria have been attained:

Control of inflammation with minimal edema, swelling, muscle spasm, and pain

Range of motion, joint flexibility, and muscular strength, endurance, and power are maintained in the general body

Cardiovascular fitness is maintained at the preinjury level

Collagenous scar formation, a natural component of the repair and regeneration of injured tissue, is less efficient and tolerant of tensile forces than the original mature tissue. The length of the inflammatory response is a key factor that influences the ultimate stability and function of scar tissue. The longer the inflammatory process progresses, the more likely the resulting scar tissue will be less dense and weaker in yielding to applied stress. Furthermore, immobilization for more than two weeks may lead to joint adhesions which inhibits muscle fiber regeneration (5). Therefore, all inflammatory symptoms need to be controlled as soon as possible. **PRICE** is a well known acronym for **p**rotect, **r**estrict activity, **i**ce, **c**ompression and **e**levation, and is the principle used to reduce acute symptoms at an injury site.

Control of Inflammation

After trauma, hemorrhage and edema cause a pooling of tissue fluids and blood products that increase pain and muscle spasm. The increased pressure decreases blood flow to the injury site leading to ischemia and hypoxia (deficiency of oxygen). As pain continues, the threshold of pain is lowered. These events lead to a cyclical pattern of pain-spasm-ischemia-hypoxia-pain. For this reason, cryotherapy (ice, compression, and elevation) is preferred during the acute inflammatory phase to decrease circulation, cellular metabolism, need for oxygen, nerve impulses and conduction velocity, to break the pain-spasm cycle. **Field Strategy 5-1** explains acute care of soft tissue injuries using the PRICE principle.

Application of cold immediately after injury leads to vasoconstriction, decreased circulation and capillary permeability, and decreased time for blood coagulation. Nerve impulses and conduction velocities are diminished leading to an **analgesic effect** and a reduction in muscle spasm. An elastic compression wrap can assist in decreasing hemorrhage and hematoma formation yet allows some expansion in cases of extreme swelling. Studies show that icebags applied with a single layer of wet elastic wrap between the skin and ice pack produce a lower skin temperature than when used with a dry elastic wrap (6,7). Elevation uses gravity to reduce pooling of fluids and pressure inside the venous and lymphatic vessels to prevent fluid from filtering into surrounding tissue spaces. The result is less tissue necrosis and local waste leading to a shorter inflammatory phase.

Cryotherapy, intermittent compression, and electrical muscle stimulation (EMS) may all be used to control hemorrhage and eliminate edema. Electrical stimulation has also been shown to retard atrophy in injured or immobilized muscles, and enhance the healing rate of injured tendons (8). Transcutaneous electrical nerve stimulation (TENS) might also be included to limit pain (See modality section). The modality of choice is determined by the size of the injured area, location, availability of the modality, and preference of the supervising health care provider. A decision to discontinue treatment and move to another modality should be based on the cessation of the inflammation. Placing the back of the hand over the injured site will show any temperature change as compared to an uninjured area. Increased heat may indicate inflammation and edema are still present. A cooler area may indicate diminished circulation restricted by edema or scar tissue.

Protect and Restrict Activity

Protecting an injured area is essential if repair and healing are to progress in a timely manner.

Field Strategy 5-1. Acute Care of Soft Tissue Injuries

Ice Application

Acute cold application should be limited to 20 to 30 minutes because of vasodilation caused by prolonged cold. This application may include ice massage, ice packs, ice immersion and cold whirlpools, commercial gel or chemical ice packs, or cryo cuffs.

Ice applications should be repeated every 11/2 to 2 hours when awake and may extend from one to 72+ hours post-injury.

Ice may be applied directly to the skin, however, because air is an insulator, a layer of wet elastic wrap between the skin and ice pack is recommended.

Skin temperature can determine when acute hemorrhage and swelling has subsided. For example, if the area (compared bilaterally) feels warm to the touch, hemorrhage and swelling continue. If in doubt, it is better to extend the time of a cold application.

Compression

On an extremity, apply the wrap in a distal to proximal direction. This will prevent extracellular fluid from moving into the distal digits.

Take a distal pulse after applying the wrap to ensure the wrap is not overly tight.

Horseshoe-pads can be placed around the malleolus in combination with an elastic wrap or tape to prevent or limit ankle swelling.

Compression can be maintained continuously on an injury. Remove the elastic wrap at night and elevate the body part above the heart to avoid pooling of fluids when body processes slow. For a lower extremity injury, place a hard suitcase between the mattress and boxspring or place the extremity on several pillows.

Elevation

Used in conjunction with cold and compression, elevation can reduce swelling. Elevate the injured site above the heart.

Restrict Activity and Protect the Area

If the individual is unable to walk without a limp, fit the person for crutches for the first 2 to 3 days following injury to allow healing to begin without complication. Apply an appropriate protective device to limit unnecessary movement of the injured joint.

If the individual has an upper extremity injury and is unable to move the limb without pain, fit the person with an appropriate sling or brace.

Moreover, muscle tension, muscle and ligament atrophy, decreased circulation, and loss of motion prolong repair and regeneration of damaged tissues. Early controlled mobilization allows for orderly formation of collagen in lines of stress and promotes healthy joint biomechanics. Continuous passive motion (CPM) can prevent joint adhesions and stiffness, and decrease joint hemarthrosis and pain (5). Early motion, and the loading and unloading of joints through partial weight-bearing maintains joint lubrication to nourish articular cartilage, meniscus, and ligaments leading to an optimal environment for proper collagen fibril formation. Tissues recover at different rates with mobilization; muscle recovers faster, and articular cartilage and bone respond least favorably (5).

The type of protection selected and length of activity modification depend on injury severity, structures damaged, and the philosophy of the supervising health care provider. Several materials can be used to protect the area including elastic wraps, tape, pads, slings, braces, splints, casts, and crutches. If an individual cannot walk without pain or walks with a limp, crutches should be recommended. Proper crutch fitting and use are summarized in **Field Strategy 5-2**.

Restricted activity does not imply cessation of activity but simply means "relative rest," i.e., decreasing activity to a level below that required in sport, but tolerated by the recently injured tissue or joint. Detraining can occur after only one to two weeks of nonactivity, with significant decreases measured in both meta-

Restricted activity implies decreasing activity to a level below that required to participate in sport, but tolerated by the injured tissue or joint

Field Strategy 5–2. Fitting and Using Crutches and Canes

Fitting Crutches

Have the individual stand erect in flat shoes

Place the tip of the crutch slightly in front, and to the side, of the involved leg

Adjust the length so the axillary pad is approximately 1 to 1½ inches (2 to 3 finger-widths) below the axilla, to avoid undue pressure on the neurovascular structures

Adjust the hand grip so the elbow is flexed at about 30°, and is at the level of the greater trochanter

Fitting for a Cane

Place the individual in the same position as above. Adjust the hand grip so the elbow is flexed at about 30°. This should place the hand grip at the level of the greater trochanter

How to use crutches. Rule of thumb is: "Crutches and the injured leg ALWAYS go together!"

For non-weight bearing on one limb:

Stand on the uninvolved leg. Lean forward and place both crutches and the involved leg approximately 12 inches in front of the body

Body weight should rest on the hands, not the axillary pads

With the good leg, step through the crutches as if taking a normal step. Repeat process

If possible, the involved leg should be extended while swinging forward to prevent atrophy of the quadriceps muscles

Going up and down stairs:

Place both crutches under the arm opposite the handrail

To go **up** the stairs, **step up with the good leg** while leaning on the rail

To go **down** the stairs, place the crutches down to the next step and **step down with the involved leg**

Progressing to partial weight bearing:

As tolerated, place as much body weight as possible onto the involved leg, taking the rest of the weight on the hands

Make sure a good heel-toe technique is used, whereby the heel strikes first, then the weight is shifted to the ball of the foot

Using One Crutch or Cane:

One crutch or cane is placed on the uninvolved side and moves forward with the involved leg.
The individual should not lean heavily on the crutch or cane

---

bolic and working capacity (9). Strengthening exercises through a weight-lifting program can be alternated with cardiovascular exercises, such as jogging, swimming, use of a stationary bike, or upper body ergometer (UBE). These exercises prevent the individual from experiencing depression as a result of inactivity, and can be done simultaneously with phase one exercises as long as the injured area is not irritated or inflamed.

Relaxation

Muscle tension can lead to a painful pain-spasm cycle. Relaxation allows an individual to consciously relieve muscle tension, thus breaking the cycle. Relaxation training can relieve both generalized and specific muscle tension, and is used in biofeedback and transcendental meditation to promote generalized body relaxation. Biofeedback monitors electrical activity associated with a muscular contraction, and converts the activity into auditory and/or visual signals. These units assist in facilitating muscle relaxation, controlling blood pressure and heart rate, reducing stress caused by tension headaches or muscular pain, and developing strength of muscle contractions (10).

Jacobson's system of progressive relaxation is often used instead of biofeedback to relax specific muscles or a body segment. It consists of an active contraction of various skeletal muscles followed by a reflex relaxation of those muscles. The stronger the contraction, the greater the relaxation. In addition, when a muscle is contracting, its corresponding antagonistic muscle is inhibited, and thus relaxed (Sherrington's law of reciprocal innervation) (11). **Field Strategy 5-3** explains Jacobson's relaxation exercises.

🔴 *Did you determine that cryotherapy, intermittent compression, EMS, and TENS can be used to control pain and inflammation on the injured elbow? If so, you are correct. Early controlled mobilization, pain-free range of motion, general strengthening and cardiovascular exercises should also be included as long as the injured area is not irritated.*

PHASE TWO: RESTORATION OF MOTION

🔴 *The acute inflammatory symptoms have been controlled using the PRICE principles. What exercises can be used to restore range of motion at the injured elbow and enhance healing?*

After inflammation is controlled, phase two begins immediately. This phase focuses on restoring range of motion and flexibility at the injured site, as well as continuing to maintain general body strength and cardiovascular endurance. If the individual is in an immobilizer or splint, remove the splint for treatment and exercise. The splint can then be replaced to support and protect the injured site. The individual can move into phase three when the following criteria have been completed:

Inflammation and pain are under control

Passive and active range of motion are within 80% of normal in the unaffected limb

Joint flexibility in the affected limb is restored compared to the unaffected limb

Cardiovascular endurance and general body strength are maintained at the preinjury level

Assessment of normal range of motion is done with a goniometer on the paired uninjured joint, as discussed in Chapter 4. Cryotherapy may be used prior to exercise to decrease perceived pain, or thermotherapy and EMS may be used to warm the tissues and increase circulation to the region. Once warmed, friction massage or joint mobilization may be helpful to break up scar tissue and adhesions to regain normal motion.

 Field Strategy 5-3. Jacobson's Progressive Relaxation Exercises.

Localized relaxation can be assisted through the application of superficial and deep heat, and massage.

Focus on the muscle and initiate an isometric muscle contraction for five to seven seconds; then relax. Imagine the muscle is heavy, warm, and relaxed. If continued muscle tension is perceived, repeat the process.

Generalized body relaxation can be done in any position. Although a reclining position is favored, a seated position provides the same result.

Locate a comfortable, quiet area and dress in comfortable nonrestrictive clothing.

Close the eyes and breathe in a deep, relaxed manner.

Picture in your mind the fingers or toes of the upper or lower extremity. Isometrically contract the musculature in that region for five to seven seconds; relax.

Imagine that the body segment is heavy, warm, and relaxed after the contraction.

Slowly progress to the next proximal segment. Repeat the process.

As the various segments of the extremity are relaxed, perform an isometric contraction of the entire extremity. Imagine that the whole unit is now very heavy, warm, and relaxed. Do not move that extremity until the entire session is complete.

Repeat the sequence for the remaining extremities, then move to the abdomen, thorax, and neck.

When the entire sequence is completed, remain in the position picturing the body in the relaxed state.

Limited joint motion may be caused by a bony block, joint adhesions, muscle tightness, tight skin or an inelastic dense scar tissue, swelling, pain, or the presence of fat or other soft tissues that block normal motion

Contracture
Adhesions occurring in an immobilized muscle leading to a shortened contractile state

Painful exercises can be facilitated by using a warm or hot whirlpool to provide an analgesic effect and relieve the stress of gravity on sensitive structures

Restoring passive range of motion prevents degenerative joint change and promotes healing

Hypomobility
Decreased motion at a joint

Hypermobility
Increased motion at a joint; joint laxity

Working the limb through available pain free motion with assistance will restore normal function more quickly than working the limb within limited voluntary motion

Flexibility
Total range of motion at a joint dependent on normal joint mechanics, mobility of soft tissues, and muscle extensibility

Progression in this phase begins gradually with restoration of range of motion and total joint flexibility. Several factors can limit joint motion including a bony block, joint adhesions, muscle tightness, tight skin or an inelastic dense scar tissue, swelling, pain, or the presence of fat or other soft tissues that block normal motion. Prolonged immobilization can lead to muscles losing their flexibility and assuming a shortened position, referred to as a **contracture**. Connective tissue around joints has no contractile properties. Although connective tissue is supple and will elongate slowly with a sustained stretch, like muscle tissue it will adaptively shorten if immobilized. Connective tissue and muscles may be lengthened through passive and active stretching, and proprioceptive neuromuscular facilitation (PNF) exercises.

Active Range of Motion (AROM)

Active range of motion exercises performed by the individual enhance circulation through a pumping action during muscular contraction and relaxation. Full pain-free active range of motion need not be achieved before strength exercises are initiated, but certain skills and drills requiring full functional motion, such as throwing, full squats, or certain agility drills, must wait until proper joint mechanics are restored. Active range of motion exercises should be relatively painless and may be facilitated during early stages of the program by completing the exercises in a warm or hot whirlpool to provide an analgesic effect and relieve the stress of gravity on sensitive structures. Examples of active range of motion exercises include spelling out the letters of the alphabet with the ankle, and using a wand or cane with the upper extremity to improve joint mobility.

Passive Range of Motion (PROM)

Passive range of motion exercises are performed by the athletic trainer or therapist, not by the injured individual. Restoring passive range of motion prevents degenerative joint changes and promotes healing. Limited passive range of motion is called **hypomobility**. These discrete limitations of motion can prevent pain-free return to competition, and predispose an individual to microtraumatic injuries reinflaming the old injury. Passive motion at hypomobile joints can be restored through joint mobilization. Joint mobilization

is an advanced stretching technique utilized by physical therapists and athletic trainers to apply an intermittent stretch to an aspect of the joint capsule. Various grades of oscillating force are applied in the loose-packed position to "free up" stiff joints and reduce pain to allow normal passive motion (5). Joint mobilization is contraindicated in cases involving arthritis, bone fractures, bone disease, neoplasm or vascular disorders of the vertebral artery, and should only be applied by trained individuals (4). Excessive passive motion, or **hypermobility** (joint laxity), cannot be reversed.

In performing passive range of motion exercises, the individual is placed in a comfortable position with the joint supported, such as lying on a table or having the body segment supported in one of your hands **(Figure 5-2)**. Casual conversation during the exercise period develops rapport between clinician and patient, and can assist in gathering subjective information about pain or discomfort occurring during the motion sequence.

Active Assisted Range of Motion (AAROM)

Frequently passive range of motion at the injured joint may be greater than active motion, perhaps due to muscle weakness. A person may be able to sit on top of a table and slide the leg across the table top away from the body to fully extend the knee. If the individual sits at the edge of the table with their legs hanging over the edge, however, then attempts to straighten the knee, the individual may be unable to move the limb into full extension voluntarily. Here, normal joint mechanics exist and full PROM is present. However, in order to attain full active range of motion the individual may require some assistance from a clinician, a mechanical device, or assistance from their opposite limb to attain full range of motion. Working the limb through available pain-free motion with assistance will more quickly restore normal active range of motion than working the limb within limited voluntary motion. **Field Strategy 5-4** illustrates selected range of motion exercises.

Flexibility

Flexibility is the total range of motion at a joint that occurs pain-free in each of the planes of motion (11). Joint flexibility is a combination of normal joint mechanics, mobility of soft tissues, and muscle extensibil-

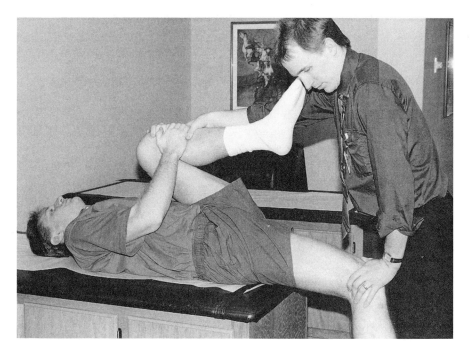

Fig. 5.2: To passively stretch a muscle group, stabilize the proximal body segment and apply a gentle, slow, sustained movement of the distal body part through the available range of motion until a point of tightness is felt, then apply a slight overpressure. Do not bounce the extremity at the end of the range of motion. This will facilitate the stretch reflex. In the stretched position, the patient should feel slight tension or tightness of the structures being stretched, but not pain.

ity. For example, the hip joint may have full passive range of motion, but when doing active hip flexion from a seated position, as in touching one's toes, resistance from tight hamstrings may limit full hip flexion. Resistance, such as this, may be generated from tension in muscle fibers or connective tissue.

Muscles contain two primary proprioceptors that can be stimulated during stretching, *muscle spindles* and *Golgi's tendon organs*. Because muscle spindles lie parallel to muscle fibers, they stretch with the muscle (**Figure 5-3**). When stimulated, the spindle sensory fibers discharge and through reflex action in the spinal cord initiate impulses to cause the muscle to contract reflexively, thus inhibiting the stretch. Muscles that perform the desired movement are called **agonists**. Unlike muscle spindles, Golgi's tendon organs are connected in a series of fibers located in tendons and joint ligaments, and respond to muscle tension rather than length. If the stretch continues for an extended time (over 6 to 8 seconds), the Golgi's tendons are stimulated. This stimulus, unlike the stimulus from muscle spindles, causes a reflex inhibition in the **antagonist** muscles. This sensory mechanism protects the musculotendinous

unit from excessive tensile forces that could damage muscle fibers.

Flexibility can be increased through ballistic or static stretching techniques. **Ballistic stretching** uses repetitive bouncing motions at the end of the available range of motion. Muscle spindles are repetitively stretched, but because the bouncing motions are of short duration, the Golgi's tendon organs do not fire. As such, the muscles resist relaxation. Because generated momentum may carry the body part beyond normal range of motion, the muscles being stretched often remain contracted to prevent overstretching, leading to microscopic tears in the musculotendinous unit. In a **static stretch**, movement is slow and deliberate. Golgi's tendon organs are able to override impulses from the muscle spindles leading to a safer, more effective muscle stretch. When the muscle is stretched to the point where a mild burn is felt, joint position is maintained statically for about 15 seconds and repeated several times (11). **Field Strategy 5-5** explains how static stretching is used to improve flexibility.

Proprioceptive neuromuscular facilitation (PNF) exercises promote and hasten the response of the neuromuscular system

Agonist
A muscle that performs the desired movement; a primary mover

Antagonist
A muscle that acts in opposition to another muscle, its agonist

Ballistic stretching
Increasing flexibility by utilizing repetitive bouncing motions at the end of the available range of motion

Static stretching
Slow and deliberate muscle stretching used to increase flexibility

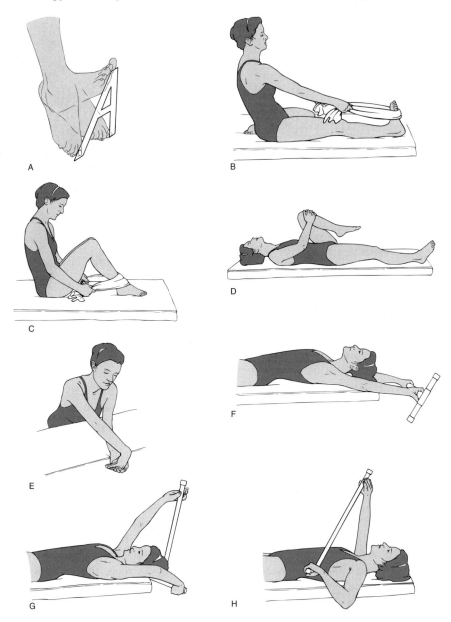

A. Ankle. Write out the letters of the alphabet using sweeping capital letters. Do all letters three times

B. Achilles tendon. In a seated position, wrap a towel around the forefoot and slowly stretch the Achilles tendon

C. Knee. In a seated position with the knee slightly bent, wrap a towel around the lower leg and slowly bring the lower leg toward the buttocks

D. Hip. Lying down, bring one knee toward the chest. Repeat with the other knee

E. Wrist or elbow. Using the unaffected hand, slowly stretch the affected hand or forearm in flexion and extension

F. Shoulder flexion. Using a wand or cane, use the unaffected arm to slowly raise the wand high above the head

G. Shoulder lateral (external) rotation. Using a wand or cane, use the unaffected arm to slowly do lateral (external) rotation of the glenohumeral joint

H. Shoulder medial (internal) rotation. Using a wand or cane, use the unaffected arm to slowly do medial (internal) rotation of the glenohumeral joint

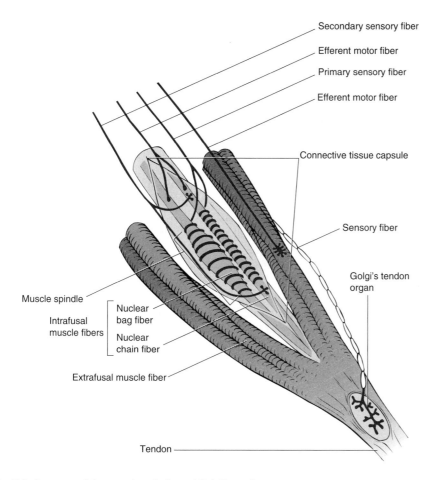

Secondary sensory fiber

Efferent motor fiber

Primary sensory fiber

Efferent motor fiber

Connective tissue capsule

Sensory fiber

Golgi's tendon organ

Muscle spindle

Intrafusal muscle fibers

Nuclear bag fiber

Nuclear chain fiber

Extrafusal muscle fiber

Tendon

Fig. 5.3: Anatomy of the muscle spindle and Golgi's tendon organ.

through stimulation of the proprioceptors. Supplemented by cutaneous and auditory input, these stretching exercises increase flexibility in one muscle group (agonist), and simultaneously improve strength in another muscle group (antagonist) (12). Furthermore, if instituted early in the exercise program, PNF stretches can aid in elongating scar tissue. As scar tissue matures and increases in density, it becomes less receptive to short-term stretches and may require prolonged stretching to achieve deformation changes in the tissue (8).

PNF technique recruits muscle contractions in a coordinated pattern as agonists and antagonists move through a movement pattern. One technique utilizes **active inhibition** whereby the muscle group reflexively relaxes prior to the stretching maneuver.. Contractions may be held for 3, 6, or 10 seconds, with similar results obtained (13). The clinician stabilizes the limb to be exercised. Alternating contractions and passive stretching of a group of muscles is then performed **(Figure 5-4)**. Common methods include

contract-relax, hold-relax, and slow reversal-hold-relax (4,11). Steady resistance is applied throughout the movement pattern for approximately 10 seconds. **Field Strategy 5-6** explains three PNF stretching techniques used in active inhibition.

A second technique known as **reciprocal inhibition** uses active agonist contractions to relax a tight antagonist muscle. In this technique, the individual contracts the muscle opposite the tight muscle against resistance. This causes a reciprocal inhibition of the tight muscle leading to muscle lengthening. An advantage to PNF exercise is the ability to stretch a tight muscle that may be painful or in the early stages of healing. In addition, movement can occur in single plane or diagonal pattern that mimics actual skill performance.

When range of motion has been achieved, repetition of motion through actual skill movements can improve coordination and joint mechanics as the individual progresses into phase three of the program. For example, a pitcher may begin throwing without

Proprioceptive neuro-muscular facilitation (PNF)
Exercises that stimulate proprioceptors in muscles, tendons, and joints to improve flexibility and strength

Active inhibition
Technique whereby an individual consciously relaxes a muscle prior to stretching it

Reciprocal inhibition
Technique using an active contraction of the agonist to cause a reflex relaxation in the antagonist allowing it to stretch; a phenomenon resulting from reciprocal innervation

Field Strategy 5–5. Using Static Stretching to Improve Flexibility

Avoid vigorous stretching of tissues in the following conditions:
   After a recent fracture
   After prolonged immobilization
   With acute inflammation or infection in or around the joint
   With a bony block that limits motion
   With muscle contractures or joint adhesions that limit motion
   With acute pain occurring during stretching
Stretching is facilitated by warm body tissues. Therefore, a brief warm-up period is recommended. If it is not possible to jog lightly, for example, stretching could be performed after a superficial heat treatment. If possible, play quiet, serene music.
In the designated stretch position, position yourself so a sensation of tension is felt, but not discomfort.
Do not bounce; hold the stretch for 10 to 30 seconds until a sense of relaxation occurs. Be aware of the feeling of relaxation, or "letting go." Repeat the stretch 6 to 8 times.
Breathe rhythmically and slowly. Exhale during the stretch.
Do not be overly aggressive in stretching. Flexibility is very individualized and may take 4 to 6 weeks before significant changes are noted.
If an area is particularly resistant to stretching, partner stretching or proprioceptive neuromuscular facilitation (PNF) stretching using the contact/relax technique may be used (see Table 5–3).

PNF exercises can stretch a tight muscle that may be painful or in the early stages of healing

resistance or force application in front of a mirror to visualize the action. This can also motivate the individual to continue to progress in the therapeutic exercise program. *In phase two, did you determine that active and passive range of motion exercises should be conducted at the elbow and wrist? Cryotherapy, thermotherapy, EMS, or massage can complement the exercise pro-*

gram. What activities can the tennis player do at home to assist recovery?

PHASE THREE: DEVELOPING MUSCULAR STRENGTH, ENDURANCE, AND POWER

The tennis player has regained normal range of motion at the elbow and wants

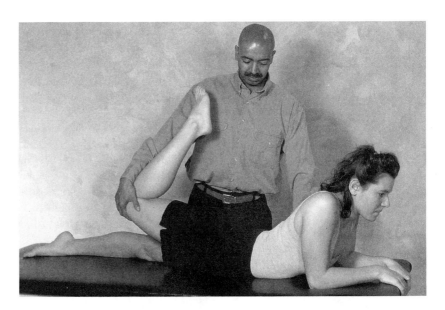

Fig. 5.4: In performing proprioceptive neuromuscular facilitation stretching techniques, the patient alternates muscular contractions and relaxations to stretch a group of muscles with the aid of a partner or clinician.

Field Strategy 5-6. Active Inhibition Techniques.

To stretch the hamstring group on a single leg using the three separate techniques, do the following:

Contract-relax

Instruct the individual to perform an isometric contraction of the hamstring muscle group for 3 seconds prior to stretching
Stabilize the thigh (do not hyperextend the knee), and flex the hip while slowly doing a passive stretch of the hamstring muscle group. Repeat the process 5 to 8 times, continuing to stretch the hamstring muscle group a few more degrees each time

Hold-relax

This is similar to contract-relax
Instruct the individual to flex the hip until resistance is felt in the hamstring. At that time "hold" the position against resistance with an isometric contraction for about 10 seconds
Allow the individual to relax approximately 5 seconds, then you move the limb to the new range either actively or passively. Repeat the sequence 3 or 4 times.

Slow reversal-hold-relax

Stabilize the thigh and flex the hip while the individual consciously relaxes the hamstring muscles. When resistance is felt in the hamstrings, instruct the individual to perform an isometric contraction of the hamstring muscle group for approximately 30 seconds or until fatigue is felt.
The individual then does a concentric contraction of the quadriceps muscles while you assist in slowly increasing hip flexion. Repeat the isometric contraction of the hamstrings, relaxation and concentric contraction of the quadriceps while you passively stretch the hamstrings a few more degrees. Repeat the sequence 5 to 8 times

to begin playing tennis again. Is this a good idea? Will reinjury occur? Why?

Phase three focuses on developing muscular strength, endurance, and power in the injured extremity as compared to the uninjured extremity. The individual can move into phase four when the following criteria have been completed:

Range of motion and joint flexibility in the affected limb equals that in the unaffected limb
Muscular strength, endurance, and power in the affected limb is equal, or near equal to the unaffected limb
Cardiovascular endurance and general body strength is at or better than the preinjury level
Sport-specific functional patterns should be completed using mild to moderate resistance

Muscular Strength

Strength is the ability of a muscle or group of muscles to produce resulting force in one maximal effort, either statically or dynamically (11). Static strength, measured with an

isometric muscle contraction, can be used during Phases 1 and 2 of the exercise program in a pain-free arc of motion. Dynamic strength is measured through a concentric or eccentric muscle contraction. Eccentric contractions provide more force than concentric contractions, and may also be used during early phases of rehabilitation. Repeated eccentric muscle contractions can lead to post-exercise muscle soreness, however.

Strength can only be increased by utilizing the **overload principle**, whereby physiological improvements occur only when an individual physically demands more of their muscles than is normally required. This philosophy is based on the **s**pecific **a**daptations to **i**mposed **d**emands (SAID) principle, which states that the body responds to a given demand with a specific and predictable adaptation (5). Overload is achieved by manipulating frequency, intensity, or duration of the exercise program. Frequency refers to the number of exercise sessions per day or week. Intensity reflects both the caloric cost of the work and specific energy systems activated. Duration refers to the length of a single exercise session. Strength gains depend primarily

Strength
The ability of a muscle to produce resulting force in one maximal effort, either statically or dynamically

Static strength is measured with an isometric muscle contraction, and dynamic strength is measured through a concentric or eccentric muscle contrac-.tion

Overload principle
Physiological improvements occur only when an individual physically demands more of the muscle than is normally required

Overload is achieved by manipulating frequency, intensity, or duration of the exercise program

on the intensity of the overload and not the specific training method used to improve strength. For example, when doing biceps curls with 50 pounds of weight, and doing three sets of twelve repetitions every other day, you can overload the muscle by increasing the following: *frequency*—do the exercise bout everyday; *intensity*—increase the weight to 75 pounds; and *duration*—increase the sets to four sets of 12 repetitions.

Knight's **d**aily **a**djusted **p**rogressive **r**esistance **e**xercise (DAPRE) is an objective method of increasing resistance as the individual's strength increases or decreases (14). A fixed percentage of the maximum weight for a single repetition (1 RM) is lifted during the first and second set. Maximum repetitions of the resistance maximum (RM) are lifted in the third set. Adaptations to the amount of weight lifted are then increased or decreased accordingly in the fourth set and in the first set of the next session. Guidelines for the DAPRE method are listed in **Table 5-3**.

Muscular strength is improved with a minimum 3 days per week of training that includes 12 to 15 repetitions/bout of 8 to 10 exercises for the major muscle groups (9). This may include isometric, isotonic, or isokinetic resistance training. Regardless of the method, the muscle must be worked at a higher level than customary.

Isometric Training

Isometric training measures a muscle's maximum potential to produce static force (15). The muscle is at a constant tension whereas muscle length and joint angle remain the same. For example, standing in a doorway and pushing outward against the doorframe produces a maximal muscle contraction, but joints of the upper extremity do not appear to move. Isometric exercise is useful in the first two phases of the exercise program when motion: (a) is contraindicated by pathology or bracing, (b) is limited because of muscle weakness at a particular angle, called a **sticking point**, or (c) when a painful arc is present. Isometric strength exercises are the least effective training method, as gains are isolated to a range of $10°$ on either side of the joint angle (5). An adverse rapid increase in blood pressure occurs when the breath is held against a closed glottis, and is referred to as the **Valsalva effect**. This can be avoided with proper breathing. To perform an isometric contraction, a maximal force is generated against an object, such as the clinician's hand, for about 10 seconds and repeated 10 times per set (11). Contractions, performed every $20°$ throughout the available range of motion, are called multiple-angle isometric exercises (11,16). **Figure 5-5** illustrates a variety of isometric exercises.

Isotonic Training (Variable Speed/Fixed Resistance)

A more common method of strength training is isotonic exercise. Here a maximal muscle contraction generates a force to move a constant load throughout the range of motion at a variable speed (17). This method is readily available with free weights, elastic tubing, and weight machines.

Table 5–3. The Daily Adjusted Progressive Resistance Exercise (DAPRE) Program.

Set	Weight	Repetitions
1	50% of RM	10
2	75% of RM	6
3	100% of RM	Maximum
4	Adjusted*	Maximum

# of Repetitions during Set 3	Adjusted working weight During Set 4	Next Day Exercise Session+
0–2	Decrease by 5–10 lb and repeat set	
3–4	Decrease by 0–5 lb	Keep the same
5–7	Keep the same	Increase by 5–10 lb
8–12	Increase by 5–10 lb	Increase by 5–15 lb
13–	Increase by 10–15 lb	Increase by 10–20 lb

*Adjusted work weight is gauged on individual differences completed in Set 3.
+Adjusted work weight for the next day is gauged on individual differences completed in Set 4.

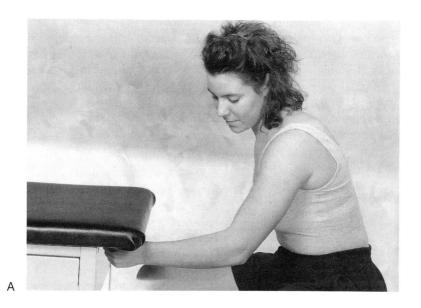

A

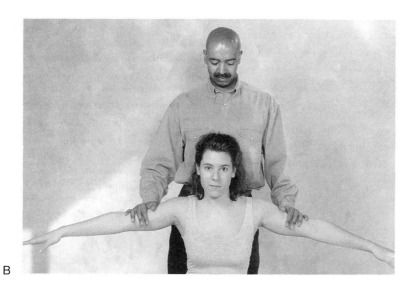

B

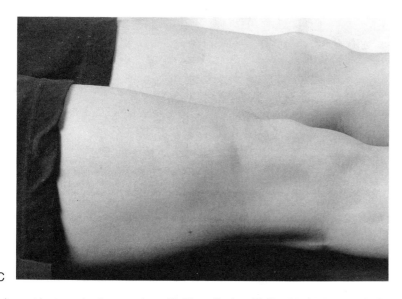

C

Fig. 5.5: Isometric strengthening exercises. (A) Elbow flexion. (B) Shoulder abduction. (C) Quad sets.

Free weights are inexpensive, can be used in diagonal patterns for sport-specific skills, but adding or removing weights from the bars can be troublesome. In addition, a spotter may be required for safety purposes to avoid dropping heavy weights. Theraband, or surgical tubing, is inexpensive, easy to set up, can be used in diagonal patterns for sport-specific skills, and can adjust to the patient's strength level by using bands of different tension (**Figure 5-6**). Weights on commercial machines can be changed quickly and easily. With several stations utilizing free weights and commercial machines, an individual can do circuit training to strengthen multiple muscle groups in a single exercise session. However, the machines are typically large, expensive, work in only a single plane of motion, and may not match the biomechanical makeup, nor body size of the individual.

Isotonic training permits exercise of multiple joints simultaneously, allows for both eccentric and concentric contractions, and permits weight bearing closed kinetic chain exercises. A disadvantage is that when a load is applied, the muscle can only move that load through the range of motion with as much force as the muscle provides at its weakest point. Nautilus and Eagle equipment are examples of variable resistance machines with an elliptical cam. The cam system provides minimal resistance where the ability to produce force is comparatively lower (early and late in the range of motion) and the greatest resistance where the muscle is at its optimal length-tension and mechanical advantage (usually the midrange) (15). The axis of rotation generates an isokinetic-like effect but angular velocity cannot be controlled.

Isokinetic Training (Fixed Speed/ Variable Resistance)

Isokinetic training, or accommodating resistance, allows an individual to provide muscular overload and angular movement to rotate a lever arm at a controlled velocity or fixed speed (**Figure 5-7**) (15). Theoretically, isokinetic training should activate the maximum number of motor units, which in consistently overloaded muscles, achieve maximum tension-developing or force output capacity at every point in the range of motion, even at the relatively "weaker" joint angles (9). Cybex, Biodex, or KinCom are examples of this strength training method. Coupled with a computer and appropriate software, torque-motion curves, total work, average power, and torque-to-body weight measurements can be instantaneously calculated to provide immediate objective measurement to the individual and clinician.

Two advantages of isokinetic training are that a muscle group can be exercised to its maximum potential throughout the full range

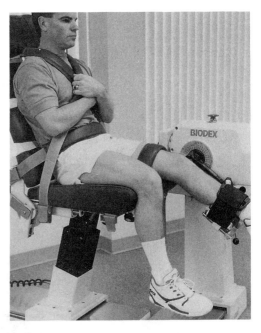

Fig. 5.7: The Biodex machine is an example of isokinetic training that utilizes a fixed speed and variable resistance to maximally work the muscles throughout the range of motion.

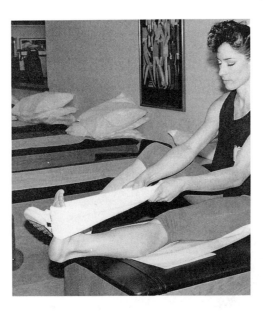

Fig. 5.6: Theraband or elastic tubing can be used in single or diagonal patterns for sport specific skills.

of motion, and, unlike isotonic training, the dynamometer's resistance mechanism essentially disengages if pain is experienced by the patient (15). Two disadvantages are the cost of the machine, computer, and software package (ranging from $25,000 to $60,000), and that nearly all available machines only do open chain exercises. For this reason, isokinetic training should be used in conjunction with other modes of resistance training.

Muscular Endurance

Muscular endurance is the ability of muscle tissue to exert repetitive tension over an extended period. The more rapid the muscle fatigues, the less endurance it has (18). A direct relationship exists between muscle strength and muscle endurance. As muscle endurance is developed, density in the capillary beds increase, providing a greater blood supply, and thus, a greater oxygen supply to the working muscle. Increases in muscle endurance may influence strength gains; however, strength development has not been shown to increase muscle endurance. Muscular endurance is gained by lifting low weights at a faster contractile velocity with more repetitions in the exercise session, or with use of stationary bikes, aquatic therapy, Stair Master, Nordic Track, or a Slide Board (5).

Muscular Power

Muscular power is the ability of muscle to produce force in a given time. Power training is started after the injured limb has regained at least 80 percent of the muscle strength in the unaffected limb. Regaining power involves weight training at higher contractile velocities or using plyometric exercises.

Plyometric training employs the inherent stretch-recoil characteristics of skeletal muscle through an initial rapid eccentric (loading) stretch of a muscle to produce tension prior to initiating an explosive concentric contraction of the muscle. This stretch produces a strong stimulus at the spinal cord level that causes a explosive reflex concentric contraction (9,19). The greater the stretch from the muscle's resting length, the greater the force the muscle can lift or overcome. Injury can result if the individual does not have full range of motion, flexibility, and near normal strength before beginning these exercises. Examples of plyometric exercises include standing jump, multiple jumps, depth jumps or drop jumping from

a height, bounding, leaps or skips, and throwing a weighted object, such as a medicine ball, in a controlled, explosive manner. Performing jumping and skipping exercises on grass will reduce impact on the lower extremity during landing. These exercises should be performed every three days to allow the muscles to recover from fatigue. **Field Strategy 5-7** lists exercises for developing muscular power and strength.

Open vs. Closed Kinetic Chain Exercises

In phase three, a common error in developing an exercise program is neglecting to assess the proximal and distal segments of the entire extremity (kinetic chain). **Kinematic chains** are a series of interrelated joints that constitute a complex motor unit constructed so that motion at one joint will produce motion at the other joints in a predictable manner (5,20). Whereas kinematics describes the appearance of motion, **kinetics** involves the forces, whether internal (e.g., muscle contractions or connective tissue restraints) or external (e.g., gravity, inertia, or segmental masses) that affect motion. A closed kinetic chain is seen in the lower extremity and pelvis when a person is weight bearing, or in a foot-fixed position. When the ends of the extremities are free to move without causing motion at another joint, such as when non-weight bearing, the system is referred to as an open kinetic chain. When force is applied, the distal joints may function independently or in unison with the other joints.

Injury and subsequent immobilization can affect the proprioceptors in the skeletal muscles, tendons, and joints. In rehabilitation it is critical that closed chain activities be used to facilitate retraining joint dynamics and muscle proprioceptors to respond to sensory input. Although open kinetic chain exercises (non-weight bearing) may produce great gains in peak force production, the exercises are usually limited to one joint in a single plane, have greater potential for joint shear, have limited functional application, and have limited eccentric and proprioceptive retraining. Closed kinetic chain exercises (weight bearing) are recommended for several reasons: (1) multiple joints are exercised through weight bearing and muscular cocontractions, (2) velocity and torque are more controlled, (3) shear forces are reduced, (4) propriocep-

Muscular endurance
The ability of muscles to exert tension over an extended period of time

Muscular power
The ability of muscles to produce force in a given time period

Plyometric training
Exercises that employ explosive movements to develop muscular power

Kinematic chains
A series of interrelated joints that constitute a complex motor unit so that motion at one joint produces motion at the other joints predictably

Kinetics
The study of forces that affect motion

A closed kinetic chain is seen when a person is weight bearing, or in a foot-fixed position

Closed chain exercises facilitate retraining of joint dynamics and muscle proprioceptors to respond to sensory input

Field Strategy 5–7. Power and Strength Exercises.

Stairs

Use a "low" walking stance and vigorously swing the arms. The exercise works the quadriceps, hamstrings, gluteals and lower back muscles
Triple stair: Walk only. One repetition is a round trip from the bottom of the stairwell to the top and back down. Use the walk down as recovery
Double stairs: Emphasize technique
Single stairs: Emphasize speed

Bounding

Technique involves one foot take off and landing for 30 to 40 yards. Swing the arms vigorously to provide a strong movement
Run-Run-Bound: Establish the number of bounds (repetitions) and the number of sets.
Distance: Establish the number of bounds in a given distance.

Hops. (Can be performed one-legged or two-legged for established distance)

Single goal: 40–50 yards.
Double goal: Sequence of 10 hops in each of 3 sets.

Uphill Running

Decrease the stride length and make sure foot strike is underneath the body rather than in front. Land on the forefoot/toes, not on the heels

Bench Steps with Barbells

Technique is similar to the Harvard step test; up, up, down, down. Begin with a light weight and add one minute daily until consecutive step-ups can be done for a preset period

---

tors are reeducated, (5) postural and stabilization mechanics are facilitated, and (6) exercises can work in spiral or diagonal movement patterns (5,21,22). **Figures 5-8** and **5-9** illustrate open and closed kinetic chain exercises.

⬤ *Are you going to allow the tennis player to resume playing after full range of motion is attained? If you determined that muscle strength, endurance, and power need to be developed prior to allowing gradual return to activity, you are correct.*

PHASE FOUR: RETURN TO SPORT ACTIVITY

⬤ *The tennis player has regained nearly normal strength in the affected limb as compared to the unaffected limb and maintained cardiovascular endurance by riding a stationary bike. What additional factors need to be considered to prepare this individual to return to full activity?*

The individual should be returned to their sport activity as soon as possible after muscle strength, endurance, and power are restored. During phase four the individual should cor-

rect any biomechanical inefficiencies in motion, restore coordination and muscle strength, endurance, and power in sport-specific skills, and improve cardiovascular endurance. The individual may be returned to activity if the following goals are attained:

Normal biomechanical function and sport-specific functional patterns are restored in the injured extremity
Muscle strength, endurance, and power in the affected limb is equal to that of the unaffected limb
Coordination and balance are normal
Cardiovascular endurance is at, or greater than, the pre-injury level
If needed, the individual wears appropriate taping, padding, braces, or protective devices to prevent reinjury
The individual receives clearance to return to participation by the supervising physician

Coordination

Coordination refers to the body's ability to execute smooth, fluid, accurate, and con-

Coordination
The body's ability to execute smooth, accurate, and controlled movements

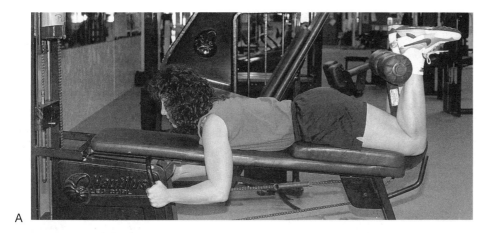

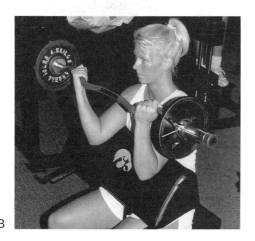

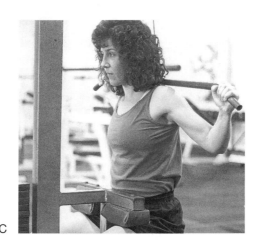

Fig. 5.8: Open chain exercises. (A) Hamstring strengthening. (B) Biceps curl. (C) Lat pull.

trolled movements. Simple movement, such as combing hair, involves a complex muscular interaction utilizing the appropriate speed, distance, direction, rhythm, and muscle tension to execute the task (23)

Coordination may be divided into two categories: gross motor movements involving large muscle groups, and fine motor movements utilizing small muscle groups. Gross motor movements involve activities such as standing, walking, skipping, and running. Fine motor movements are seen in precise actions, particularly with fingers, such as picking up a coin off a table, clutching an opponent's jersey, or picking up a ground ball with a glove. Coordination and proprioception are directly linked. When an injury occurs and the limb is immobilized, sensory input from proprioceptors is disrupted, as are motor commands, altering coordination.

Performing closed kinetic chain activities in phase three of the exercise program can help restore proprioceptive input and improve coordination. Constant repetition of

motor activities, using sensory cues (tactile, visual, or proprioceptive), or increasing the speed of the activity over time can continue to develop coordination in phase four (13). A wobble board, teeter board, ProFitter, and BAPS (Biomechanical Ankle Platform System) board are often used to improve sensory cues and balance in the lower extremity. PNF patterns and the ProFitter may also be used to improve sensory cues in the upper and lower extremities. **Field Strategy 5-8** lists several lower extremity exercises used to improve coordination and balance.

Sport-specific Skill Conditioning

Because sports require different skills, therapeutic exercise should progress to the load and speed expected for the individual's sport. For example, a baseball player performs skills at different speeds and intensities than a football lineman. Therefore, exercises must be coupled with functional training, or specificity of training related to the physical demands of the sport.

Coordination is divided into gross motor movements involving large muscle groups, and fine motor movements utilizing small muscle groups

Coordination can be restored with constant repetition of motor activities, using sensory cues, or increasing the speed of the activity over time

Specificity of training relates to the physical demands of the sport

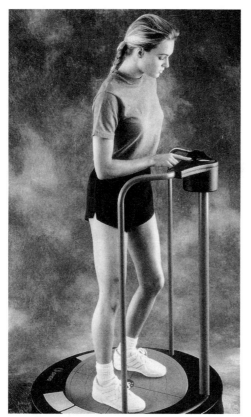
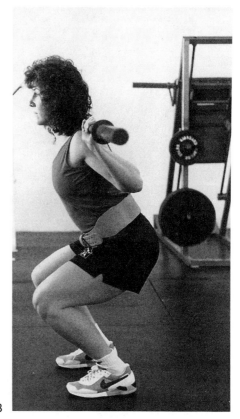

A

B

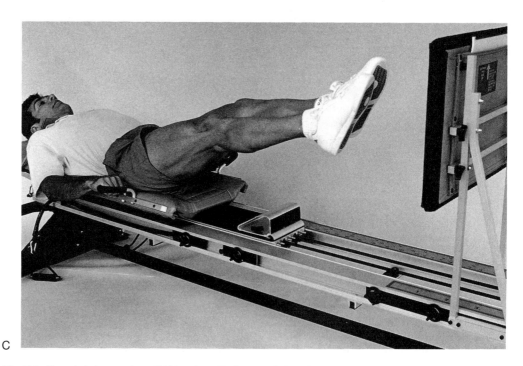

C

Fig. 5.9: Closed chain exercises. (A) Kat 1000. (B) Squats. (C) The Shuttle 2000 may be adapted for closed chain exercises including plyometric training (as shown), or open chain exercises

As range and motion, muscular strength, and coordination are restored, the individual should work the affected extremity through functional diagonal or sport-specific patterns. For example, in phase three a baseball pitcher may have been moving the injured arm

Field Strategy 5–8. Lower Extremity Exercises to Improve Balance and Proprioception.

Flat foot balance exercises

Stand on one foot (stork stand) and maintain balance for 3 to 5 minutes
Stand on one foot and maintain balance while performing daily living activities, such as washing
the dishes, toothbrushing, or blow drying hair
Stand on one foot with the toes off the floor and maintain balance for 3 to 5 minutes

Balancing on the toes

Balance on the toes/forefoot using both feet for 3 to 5 minutes
Balance on the toes while performing an activity
Stand on one foot, rise up onto the toes, and maintain balance for 3 to 5 minutes
Stand on one foot, rise up onto the toes, and maintain balance while performing the above activities

ProFitter exercises

In a location with a sturdy hand rail, stand on the ProFitter with the feet perpendicular to the long
axis of the rails. Gently slide side-to-side placing pressure first on the toes, then on the heels
Progress to more rapid movement. When you feel comfortable, do the sliding motion without
hand support. Keep track of the repetitions and sets

Sand walking

In a clean, safe sandy area, initiate a barefoot walking program focusing on proper gait
mechanics. Feel the heel hit firmly in the sand. Focus on shifting weight from the heel toward
the toes during the contact with the sand. A firm pushoff should occur from the ball of the foot

BAPS board exercises

Begin in a seated position by rotating the foot clockwise and counterclockwise
Stand and perform the exercises while holding onto a sturdy support
Progress to a free standing position and control the board through the range of motion

---

through the throwing pattern with mild to moderate resistance. In phase four the individual should increase resistance and speed of motion. Working with a ball attached to surgical tubing, the individual can develop a kinesthetic awareness in a functional pattern. When controlled motion is done pain free, actual throwing can begin. Initially, short throws with low intensity can be used, progressing to longer throws and low intensity. As the player feels more comfortable with the action, the number of throws and their intensity are increased. Similar programs can be developed for other sports.

Cardiovascular Endurance

Cardiovascular endurance, commonly called aerobic capacity, is the body's ability to sustain submaximal exercise over an extended period, and depends on the efficiency of the pulmonary and cardiovascular systems. When an injured individual is unable to continue,

or chooses to stop, aerobic training, detraining occurs within one to two weeks (9). If the individual returns to activity without high cardiovascular endurance, fatigue sets in quickly and places the individual at risk for reinjury.

Like strength training, maintaining and improving cardiovascular endurance are influenced by an interaction of frequency, duration, and intensity. The American College of Sports Medicine recommends that aerobic training include activity 3 to 5 days per week lasting more than 20 minutes at an intensity of 60% to 90% of maximal heart rate (24). Non-weight bearing exercises, such as swimming, rowing, biking, or use of the UBE can be helpful early in the therapeutic program, particularly if the individual has a lower extremity injury. Walking, cross-country skiing, jumping rope, or running can be performed as the condition improves. **Field Strategy 5-9** lists cardiovascular conditioning exercises. **Field Strategy 5-10** lists exer-

Cardiovascular endurance
The body's ability to sustain submaximal exercise over an extended period

Cardiovascular endurance training should include activity 3 to 5 days per week lasting over 20 minutes at an intensity of 60% to 90% of maximal heart rate

cises in the various phases that might be incorporated into the rehabilitation program for the tennis player.

● *The documentation needed to clear the tennis player for return to full activity includes successful completion of the goals listed in Phase 4, and a doctor's medical clearance. The individual should also agree to wear any appropriate taping, bracing or protective device to ensure safe return. Remember that*

all written documentation of the exercise program and written medical clearance should be placed in the individual's file and stored in a safe, secure location for 3 to 5 years.

THERAPEUTIC MODALITIES AND MEDICATIONS

● *You are developing a treatment plan for the injured tennis player. Your first task is to control inflammation, muscle spasm, and*

 Field Strategy 5–9. Cardiovascular Conditioning Exercises.

1. Jumping rope. The rope should pass from one armpit, under the feet, to the other armpit. Jump with the forearms near the ribs at a 45° angle. Rotation occurs at the hand and wrist. Jump with minimal ground clearance

   Two Footed Jumps
   a. Two feet. Bounce on the balls of the feet
   b. Tap heel of one foot to toe of the other foot on one jump. Variation: tap toe of same foot to heel of other foot
   c. Pepper.
   d. Arm crossovers and foot crossovers.

   One Footed Jumps
   a. One foot hop
   b. Rocker step. Rock forward and backward with feet in a forward straddle
   c. Heel strikes and toe taps
   d. Jogging steps

2. Stair Master. Twenty minutes of exercise is recommended three or four times a week
   a. Beginner level. Manual or Pike's Peak mode at Level 2 or 3 for 5 minutes. Increase time to 8, 10, 15, and 20 minutes.
   b. Advanced level. When 20 minutes are comfortable, decrease time to 5 to 8 minutes, and increase intensity level for 5 to 8 minutes, then increase time again. As intensity increases, include warm-up and cool-down periods

3. Treadmill
   a. Beginner level. Begin with a manual mode with a ground level (0° incline) for 5 minutes at approximately 2.5 mph. Increase time to 8, 10, 15, and 20 minutes.
   b. When 20 minutes is comfortable, increase speed to 3.0–5.0 mph, and progress to 8, 10, 15, and 20 minutes. Allow for warm-up and cool-down periods.
       For example:
       Warm-up at 2.5 mph for 5 min
       Increase speed to 4.0 to 5.0 mph for 10 min
       Cool-down at 2.5 mph for 5 min
       Total workout = 20 min
   c. Advanced level. Increase incline during the warm-up and decrease incline during the cool-down

4. Upper body ergometer (UBE)
   a. Beginner level. Start at 120 RPM for 4 minutes in alternating directions; 2 minutes forward—2 minutes backward
   b. Progress to 90 RPM and increase time to 6, 8, and 10 minutes
   c. Advanced level. Alternate directions as tolerated, however, duration should not exceed 12 minutes
       Warm-up at 90 RPM for 2.5 minutes
       Workout at 60 RPM for 5 minutes
       Cool-down at 120 RPM for 2.5 minutes

Field Strategy 5–10. Therapeutic Exercise Program for Wrist Extensor Strain

Phase one: Control of inflammation

Ice, compression, and elevation for 10 to 15 minutes for local effect
Gentle massage with the arm elevated to facilitate venous return

Phase two: Regaining range of motion

AROM through full range. AAROM at end ranges if limited—three sets with ten repetitions or as tolerated
PROM at end ranges—three sets with ten repetitions
Begin contract-relax stretching at end ranges—two sets with ten repetitions
Seated wrist flexion and extension stretching with a 20 second hold for five repetitions
Elbow flexor stretching in a quadruped position with a 20 second hold for five repetitions

Phase three: Regaining strength, endurance, and power

Continue with above stretching.
Upper body ergometer (UBE). Warm-up at 90 to 120 RPMs at 5 minutes—no load
Multiangle isometric. 10 second holds with wrist flexion and extension, and radial and ulnar deviation for 3 sets with five repetitions
Isotonics with wrist roll bar. 1½ lbs for 3 sets with ten repetitions in both directions, progressing to 4 to 5 lbs.
Theraband or Thera-tubing exercises. In a standing racquet-ready position in varying positions, do 3 sets with ten repetitions progressing to multiple sets of 20 to 30 repetitions for endurance. (Note: use pain and fatigue as guidelines to end exercise)
Theraputty grip strengthening exercises. Begin at 20 repetitions progressing as tolerance allows. Yellow or light blue putty is recommended
Swedish ball exercises. In standing position facing a wall, use both hands to tap the ball against the wall beginning at shoulder level; then move upward and add diagonal patterns, as tolerated
Proprioception exercise. Toss a tennis ball against the wall at designated targets
Closed chain exercises:
    Do floor push-ups in a partial weight-bearing knee position for 2 sets with ten repetitions progressing to 3 sets with ten repetitions. Increase to one arm push-ups or use varying hand positions
    Multidirectional balance board exercises. Control balance activity while in a push-up position either in partial or full weight bearing position for 30 second bouts with five to ten repetitions
    Wall push-ups 3 to 5 sets with fifteen to twenty repetitions
Plyometric wall push-ups for 3 to 5 sets with fifteen to twenty repetitions. Use caution with younger and older patients

Phase four: Return to sport activity

Isokinetic strengthening. Begin with wrist extension and flexion exercises using a concentric/eccentric muscle contraction at 60°, 75°, and 90° per second at 3 sets with ten repetitions
Kin Com strengthening in an isotonic mode for muscular control. Wrist flexion and extension using a concentric/concentric muscle contraction progressing to concentric/eccentric at 70° per second with a load of approximately 5 lbs.
Return to Sport Activities
    Check racquet size, string tightness and grip size of racquet
    Functional activities started earlier can be progressed to hitting easy against a wall board for 15 minutes using a forehand and progressing to backhand as tolerated. Increase speed of stroke as tolerated
Ice should be applied following all exercises for 15 to 20 minutes

pain, to enhance the healing process. Think for a minute or two about what therapeutic modalities can be used to assist the therapeutic exercise program?

Therapeutic modalities create an optimal environment for injury repair by limiting inflammation and breaking the pain-spasm cycle

Indication
A condition that could benefit from use of a specific modality

Contraindication
A condition adversely affected if a particular modality is used

Cryotherapy
Cold or ice application

Cold application leads to vasoconstriction and a decrease in cellular metabolism, capillary permeability, and pain

Counterirritant
A substance causing irritation of superficial sensory nerves so as to reduce pain transmission from another underlying irritation

Hunting response
Cyclical periods of vasoconstriction and vasodilation after ice application

Cryotherapy is the modality of choice during the acute inflammatory stage

Raynaud's phenomenon
Intermittent bilateral attacks of ischemia in the digits, marked by severe pallor, burning, and pain brought on by cold

Cold allergies
Hypersensitivity to cold leading to superficial vascular reaction manifested by transient itching, erythema, hives or wheals

Therapeutic modalities, or physical agents, can create an optimal environment for injury repair by limiting the inflammatory processs and breaking the pain-spasm cycle. As the exercise program progresses, selection of appropriate modalities and medications can inhibit inflammation by increasing localized circulation and transfer of nutrients, thus aiding the healing process. Use of any modality is dependent on the supervising physician's exercise prescription, injury site, type, and severity of injury. An **indication** is a condition that could benefit from a specific modality, whereas a **contraindication** is a condition that could be adversely affected if a particular modality is used. At times, a modality may be indicated and contraindicated for the same condition. For example, thermotherapy (heat therapy) may be contraindicated for tendinitis during phase one of the exercise program. Once acute inflammation is controlled, however, heat therapy may be indicated. Frequent assessment of the individual's progress can indicate if the appropriate modality is being used.

Licensure laws vary from state to state regarding the authorization and administration of modalities. For this reason, always check state laws and document modality use in the athletic training/clinic setting.

Several categories of modalities are available, and include the following:

1. Cryotherapy/cryokinetics including ice massage, ice and contoured cryo packs, ice immersion and cold whirlpools, commercial gel and chemical cold packs, and vapocoolant sprays
2. Thermotherapy including whirlpool and immersion baths, contrast baths, hydrocollator packs, paraffin baths, diathermy, ultrasound, and phonophoresis
3. Electrical stimulation including transcutaneous electrical nerve stimulation (TENS), high-voltage and low-voltage muscle stimulation (EMS), iontophoresis, and interferential current
4. Intermittent compression
5. Continuous passive motion
6. Massage.

Cryotherapy

Cryotherapy is an umbrella term that describes multiple types of cold application. Cold application for less than 15 minutes causes immediate skin cooling, a slight delay in cooling subcutaneous tissue, and a longer delay in cooling muscle tissue. Depth of cold penetration can reach 5 cm (10). Muscle temperature changes depend on the amount of subcutaneous insulation, vascular response to skin cooling, limb circumference, and temperature and duration of application (25).

Cold application leads to vasoconstriction at the cellular level decreasing the need for oxygen in the area being treated. Reducing the number of cells destroyed by the absence of oxygen limits the level of secondary hypoxic injury, and smaller amounts of inflammatory substances are released in the region. Localized cellular metabolism, capillary permeability, and pain are decreased. In addition, the release of inflammatory mediators and prostaglandin synthesis is inhibited (10).

As the temperature of peripheral nerves decrease, a corresponding decrease is seen in nerve conduction velocity across the nerve synapse, thus increasing the threshold required to fire the nerves. The gate theory of pain hypothesizes that cold inhibits pain transmission by stimulating large-diameter neurons in the spinal cord, acting as a **counterirritant**, which blocks pain perception (10,26,27). With nerve impulses inhibited and muscles spindle activity decreased, muscles in spasm are relaxed breaking the pain-spasm cycle leading to an analgesic, or pain free, effect.

When cold application is maintained over a longer period of time, or skin temperature is reduced below 10° C (50° F), it is believed a cold-induced vasodilation occurs. Although not totally understood nor universally accepted, the vasodilation is thought to occur by activation of an axon reflex, inhibition of smooth muscle activity, or reduction of sensitivity in blood vessels to chemicals that cause vasoconstriction. Each factor leads to vasodilation (27). As tissue temperature rises above 10° C, the vasoconstriction properties of cold take over once again. The cyclical periods are called the "**hunting response**," and are typically seen in isolated regions of high arteriovenous circulation, such as the ears, hands, and feet (6,27).

Because vasoconstriction leads to a decrease in metabolic rate, inflammation, and pain, cryotherapy is the modality of choice during phase one of the therapeutic exercise program. Cryotherapy is contraindicated in individuals with **Raynaud's phenomenon**, **cold allergies**, sensitivity to cold, leukemia, systemic lupus, high blood pressure, or over areas that have a compromised circulatory supply or anesthetized skin (26). **Table 5-4** lists indications and contraindications for cryotherapy application.

Cryotherapy is usually applied for 15 to 30 minutes per treatment, and can be applied hourly during the first 24 to 72 hours after injury. In addition, certain methods of cryotherapy may be used prior to range-of-motion exercises during phase two of the therapeutic exercise program and at the conclusion of an exercise bout. Use of cold treatments prior to exercise is called **cryokinetics**. An example of a cryokinetic program is listed in **Field Strategy 5-11**. Methods of cryotherapy include ice massage, ice and cryo packs, ice immersion and cold whirlpools, commercial gel and chemical packs, and vapocoolant sprays. With each method, the individual will experience four progressive sensations: cold, burning, aching, and finally analgesia.

Ice Massage

Ice massage is an inexpensive and effective method of cold application. Done over a relatively small area, it produces significant cooling of the skin and a large reactive **hyperemia**, or increase of blood flow into the region once the treatment has ended (26). As such, it is not the treatment of choice in acute injuries. Ice massage is particularly useful for its analgesic effect in relieving pain that may inhibit stretching of a muscle, and has been shown to decrease muscle soreness when combined with stretching (27). It is com-

monly used prior to range of motion exercises and friction massage when treating chronic tendinitis and muscle strains.

Treatment consists of water frozen in a cup, then rubbed over the skin in small circular motions for 7 to 10 minutes (**Figure 5-10**). A wooden tongue depressor frozen in the cup provides a handle for easy application.

Ice Packs and Contoured Cryo Cuffs

Ice packs are also inexpensive and maintain a constant temperature making them more effective in tissue cooling. When filled with flaked ice or small cubes, the ice packs can be safely applied to the skin for 20 to 30 minutes without danger of frostbite. Furthermore, ice packs can be molded to the body's contours, held in place by a cold compression wrap, and elevated above the heart to minimize swelling and pooling of fluids in the interstitial tissue spaces (**Figure 5-11A**). During the initial treatments, check the skin frequently for **wheal** or blister formation (**Figure 5-11B**).

Contoured cryo cuffs utilize ice water placed in an insulated thermos. When the thermos is raised above the body part, water flows into the cryo pack maintaining cold compression for five to seven hours (**Figure 5-12**). Although more expensive, the devices combine ice and compression over a longer period without threat of frostbite (26).

Ice Immersion and Cold Whirlpools

Ice immersion and cold whirlpools are used to quickly reduce temperature over the entire surface of a distal extremity, i.e., fore-

Cryokinetics
Use of cold treatments prior to an exercise session

Hyperemia
Increase of blood flow into a region once treatment has ended

> Ice massage is commonly used prior to range of motion exercises. Friction massage is used when treating chronic tendinitis and muscle strains.

Wheal
A smooth, slightly elevated area on the body, that appears red or white, and is accompanied by severe itching; commonly seen in allergies to mechanical or chemical irritants

---

Table 5–4. Cryotherapy Application.

Indications	Contraindications
Acute or chronic pain	Decreased cold sensitivity and/or hypersensitivity
Acute or chronic muscle spasm/guarding	Cold allergy
Acute inflammation or injury	Circulatory impairment
Postsurgical pain and edema	Raynaud's phenomenon
Superficial first degree burns	Hypertension
Used with exercises to:	Uncovered open wounds
Facilitate mobilization	Anesthetized skin
Relieve pain	Possible frostbite
Decrease muscle spasticity	Arthritis
Increase ROM	Cardiac or respiratory disorders
	Nerve palsy
	Leukemia or systemic lupus
	Multiple myeloma (tumors in bone marrow)

Field Strategy 5–11. Cryokinetics for an Ankle Sprain.

1. Immerse ankle in ice water until numb (12 to 20 min)
2. Exercise within limits of pain (see progression below) (3 to 5 min)
3. Renumb ankle by immersion (3 to 5 min)
4. Exercise within limits of pain (3 to 5 min)
5. Repeat steps 3 and 4 three times
6. Principles of exercising:
   a. All exercise should be active, i.e., performed by the individual
   b. All exercise must be pain-free
   c. All exercise is performed smoothly, without limping, twitching, or any abnormal motion
   d. The exercise must be aggressive and progress in complexity and difficulty as quickly as possible while remaining pain-free
7. Exercise progression for the ankle:
   a. Active range of motion
   b. Shift weight from foot to foot
   c. Weight-bearing plantar and dorsiflexion
   d. Walk with short steps
   e. Walk with long steps
   f. Walk in circles, figure eights, or other weaving pattern
   g. Jog straight ahead
   h. Jog in lazy S or big figure eight pattern
   i. Jog in sharp Z or smaller figure eight pattern
   j. Sprint 5 to 10 yards with slow starts and stops
   k. Sprint 5 to 10 yards with quick starts and stops
   l. Begin the DAPRE technique to strengthen ankle musculature
   m. Half-speed team drills (with ankle taped or braced)
   n. Three quarter-speed team drills (with ankle taped or braced)
   o. Full-speed team drills (with ankle taped or braced)
   p. Full team practice (with ankle taped or braced)

---

arm, hand, ankle, or foot. Because of the analgesic effect and buoyancy of the water, both modalities are often used during the inflammatory phase and combined with range of motion exercises. Cold whirlpool baths also provide a hydromassaging effect. This is controlled by the amount of air emitted through the electrical turbine. The turbine can be moved up and down, or directed at a specific angle and locked in place. In addition to controlling acute inflammation, cold whirlpools can be used to decrease soft tissue trauma and increase active range of motion after prolonged immobilization.

If the goal is to reduce edema, placing the body part in a stationary position below the level of the heart keeps fluid in the body segment, and is contraindicated. This can be avoided by placing a compression wrap over the body part prior to submersion and doing active muscle contractions (26). Neoprene toe caps may be used to reduce discomfort on the toes. A bucket or cold whirlpool is filled with water and ice, and maintained at a temperature between 13 and 18° C (55 and 65° F) (**Figure 5-13**) (27). The lower the tempera-

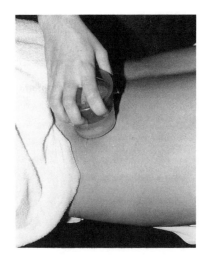

Fig. 5.10: Ice massage is an easy and inexpensive method of cryotherapy that can be self-administered.

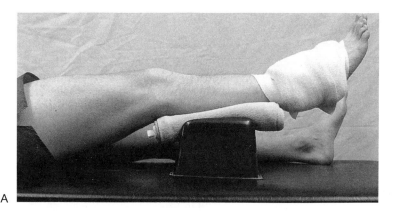

A

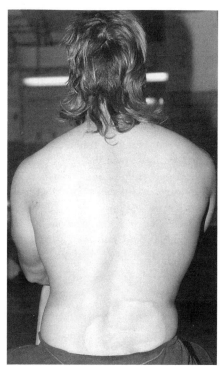

B

Fig. 5.11: A. Ice, compression, and elevation can reduce acute inflammation. B. A slightly raised wheal formation may appear shortly after cold application in individuals who are sensitive to cold or have cold allergies.

ture, the shorter the immersion should be. Treatment lasts from 5 to 15 minutes. When pain is relieved, the part is removed from the water and functional movement patterns are performed. As pain returns, the area is reimmersed. The cycle continues three to four times.

Commercial Gel and Chemical Packs

Commercial gel packs are composed of flexible silicone enclosed in a strong vinyl case, and come in a variety of sizes to conform to the body's natural contours **(Figure 5-14)**. Used with compression and elevation, they are an effective cold application. The packs are stored at a temperature of about −5° C for at least 2 hours prior to application (27). A wet towel is placed between the pack and

skin to prevent frostbite and maintain a hygienic surface for the reusable packs. Treatment time is 15 to 20 minutes.

Chemical packs are convenient to carry in a training kit, are disposable after a single use, can conform to the body part, but can be expensive. The packs are activated by squeezing or hitting the pack against a hard area. The chemical reaction is at an alkaline pH and can cause skin burns if the package breaks and the contents spill **(Figure 5-15)**. As such, the packs should never be squeezed in front of the face, and if possible, should be placed inside another plastic bag. Treatment ranges from 15 to 20 minutes. With longer treatments, the pack warms and becomes ineffective as a cold treatment. Some commercial packs can be refrozen and reused.

A wet towel is placed between the pack and skin to prevent frostbite and maintain a clean surface for the reusable packs

Thermotherapy
Heat application

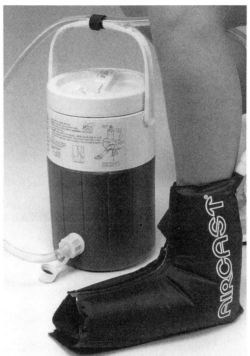

Fig. 5.12: Contoured cryo cuffs are an effective means of cold application. When the thermos is raised above the body part, water flows into the cryo pack maintaining cold compression for 5 to 7 hours.

Vapocoolant Sprays

Fluori-Methane spray uses rapid evaporation of chemicals on the skin area to freeze the skin prior to stretching a muscle (**Figure 5-16**). The effects are temporary and superficial. The patient is comfortably positioned with the muscle passively stretched. The bottle of vapocoolant spray is then inverted and sprayed in a unidirectional parallel sweeping pattern over the involved site. The clinician then provides further stretch as tolerated by the patient (5).

Thermotherapy

Thermotherapy, or heat application, is typically used in phase two to increase blood flow and promote healing in the injured area. If used during the acute inflammatory stage, heat application may overwhelm the injured blood and lymphatic vessels leading to increased hemorrhage and edema. When applied at the appropriate time, however, heat can increase circulation and cellular metabolism, and decrease muscle spasm and pain. Heat application also has an analgesic, or sedative, effect. With vasodilation and increased circulation, an influx of oxygen and nutrients move into the area to promote healing of damaged tissues.

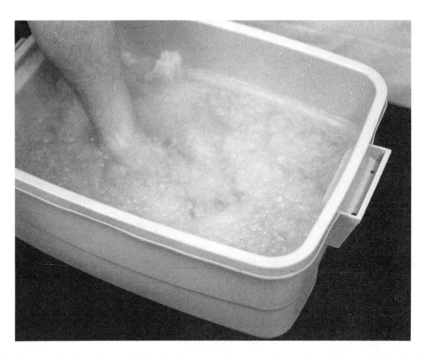

Fig. 5.13: Ice immersion is used to quickly reduce temperature over the entire surface area of a distal extremity. Toe caps may be used to prevent frostbite of the toes during the treatment.

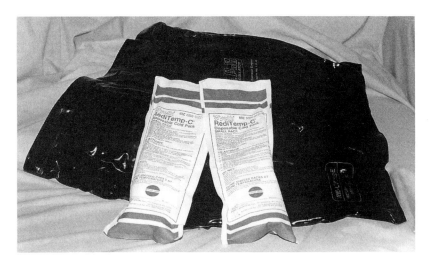

Fig. 5.14: Commercial gel packs can be molded around bony segments, and combined with compression and elevation, provide an excellent cryotherapy treatment. Chemical ice packs are convenient to carry in a training kit, are disposable after a single use, and conform to the body part.

Debris and waste products are then removed from the injury site. Used prior to stretching exercises, thermotherapy can increase extensibility of connective tissue leading to increased range of motion (28). Heat may be applied using superficial thermotherapy including warm and hot whirlpools, hydrocollator packs, and paraffin baths, or with penetrating thermotherapy including diathermy, ultrasound, and phonophoresis. Depth of penetration ranges from 2 cm with superficial thermotherapy, and 2 to 5 cm with penetrating thermotherapy (10). **Table 5-5** lists indications and contraindications for thermotherapy.

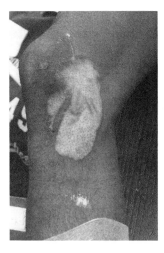

Fig. 5.15: This intercollegiate soccer player fell asleep with a chemical ice bag on his leg, unaware of a small leak in the bag. The resulting irritation led to a second degree burn to the skin.

Whirlpool and Immersion Baths

Whirlpool or immersion baths combine warm or hot water with a hydromassaging effect to increase superficial skin temperature **(Figure 5-17)**. Like cold whirlpools and immersion baths, buoyancy facilitates increased range of motion. This modality is used for relaxation to decrease muscle spasm and pain, and facilitate range of motion exercises after prolonged immobilization. Treatment time ranges from 20 to 30 minutes. Total body immersion exceeding 20 to 30 minutes can dehydrate the athlete, leading to dizziness and high body core temperature (25). Only the body parts being treated should be immersed. **Field Strategy 5-12** lists indications, contraindications, technique, and suggested temperatures used with this modality.

Hydrocollator Packs

Hydrocollator packs provide superficial moist heat to a slightly deeper tissue level than a whirlpool (25,27). The packs consist of several silicone gel compartments encased in a canvas fabric **(Figure 5-18)**. The packs are stored in a hot water unit at a temperature of approximately 71.1° C (160° F) (5). When removed from the water the pack is wrapped in a commercial padded hot-pack cover or in six to eight layers of toweling, and placed directly over the injury site for 20 minutes. The pack should completely cover the area being treated and be secured. The patient should never lie on top of the pack, as this

Thermotherapy can increase extensibility of connective tissue leading to increased range of motion

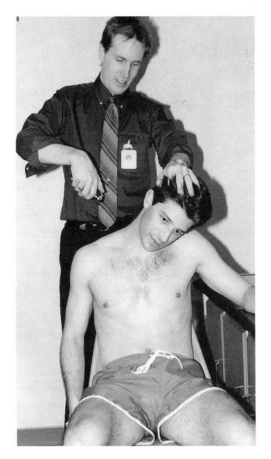

Fig. 5.16: Vapocoolant sprays temporarily freeze superficial tissues and aid the clinician in reducing the pain-spasm cycle prior to stretching exercises.

Contrast baths combine cryotherapy and thermotherapy in subacute or chronic injuries to reduce edema and restore range of motion

Diathermy can decrease joint stiffness, pain, muscle spasm, and facilitate healing of soft tissue injuries in the postacute stage

may accelerate the rate of heat transfer leading to burns on sensitive skin. After 5 minutes of treatment, the area should be checked for any redness or signs of burning.

Paraffin Baths

Paraffin baths provide heat to contoured bony areas of the body (feet, hands, or wrists). A paraffin and mineral oil mixture (8:1 ratio) is heated in a unit at 47.0 to 54.4° C (125 to 130° F) (27). The body part is thoroughly cleansed and all jewelry removed. The body part is then dipped into the bath several times, each time allowing the previous coat to dry. Outer layers of paraffin should not extend over new skin, as burning may occur. When completed, the body part is wrapped in a plastic bag and towel to maintain heat, then elevated for 15 to 20 minutes (**Figure 5-19**). When treatment is completed, the wax is peeled off and returned to the bath where it can be reused. The mineral oil in the wax helps keep skin soft and pliable during massage when treating a variety of hand and foot conditions.

Contrast Baths

Contrast baths combine cryotherapy and thermotherapy in subacute or chronic injuries to reduce edema and restore range of motion. Two whirlpools or containers are placed next to each other. One is filled with cold water and ice at 10 to 18° C (50 to 65° F), and the other is filled with hot water at 37 to 44° C (98.6 to 111° F) (27). The injured extremity is alternated between the two tubs at a 3:1 or 4:1 ratio (hot water to cold water) for approximately 20 minutes. The treatment begins and ends in cold water prior to starting therapeutic exercise in subacute conditions. In chronic conditions, treatment is more often concluded in warm immersion.

Diathermy

Diathermy uses electromagnetic energy to elicit deep penetrating thermal effects. This modality can decrease joint stiffness, pain, muscle spasm, and facilitate healing of soft tissue injuries in the postacute stage. The depth of penetration and extent of heat pro-

Table 5–5. Thermotherapy Application.	
Indications	**Contraindications**
Subacute or chronic injuries to:	Acute inflammation or injuries
Reduce swelling, edema and ecchymosis	Impaired or poor circulation
Reduce muscle spasm/guarding	Subacute or chronic pain
Increase blood flow to:	Impaired or poor sensation
Increase ROM prior to activity	Impaired thermal regulation
Resolve hematoma	Malignancy
Increase tissue healing	Patients, either elderly or infants who
Relieve joint contractures	cannot report their reactions
Fight infection	

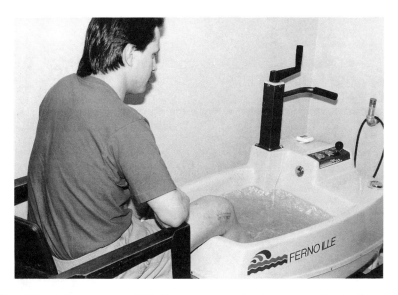

Fig. 5.17: Hot whirlpools increase superficial skin temperatures leading to an analgesic effect which can reduce muscle spasm and pain, facilitate range of motion exercises, and promote healing.

Field Strategy 5–12. Techniques for Using a Whirlpool Bath.

Indications	Contraindications
Subacute and chronic inflammation	Acute injuries
Peripheral nerve injuries	Fever
Peripheral vascular injuries	Certain skin conditions
Increase range of motion	

Inspect the electrical system. To avoid electrical surges, make sure that ground-fault circuit breakers are used in the electrical outlet or are in the circuit-breaker box

Apply a povidone-iodine (Betadine) additive, or a 5% bleach (Dakin's) solution to the water as an antibacterial agent, especially if anyone has an open wound

Recommended temperature and treatment time include:

Cold whirlpools	55 to 65°F	5 to 15 mins
Hot whirlpools		
Extremity	98 to 110°F	20 to 30 mins
Full body	98 to 102°F	10 to 12 mins

Assist the patient into the water and provide towels for padding and drying off

Turn the turbine on and adjust the height to direct the water flow 6 to 8 inches away from the injury site

Instruct the patient to move the body part through the available range of motion. This will increase blood flow to the area, aid in removal of debris, and improve proprioception

Turn the turbine off and remove the patient from the water. Dry the treated area and assist the individual from the whirlpool area

Drain and cleanse the whirlpool tub after each use

Cultures for bacterial and fungal agents should be conducted monthly from water samples in the whirlpool turbine and drain

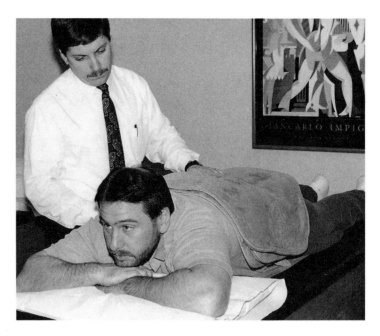

Fig. 5.18: Moist heat treatments can produce burns to sensitive skin. To avoid this, place the hydrocollator pack in a commercial padded towel, or six to eight layers of towel and periodically check the skin surface for any redness or signs of burning.

duction depends on wave frequency, the electrical properties of the tissues receiving the energy, and the type of applicator used (27). There are two forms of diathermy: shortwave and microwave.

Shortwave diathermy uses a pulsed high-frequency current at 27.12 MHz per second. There are two methods for heating. One places two condensor plates on either side of the injured area, thus placing the patient in the electrical circuit. The other method uses an induction coil wrapped around the body part that places the patient in an electromagnetic field. Tissues with a high fluid content, such as skeletal muscle and areas surrounding joints, absorb more of the energy and are heated to a greater extent, whereas fat is not heated as much (26,27). Because the applicators are not in contact with the skin, shortwave diathermy can be used for heating skeletal muscle when the skin is abraded, as long as edema is not present (26).

Microwave diathermy relies upon a specialized amplifying component called a magnetron to apply a high-oscillating electrical current at 2,450 megacycles per second. The electromagnetic energy is also absorbed in tissues with a high fluid content. The amount of heating in deep structures is diminished with increasing depth, however. Any moisture on the skin should be removed, as superficial structures can receive excessive radiation,

causing blistered skin and burns to the underlying fat tissue (27). In addition, no metal can be in or near the electrical fields, neither internal (surgical implants) nor external (jewelry, watches, tables, or stools). Dosage for both shortwave and microwave diathermy is determined by the patient's feeling a warming, but not excessively hot, sensation. Treatment time is usually 20 minutes.

Ultrasound

Ultrasound uses high frequency sound waves to elicit thermal and nonthermal effects in deep tissue. Thermal effects elevate tissue temperature and are used to increase collagen tissue extensibility, blood flow, sensory and motor nerve conduction velocity, enzymatic activity, and to reduce muscle spasm and pain. Nonthermal effects caused by the mechanical effect of ultrasound increase cell membrane and vascular wall permeability, blood flow, tissue regeneration, synthesis of protein, and reduction of edema (10,27). Ultrasound is used to manage several soft tissue conditions, such as tendinitis, bursitis, muscle spasm, calcium deposits in soft tissue, and to reduce joint contractures, pain, and scar tissue. **Table 5-6** lists indications and contraindications for ultrasound.

Ultrasound waves are applied in a pulsed wave or continuous mode. Pulsed ultrasound

Ultrasound uses high frequency sound waves to elicit thermal and nonthermal effects in deep tissues

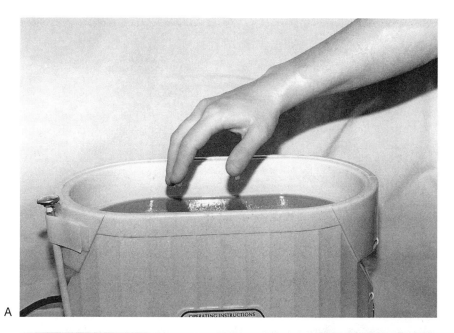

A

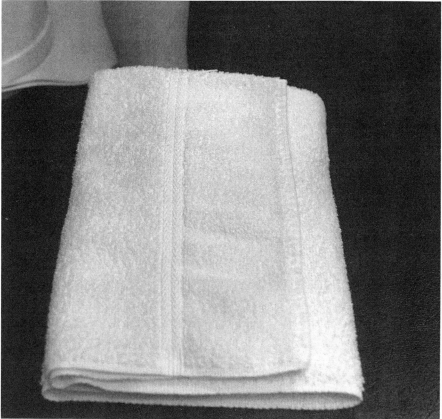

B

Fig. 5.19: In a paraffin-bath treatment, the limb is thoroughly cleansed and dipped several times into the solution (A). The limb is then wrapped in plastic and towel to maintain heat (B).

or low intensity continuous ultrasound produce primarily nonthermal effects and are used to facilitate repair and healing when a high increase in tissue temperature is not desired. Continuous ultrasound provides both thermal and nonthermal effects and is used when a deep elevated tissue temperature is advisable. Sound wave intensity is expressed in watts per square centimeter (W/cm^2). In a clinical setting, intensities range from 0.25 to 3.0 W/cm^2. The greater the intensity, the greater the resulting temperature elevation.

Table 5–6. Ultrasound Application.

Indications	Contraindications
Increase deep tissue heating	Acute and postacute hemorrhage
Decrease inflammation and resolve hematomas	Infection
Decrease muscle spasm/spasticity	Thrombophlebitis
Decrease pain	Over suspected malignancy/cancer
Increase extensibility of collagen tissue	Areas of impaired circulation or sensation
Decrease pain of neuromas	Over stress fracture sites
Decrease joint adhesions and/or joint contractures	Over epiphyseal growth plates
Postacute myositis ossificans	Over the eyes, heart, spine, or genitals
Plantar warts	Over pelvic area in pregnant or menstruating person

Cavitation
Gas bubble formation due to nonthermal effects of ultrasound

Phonophoresis
The introduction of anti-inflammatory drugs through the skin with ultrasound

Anesthetic
A drug or agent that leads to an inability to perceive pain and/or other sensations

Analgesic
A drug or agent that reduces the response to pain, and is usually accompanied by sedation without loss of consciousness

Salicylate
Any salt of salicylic acid; used in aspirin

Neuromuscular electrical stimulation (NMES) can relieve pain; reduce swelling, muscle spasm and atrophy; increase blood flow, range of motion, and muscle strength; enhance wound healing; re-educate muscle; and through iontophoresis, introduce anti-inflammatory, analgesic, or anesthetic drugs to an injured area.

Thermal temperature can increase 7 to 8° F up to a depth of 5 cm (27). Ultrasound waves are absorbed in tissues highest in collagen content and reflected at tissue interfaces, particularly between bone and muscle. The greater the intensity, the greater the resulting temperature elevation (27). Treatment time is 5 to 10 minutes over a 3- to 4-square inch area. Research has shown that low wattage pulsed ultrasound used on tendons on the 2nd and 4th days after surgery can increase tensile strength of tendons, however, after the 5th day, application decreases tensile strength (8).

Because ultrasound waves cannot travel through air, a coupling agent is used between the transducer head and tissue to facilitate passage of the waves. Coupling gels are applied liberally over the area to be treated. The transducer head is then stroked slowly over the area (**Figure 5-20**). Strokes are applied in small continuous circles or longitudinal patterns to distribute the energy as evenly as possible, and to prevent **cavitation** (gas bubble formation) in deep tissues (27). An alternate method for irregularly shaped areas, such as the wrist, hand, ankle, or foot is application under water. Intensity is increased .5 W/cm^2 to compensate for air and minerals in the water (10). Intensity for both gel and underwater treatment is determined by the stage of injury, mode used (pulsed or continuous), and desired depth of penetration. The patient should feel a mild, warm sensation.

Phonophoresis

Phonophoresis is a technique, whereby ultrasound is used to drive anti-inflammatory drugs, such as a 10 percent hydrocortisone ointment, **anesthetics**, such as lidocaine, or **analgesics**, such as **salicylates** through the skin to the underlying tissues. One advantage of this modality is that the drug is delivered directly to the site where the effect is sought (10,27). This technique is used in the postacute stage in conditions such as tendinitis, bursitis, or contusions. The standard coupling gel is replaced by a gel or cream containing the medication. Treatment occurs at a lower intensity (1 to 1.5 W/cm^2) for 5 to 15 minutes.

Neuromuscular Electrical Stimulation

Neuromuscular electrical stimulation (NMES) is used to relieve pain; reduce swelling, muscle spasm and atrophy; increase blood flow, range of motion, and muscle strength; enhance wound healing; reeducate muscle; and through iontophoresis, introduce anti-inflammatory, analgesic, or anesthetic drugs to an injured area (26,29,30). Electrical stimulation can be applied to injured or immobilized muscles in the early stages of exercise when the muscle is at its weakest (8). To understand how electrical stimulation is clinically used, you must review the basic principles of electricity.

Electrical energy flows between two points. In an atom, protons are positively charged, electrons are negatively charged, and neutrons have no charge. Equal numbers of protons and electrons produce a balanced neutrality in the atom. To transfer energy from one atom to the next, only electrons are moved from the nucleus, creating an electrical imbalance. This subtraction and addition of electrons causes atoms to become electrically charged, and the atom is then called an ion. An ion that has more electrons is said to be negatively charged; an ion with more protons is positively charged. Ions of similar charge repel one another, whereas ions of dissimilar charge attract one

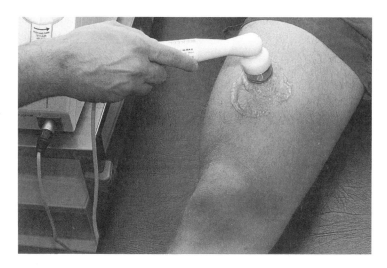

Fig. 5.20: In an ultrasound treatment, a coupling agent is used between the transducer head and area being treated. The head is moved in small circles or longitudinal strokes to distribute the energy as evenly as possible, and to prevent damage to the underlying tissues.

another (26). The strength of the force and distance between the ions determines how quickly the transfer of energy occurs.

Voltage is the force that causes ions to move. The actual movement is called **current**. Current intensity is measured in amperes, with 1 ampere (amp) equal to the rate of 1 coulomb of electrons moving past a specific point in 1 second. Voltage and current are proportional, in that high voltage produces a high movement of ions, representing a high current flow. Mediums that facilitate movement of the ions are called conductors and include water, blood, and electrolyte solutions such as sweat. Mediums that inhibit movement of the ions are called resistors and include skin, fat, and lotion. The combination of voltage, current, and resistance is measured in ohms. Ohm's law (I = V/R) states that current (I) in a conductor increases as the driving force (V) becomes larger, or resistance (R) is decreased (26).

Three types of electrical current can be applied to tissues: direct, alternating, and pulsed **(Figure 5-21)**. Direct current (DC), or galvanic current, is a continuous one-directional flow of ions. Alternating current (AC), or faradic current, is a continuous two-directional flow of ions. Pulsed current is a flow of ions in direct or alternating current that is briefly interrupted periodically, and may be one-directional or two-directional depending on the type of current used (26). In therapeutic use each current can be manipulated by altering the frequency, intensity, and duration of the wave or pulse.

Electrical currents are introduced into the body through electrodes and a conducting medium. At the positive electrode, called an **anode**, positive ions are repelled and negative ions attracted. At the negative electrode, called a **cathode**, the negative ions are repelled and positive ions attracted. Water or

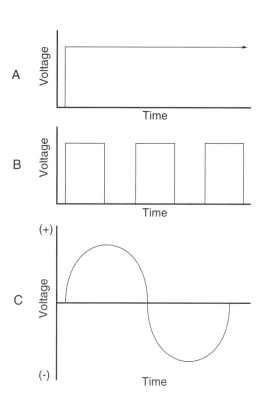

Fig. 5.21: Graphic drawing of the three types of electrical current. (A) Direct current. (B) Alternating current. (C) Pulse currents.

Voltage
The force that causes ions to move

Current
The actual movement of ions

Mediums that facilitate movement of ions are called conductors; mediums that inhibit movement of ions are called resistors

Anode
Positively charged electrode in a direct current system

Cathode
Negatively charged electrode in a direct current system

an electrolyte gel are used because of their high conductive values. When the current reaches a certain magnitude, called the threshold, ions are transferred through nerve and muscle fibers to cause an electrical impulse or muscle contraction. This is called the all-or-none response, and is not dependent on the strength of the stimulus. Modalities using therapeutic electricity principles are high voltage electrical stimulators which can be used with iontophoresis, interferential current, and transcutaneous electrical nerve stimulation (TENS). **Table 5-7** lists indications and contraindications for the electrical modalities.

High Voltage Electrical Stimulation

High voltage electrical stimulation uses an output between 100V to 500V to reduce edema, pain, and muscle spasm during the acute phase (28,30). It is also used to exercise

muscle to maintain muscle size and strength during periods of immobilization, to re-educate muscles, and increase blood flow to tissues (**Figure 5-22**). Direct current is used primarily to stimulate denervated muscle, enhance wound healing, and during iontophoresis (26).

Iontophoresis

Iontophoresis uses direct current to drive charged molecules from certain medications, such as anti-inflammatories (hydrocortisone), anesthetics (lidocaine), or analgesics (aspirin or acetaminophen) into damaged tissue. The polarity of the medication determines which electrode is used to drive the molecules into the skin. The medication is placed under the electrode with the same polarity. When the current is applied, the molecules are pushed away from the electrode and driven into the skin toward the injured site. This localized

Table 5–7. Application of Neuromuscular Electrical Stimulation.

High Voltage EMS	Indications	Contraindications
	Increase circulation and ROM	Patients with pacemakers
	Decrease pain and edema	Pain of unknown origin
	Denervate peripheral nerve injuries	Pregnancy (abdominal and/or pelvic area)
	Decrease muscle spasm/spasticity	Thrombophlebitis
	Facilitate nonunion fracture healing	Superficial skin lesions or infections
	Delay disuse atrophy	Cancerous lesions
	Muscle strengthening and re-education	Over suspected fracture sites
Low voltage EMS	**Indications**	**Contraindications**
	Facilitate nonunion wound healing	Malignancy
	Facilitate fracture healing	Hypersensitive skin
	Iontophoresis	Allergies to certain drugs
TENS	**Indications**	**Contraindications**
	Reduce post traumatic and chronic pain	Patients with pacemakers
	Manage postsurgical pain	Pregnancy (abdominal and/or pelvic area)
	Analgesia	Pain of unknown origin
Interferential	**Indications**	**Contraindications**
	Posttraumatic and chronic edema	Patients with pacemakers
	Acute and chronic pain	Pregnancy (abdominal and/or pelvic area)
	Increase circulation	Pain of unknown origin
	Reduce muscle spasm/guarding	Prolonged use may increase muscle soreness or spasm
	Aid in healing chronic wounds	
	Relieve abdominal organ dysfunction	

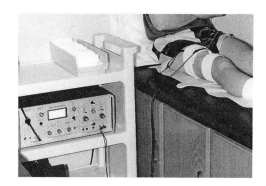

Fig. 5.22: Electrical muscle stimulation is used to exercise muscle to maintain muscle size and strength during immobilization, re-educate muscles, prevent muscle atrophy, and increase blood flow to tissues to decrease pain and spasm.

treatment is often preferred over more disruptive systemic treatments.

Interferential Current

Interferential current utilizes two separate generators and a quadripolar electrode arrangement to produce two simultaneous electrical currents acting on the tissues. The two paired pads are placed in a diagonal pattern (**Figure 5-23**). Currents range from 1000 to 10,000 Hz, with the paired pads differing from each other by about 100 to 200 Hz (26,31). The higher currents lower skin resistance, thus eliciting a stronger response with less current intensity. Furthermore, sensory perception is decreased between the pads allowing for a higher current to be used leading to increased stimulation. This modality is used to decrease pain, acute and chronic edema, muscle spasm, strengthen weakened muscles, improve blood flow to an area, heal chronic wounds, and relieve abdominal organ dysfunction (26,29,31).

Transcutaneous Electrical Nerve Stimulation (TENS)

TENS is used to produce analgesia and decrease acute and chronic pain, and is often used continuously after surgery, or in a 30 to 60 minute session several times a day (26,29). It is thought that TENS works to override the body's internal signals of pain (gate theory of pain), and stimulates the release of endomorphins, a strong opiate-like substance produced by the body. The unit utilizes small carbonized silicone electrodes to transmit electrical pulses through the skin (**Figure 5-**

24). Most units are small enough to be worn on a belt and are battery powered. The electrodes are taped on the skin over or around the painful site, but may be secured along the peripheral or spinal nerve pathways. For individuals who have allergic reactions to the tape adhesive or who develop skin abrasions from repeated applications, electrodes with a self-adhering adhesive are available.

Intermittent Compression Units

Intermittent compression uses compression and elevation to decrease blood flow to an extremity and assist venous return, thus decreasing edema. A boot or sleeve is applied around the injured extremity. Compression is formed when air or cold water inflates and deflates the unit intermittently for 20 to 30 minutes, several times a day (**Figure 5-25**). During deflation, the patient can do active range of motion exercises to enhance blood flow to the injured area. **Table 5-8** lists indications and contraindications for intermittent compression.

Continuous Passive Motion (CPM)

Continuous passive motion is a modality that applies an external force to move the joint

> Intermittent compression decreases blood flow to an extremity and assists in venous return, thus decreasing edema

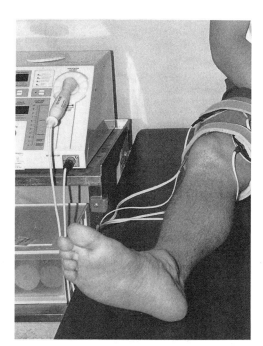

> TENS is used to produce analgesia and decrease all levels of pain

Fig. 5.23: Interferential current is used to decrease pain, acute and chronic edema, muscle spasm, strengthen weakened muscles, improve blood flow to an area, and heal chronic wounds.

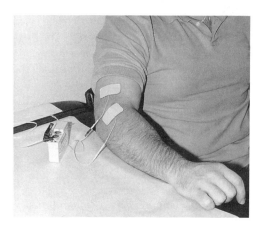

Fig. 5.24: Transcutaneous Electrical Nerve Stimulation (TENS) is used to decrease acute and chronic pain to an injured area.

through a limited range of motion (**Figure 5-26**). It is primarily used post-surgically at the knee, after knee manipulation, or after stable fixation of intra-articular and extra-articular fractures of most joints. The application is relatively pain-free and has been shown to stimulate the intrinsic healing process, maintain articular cartilage nutrition, reduce disuse effects, retard joint stiffness and the pain-spasm cycle, and benefit collagen remodeling, joint dynamics, and pain reduction (10,32). **Table 5-8** lists indications and contraindications for use of continuous passive motion.

Massage

Soft tissue massage is an excellent means to increase cutaneous circulation, cell metabolism, venous and lymphatic flow to assist in the removal of edema, stretch superficial scar

tissue and decrease neuromuscular excitability (10). To reduce friction between the patient's skin and hand, particularly over hairy areas, lubricants are often used, i.e., massage lotion, peanut oil, coconut oil, or powder. Gentle massage can be initiated in the acute phase, however, it is typically used in phase two of the therapeutic exercise program. Friction massage performed at right angles to the involved tissue is used to loosen adherent fibrous tissue (scar), aid in absorption of edema, and reduce localized muscular spasm.

Massage over a larger area involves effleurage, pétrissage, tapotement, and vibration to treat muscle, tendon, and joint conditions. Effleurage, or stroking, relaxes the patient, and when applied toward the heart, reduces swelling and aids venous return. Pétrissage, or kneading, consists of pressing and rolling the muscles under the fingers and hands. This increases venous and lymphatic return, and removes metabolic waste products from the injured area. Furthermore, it breaks up adhesions within the underlying tissues, loosens fibrous tissue, and increases elasticity of the skin (10). Tapotement, or percussion, uses sharp alternating hand movements to increase blood flow and stimulate peripheral nerve endings. Hacking, slapping, beating, cupping, and clapping are various techniques used. Vibration uses finite movement of the fingers to vibrate the underlying tissues. **Field Strategy 5-13** lists techniques, indications, contraindications, and mode of application for therapeutic massage.

Medications

Therapeutic drugs are either prescription or over-the-counter medications used to treat

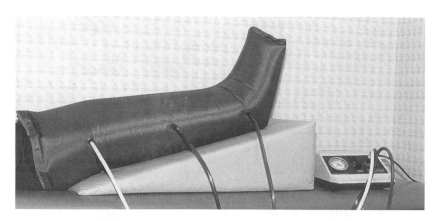

Fig. 5.25: An air-filled boot or sleeve can provide pressure or intermittent compression to an injured area to decrease edema.

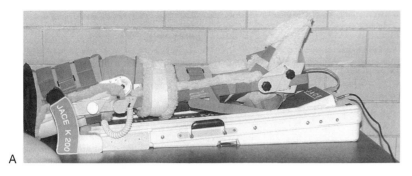

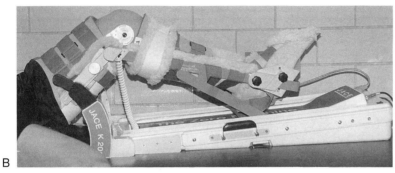

Fig. 5.26: Continuous passive motion machines are often used postsurgically to apply an external force to move the joint through a limited range of motion. (A) Starting position. (B) Ending position.

an injury or illness. Common drugs used to control pain, inflammation, and muscle spasm include anesthetics, analgesics, nonsteroidal anti-inflammatory drugs (NSAIDs), adrenocorticosteroids, and muscle relaxants.

Local anesthetics eliminate short-term pain sensation in a specific body part or region by blocking afferent (sensory) neural transmissions along peripheral nerves. These drugs can be identified by their "-caine" suffix (i.e., lidocaine, procaine, and benzocaine). The drugs may be topically applied to skin for minor irritations (burns, abrasions, mild inflammation), introduced into subcutaneous

> Local anesthetics produce analgesia and short-term pain relief in a body part by blocking afferent neural transmissions along peripheral nerves.

Table 5–8. Application of Intermittent Compression and Continuous Passive Motion (CPM).

Intermittent compression	Indications	Contraindications
	Acute hemorrhage/edema	Circulatory impairment
	Acute inflammation and pain	Possible fracture site
	Postsurgical edema	Compartment syndrome
	Swelling of the lymph nodes	Peripheral vascular disease

CPM	Indications	Contraindications
	Postoperative rehabilitation to:	Noncompliant patient
	Reduce pain	If use would disrupt surgical
	Improve general circulation	repair, fracture fixation, or lead
	Enhance joint nutrition	to hemorrhage in postoperative
	Prevent joint contractures	period
	Benefit collagen remodeling	Malfunction of device
	Following knee manipulation	
	Following joint débridement	
	Following meniscal or osteochondral repair	
	Tendon lacerations	

Field Strategy 5–13. Techniques Used in Therapeutic Massage.

Indications	Contraindications
Increase local circulation	Acute contusions, sprains, and strains
Increase venous and lymphatic flow	Over fracture sites
Reduce pain (analgesia)	Over open lesions or skin conditions
Reduce muscle spasm	Conditions such as: acute phlebitis, thrombosis, severe
Stretch superficial scar tissue	varicose veins, cellulitis, synovitis, arteriosclerosis, and
Improve systemic relaxation	cancer
Chronic myositis, bursitis, tendinitis, tenosynovitis, fibrositis	

Technique	Use	Method of Application
Effleurage (stroking)	Relaxes patient	Gliding motion over the skin without any attempt to move deep muscles
	Evenly distributes any lubricant	Apply pressure with the flat of the hand, fingers and thumbs spread, stroke toward the heart
	Increases surface circulation	Massage begins and ends with stroking
Pétrissage (kneading)	Increases circulation	Kneading manipulation that grasps and rolls the muscles under the fingers or hands
	Promotes venous and lymphatic return	
	Breaks up adhesions in superficial connective tissue	
	Increases elasticity of skin	
Tapotement (percussion)	Increases circulation	Brisk blows in rapid succession with hand:
	Stimulates subcutaneous structures	hacking—with ulnar border slapping—with flat hand beating—with half-closed fist tapping—with finger tips cupping—with arched hand
Vibration	Relaxes limb	Fine vibrations made with fingers pressed into a specific body part
Friction (rubbing)	Loosens fibrous scar tissue	Small circular motions with the fingers, thumb or heel of the hand
	Aids in absorption of edema	Transverse friction is done
	Reduces inflammation	perpendicularly to the fibers being
	Reduces muscular spasm	massaged.

Antipyresis
Action whereby body temperature associated with a fever is reduced

tissues via phonophoresis or iontophoresis (bursitis, tendinitis, contusions), injected by a physician into soft tissue around a laceration for surgical repair (suturing), or injected by a physician near a peripheral nerve to interrupt nerve transmission (nerve block) (33).

Analgesics and nonsteroidal anti-inflammatory drugs (NSAIDs) are commonly used to vasodilate blood vessels and inhibit production of prostaglandins. Certain prostaglandins increase local blood flow, capillary permeabil-ity, erythema, and edema associated with inflammation, and are believed to increase the sensitivity of pain receptors to the effects of other pain producing substances, such as bradykinin (8,33). Therefore, these drugs decrease inflammation, relieve mild to moderate pain (analgesia), decrease body temperature associated with fever (**antipyresis**), increase collagen strength, and inhibit coagulation and blood clotting. The most important time to administer NSAIDs is during the early stages of healing when prostaglandins produce the most detrimental effects of pain and edema (8). Prolonged use (2 or more weeks) may actually retard the healing process. Examples of analgesics and NSAIDs include aspirin (acetylsalicylic acid), acetaminophen (Tylenol), ibuprofen (Advil, Nuprin, Motrin), diflunicsal (Dolobid), Indocin, Butazolidin, Feldene, and Clinoril.

Acetaminophen reduces pain and fever, but does not have any appreciable anti-inflammatory or anticoagulant effects. Unlike aspirin, acetaminophen is not associated with gastrointestinal irritation. However, high doses can be toxic to the liver and may be fatal (33).

Aspirin is the most commonly used drug to relieve pain and inflammation. Because of its anticoagulant properties, it is not used during the acute phase. Aspirin is associated with a number of adverse side effects including gastrointestinal irritation. Stomach distress can be limited by coating the aspirin to delay release of the drug until it reaches the small intestine, or by taking a buffered aspirin to blunt the acidic effects of aspirin in the stomach. With chronic use or high doses (10 to 30 grams), renal problems, liver toxicity, congestive heart failure, hypertension, aspirin intoxication or poisoning may occur (11). Normal dosage is 325 to 650 mg every 4 hr.

Ibuprofen and the other NSAIDs are administered primarily for pain relief and anti-inflammatory effects. However, they are more expensive than aspirin. Although many are still associated with some stomach discomfort, they provide better effects in some patients. Taking the medication after a meal or with a glass of milk or water will greatly reduce stomach discomfort.

Adrenocorticosteroids are steroid hormones produced by the adrenal cortex. Higher doses, referred to as a pharmacological dose, are typically used to treat endocrine disorders, but can be used to decrease edema, inflammation, erythema, and tenderness in a region, or as an immunosuppressant in nonendocrine disorders. These drugs may be topically applied, given orally, or injected by a physician into a specific area, such as a tendon or joint (33). Examples of these drugs include cortisone, prednisone, and hydrocortisone. Because many of these drugs can lead to breakdown and rupture of structures, long-term use is contraindicated.

Skeletal muscle relaxants are used to relieve muscle spasms. Muscle spasms can result from certain musculoskeletal injuries or inflammation. When involuntary tension in the muscle cannot be relaxed, it leads to intense pain and a buildup of pain-mediating metabolites (e.g., lactate) (33). A vicious cycle is created with the increased pain leading to more spasm, more pain, more spasm, and so on. Skeletal muscle relaxants break the pain-spasm cycle by depressing tonic and somatic motor activity at the brain stem, thus reducing muscle excitability. Muscle relaxants do not prevent muscle contraction, but rather attempt to normalize muscle excitability to decrease pain and improve motor function (33). Examples of muscle relaxants include Flexeril, Soma, and Dantrium.

After reading this section, did you determine that NSAIDs, cryotherapy, intermittent compression, EMS, and TENs can be used in the early phases of healing? Thermotherapy, cryotherapy, ultrasound, and EMS can be used in the later stages of repair. What can the tennis player do at home to assist treatments provided in the athletic training room or clinic setting?

NUTRITION

Think for a minute or two about how nutrition can influence the repair and healing process of damaged tissue. Can an individual return to peak performance without the necessary energy sources?

Proper nutrition for an active individual is essential to provide the necessary nutrients to perform work. In addition, extended inactivity can result in a slight weight gain placing additional stress on injured joint structures. This factor adds strength to initiating cardiovascular endurance activities as soon as possible if only designed to burn calories.

After cellular injury, energy and protein metabolism increase due to hormonal changes, and is often depicted as an *ebb and flow pattern*. Initially in the *ebb*, circulatory insufficiency of protein and energy is seen. This is followed by the *flow*, an increased metabolism or hypermetabolic state coupled with depletion of body protein within 24 to 48 hours after injury (34).

Carbohydrates are the main energy fuel for the body. In addition, the brain uses blood glucose almost exclusively as its fuel and does not have a stored supply of this nutrient. Although fat does provide a large store of potential energy, and serves as a cushion to protect the vital organs and provide thermal

Adenocorticosteroids decrease edema, inflammation, erythema, and tenderness in a region insulation, it has little function in wound healing. Proteins serve a vital role in the maintenance, repair, and growth of body tissues. When carbohydrate reserves are low, the synthesis of glucose will draw upon protein or the glycerol portion of fat, thus further draining the body's protein "stores," especially muscle protein. In extreme conditions, this can lead to a reduction in lean tissue and place an excessive load on the kidneys as they excrete the nitrogen-containing byproducts of protein breakdown (9). Without an adequate carbohydrate and protein intake, repair and healing of damaged tissues will be prolonged.

Vitamins also play an important role in wound healing. Riboflavin (vitamin B_2), pyridoxine (vitamin B_6), pantothenic acid, folacin, and vitamin B_{12} all aid in energy metabolism. Vitamin C maintains the intercellular matrix of cartilage, bone, and dentine, and is required for collagen secretion. A lack of Vitamin C can result in deficient wound healing evident in inferior vascularization and scanty collagen deposition. Vitamin A is necessary to maintain epithelial tissue, and Vitamin D promotes growth and mineralization of bones, and aids in the absorption of calcium. Vitamin E prevents cell-membrane damage, and Vitamin K is essential in blood clotting (9).

Calcium also aids in blood clotting, and, coupled with sodium, is necessary for proper nerve function. Zinc is also known to promote faster healing (35). Water is essential to transport nutrients, control thermoregulation, and aid in metabolic reactions (9).

The U.S. Department of Agriculture (USDA) has adopted a food guide pyramid to replace the traditional four food groups. It is now recommended that a diet should be high in fruits, vegetables, and grains, and low in fat and sugar **(Figure 5-27)**. The pyramid includes 6 to 11 daily servings in the bread, cereal, rice and pasta group; 2 to 4 servings in the fruit group; 3 to 5 servings of vegetables; 2 to 3 servings in the milk, yogurt, and cheese group; 2 to 3 servings of meat, poultry, fish, dry beans, eggs, and nuts group; and limited use of fats, oils, and sweets (36). Under normal circumstances, this diet should provide an adequate source of carbohydrates, protein, fat, vitamins, minerals and water to promote wound healing and prevent unnecessary weight gain. Dietary supplements are not necessary if the individual's diet is nutritionally balanced.

An injured individual must have an adequate diet that provides the nutrients necessary to enhance wound healing. In addition, a diet high in carbohydrates should supply the energy necessary to compete on a highly competitive level.

SUMMARY

Rehabilitation begins immediately after injury assessment. The level of function and dysfunction is assessed, results are organized and interpreted, a list of patient problems is formulated, long- and short-term goals are established, and a course of action is developed including therapeutic exercises, modalities, and medications. The program is then supervised and periodically reassessed with appropriate changes made.

Phase one of the therapeutic exercise program should focus on patient education and control of inflammation, muscle spasm, and pain. Phase two should regain any deficits in active and passive range of motion at the affected joint as compared to the unaffected joint. Phase three should regain muscular strength, endurance, and power in the affected limb. Phase four prepares the individual to return to activity and includes analysis of motion, sport-specific skill training, regaining coordination, and cardiovascular conditioning. Throughout the total therapeutic exercise program, nutritional and psychological needs of the injured individual should be addressed.

Therapeutic modalities including cryotherapy, thermotherapy, electrical stimulation, intermittent compression, continuous passive motion, massage, and medications can supplement the exercise program to control inflammation and enhance healing. At the conclusion of the exercise program, the supervising physician will determine if the individual is ready to return to full activity. This decision should be based on review of the individual's range of motion, flexibility, muscular strength, endurance, power, biomechanical skill analysis, coordination, and cardiovascular endurance. If additional protective bracing, padding, or taping is necessary to enable the individual to return safely to activity, this should be documented in the individual's file. In addition, it should be stressed that use of any protective device should not replace a maintenance program of condition-

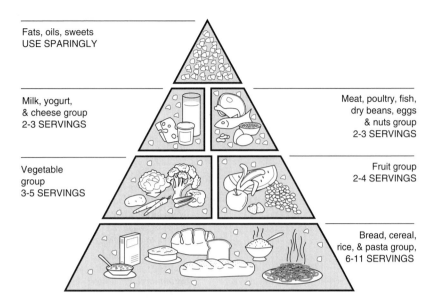

Fig. 5.27: The US Department of Agriculture (USDA) now recommends a diet high in fruits, vegetables, and grains, and low in fat and sugar.

ing exercises. Year-round conditioning can prevent many injuries from recurring.

The athletic trainer and sport supervisor can keep a watchful eye on the individual as the person gradually re-enters activity. If the individual begins to show signs of pain, swelling, discomfort, or skill performance deteriorates, the individual should be re-evaluated to determine if activity should continue or the therapeutic exercise program needs to be reinstituted.

REFERENCES

1. Kubler-Ross, E. *On death and dying*. New York: MacMillan, 1969.
2. O'Sullivan, SB. "Clinical decision making: Planning effective treatments." In *Physical rehabilitation: Assessment and treatment*, edited by SB O'Sullivan and TJ Schmitz. Philadelphia: FA Davis, 1988.
3. DePalma, MT, and DePalma, B. 1989. The use of instruction and the behavioral approach to facilitate injury rehabilitation. Ath Tr (JNATA), 24(3):217–219.
4. Prentice, WE. *Rehabilitation techniques in sports medicine*. St. Louis: Times Mirror/Mosby College, 1994.
5. Harrelson, GL. "Introduction to rehabilitation." In *Physical rehabilitation of the injured athlete*, edited by JR Andrews and GL Harrelson. Philadelphia: WB Saunders, 1991.
6. Knight, KL. *Cryotherapy, theory, technique, and physiology*. Chattanooga: Chattanooga Corporation, 1985.
7. Wilkerson, GB. 1985. External compression for controlling traumatic edema. Phys Sportsmed 13(6):97–106.
8. Houglum, PA. 1992. Soft tissue healing and its impact on rehabilitation. J Sport Rehab, 1(1):19–39.
9. McArdle, WD, Katch FI, and Katch, VL. *Exercise physiology: Energy, nutrition, and human performance*. Philadelphia: Lea & Febiger, 1991.
10. Starkey, C. *Therapeutic modalities for athletic trainers*. Philadelphia: FA Davis, 1993.
11. Kisner, C, and Colby, LA. *Therapeutic exercise: Foundations and techniques*. Philadelphia: FA Davis, 1990.
12. Voss, DE, Ionta, MK, and Myers, BJ. *Proprioceptive neuromuscular facilitation: Patterns and techniques*. Philadelphia: Harper & Row, 1985.
13. Nelson, KC, and Cornelius, WL. 1991. The relationship between isometric contraction durations and improvement in shoulder joint range of motion. J Sports Med Phys Fitness, 31(3):385–388.
14. Knight, KL. 1979. Rehabilitating chondromalacia patellae. Phys Sportsmed, 7(10):147–148.
15. Perrin, DH. *Isokinetic exercise and assessment*. Champaign, IL: Human Kinetics, 1993.
16. Gould, JA, and Davies, GJ. "Orthopaedic and sports rehabilitation concepts." In *Orthopaedic and sports physical therapy*, edited by JA Gould and GJ Davies. St. Louis: CV Mosby, 1990.
17. IOC Medical Commission. 1991. Terminology and units of measurement for the description of exercise and sport. J Appl Spt Sci Res, 5(2):108.
18. Hall, SJ. *Basic biomechanics*. St. Louis: Mosby-Year, 1991.
19. Radcliffe, JC, and Farentino, RC. *Plyometrics*. Champaign, IL, Human Kinetics, 1985.

20. Norkin, CC, and Levangie, PK. *Joint structure & function: A comprehensive analysis*. Philadelphia: FA Davis, 1989.

21. Albert, MS. "Principles of exercise progression." In *Rehabilitation of the knee: A problem-solving approach*, edited by BH Greenfield. Philadelphia: FA Davis, 1993.

22. Stone, JA, Lueken, JS, Partin, NB, Timm, KE, and Ryan, EJ. 1993. Closed kinetic chain rehabilitation for the glenohumeral joint. J Ath Tr, 28(1):34–37.

23. Schmitz, TJ. "Coordination assessment." In *Physical rehabilitation: Assessment and treatment*, edited by SB O'Sullivan and TJ Schmitz. Philadelphia: FA Davis, 1988.

24. American College of Sports Medicine. 1990. The recommended quantity and quality of exercise for developing and maintaining cardiorespiratory and muscular fitness in healthy adults. Sports Med Bull, 13(3):1–4.

25. Halvorson, GA. 1990. Therapeutic heat and cold for athletic injuries. Phys Sportsmed, 18(5):87–94.

26. Cooper, M. "Use of modalities in rehabilitation." In *Physical rehabilitation of the injured athlete*, edited by JR Andrews and GL Harrelson. Philadelphia: WB Saunders, 1991.

27. Michlovitz, SL. "Cryotherapy: The use of cold as a therapeutic agent." In *Thermal agents in rehabilitation*, edited by SL Michlovitz. Philadelphia: FA Davis, 1990.

28. Leadbetter, WB, Buckwalter, JA, and Gordon, SL. *Sports-induced inflammation*. Park Ridge, IL: American Academy of Orthopaedic Surgeons, 1990.

29. Windsor, RE, Lester, JP, and Herring, SA. 1993. Electrical stimulation in clinical practice. Phys and Sportsmed, 21(2):85–93.

30. Alon, D. *High voltage stimulation: A monograph*. Chattanooga, TN: Chattanooga Corporation, 1984.

31. DeDomenico, G. *Interferential stimulation: A monograph*. Chattanooga, TN: Chattanooga Corporation, 1988.

32. O'Donoghue, PC, McCarthy, MR, Gieck, JH, and Yates, CK. 1991. Clinical use of continuous passive motion in athletic training. Ath Tr (JNATA), 26(3):200–208.

33. Ciccone, CD, and Wolf, SL. *Pharmacology in rehabilitation*. Philadelphia: FA Davis, 1990.

34. Frank, GC. "Nutritional requirements for patients with chronic wounds." In *Wound healing: Alternatives to management*, edited by LC Kloth, JM McCullock, and JA Feedar. Philadelphia: FA Davis, 1990.

35. Martinez-Hernandez, A, and Amenta, PS. "Basic concepts in wound healing." In *Sports-induced inflammation*, edited by WB Leadbetter, JA Buckwalter, and SL Gordon. Park Ridge, IL: American Academy of Orthopaedic Surgeons, 1990.

36. US Department of Agriculture. Food group pyramid. Hyattsville, MD: US Department of Agriculture, 1992.

Chapter 6

Protective Equipment

After you have completed this chapter, you should be able to:

- Identify the principles used to design protective equipment
- Explain the types of materials used in the development of padding
- List the organizations responsible for establishing standards for protective devices
- Fit selected equipment (i.e., football helmets, mouth guards, and shoulder pads)
- Identify and discuss common protective equipment for the head and face, torso, and the upper and lower body

Protective equipment, when properly used, can protect the sport participant from accidental or routine injuries associated with a particular sport. However, there are limitations to its effectiveness. Today's players are faster, stronger, and more skilled. A natural outcome of wearing protective equipment is to feel more secure. Unfortunately, this often leads to more aggressive play, which can result in injury to the participant or an opponent. Protective equipment will not be effective if ill-fitted, worn-out, under-utilized, or used in an unintended manner. Several of these factors were presented in the section on Legal Liability in Chapter 1. It is your responsibility to ensure that protective equipment meets minimum standards of protection, is in good condition, clean, properly fitted, and used regularly.

In this chapter, principles of protective equipment and materials used in the development of padding will be discussed first. Secondly, protective equipment for the head and face is followed by equipment commonly used to protect the upper body and lower body. Where appropriate, guidelines for fitting specific equipment are listed in field strategies. Although several commercial braces and support devices are illustrated, these are intended to only demonstrate a variety of products available to protect a body region.

PRINCIPLES OF PROTECTIVE EQUIPMENT

What type of energy-absorbing material can best protect a body region from a single blow? What material can best protect an area subject to repeated blows?

In athletic events involving impact and collisions, the sport participant must be protected from high velocity-low mass forces, and low velocity-high mass forces. High velocity-low mass forces occur when an individual is struck by a ball, puck, bat, or hockey stick. The low mass and high speed of impact lead to forces concentrated in a smaller area, resulting in **focal injuries**. Low velocity-high mass forces occur when an individual falls on the ground or ice, or is checked into the sideboards of an ice hockey rink, thereby absorbing the forces over a larger area leading to **diffuse injuries**. Techniques and equipment to prevent or protect an injury site are called **prophylactic** devices.

Sport related injuries can result from a variety of factors, including:

Illegal play
Poor technique
Inadequate conditioning
Poorly matched player levels
A previously injured area that is now vulnerable to reinjury
Low tolerance of a player to injury
Inability to adequately protect an area without restricting motion
Poor quality, maintenance, or cleanliness of protective equipment

Protective equipment can protect an area from accidental or routine injuries associated with a particular sport. This is accomplished through several means, many of which are

Sport participants must be protected from high velocity-low mass forces, and low velocity-high mass forces

Focal injury
Injury in a small concentrated area, usually due to high velocity-low mass forces

Diffuse injury
Injury over a large body area, usually due to low velocity-high mass forces

Prophylactic
Preventive or protective

Low-density material
Materials that absorb energy
from low-impact intensity
levels

High-density material
Materials that absorb more
energy from high-impact
intensity levels through
deformation, thus transferring less stress to a body
part.

Resilience
The ability to bounce or
spring back into shape or
position after being
stretched, bent, or impacted

listed in **Table 6-1** (1). Equipment design extends beyond the physical protective properties to include size, comfort, style, tradition, and initial and long term maintenance costs. Individuals responsible for the selection and purchase of equipment should be less concerned about looks, style, and cost, and more concerned about the ability of equipment to prevent injury.

The design and selection of protective equipment is based on the optimal level of impact intensity afforded by the given thickness, density, and temperature of energy-absorbing material. Soft, **low-density material** is light and comfortable to wear, but is only effective at low levels of impact intensity. Examples of low-density material include gauze padding, foam, neoprene, sorbothane, felt, and moleskin. In contrast, firmer, **high-density material** of the same thickness tends to be less comfortable, offers less cushioning of low-level impact, but can absorb more energy by deformation and thus, transfers less stress to an area at higher impact intensity levels (1). Examples of high-density material include thermomoldable plastics, such as orthoplast and thermoplast, and casting materials, such as fiberglass or plaster. Many of these materials are demonstrated in **Figure 6-1**.

Soft foam over a bruised area will not absorb high level impact forces as effectively as a denser foam. To address this factor, many equipment designers layer materials of varying density. Soft, lower density material is placed next to the skin covered by increasingly more dense, firmer material away from the skin to absorb and disperse higher-intensity blows.

Another factor to consider in energy-absorbing material is **resilience** to impact forces. Highly resilient materials regain their shape after impact and are commonly used over areas subject to repeated impact. Nonresilient or slow-recovery resilient material offers the best protection, and is used over areas that are subject to one-time or occasional impact (1). It is important to select equipment that will absorb impact and disperse it before injury occurs to the underlying body part.

Nonresilient or slow-recovery resilient materials are best for protecting a body region subjected to a one-time or occasional blow. High resilient materials are used over an area subjected to repeated blows. In addition, a laminated layering of soft, lower density material covered by a firmer, higher density material will absorb high impact forces to prevent further injury.

PROTECTIVE EQUIPMENT FOR THE HEAD AND FACE

Preseason football camp has just begun. What guidelines should be used to properly fit a football helmet?

Many head and facial injuries can be prevented with regular use of properly fitted helmets and facial protective devices, such as face guards, mouth guards, eye wear, ear wear, and throat protectors. Collision sports, such as football and ice hockey, require special protection of the head and face. Standards of protection have been vastly improved through the combined efforts of athletic governing bodies, the American Society for Testing and Materials (ASTM), the National Operating Committee on Standards for Athletic Equipment (NOCSAE), and the Hockey Equipment Certification Council (HECC) of the Canadian Standards Association (CSA). NOCSAE, working since 1969, has defined impact standards for football and baseball/softball helmets to minimize injury. Since 1974 when the first football helmet was tested, head injuries have declined significantly with only .23 per 1000 participants

---

Table 6–1. Equipment Design Factors that can Reduce Potential Injury.

1. Increase the impact area
2. Transfer or disperse the impact area to another body part
3. Limit the relative motion of a body part
4. Add mass to the body part to limit deformation and displacement
5. Reduce friction between contacting surfaces
6. Absorb energy
7. Use materials resistant to the absorption of bacteria, fungus, and viruses that can be easily cleaned and disinfected

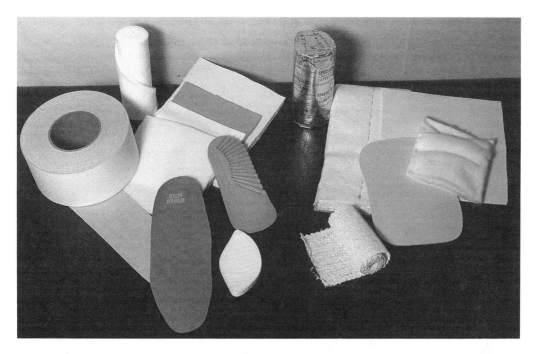

Fig. 6.1: On the left are examples of low density material used to cushion low-level impact forces. These include moleskin, gauze padding, foam materials, neoprene, sorbothane, and felt. On the right are high density materials, such as thermomoldable plastics and casting materials that can absorb more energy by deformation and thus transfer less stress to an injured area.

injured during the 1992–1993 intercollegiate football season (2).

Football Helmets

Football helmets typically are air- and fluid-filled, foam padded, or a combination of the two. All helmets must protect the cranium from low velocity-high mass impact forces that could conceivably fracture the skull, and must be NOCSAE approved. Heat, as an environmental factor, can alter the effectiveness of shock absorption in the liner and some shell materials. As a result, materials bottom out more easily and absorb less shock at higher temperatures than lower. To compensate, NOCSAE drops the helmet twice within one minute from a height of 152 cm (60 inches) on the right frontal boss in ambient temperature. The process is repeated after soaking the helmet for 4 hours at 49° C (120° F). The helmet must meet the same criterion at both temperatures (3). The NOCSAE mark on a helmet indicates it meets minimum impact standards, and can tolerate forces applied to several different areas of the helmet. NOCSAE also includes a warning label regarding risk of injury on each helmet that states:

Warning: Do not strike an opponent with any part of this helmet or face mask. This is a violation of football rules and may cause you to suffer severe brain or neck injury, including paralysis or death. Severe brain or neck injury may also occur accidentally while playing football. NO HELMET CAN PREVENT ALL SUCH INJURIES. USE THIS HELMET AT YOUR OWN RISK.

This warning label must be clearly visible on the exterior shell of all new and reconditioned helmets (4). In addition, the athletic trainer and coach should continually warn athletes of the risks involved in football and ensure the helmet is properly used within the guidelines and rules of the game.

Always follow manufacturer's guidelines when fitting a football helmet. Prior to fitting, the athletes should have haircuts in the style that will be worn during the athletic season, and wet their heads to simulate game conditions. **Field Strategy 6-1** lists the general steps in fitting a football helmet. Once fitted, the helmet should be checked periodically for proper fit that could be altered by hair length, deterioration of internal padding, loss of air from cells, and spread of the face mask (5). This is performed by inserting a tongue depressor between the pads and face. When

All helmets must protect the cranium from low velocity-high mass impact forces that could conceivably fracture the skull

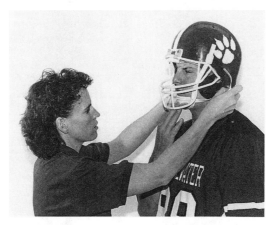

A. The player should have a haircut in the style that will be worn during the competitive season and should wet his hair to simulate game conditions. The helmet should fit snugly all around the player's head with the cheek pads snug against the sides of the face. The chin pad should be an equal distance from each side of the helmet.

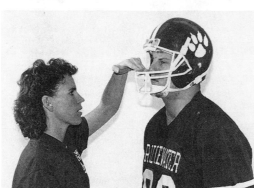

B. The helmet should set three-quarters of an inch above the player's eyebrows, and the face mask should extend two finger widths away from the forehead and nose.

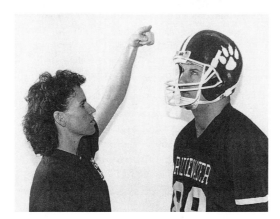

C. The face mask should allow for complete field of vision.

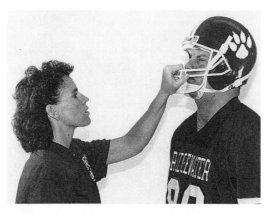

D. The back of the helmet should cover the base of the skull, and the ear holes should match up with the external auditory ear canal. With the chin strap secured, the helmet should not move when you pull the face guard up and down or side to side.

moved back and forth, a firm resistance should be felt. A snug-fitting helmet should not move in one direction when the head moves in another. If air- and fluid-filled helmets are used, and the team travels to a different altitude, always recheck the fit prior to use.

Ice Hockey Helmets

Ice hockey helmet standards are monitored by the American Society for Testing and Materials (ASTM) and the Hockey Equipment Certification Council (HECC). These helmets must absorb and disperse high velocity-low mass forces, i.e., being struck by a stick or puck, and low velocity-high mass forces, i.e., being checked into the sideboard or falling on the ice. All helmets are required to meet HECC standards and carry the stamp of approval from the Canadian Standards Association (CSA) (**Figure 6-2**). As with a football helmet, proper fit is achieved when a snug-fitting helmet does not move in one direction when the head is turned in the other.

Batting Helmets

Batting helmets used in baseball and softball require the NOCSAE mark and must be a double ear-flap design (**Figure 6-3**) (4). It is best to have a thick layer of foam between the primary energy absorber and the head to allow the shell to move slightly and deform. This maximizes its ability to absorb missile kinetic energy from a high velocity-low mass projectile, such as a ball or bat, and prevents

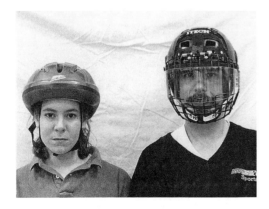

Fig. 6.2: Ice hockey helmets (right) must absorb and disperse high velocity—low mass forces (being hit by a high stick or puck), and low velocity—high mass forces (being checked into the boards). Full face guards may be clear or wire mesh. Bicycle helmets (left) have been shown to reduce the severity of head injuries, and protect against serious upper facial injuries.

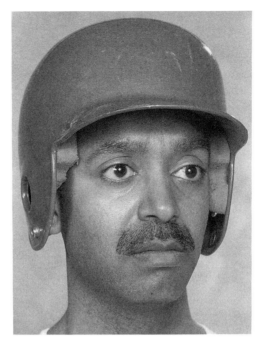

Fig. 6.3: Batting helmets should always be worn during batting and base-running.

excessive pressure on the cranium (1). The helmet should be snug enough so it does not move or fall off during batting and running bases.

Other Helmets

Lacrosse helmets are mandatory in the men's game, optional in the women's game, and are also worn by field hockey goalies. The helmet is made of a high resistant plastic or fiberglass shell, and must meet NOCSAE standards and carry the NOCSAE mark. The helmet, wire face guard, and chin pad are secured with a four-point chin strap (**Figure 6-4**). The helmet should not move in one direction when the head moves in another.

Standards for bicycle helmets changed in 1990 to include resistance testing to localized loading, thereby allowing the use of soft-shell helmets. Laboratory and field testing showed that the effectiveness of both hard shell and soft shell helmets are comparable (6). Helmet drop tests have concluded that bicycle helmets provide little protection against axial compressive loading on the cervical spine (7). They may have some protective effect, however, against serious upper facial injuries (8).

An effective bicycle helmet has a plastic or fiberglass rigid shell with a chin strap and an energy-absorbing foam liner (**Figure 6-4**). A

> It is best to have a thick layer of foam between the primary energy absorber and the head to allow the shell to move slightly and deform

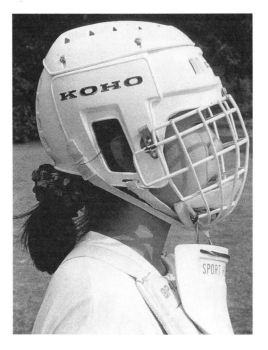

Fig. 6.4: Lacrosse helmets provide full face and neck protection.

stiffer shell results in better diffusion and resilience to impact. A firmer, denser foam liner is more effective at higher velocities, whereas a less stiff foam provides more protection at lower velocities. Increasing the thickness of the liner may lead to a more effective level of protection, but the increased mass and weight of the helmet may make it more uncomfortable (6). As in other helmets, a snug-fit is necessary for a proper fit.

Face Guards

Face guards come in a variety of sizes and configurations, and protect and shield the facial region from flying projectiles. Football face guards are made of heavy-gauge, plastic-coated steel rod, designed to withstand impacts from blunt surfaces, such as the turf or another player's knee or elbow. When properly fitted, the face mask should extend two finger widths away from the forehead and allow for complete field of vision (**Field Strategy 6-1B**). No face protection should be less than two bars. The effectiveness of a football face guard depends on the strength of the guard itself, the helmet attachments, and the four-point chin strap on the helmet. NOCSAE has set standards for strength and deflection for football face guards worn at the high school and college levels (3).

Ice hockey face guards are made of clear plastic (polycarbonate), steel wire, or a combination of the two (**Figure 6-2**). The guard stands away from the nose approximately 1 to 1½ inches. If a wire mesh is used, the holes should be small enough to prevent penetration by a hockey stick. Face guards must meet eye and face protective equipment standards for hockey players established by the HECC and ASTM (4). Hockey face guards primarily prevent penetration of the hockey stick, but are also effective against flying pucks and collisions with helmets, elbows, side boards, or the ice. It has been estimated that through the use of these devices, players have saved a projected 10 million dollars annually in medical expenses (9).

Lacrosse face guards must meet NOCSAE lacrosse helmet/faceguard standards. The wire mesh guard stands away from the face, but has a padded chin region in case the guard is driven back during a collision with another player (**Figure 6-4**). Face masks used by catchers and the home plate umpire in baseball and softball should fit snugly to the cheeks and forehead, but should not impair vision (**Figure 6-5**). Men's and women's fencing masks have an adjustable spring to prevent the mask from moving during competition.

Mouth Guards

An intraoral mouth guard and tooth protector is required in all interscholastic and intercollegiate football, ice hockey, field hockey, and men's and women's lacrosse. A properly fitted mouth guard can absorb energy, disperse

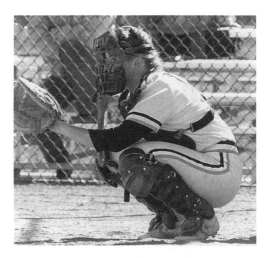

Fig. 6.5: Baseball and softball catchers must wear full face and neck protection.

impact, cushion contact between the upper and lower teeth, and keep the upper lip away from the incisal edges of the teeth (10). This action significantly reduces dental and oral soft tissue injuries, and to a lesser extent jaw fractures, cerebral concussions, and temporomandibular joint (TMJ) injuries (10,11).

Mouth guards should be durable, resilient, resistant to tear, inexpensive, easy to fabricate, tasteless, odorless, and be clearly visible to officials (10,12). Although players may complain that use of a mouth guard interferes with speech, and has been shown to reduce forced expiratory air volume and peak expiratory flow rates, the benefits of preventing oral injuries far outweigh the disadvantages (13).

Mouth guards are available in three basic types: stock (ready-made), mouth-formed, and custom-made over a model made from an impression of the athlete's maxillary arch (10,14). The NCAA and many high school sports now require an intraoral yellow or readily visible colored mouth guard that covers all upper teeth (4). The practice of cutting down mouth guards to cover only the front four teeth invalidates the manufacturer's warranty, cannot prevent many dental injuries, and can lead to airway obstruction should the individual choke. This practice should not be tolerated.

Stock mouth guards are usually made of latex rubber or plastic, and are available in small, medium, and large sizes. Because they are not formed around the teeth, constant occlusal pressure must be exerted to hold the mouth guard in place. Due to the bulky size, they often interfere with speech and breathing, and are easily ejected from the mouth onto the ground. As such, the stock protectors are the least favored among sport participants (10).

The most popular type is the thermal set, mouth-formed mouth guard (**Figure 6-6**).

Although not as effective as the custom-made mouth guard, when properly fitted, the mouth-formed guard can virtually match the efficacy and comfort of the custom-made guard. This type of guard is readily available, inexpensive, and has a loop strap for attachment to a face mask. The loop strap has two advantages in that it prevents individuals from choking on the mouth guard in an emergency, and prevents the individual from losing the mouth guard when it is ejected from the mouth (15).

The mouth-formed guard usually consists of a firm outer shell, fitted with a softer inner material. The softer material is thermally or chemically set after being molded to the player's teeth (15). **Field Strategy 6-2** demonstrates how to fit a thermoplastic mouth-formed mouthguard. The thermoplastic mouth guards often lack full extension into the labial and buccal vestibules. Therefore, they do not provide adequate protection against oral soft tissue injuries. Furthermore, the thermoplastic inner material loses its elasticity at mouth temperature, and may cause the protector to loosen (10).

The most effective type of mouth protector is the custom-made mouthguard. These protectors require fabrication by a dentist, making them more expensive. The dentist takes an impression of the maxillary teeth of each player and makes a model over which a material such as thermoplastic vinyl (i.e., polyvinyl acetate-polyethylene), is then vacuum adapted. Custom fitted mouth guards are more comfortable, retentive, tasteless, odorless, tear resistant, resilient, of uniform thickness, and have little effect on speaking, drinking, or breathing (10).

Another type of custom-made mouth protector is the bimaxillary mouth guard that covers both upper and lower dental arches. The mandible is opened to a predetermined

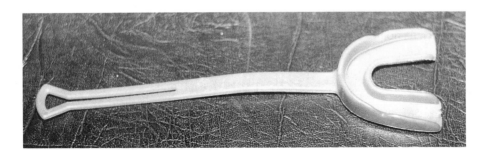

Fig. 6.6: The thermal set, mouth-formed mouthguard is the most frequently used because it is inexpensive, readily available, and has a loop strap for attachment to a face mask.

Field Strategy 6–2. Fitting Mouth-Formed Mouthguards.

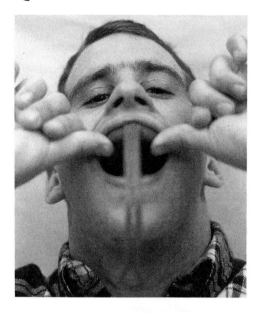

A. Submerge the mouthguard only, not the loop strap, in boiling water for 20 to 25 seconds, or until soft and pliable. Shake off any excess water, but do not rinse the mouthguard in cold water as this decreases pliability

B. Place the mouthguard directly in the mouth over the upper dental arch. Center the mouthguard with your thumbs using the loop strap as a guide

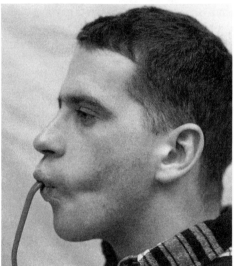

C. Close the mouth, but do not bring the teeth together or bite down on the mouthguard. Place the tongue on the roof of the mouth and *suck* as hard as possible for 15 to 25 seconds. The sucking mechanism acts a vacuum to mold the mouthguard around the teeth and gums

D. Rinse the mouthguard in cold water to harden the material. Check the finished product for any significant indentations on the bottom and to ensure it is centered correctly. If any imperfections or errors are noted, do not reheat the mouthguard because this decreases its effectiveness. Select a new mouthguard and repeat the process

position, i.e, position of heavy breathing. This guard does not interfere with breathing, provides protection for the lower teeth as well as the upper, and stabilizes the mandible to the head to reduce mandibulocranial force transmission (10).

Eye Wear

Eye injuries are relatively frequent and almost always preventable, yet no interscholastic or intercollegiate sport requires their use. In a 10 year Canadian study from 1982 to 1991, over 710 eye injuries occurred in racquet sports ranging from lid lacerations and irritation of the iris, to corneal abrasions, lid hemorrhage, and hyphemas (hemorrhage within the anterior chamber of the eye) (16). The most common eye injury in recreational sports is rupture of the sclera caused by a ball squarely hitting the eye (17). Glass lenses, ordinary plastic lenses, and open eye guards do not provide adequate protection. In many situations, their use increases the risk and severity of injury. In a separate study of 80 Canadian racquet sport players wearing open eye guards, 77 injuries (96%) involved the ball penetrating the open eye guard (18). Sev-

Glass lenses, ordinary plastic lenses, and open eye guards do not provide adequate protection against eye injuries

eral types of approved eye protectors are commercially available for the sport participant (**Figure 6-7**).

Eye protectors are made from polycarbonate, the plastic used in making jet canopies and police riot gear. Polycarbonate is lightweight, scratch- and impact-resistant, and can have an antifog and ultraviolet inhibitor incorporated into the lens (19). The frame should be constructed of a resilient plastic, with reinforced temples, hinges, and nose piece. Adequate cushioning should protect the eyebrow and nasal bridge from sharp edges. Lenses should be 3 mm thick. Only polycarbonate eye protectors and eye frames that meet the standards of the American Society for Testing and Materials (ASTM), and parallel Canadian Standards Association (CSA), offer enough protection for a sport participant. Approved eye guards protect the eye when impacted with a racquet ball traveling at 90 mph (40 meters per second) or a racquet going 50 mph (22.2 meters per second) (20). Approved eye guards will state so on the package.

Any person with good vision in only one eye should consult with an ophthalmologist on whether to participate in a given sport. One-eyed athletes have reduced visual fields and depth perception. If a decision is made to participate, the individual should wear maximum eye protection during all practices and competitions (21). Sport participants should wear a sweatband to keep sweat out of the eye guard, and should remove the eye guard when not participating.

For collision sports, such as football, hockey, lacrosse, baseball, downhill racing, motorcycle racing, and bike racing, wearing eye protectors is insufficient. The force of a collision could break not only the eye protector, but also the facial bones. As previously mentioned, face guards in combination with a helmet, or full face mask, protect the entire facial region. The space between the bars or wire mesh must be small enough to prevent objects, such as a stick, puck, ball, or fencing foil from penetrating the eye region.

Although sport participants often wear contact lenses because they improve peripheral vision, astigmatism, and do not normally cloud during temperature changes, they do not protect against eye injury. Contact lenses come in two types: hard, or corneal type lens, which covers only the iris of the eye; and soft, or scleral type, which covers the entire front of the eye. Hard contact lenses often become dislodged, and are associated more frequently with irritation from foreign bodies. Dust and other foreign matter may get underneath the lens and damage the cornea, or the cornea may be scratched while inserting or removing the lens.

Soft contact lenses have been shown to protect the eye from irritation by chlorine in pools (22). Although research has shown that pool water causes soft lenses to adhere to the cornea reducing the risk of loss, this practice is not recommended (23). Micro-organisms, especially *Acanthamoeba*, are responsible for a rare, but serious, corneal infection, *Acanthamoeba* keratitis. It is recommended that goggles should always be worn in water, with or without contact lenses, to protect against organisms in the water and irritation from chlorine. Swimmers should wait 20 to 30 minutes after leaving the water to remove the contact lenses. This allows time for the lenses to stop sticking to the cornea. Lenses should then be immediately disinfected. Removing the lenses too soon may cause corneal surface damage, leaving the cornea susceptible to infection (22).

> Polycarbonate is lightweight, scratch- and impact-resistant, and can have an antifog and ultraviolet inhibitor incorporated into the lens

> Contact lenses improve peripheral vision, astigmatism, and do not normally cloud during temperature changes. However, they do not protect against eye injury

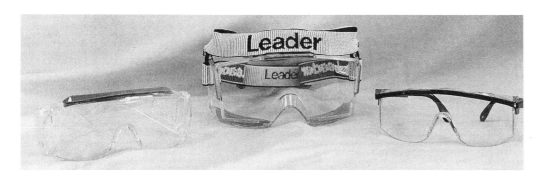

Fig. 6.7: Eye protectors should be made from polycarbonate, which is lightweight, scratch- and impact-resistant.

Ear Wear

With the exception of boxing, wrestling, and water polo, few sports have specialized ear protection **(Figure 6-8)**. Repeated friction and trauma to the ear can lead to a permanent deformity, called hematoma auris or cauliflower ear (see Chapter 13). For this reason, ear protection should be worn regularly in these sports. Fit is determined by the individual. The chin strap should provide a snug fit. The head gear should not move during contact with another player, nor should the protective ear cup compress the external ear.

Throat and Neck Protectors

Blows to the anterior throat can cause serious airway compromise as a result of a crushed larynx and/or upper trachea, edema of the glottic structures, vocal cord disarticulation, hemorrhage, or laryngospasm (24). The NCAA requires that catchers in baseball and softball wear a built-in or attachable throat guard on their masks **(Figure 6-5)** (4). Fencing masks and helmets used in field hockey, lacrosse, and ice hockey also provide anterior neck protectors to protect this vulnerable area.

Cervical neck rolls and collars are designed to limit motion of the cervical spine and have been shown to be effective in protecting players with a history of repetitive burners or stingers (see Chapter 14) (25). The majority of neck rolls are inadequate, however, in that they are attached to the top of shoulder pads and can pull away from the neck on impact (26). A higher, thicker, and stiffer posterolateral pad at the base of the neck can offer better fixation of the cervical spine **(Figure 6-9)**. Cervical collars do not decrease axial loading on the cervical spine when the neck is flexed during a tackle.

In fitting a football helmet, the helmet should be snug enough to prevent movement of the helmet in one direction when the head moves in another. Proper fit may be altered by hair length, deterioration of internal padding, loss of air from cells, and spread of the face mask necessitating periodic checks for proper fit.

PROTECTIVE EQUIPMENT FOR THE UPPER BODY

You have successfully fitted the football player with a helmet. What guidelines are used to properly fit the shoulder pads for the player?

In the upper body, special pads and braces are often used to protect the shoulder region, ribs, thorax, breasts, arm, elbow, wrist and hands. Depending on the sport, special design modifications are needed to allow maximum protection while providing maximal performance.

Shoulder Protection

The shoulder girdle must be protected against high velocity-low mass forces, and low velocity-high mass forces. For example, in football, hockey, and lacrosse, shoulder pads

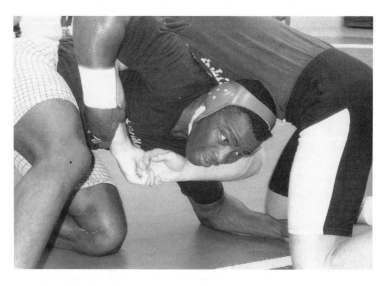

Fig. 6.8: Protective ear wear can prevent friction and trauma to the ear that may lead to permanent deformity.

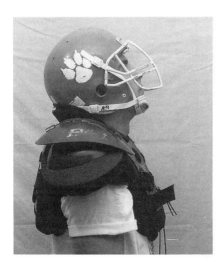

Fig. 6.9: A high, thick stiff posterolateral pad at the base of the neck can provide added protection to the cervical spine, but cannot reduce axial loading during a tackle when the head is lowered.

Commercial football shoulder pads can be supplemented with other pads to protect vulnerable areas. For example, ice hockey shoulder pads can fit under the football pads to further protect the acromion process. Detachable shoulder pad extensions protect soft tissue structures over the deltoid and upper arm region enhancing comfort and fit. Biceps pads give linemen and linebackers additional upper arm protection. **Field Strategy 6-3** lists the general steps used in fitting football shoulder pads.

Shoulder pads do not protect the glenohumeral joint from excessive motion. As a result, sprains to the glenohumeral joint may occur. Tape restraints or commercial protective braces, such as the one shown in **Figure 6-10** can be used to limit abduction of the glenohumeral joint.

Elbow, Forearm, Wrist, and Hand Protection

The entire arm is constantly subjected to compressive and shearing forces, such as those seen in blocking and tackling an opponent, deflecting projectiles, pushing opponents away to prevent collisions, or to break a fall. Goalies and field players in many sports are required to have arm, elbow, wrist and hand protection. It is important, however, that equipment or pads not pose any danger to another player. Hard, abrasive, nonyielding substances on the elbow, forearm, wrist or hand are prohibited unless covered on all sides by closed-cell foam padding (4).

Many players diagnosed with lateral epicondylitis ("tennis elbow") use a counterforce forearm brace as part of the rehabilitation program to reduce tensile forces in the wrist extensors, particularly the extensor carpi radialis brevis **(Figure 6-11)**. In some cases, these braces are also worn during activities of daily living. In two 1989 studies, a pneumatic armband was found to reduce muscular tension more effectively than a standard tennis elbow strap or nonbraced arm (28,29). In a more recent 1992 study, a pneumatic armband and standard tennis elbow strap were analyzed to determine concentric torque output and maximum repetition work produced by the right wrist extensors. Results were compared to a nonbraced control group. No significant decrease in torque output was seen in all test conditions except when the pneumatic armband was applied to the fore-

In football, the greatest amount of force exerted on the shoulder region occurs on the acromion process

must absorb and disperse excessive forces from impact with a ball, puck or stick, and a collision with an opponent or hard surface.

In a 1992 study, football shoulder pads consisting of both closed-cell and open-cell (one and three layer foam) were subjected to impact forces in field and laboratory tests. Results indicated that in all instances, the greatest force was placed on the acromion process. The player-preferred pad in both field and laboratory tests was an open-cell air management system which resulted in lower peak impact forces when compared with closed-cell pads. Three-layer open-cell foam pads were not superior to those using one layer open-cell foam in preventing peak impact forces (26).

Shoulder pads should protect the soft and bony tissue structures in the shoulder, upper back, and chest. When these pads are used with a neck guard, motion in the midcervical spinal region may be inhibited, reducing the risk of brachial plexus nerve injuries (27). Football shoulder pads are available in two general types; flat and cantilevered. Flat shoulder pads provide less protection to the shoulder region, but allow more motion at the glenohumeral joint. These pads are often used by the quarterback or receivers who must raise their arms above the head to throw or catch a pass. Cantilevered pads limit motion at the glenohumeral joint, but provide more protection against high impact forces. These pads are used by linemen or linebackers who do a great deal of blocking and tackling.

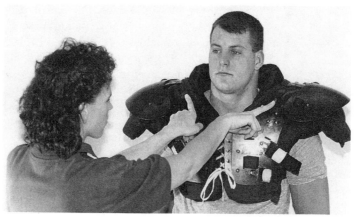

A. Determine the player's chest size by measuring circumference at the nipple line. Place the pads on the shoulders. The straps should be snug enough to prevent no more than a two-finger-width distance between the pads and body. The entire clavicle should be covered and protected by the pads.

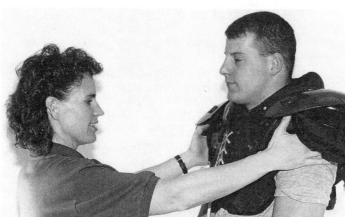

B. The acromioclavicular joint should be adequately covered and protected by the upper portion of the arch and deltoid padding. The entire deltoid should be adequately covered and protected by the extension arch padding.

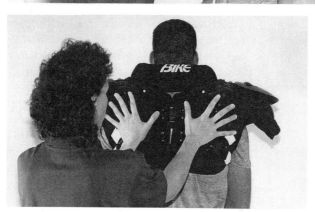

C. The entire scapula should be covered with the lower pad arch extending below the inferior angle of the scapula.

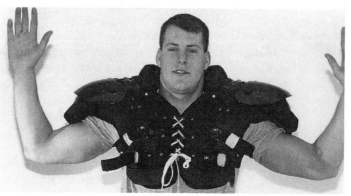

D. With the arms abducted, the neck opening should not be uncomfortable nor pinch the neck.

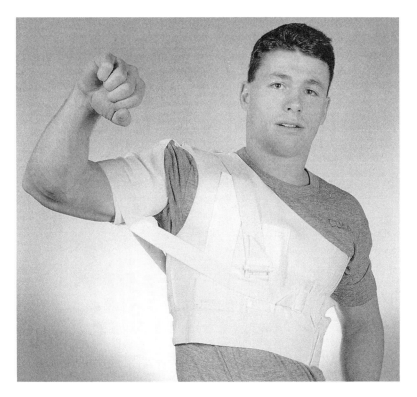

Fig. 6.10: The Sawa shoulder brace can limit glenohumeral motion in chronic shoulder injuries.

arm at 30°/s in which an increase in torque was noted (30). Although supports may relieve an individual's pain upon return to activity, debate continues about the effectiveness of counterforce forearm straps. These straps should not be used for other causes of elbow pain, such as growth plate problems in children and adolescents, or medial elbow instability in adults (31). Examples of other specialized pads and braces for the elbow can be seen in **Figure 6-12**.

The forearm, wrist, and hand are especially vulnerable to external forces and often neglected when considering protective equipment. In collision and contact sports, this area should be protected with specialized gloves and pads, such as those seen in **Figure 6-13**. In more recent years, silicone rubber

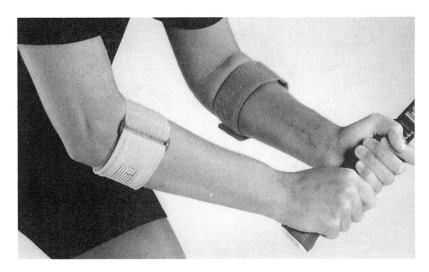

Fig. 6.11: The counterforce forearm band is often used with tennis elbow to reduce tensile forces in the wrist extensors.

and thermomoldable foam has been used to customize protective pads for the forearm, wrist, and hand (**Figure 6-14**).

Thorax, Rib, and Abdominal Protection

Many collision and contact sports require special protection of the thorax, rib, and abdominal areas. Catchers in baseball and softball wear full thoracic and abdominal protectors to prevent high speed blows from a bat or ball. Individuals in fencing, and goalies in many sports, also wear full thoracic protectors (**Figure 6-15A**). Quarterbacks and wide receivers in football often wear rib protectors composed of air-inflated, interconnected cylinders to absorb impact forces caused during tackling (**Figure 6-15B**). These protectors should be fitted according to the manufacturer's instructions.

Sport Bras

Sport bras provide added support to prevent excessive vertical and horizontal breast motion during exercise. Although sport bras are designed to limit motion, studies indicate that few bras on the market actually do so. As a result, many women continue to experience sore or tender breasts after exercise (32,33). Sport bras fall into three categories (34):

1. Bras made from nonelastic material with wide shoulder straps and wide bands under the breasts to provide upward support (**Figure 6-16A**). Waist-length designs can prevent cutting in below the breasts.
2. Compressive bras that bind the breasts to the chest wall (**Figure 6-16B**). Women with medium sized breasts prefer this type.
3. Bras with minor modifications, usually with less elasticity. These are not considered true sport bras, although they are marketed as such.

Girls and women with small breasts may not need a special bra. Women with a size C cup or larger need a firm, supportive type bra. The bra should have no irritating seams or fasteners next to the skin, have nonslip straps, and be firm and durable. Choice of fabric will depend on the intensity of activity, support needs, sensitivity to fiber, and climatic and seasonal conditions (34). A cotton/poly/lycra fabric is a pop-

> Girls and women with a bra size C cup or larger need a firm, supportive type bra

A

B

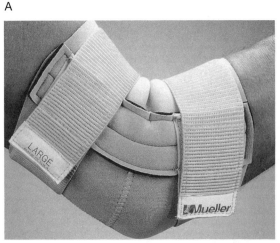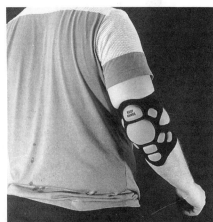

Fig. 6.12A & B: Specialized braces and pads can be utilized to protect the elbow from excessive forces.

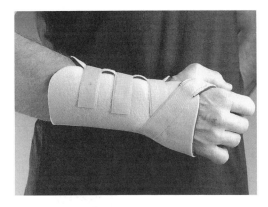

A

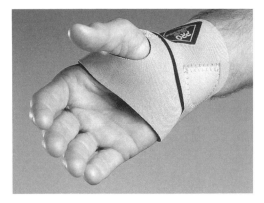

B

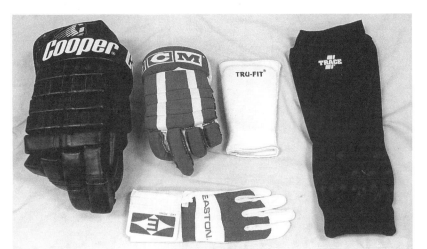

C

Fig. 6.13: Specialized braces and gloves are used in several sports to protect the wrist and hand for trauma. A–wrist splint. B–Thumb spica. C–Specialized gloves.

ular blend commonly seen in sport bras. In hot weather, an additional outer layer of textured nylon mesh can promote natural cooling of the skin. In sports requiring significant overhead motion, bra straps should stretch so as to prevent the bra from riding up over the breasts. In activities where overhead motion is not a significant part of the activity, nonstretch straps connected directly to a non-elastic cup are preferable.

Lumbar/Sacral Protection

Lumbar/sacral protection includes weight training belts used during heavy weight lifting, abdominal binders, and other similar supportive devices **(Figure 6-17)**. In general, each should support the abdominal contents, stabilize the trunk, and prevent spinal deformity or damage during heavy lifting (35). Use of belts or binders can support the low back in a more vertical lifting posture and can significantly increase intra-abdominal pressure to reduce compressive forces in the vertebral bodies (36). In two 1990 studies measuring the effects of a modified weight training belt with a rigid abdominal pad, and an elastic binder, Proflex, on selected isokinetic parameters, results indicated no statistically significant isokinetic changes relative to improving functional lifting capacity between subjects wearing the supports against the control condition (35,37). While statistical significance was limited, results did demonstrate a reduction in peak trunk lifting force

Use of belts or binders can support the lower back in a more vertical lifting posture and can significantly increase intra-abdominal pressure to reduce compressive forces in the vertebral bodies

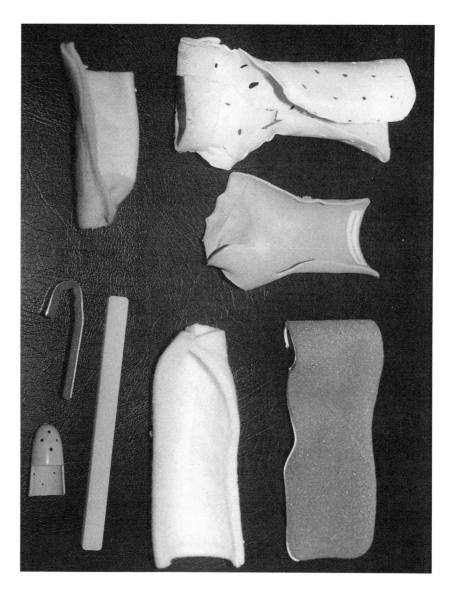

Fig. 6.14: Silicone rubber and thermomoldable foam can be used to customize protective pads for the forearm, wrist, and hand.

and rotational torque, total work, and average power. The highest averages were seen in individuals wearing a type of lumbar/sacral support as opposed to not wearing a supportive device during the simulated lifting tasks (35,37). Similar results were obtained in a 1993 study (38). These results suggest that wearing a lumbar/sacral support during trunk movements, such as in weight lifting, can prevent back-related trauma.

In fitting the shoulder pads, did you adequately protect the acromion process, deltoid musculature, pectoral, and scapular region? When the player raised his arms, was *the neck opening comfortable and nonconstrictive? If so, the pads are fitted correctly.*

PROTECTIVE EQUIPMENT FOR THE LOWER BODY

A baseball player has a chronic ankle sprain that requires external support. What method of support can provide a higher level of protection for this player?

In the lower body, commercial braces are commonly used to protect the knee and ankle. In addition, special pads are used to protect bony and soft tissue structures in the

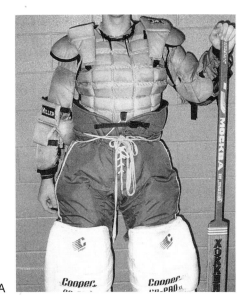
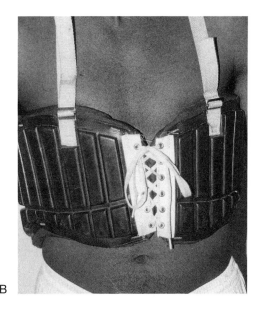

Fig. 6.15: (A) Several sports require extensive chest protection (ice hockey). (B) Rib protectors absorb impact forces caused during tackling.

hip and thigh region. Depending on the sport, special design modifications are needed to allow maximum protection while providing maximal performance.

Hip and Buttock Protection

In collision and contact sports, the hip and buttock region require special pads to protect the iliac crest, sacrum and coccyx, and the genital region. Football, hockey, and boxing have specially designed girdle type pads to protect the hip and buttock region **(Figure 6-18A)**. Hip spica braces are used to limit excessive hip abduction after a muscular strain in a groin injury **(Figure 6-18B)**. The male genital region is best protected by a protective cup placed in the athletic supporter **(Figure 6-18C)**.

Thigh Protection

The thigh and upper leg require special padding in collision sports, such as football and hockey. Pads, such as those illustrated in **Figure 6-18A** slip into ready-made pockets in the uniform to prevent injury to the quadriceps area, and can be used in other

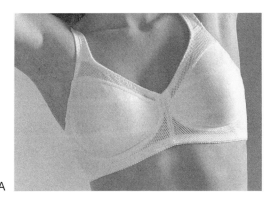
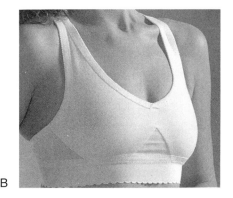

Fig. 6.16: (A) Sport bras. Nonelastic material with wide shoulder straps and wide bands under the breasts provide upward support for larger breasted girls and women. (B) Compressive bras bind the breasts to the chest wall.

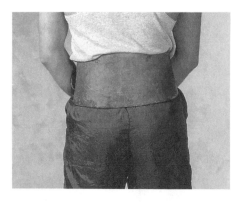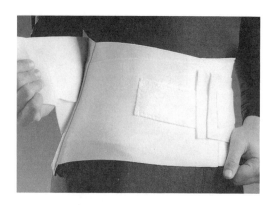

Fig. 6.17: Weight training belts, (A) abdominal binders, (B) and other lumbar devices support the abdominal contents, stabilize the trunk, and prevent spinal deformity or damage.

sports to prevent a quadriceps contusion (39). In addition, neoprene sleeves can provide uniform compression, therapeutic warmth, and support for a quadriceps or hamstrings strain.

Knee and Patella Protection

The knee is second only to the ankle and foot in incidence of injury (5). Commercially available knee pads can protect the area from high-velocity projectiles, and impact during a

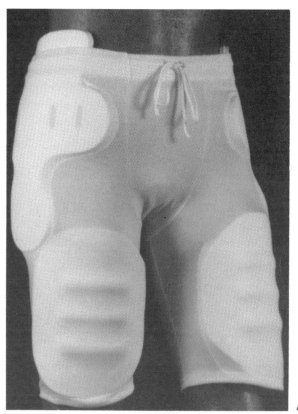

Fig. 6.18: Hip protection. (A) Girdle pads protect the gluteal and sacral area from high velocity forces. Thigh pads can also be inserted to protect the quadriceps area. (B) Hip spica braces limit excessive hip abduction after a muscular strain to the groin. (C) Protective cups placed inside an athletic supporter can reduce trauma to the male genital region.

A

collision or fall, such as in soccer, volleyball, or basketball (**Figure 6-19**). In wrestling, pads protect the prepatellar and infrapatellar bursa from friction injuries.

Knee braces fall into three broad groups: prophylactic or preventive, functional, and rehabilitative. Since 1980, several studies have investigated biomechanical and epidemiological concerns on the effectiveness of knee braces in the prevention and management of knee injuries. Results are often conflicting and misleading. Changes in coaching technique and philosophy, conditioning programs, footwear, playing surfaces, brace selection bias, environmental factors, and rule changes are all factors that can influence test results, making comparisons difficult at best (40).

Knee braces fall into three broad groups: prophylactic, functional, and rehabilitative

Fig. 6.18: *continued*

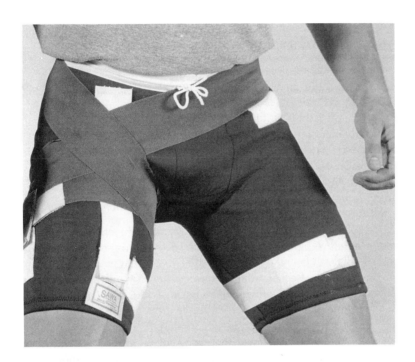

B

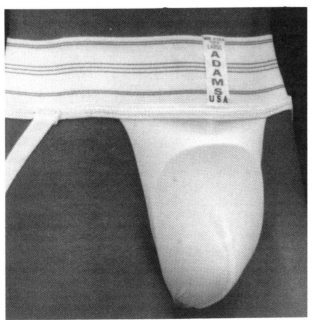

C

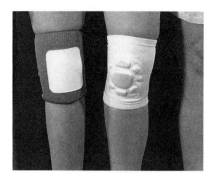

Fig. 6.19: Knee pads can protect the area from high-velocity projectiles, and impact from a fall.

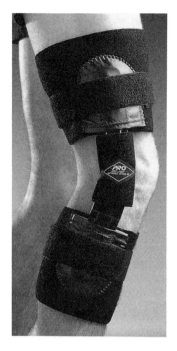

Fig. 6.20: Prophylactic knee braces may be a single or bilateral bar design.

Prophylactic Knee Braces

Prophylactic knee braces (PKBs) are designed to protect the medial collateral ligament (MCL) by redirecting a lateral valgus force away from the joint itself to points more distal to the tibia and femur. Two general types of PKBs are the lateral and bilateral bar designs **(Figure 6-20)**. The lateral bar PKBs are constructed with single, dual, or polycentric hinge designs. Each model has a knee hyperextension stop, and is applied using a combination of neoprene wraps, Velcro straps, and/or adhesive tape. The bilateral bar PKB has a medial and lateral upright bar with biaxial hinges (40). Recent studies have concluded, that although individual PKBs may provide some increases in MCL failure loading, knee ligament protection is only modest (41,42). One study has shown that at 30° of flexion, the braces tested did offer some protection to the MCL by reducing peak strain values, but at 0° the braces were unable to afford the same protection (43). Lateral knee braces have also been shown to inhibit isokinetic muscular strength parameters and sprint speed in players unaccustomed to wearing the brace (44).

After comprehensive review of available research, the American Academy of Orthopedic Surgeons (AAOS) in 1987 stated that the routine use of available PKBs had not been proven effective in reducing either the number or severity of knee injuries, and in some instances may have been a contributing factor to the injury (45). As future innovations and design modifications are made in PKBs, benefits in injury prevention may become more cost effective. Until then, clinicians should base decisions on PKB use on the individual needs of the athlete.

Functional knee braces, commonly called derotation or ACL braces, are designed to control tibial translation and rotational stress relative to the femur with a rigid snug fit, and extension limitations

In vivo
Occurring within the living organism or body

Functional Knee Braces

Functional knee braces are widely used to protect moderate anterior cruciate ligament (ACL) injuries, or in post-surgical ACL ligament repair or reconstruction cases **(Figure 6-21)**. These braces, commonly called derotation or ACL braces, are designed to control tibial translation and rotational stress relative to the femur with a rigid snug fit, and extension limitations (46). Performance of the brace depends on the magnitude of anterior shear load, and the internal torque applied across the tibiofemoral joint (47). Much of the early research was based on hearsay and cadaver studies which produced conflicting results. Recent studies **in vivo** have demonstrated a strain-shielding effect on the anterior cruciate ligament or its replacement at only relatively low anterior shear loads (less than 100-newtons) (47–50). Functional knee braces have been found to increase intramuscular pressures in the anterior compartment of the leg (51). In situations involving high loads encountered by the knee, or when the load is applied unpredictably, the brace may fail to protect the injured ligament (50,52).

Levels of protection differ among braces, and may be affected by several factors, such as (47):

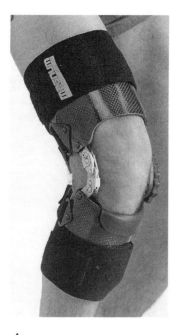

A

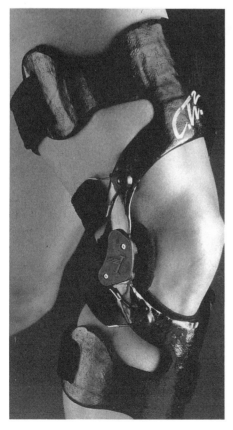

C

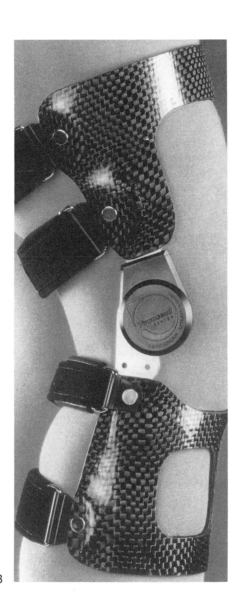

B

Fig. 6.21: Functional knee braces are designed for snug fit to control tibial translation and rotational stress relative to the femur, and can provide extension limitations.

1. The technique of attachment
2. The design of the brace, including:
   a. Hinge design
   b. Materials of fabrication
   c. Geometry of the attachment interface
   d. Mechanism of attachment
3. Variables in the attachment interface, including
   a. How the interface molds around the soft tissue contours of the limb
   b. How much displacement occurs between the rigid brace and compliant soft tissues surrounding the distal femur and proximal tibia while loads are applied across the knee.

Derotation braces may be prescribed by a physician in individuals with a moderate degree of instability who participate in activities with low or moderate load potential. In addition, these braces may also be effective following ligament repair or reconstructive surgery in reducing repetitive low loads during activities of daily living as part of a total rehabilitation program (50).

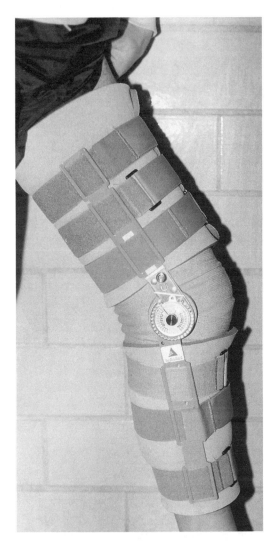

Fig. 6.22: Rehabilitative braces provide absolute or relative immobilization following surgery.

Rehabilitative Braces

Rehabilitative braces provide absolute or relative immobilization following surgery **(Figure 6-22)**. The amount of protection required by the graft will vary depending upon the type of graft used, and the quality of fixation obtained intraoperatively (53). As the individual progresses in the rehabilitation program, the allowable range of motion is adjusted periodically by the clinician. Research has shown that most rehabilitative braces which integrate and function as a single unit significantly reduce the amount of rotation and translations at the knee (54). Newer braces are lighter in weight, adjustable for optimal fit, and can be easily removed and reapplied for wound inspection and rehabilitation. In varying degrees, these braces allow the individual to perform passive or active motion through predetermined arcs to allow functional activities, such as standing or walking while protecting the injury site (46,55). Early motion prevents joint adhesions from forming, enhances proprioception, and increases synovial nutrient flow to promote healing of cartilage and collagen tissue.

Decisions to use any of the three major categories of knee braces should rest with the supervising physician or surgeon. Selection should be based on the projected objectives, needs of the sport participant relative to sport demands, cost effectiveness, durability, fit, and comfort (46).

Patellofemoral Protection

Use of braces in the treatment of recurring patellofemoral subluxation or dislocation has been found to relieve pain and tension on the quadriceps extensor mechanism (56). These braces typically have a horseshoe type pad sewn into an elastic or neoprene sleeve **(Figure 6-23A)**. These braces may also be helpful in relieving chronic patellar pain. An alternative brace for treating patellar pain is a strap worn over the infrapatellar ligament **(Figure 6-23B)**.

> Newer rehabilitative braces are lighter in weight, adjustable for optimal fit, and can be easily removed and reapplied for wound inspection and rehabilitation

Lower Leg Protection

Pads for the anterior tibia area should protect against impact from a ball, bat, stick, or kick from a foot. Sports such as baseball, softball, soccer, ice and field hockey require such protection. Several commercial designs are available **(Figure 6-24)**. These pads involve a high density padding covered by a molded hard shell. Additional supplemental padding may also be added to protect a highly sensitive area.

Ankle and Foot Protection

Commercial ankle protections prevent excessive inversion and eversion at the ankle joint, and typically involve a lace-up brace, semirigid orthrosis, or air bladder brace **(Figure 6-25)**. These braces, along with adhesive ankle taping, are commonly used as prophylactic devices, and are used post-injury to provide additional stabilization to the joint. Studies have shown that ankle strapping, lace-up braces, semirigid orthrosis, and air bladder braces do limit ankle range of motion. Use of a lace-up brace has been shown to limit all ankle motions, whereas a semirigid orthrosis and air bladder brace limit only inversion and eversion (57,58). In addition, lace-up braces and semirigid orthroses have been shown to decrease force production and total work (57,58). Semirigid devices have not been shown to affect vertical jump (59). In several studies, it was found that after exercise, semirigid orthosis and air bladder devices provided the most inversion restraint, followed by the lace-up brace (59-62). Maximal loss in taping restriction for both inversion and eversion has been found to occur after 20 minutes or more of exercise (59,62–65). Semirigid and air bladder braces are more effective in reducing the frequency of ankle injuries, are easier for the wearer to apply independently, do not produce some of the skin irritation problems associated with adhesive tape, provide better comfort and fit, and may be more cost effective (66–68). In basketball, high-top shoes with inflatable air chambers have not been shown to reduce the incidence of ankle sprains (69).

Specific foot conditions can also be padded and supported with a variety of products. Innersoles made of Poron provide a porous structure to absorb and disperse shock during activities of daily living, and can be used for an arthritic or diabetic foot **(Figure 6-26A)**. Semirigid orthotics provide more stable and durable support to the

> A lace-up ankle brace limits all ankle motion, whereas a semirigid orthrosis and an air bladder brace limit only inversion and eversion

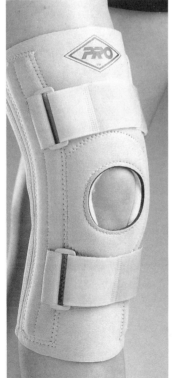

A

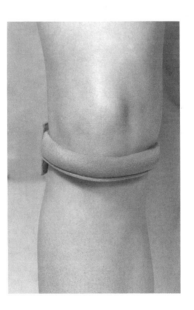

B

Fig. 6.23: Patellofermoral braces are helpful in relieving chronic patella pain (A). A strap worn over the infrapatellar ligament may also relieve patellar pain (B).

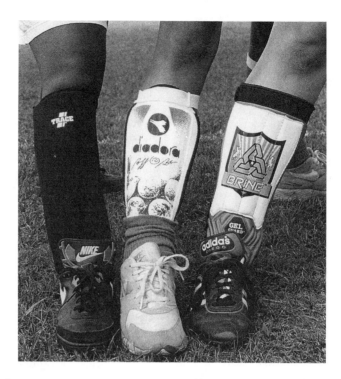

Fig. 6.24: Shin guards.

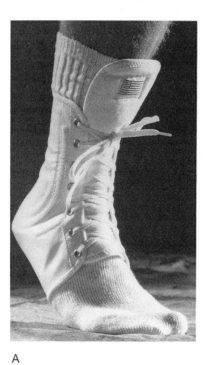

A

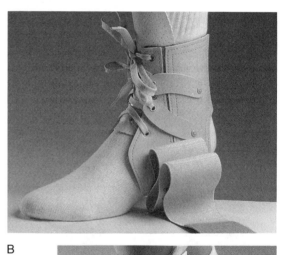

B

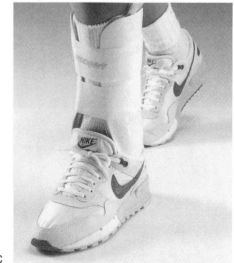

C

Fig. 6.25: Ankle protectors can prevent ankle sprains, and include the lace-up brace (A), semi-rigid orthrosis (B), and air bladder brace (C).

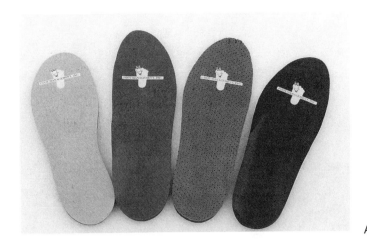

A

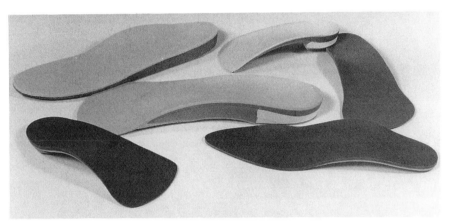

B

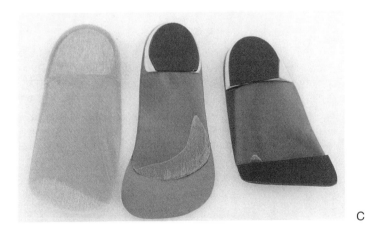

C

Fig. 6.26: Foot protection. (A) Inner soles can absorb and disperse shock during activities of daily living. (B) Semi-rigid orthotics provide more stability and support to the intrinsic structures of the foot. (C) Rigid orthotics are more effective at correcting biomechanical malalignment in the foot region.

intrinsic structures of the foot, and are often used for fallen arches, pronated feet, or medial tibial stress syndrome **(Figure 6-26B)**. Rigid orthotics have additional support and padding to more effectively correct biomechanical malalignment **(Figure 6-26C)**. Antishock heel lifts use a dense silicone mixture to cushion heel impact and may be angled to correct some biomechanical alignment of the foot, and relieve strain on the Achilles tendon **(Figure 6-27A)**. Heel cups are used to reduce tissue shearing and shock

in the calcaneal region **(Figure 6-27B)**. Other pads may be used to protect the forefoot region, bunions, and toes. Commercially available pads and devices are readily accessible and easy to apply when treating specific foot conditions. Adhesive felt (moleskin), felt, and foam can be cut to construct similar pads to protect the specified areas.

Selection and fit of shoes may also affect injuries to the lower extremity. Demands of the sport require adaptations in shoe design. For example, in sports requiring repeated

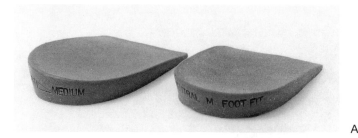

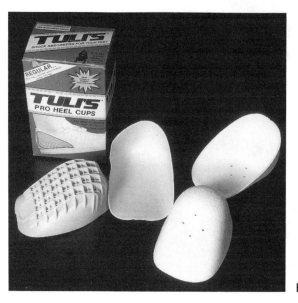

Fig. 6.27: Heel protection. (A) Heel lifts cushion heel impact and may be angled to correct some biomechanical alignment of the foot. (B) Heel cups are used to reduce tissue shearing and shock in the calcaneal region.

> Cleats should be positioned under the major weight-bearing joints of the foot, and should not be felt through the sole of the shoe

push-off, additional forefoot cushioning with greater control on the medial aspect of the shoe should be present. The least amount of pronation in the forefoot takes place while running barefoot. Excessive or prolonged pronation while running in shoes, however, is a major indicator in many running injuries. Although great progress has been made in the past decade in shoe design, recent studies indicate that improved shoe design is still needed with respect to forefoot torsional stiffness and rearfoot construction (70–72). Shoes should adequately cushion impact forces, and support and guide the foot during the stance and final push-off phase of running. In sports requiring repeated heel impact, additional heel cushioning should be present. Length should be sufficient to allow all toes to be fully extended. Individuals with toe abnormalities or bunions may also require a wider toe box. Always fit shoes late in the the day to accommodate any increase in size which may have occurred since awakening. During walking, the shoe should "break" at the widest part

(73). **Field Strategy 6-4** lists several important points to remember when purchasing athletic shoes.

In field sports, the cleated shoe may have long cleats, short cleats, or a multicleated design (**Figure 6-28**). The cleats should be properly positioned under the major weight-bearing joints of the foot, and should not be felt through the sole of the shoe. In individuals with arch problems, the shoe should include adequate forefoot, arch, and heel support. In all cases, individuals should select shoes based on the demands of the activity, not on the color, style, or price.

Did you determine that the baseball player could benefit from an external ankle supportive device, such as a lace-up, semirigid, or air bladder model? These devices are easier for the wearer to apply, do not irritate the skin as much, provide better comfort and fit, and are more cost effective. Use of any external supportive device should be combined with a full rehabilitation program to strengthen the muscles around the injured joint.

Field Strategy 6–4. Factors in the Selection and Fit of Athletic Shoes.

1. Shop with retailers who employ a professional shoe fitter, or pedorthist, who knows about foot biomechanics and foot problems. If one is unavailable in your area, go to stores staffed and patronized by serious recreational athletes.
2. Always fit shoes toward late afternoon or evening, preferably after a workout, to accommodate any increase in shoe size from the start of the day.
3. Wear socks typically worn during sport participation.
4. Fit shoes to the longest toe of the largest foot. The shoe should provide one thumb's width from the longest toe to the end of the toe box. Shoes should feel snug around the foot, but not too tight.
5. With both shoes on, approximate athletic skills in the shoes, i.e., walking, running, jumping, and changing directions.
6. The widest part of the shoe should coincide with the widest part of the foot. While standing, draw an outline of your foot on an index card. Insert the card into the shoe. If the card bends, the shoe is not wide enough.
7. Women with big or wide feet should consider purchasing boy's or men's shoes.
8. Running shoes need more flexibility in the forefoot and toe area for the push-off phase of running. In runners who overpronate, greater control on the medial side is needed. Individuals with Achilles tendinitis should have at least a 15mm heel wedge to protect the tendon.
9. In activities such as tennis, racquetball, and basketball, added side-to-side stability is recommended.
10. Individuals with rigid, high arches may prefer shoes with soft midsoles, curved lasts, and low or moderate hindfoot stability. (The last is the mold around which a shoe is designed, and is responsible for the shape and fit of the shoe.)
11. Individuals with normal arches may prefer shoes with firm midsoles, semicurved lasts, and moderate hindfoot stability.
12. Individuals with a flexible, low arch need a very firm midsole, a straight last, a high degree of hindfoot stability, and an upper shoe with very strong medial and lateral support.
13. After purchasing shoes, walk in them for two or three days to allow them to adapt to the feet. Then begin running or practicing in the shoes for about 25 to 30% of the workout. Gradually extend the length of time the shoes are worn. This will prevent blisters from forming.
14. Avid runners should replace shoes every 3 months, recreational runners every 6 months.

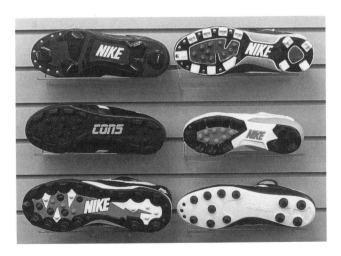

Fig. 6.28: Cleated shoes may have long cleats, short cleats, or a multi-cleated design. Selection will depend on the surface and weather conditions.

SUMMARY

Protective equipment is only effective when it is designed to meet the needs of the sport, is properly fitted and maintained, periodically cleaned and disinfected, and utilized as it was intended to be. In athletic events involving impact and collisions, the sport participant must be protected from high velocity-low mass forces, and low velocity-high mass forces. The design and selection of protective equipment is based on the optimal level of impact intensity afforded by the given thickness, density, resilience, and temperature of energy-absorbing material. Many sports, such as football and ice hockey, require full body protection against collision and impact. Many other sports also require protection over specified body areas at risk for injury. It is imperative that the athletic trainer, coach, and sport supervisor be fully aware of rules and standards governing the selection and fitting of protective equipment to ensure safe participation in the sport.

REFERENCES

1. Hodgson, VR. "Athletic equipment and injury prevention." In *Prevention of athletic injuries: The role of the sport medicine team*, edited by JO Mueller and AJ Ryan. Philadelphia: F. Davis, 1991.
2. The National Collegiate Athletic Association. *NCAA injury surveillance system: 1992–1993*. Overland Park, KS: The National Collegiate Athletic Association, 1993.
3. Hodgson, VR. Impact standards for protective equipment. In *Athletic injuries to the head, neck, and face*, edited by JS Torg. St. Louis: Mosby Year Book, 1991.
4. Committee on Competitive Safeguards and Medical Aspects of Sports. "Protective equipment." *NCAA Sports Medicine Handbook*. Overland Park, KS: The National Collegiate Athletic Association, 1993.
5. American Academy of Orthopaedic Surgeons. *Athletic training and sports medicine*. Park Ridge, IL: American Academy of Orthopaedic Surgeons, 1991.
6. Hadden, RA, and Benzel, EC. 1993. Preventive aspects of helmet safety. West J Med, 158(1):69–70.
7. Bishop, PJ, and Wells, RP. 1990. The inappropriateness of helmet drop tests in assessing neck protection in head-first impacts. Am J Spts Med, 18(2):201–205.
8. Thompson, DC, Thompson, RS, Rivara, FP, and Wolf, ME. 1990. A case-control study of the effectiveness of bicycle safety helmets in preventing facial injury. Am J Pub Health, 80(12):1471–1474.
9. Murphy, P. 1985. Hockey face guards required for 1985–86. Phys Sportsmed, 13(1):29–30.
10. Greenberg, MS, and Springer, PS. "Diagnosis and management of oral injuries." In *Athletic injuries to the head, neck, and face* , edited by JS Torg. St. Louis: Mosby Year Book, 1991.
11. Morrow, RM, Seals, RR, Barnwell, G, Day, EA, Moore, RN, and Stephens, MK. 1991. Report of a survey of oral injuries in male college and university athletes. Ath Train (JNATA), 26(4):338–342.
12. Wilkinson, EE, and Powers, JM. 1986. Properties of custom-made mouth-protector materials. Phys Sportsmed, 14(6):77–84.
13. Francis, KT, and Brasher, J. 1991. Physiological effects of wearing mouthguards. Br J of Spts Med, 25(4):227–31.
14. Kuebker, WA, Morrow, RM, and Cohen, PA. 1986. Do mouth-formed mouth guards meet the NCAA rules? Phys Sportsmed, 14(6):69–74.
15. Doberstein, ST. 1990. A procedure for fitting mouth-formed mouthguards. Ath Train (JNATA), 25(3):244–251.
16. Easterbrook, M. 1992. Getting patients to protect their eyes during sports. Phys Sportsmed, 20(7):165–170.
17. La Forge R. 1990. Preventing eye injuries. Exec Health Report, 3(26):7–9.
18. Easterbrook, M. 1988. Eye protection in racquet sports. Clin Sports Med, 7(2):253–266.
19. Pine, D. 1991. Preventing sports-related eye injuries. Phys Sportsmed, 19(2):129–134.
20. Easterbrook, M. "Eye protection in racquet sports." In *Clinics in Sports Medicine*, vol. 7, no. 2, edited by RC Lehman. Philadelphia: WB Saunders, 1988.
21. Vinger, PE, and Knuttgen, HG. 1988. International Federation of Sports Medicine position statement: Eye injuries and eye protection in sports. Phys Sportsmed, 15(11):49–51.
22. Samples, P. 1989. Experts: Don't swim with soft contacts in. Phys Sportsmed, 17(9):34–35.
23. Diefenback, CB, Soni, PS, Gillespie, BJ, et al. 1988. Extended wear contact lens movement under swimming pool conditions. Am J Optom Physiol Opt, 65(9):710–716.
24. Storey, MD, Schatz, CF, and Brown, KW. 1989. Anterior neck trauma. Phys Sportsmed, 17(9):85–96.
25. Gibbs, R. 1984. A protective collar cervical radiculopathy. Phys Sportsmed 12(5):139.
26. Deppen, D, Nobel, L, Walker, H, and Dorgan, R. 1993. Force absorption in football shoulder pads: A biomechanical assessment. J Ath Train, 28(2):155.
27. Watkins, RG, Dillin, WH, and Maxwell, J. "Cervical spine injuries in football players." In *The spine in sports*, edited by SH Hochschuler. Philadelphia: Hanley & Belfus, 1990.
28. Snyder-Mackler, L, and Epler, M. 1989. Effect of standard and Aircast tennis elbow bands on integrated electromyography of forearm extensor musculature proximal to the bands. Am J Sports Med, 17(0):278–281.
29. Wadsworth CT, Nielsen, DH, Burns LT, Krull, JD, and Thompson, CG. 1989. Effect of the counterforce armband on wrist extension and grip strength and pain in subjects with tennis elbow. J Orthop Sports Phys Ther, 11(1):197–197.
30. Wolf, BE, Kimura, IF, Sitler M, and Kenrick, Z. 1993. Effect of the Aircast pneumatic armband and Pro tennis elbow strap on torque output during concentric wrist extension. J Ath Train, 28(2):170–171.
31. Harding, WG. 1992. Use and misuse of the tennis elbow strap. Phys Sportsmed, 20(8):65–74.

32. Lorentzen, D, and Lawson, L. 1987. Selected sports bras: A biomechanical analysis of breast motion while jogging. Phys Sportsmed, 15(5):128–139.

33. Gehlsen, G, and Albohm, M. 1980. Evaluation of sports bras. Phys Sportsmed, 8(10):89–96.

34. Haycock, CE. 1987. How I manage breast problems in athletes. Phys Sportsmed, 15(3):89–95.

35. Woodhouse, ML, Heinen, JRK, Shall, L, and Bragg, K. 1990. Selected isokinetic lifting parameters of adult male athletes utilizing lumbar/sacral supports. J Ortho Sports Phy Ther, 11(10):467–473.

36. Morris, JM, Lucas, DB, and Bresler, B. 1961. Role of the trunk in stability of the spine. J Bone Joint Surg (Am), 43(2):327–350.

37. Woodhouse, ML, Heinen, JRK, Shall, L, and Bragg, K. 1990. Isokinetic trunk rotation parameters of athletes utilizing lumbar/sacral supports. Ath Train (JNATA), 25(3):240–243.

38. Woodhouse, ML, Heinen, JRK, Shall, L, and Bragg, K. 1993. Concentric isokinetic trunk extension/flexion testing of rigid and semirigid lumbar/sacral supports. J Ath Train, 28(2):106–111.

39. Aronen, JG, and Chronister, RD. 1992. Quadriceps contusions: Hastening the return to play. Phys Sportsmed, 20(7):130–136.

40. Sitler, MR 1992. Role of prophylactic knee and ankle bracing in injury reduction. J Sport Rehab, 1(3):223–236.

41. Salvaterra, GF, Wang, M, Morehouse, CA, and Buckley, WE. 1993. An in vitro biomechanical study of the static stabilizing effect of lateral prophylactic knee bracing on medial stability. Ath Train (JNATA), 28(20):113–119.

42. Brown, TD, Hoeck, JE, and Brand, RA. "Laboratory evaluation of prophylactic knee brace performance under dynamic valgus loading using a surrogate leg model." In Clinics in Sports Medicine, vol. 9, no. 4, edited by LE Paulos. Philadelphia: WB Saunders, 1990.

43. Erickson, AR, Yasuda, K, Beynnon, B, Johnson, R, and Pope, M. 1993. An in vitro dynamic evaluation of prophylactic knee braces during lateral impact loading. Am J Sports Med, 21(1):26–35.

44. Borsa, PA, Lephart, SM, and Fu, FH. 1993. Muscular and functional performance characteristics of individuals wearing prophylactic knee braces. Ath Train (JNATA), 28(4):336–342.

45. American Academy of Orthopaedic Surgeons. A position statement: The use of knee braces. Park Ridge, IL: American Academy of Orthopaedic Surgeons, 1987.

46. Zachazewski, JE, and Geissler, G. 1992. When to prescribe a knee brace. Phys Sportsmed, 20(11):91–99.

47. Beynnon, BD, Pope, MH, Wertheimer, CM, Johnson, RJ, Fleming, BC, Nichols, CE, and Howe, JG. 1992. The effect of functional knee-braces on strain on the anterior cruciate ligament in vivo. J Bone and Joint Surg, 74(9):1298–1312.

48. Woodhouse, ML, Shall, L, Henderson, L, Lambert, S, and Moses, T. 1991. Evaluative testing of functional knee braces in anterior cruciate ligament deficient limbs: An in vivo study. Ath Train (JNATA), 26(2):154.

49. Mortensen, WW, Foreman, K, Focht, L, and Daniel, D. 1988. An invitro study of functional orthoses in the ACL disrupted knee, Trans Orthop Res Soc, 13(4):520–528.

50. Branch, TP, and Hunter, RE. "Functional analysis of anterior cruciate ligament braces." In Clinics in Sports Medicine, vol. 9, no. 4, edited by LE Paulos. Philadelphia: WB Saunders, 1990.

51. Styf, JR, Nakhostine, M, and Gershuni, DH. 1992. Functional knee braces increase intramuscular pressures in the anterior compartment of the leg. Am J Sports Med, 20(1):46–49.

52. Swain, RA, and Wilson, FD. 1993. Diagnosing posterolateral rotatory knee instability, Phys Sportsmed, 21(4):95–102.

53. Frndak, PA. 1991. Rehabiliation concerns following anterior cruciate ligament reconstruction. Sports Med, 12(5):338–346.

54. Cawley, PW, France, EP, and Paulos, LE. 1989. Comparison of rehabilitative knee braces: A biomechanical investigation. Am J Sports Med, 17(2):141–146.

55. Cawley, PW. "Postoperative knee bracing." In Clinics in Sports Medicine, vol. 9, no. 4, edited by LE Paulos. Philadelphia: WB Saunders, 1990.

56. Henry, JH. "Conservative treatment of patellofemoral subluxation." In Clinics in sports medicine, vol. 8, no. 2, edited by JH Henry. Philadelphia: WB Saunders, 1989.

57. Kimura, I, Beninoato, P, and Sitler, M. 1992. Effect of sport ankle orthoses on range of motion and torque production during ankle motion. J Ath Train, 27(2):150.

58. Gehlsen, GM, Pearson, D, and Bahamonde, R. 1991. Ankle joint strength, total work, and rom: Comparison between prophylactic devices. Ath Train (JNATA), 26(1):62–65.

59. Greene, TA, and Hillman, SK. 1990. Comparison of support provided by a semirigid orthosis and adhesive ankle taping before, during, and after exercise. Am J Sports Med, 18(5):498–506.

60. Carroll, MJ, Rijke, AM, and Perrin, DH. 1993. Effect of the Swede-O ankle brace on subtalar joint displacement in subjects with unstable ankles. J Ath Train, 28(2):154.

61. Lyle, TD, and Corbin, CB. 1992. Restriction of ankle inversion: Taping versus an ankle brace. Phys Edu, 49(2):88–94.

62. Martin, N, and Harter, RA. 1993. Comparison of inversion restraint provided by ankle prophylactic devices before and after exercise. Ath Train (JNATA), 28(4):324–329.

63. Mack, KS, Douglas, MS, Kum, SKC, and Haskvits, EM. 1993. Effects of Sport-stirrup and taping on ankle inversion before and after exercise. J Ath Train, 28(2):167.

64. Gross, MT, Lapp, AK, and Davis, JM. 1991. Comparison of Swede-O Universal ankle support and Aircast Sport-stirrup, orthoses and ankle tape in restricting eversion-inversion before and after exercise. J Ortho Sports Phys Ther, 13(1):11–19.

65. Gross, MT, Bradshaw, MK, Ventry, LC, and Weller, KH. 1987. J Ortho Sports Phys Ther, 9(1):33–39.

66. Sitler, M, Ryan, J, Wheeler, B, McBride, J, Arciero, R, Anderson, J, and Horodyski, M. 1993. The clinical effectiveness of a semirigid ankle brace to reduce

acute ankle injuries in basketball. J Ath Train, 28(2):152-153.

67. Feuerback JW, and Grabiner, MD. 1993. Effect of the Aircast on unilateral postural control: amplitude and frequency variables. J Ortho Sports Phys Ther, 17(3):149-154.

68. Lepp, TM, and Teal, SW. 1991. The effectiveness of a semirigid orthosis as a phophylaxis for ankle injuries: A retrospective study. Ath Train (JNATA), 26(2):158.

69. Barrett, JR, Tanhi, JL, Drake, C, Fuller, D, Kawasaki, RI, and Fenton, RM. 1993. High- versus low-top shoes for the prevention of ankle sprains in basketball players: A prospective randomized study. Am J Sports Med, 21(4):582-585.

70. Stacoff, A, Kälin, X, and Stüssi, E. 1991. The effects of shoes on the torsion and rearfoot motion in running. Med Sci Sports Exerc, 23(4):482-490.

71. Stephens, MM, and Sammarco, GJ. 1992. Heel pain: Shoes, exertion, and Haglund's deformity. Phys Sportsmed, 20(4):87-95.

72. Nigg, BM, and Segesser, B. 1992. Biomechanical and orthopedic concepts in sport shoe construction. Med Sci Sports Exerc, 24(5):595-602.

73. Wichmann, S, and Martin, DR. 1993. Athletic shoes: Finding the right fit. Phys Sportsmed, 21(3)204–211.

Injuries to the Lower Extremity

Injuries to the Lower Extremity

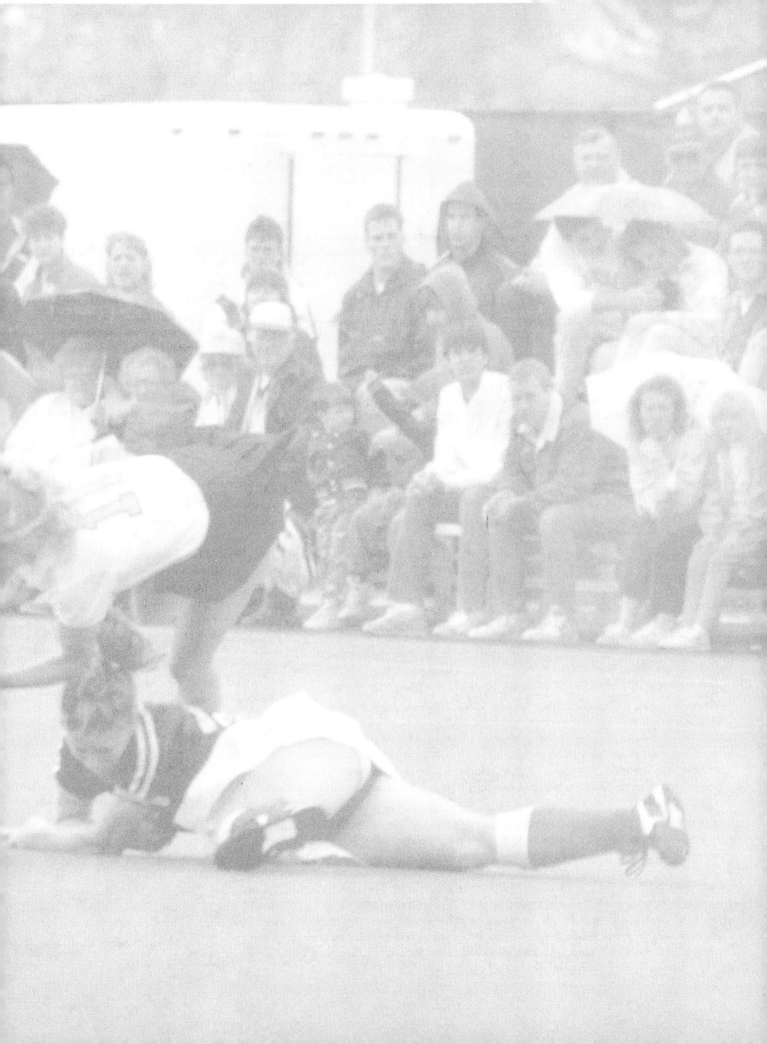

Ron O'Neil, B.S., A.T.,C.

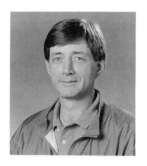

Ron O'Neil is the Head Athletic Trainer for the New England Patriots Professional Football Team in Foxboro, Massachusetts. As an athletic trainer for over two decades, Ron has distinguished himself as an educator and professional committed to providing comprehensive health care to his players.

Although I started college studying to be an architect, I got interested in athletic training after an ankle injury occurred just prior to the baseball season. The two trainers who worked daily on my ankle took time to explain what they were doing and told me exactly what I needed to do to get ready for the season. When I showed an interest in their work, they invited me to observe during the football season. It wasn't long before I knew that was what I wanted to do.

In my position as a professional football trainer, I work 12 months a year. A large part of the off-season in January through February involves supervising the rehabilitation of players who may have been injured during the season or who have just had surgery. In late February, the medical staff travels to Indianapolis to evaluate the health status of over 350 college players. We see 110+ men a day as they complete a comprehensive physical examination. From that data, my staff and I call several colleges and universities to verify the athlete's health records. In April, we fly back to Indianapolis to re-evaluate those individuals who may not have had a complete exam in February due to an injury. All of this has to be done before the draft.

Starting in March, we have over 50 men training at the stadium. Our weight room is open from 6am to 6pm. Once training camp begins in mid-July through the end of August, I work 18 to 20 hours every day of the week, and when the regular season starts in September, I work 12 to 14 hours every day. To say you have to be committed to this job is an understatement. There is very little down time, but I wouldn't give it up for the world.

It is so exciting to work with these elite athletes, especially when you realize that fewer than 0.5% of all men can play professional sports, and you're the one entrusted to keep these individuals healthy. It is really special, very gratifying. The players really appreciate what you do for them, not just taking care of the physical injury, but taking the time to talk to them, counsel them, and taking a sincere interest in their personal welfare. Our team physician and medical staff are totally committed to providing quality care to our players to increase their longevity, not only during the time they are with us, but more importantly, when they leave us. We want these individuals to have a healthy, long life, and we know that what we do everyday for them will impact that goal.

Working on the professional level is hard work, and there is a certain amount of stress to return these players to competition quickly. But you get to see a variety of injuries and can follow the player through the entire course of the rehabilitation. Because the medical staff is so extensive, we can have these players seen by a specialist almost immediately after injury. The team physician, Dr. Bert Zarins, is present at the stadium two days of the week and on game day. It is just a remarkably talented and complete medical staff.

For those of you thinking of working at the professional level, I recommend you develop a broad background in athletic training and personnel management. It's not enough just to know about prevention, treatment, rehabilitation, conditioning, weight training, and nutrition. You have to communicate this knowledge in daily interaction with your athletes. That means being physically fit, being a professional, and taking a sincere personal interest in your players. Working on the professional level is great, but you need to be willing to put in the long hours needed to provide total health care for your players. You need to volunteer at your area team locations to get your foot in the door, and you have to show initiative and commitment to your profession. Without commitment and dedication to the total health care of your athlete, you're in the wrong profession.

Chapter 7

Foot, Ankle, and Lower Leg

After you have completed this chapter, you should be able to:

■ Locate the important bony and soft tissue structures of the foot, ankle, and lower leg

■ Analyze the function of the plantar arches and their role in supporting and distributing body weight

■ Describe the motions of the foot and ankle and identify the muscles that produce them

■ Explain what forces produce the loading patterns responsible for common injuries in the foot, ankle, and lower leg

■ Identify basic principles in the prevention of injuries to the foot, ankle, and lower leg

■ Recognize and manage specific injuries of the foot, ankle, and lower leg

■ Demonstrate a thorough assessment of the foot, ankle, and lower leg

■ Demonstrate general rehabilitation exercises for the region

Because of the essential roles played by the foot, ankle, and lower leg in all sport activities, injuries to this region are common. Sport participation often places both acute and chronic overloads on the lower extremity, leading to sprains, strains, and overuse injuries. Ankle injuries, in particular, comprise 20 to 25% of all injuries associated with running and jumping sports resulting in a loss of training time (1).

This chapter begins with an anatomical review and biomechanical overview of the foot, ankle, and lower leg. Next, prevention of injuries will be followed by discussion on specific sports injuries and their management. Finally, a step-by-step injury assessment of the region will be presented, and examples of rehabilitative exercises will be provided.

ANATOMY REVIEW OF THE FOOT, ANKLE, AND LOWER LEG

● *A volleyball player has pain on the plantar side of the midfoot during jumping drills. Although the pain is not too severe, it has worsened over the past week. What anatomical structures might be the source of pain?*

The foot, ankle, and lower leg provide a foundation of support for the upright body, propulsion through space, adaptation for uneven terrain, and absorption of shock. Dis-

cussion of the anatomical structures that contribute to these abilities is organized, beginning with bone and ligamentous structures of the leg and the three major regions of the foot—the forefoot, midfoot, and hindfoot **(Figure 7-1)**. Next, the plantar arches are discussed, and finally, the muscles, nerves, and blood vessels of the region.

Forefoot

The forefoot is composed of five metatarsals and fourteen phalanges along with numerous joints. Together they work with the midfoot region to form interdependent longitudinal and transverse arches to support and distribute body weight throughout the foot.

Metatarsophalangeal and Interphalangeal Joints

The metatarsophalangeal (MTP), proximal interphalangeal (PIP), and distal interphalangeal (DIP) joints are condyloid and hinge joints, respectively, with close packed positions in full extension **(Figure 7-1)**. Both sets of joints are reinforced by numerous ligaments. The deep transverse metatarsal ligament interconnects all five metatarsals. The toes function to smooth the weight shift to the opposite foot during walking and help maintain stability during weight bearing by

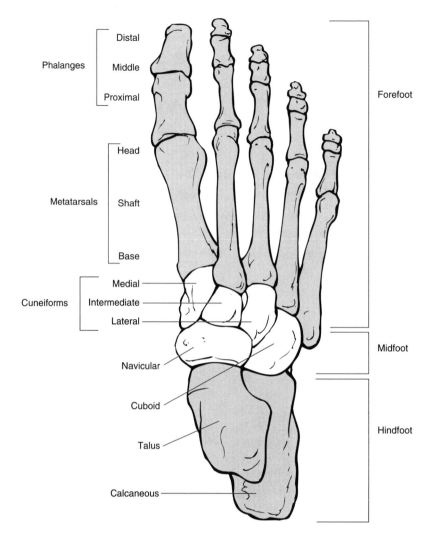

Phalanges
Distal
Middle
Proximal

Metatarsals
Head
Shaft
Base

Cuneiforms
Medial
Intermediate
Lateral

Navicular

Cuboid

Talus

Calcaneous

Forefoot

Midfoot

Hindfoot

Fig. 7.1: The bones of the foot are divided into three major regions—the hindfoot, midfoot, and forefoot.

Hallux
The first, or great toe

pressing against the ground when necessary. The first digit is referred to as the **hallux**, or "great toe," and is the main body support during walking or running.

The first MTP joint has two sesamoid bones located on the plantar surface of the joint to share in weight bearing. The sesamoid bones serve as anatomic pulleys for the flexor hallucis brevis muscle and protect the flexor hallucis longus muscle tendon from weight-bearing trauma as it passes between the two bones.

Tarsometatarsal and Intermetatarsal Joints

Both the tarsometatarsal (TM) and intermetatarsal (IM) joints are of the gliding type with the close packed position in supination. These joints enable the foot to adapt to uneven surfaces during gait (**Figure 7-1**).

The long plantar ligament contributes to transverse tarsal joint stability and supports the medial and lateral longitudinal arches

Midfoot

The midfoot region encompasses the navicular, cuboid, three cuneiform bones, and their articulations. The navicular, like its counterpart in the wrist (the scaphoid), helps to bridge movements between the hindfoot and forefoot.

Transverse Tarsal Joint

The transverse tarsal (or midtarsal) joint consists of two side-by-side articulations—calcaneocuboid on the lateral side and the talonavicular joint on the medial side (**Figure 7-2**). These two joints are collectively called the transverse tarsal joint because they are adjacent and function as a unit.

The calcaneocuboid joint is a saddle shaped joint with a close packed position in supination. The joint is nonaxial and permits

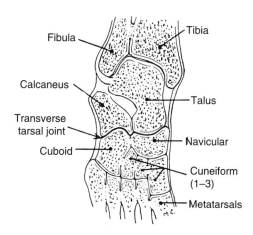

Fig. 7.2: The transverse tarsal joint consists of the adjacent talonavicular and calcaneocuboid articulations.

only limited gliding motion. It is supported by the bifurcate ligament, calcaneocuboid ligament, and long plantar ligament. The most important of these, the long plantar ligament, extends inferiorly between the calcaneus and the cuboid, and then continues distally to the base of the second, third, and fourth metatarsals, contributing significantly to transverse tarsal joint stability.

Because the talus moves simultaneously on the calcaneus and navicular, the term *talo-calcaneonavicular joint* (TCN) is often used to describe the combined action of the talonavicular and subtalar joint. The TCN is a modified ball-and-socket joint with a close packed position in supination. Movements at the joint include gliding and rotation. Three ligaments support the joint—the plantar calcaneonavicular (spring) ligament inferiorly, deltoid ligament medially, and the bifurcate ligament laterally (**Figure 7-3**).

Because the subtalar joint is mechanically linked to the TCN and transverse tarsal joints, any motion at the subtalar joint produces like motions at the transverse tarsal joints. For example, when the TCN is fully supinated and locked, the midfoot region is also supinated and rigid. When the TCN is pronated and loose packed, the midfoot region is also mobile and loose.

Other Midtarsal Joints

The remaining joints of the midfoot region include the cuneonavicular, cuboideonavicular, cuneocuboid, and the intercuneiform.

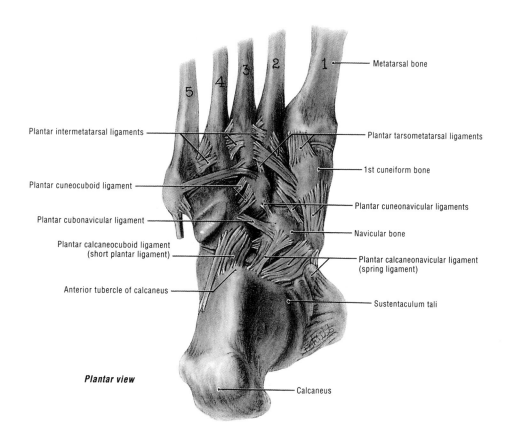

Plantar view

Fig. 7.3: The plantar ligaments provide integrity for the numerous bones and articulations of the foot.

These joints provide gliding and rotation for the midfoot with a close packed position in supination. They are bound together by several ligaments **(Figure 7-4)**. When the midfoot (TCN) is locked in supination, these joints function in a compensatory manner to pronate the forefoot to increase stability. When the hindfoot is pronated, these joints supinate the forefoot to keep the foot flat on the surface (2).

Hindfoot

The hindfoot includes the calcaneus and talus. Moveable joints in the hindfoot region include the talocrural joint (ankle joint), and subtalar joint. Both serve a unique role in the integrated function of the foot, ankle, and lower leg.

Talocrural Joint

The talocrural joint (ankle joint) is a uniaxial, modified hinge joint formed by the talus, the tibia, and the lateral malleolus of the fibula **(Figure 7-4)**. The concave end of the weight-bearing tibia mates with the convex superior surface of the talus, providing great bony stability. Because the talus is wider anteriorly than posteriorly, the joint's close packed position is maximum dorsiflexion.

Although the joint capsule is thin and especially weak anteriorly and posteriorly, the ankle is crossed by a number of strong ligaments that enhance its stability. The four separate bands of the medial collateral ligament, more commonly called the deltoid ligament, cross the ankle medially. Forces producing stress on the medial aspect of the ankle typi-

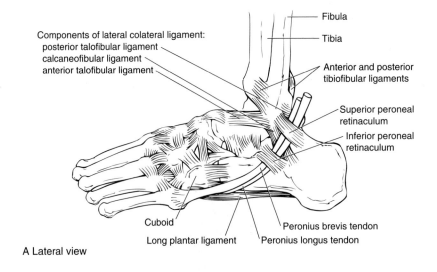

A Lateral view

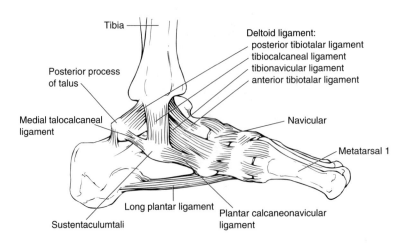

B Medial view

Fig. 7.4: Ligaments supporting the midfoot and hindfoot region.

cally cause an avulsion fracture of the medial malleolus rather than a tear of the deltoid ligament. The lateral side of the ankle is supported by three ligaments—the anterior and posterior talofibular, and the calcaneofibular. The relative weakness of these lateral ligaments as compared to the deltoid ligament, coupled with less bony stability laterally than medially, contributes to a higher frequency of lateral ankle sprains.

Subtalar Joint

As the name suggests, the subtalar joint lies beneath the talus where facets of the talus articulate with the sustentaculum tali on the superior calcaneus. The joint, also referred to as the talocalcaneal joint, is crossed by four small talocalcaneal ligaments that connect the talus to the calcaneus. The joint functions basically as a hinge joint with the axis aligned in an oblique direction (**Figure 7-5**). The orientation of the subtalar joint axis varies appreciably among individuals (2,3).

Tibiofibular Joints

The tibia is the weight-bearing bone of the leg and articulates with the fibula at both proximal and distal ends (**Figure 7-6**). The fibula, which does not assist with weight bearing, serves as a site for muscle attachments and contributes to stability at the ankle. The superior, or proximal tibiofibular joint, is a plane synovial joint that is tightly reinforced with anterior and posterior ligaments. The inferior, or distal, tibiofibular joint is a **syndesmosis**, where dense fibrous tissue binds the bones together. There is no joint capsule, but the joint is supported by the anterior and posterior tibiofibular ligaments, as well as by the crural interosseous tibiofibular ligament (**Figure 7-6**). The tibia and fibula are also joined throughout most of their length by the interosseus membrane. This membrane is of such strength that strong lateral stresses will fracture the fibula rather than tear the membrane.

Plantar Arches

The bones and supporting ligamentous structures in the tarsal and metatarsal regions of the foot form interdependent longitudinal and transverse arches (**Figure 7-7**). They function to support and distribute body weight from the talus through the foot across changing weight-bearing conditions and over varying terrains.

The longitudinal arch runs from the anterior, inferior calcaneus to the metatarsal heads. Because the arch is higher medially than laterally, the medial side is usually the point of reference.

The transverse arch runs across the anterior tarsals and the anterior metatarsals. The foundation of the arch is the medial cuneiform with the apex of the arch formed by the second metatarsal. At the level of the metatarsal heads the arch is reduced with all metatarsals aligned parallel to the weight bearing surface for even distribution of body weight (2).

The primary ligaments supporting the plantar arches are, in order of importance, the spring (calcaneonavicular), long plantar, plantar fascia (plantar aponeurosis), and the short plantar (plantar calcaneocuboid) (**Figure 7-8**). The spring ligament is the primary

> The tibiofibular interosseous ligament is so strong that excessive stress will fracture the fibula rather than rupture the ligament

> The spring ligament is the primary supporter for the medial longitudinal arch

Syndesmosis
A joint where the opposing surfaces are joined together by fibrous connective tissue

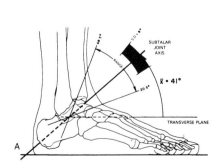
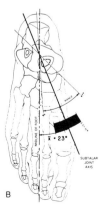

Fig. 7.5: The axis of rotation at the subtalar joint lies oblique to the sagittal and frontal planes.

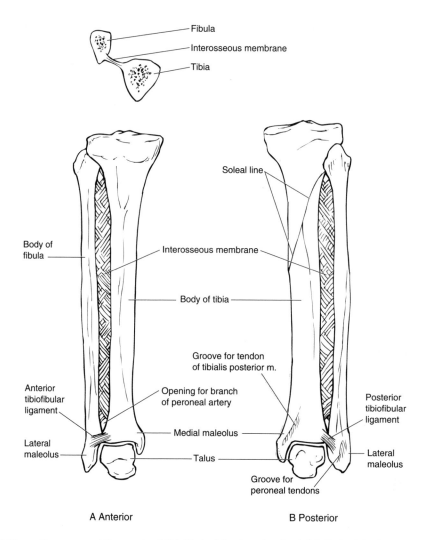

Fibula
Interosseous membrane
Tibia

Soleal line

Body of fibula

Interosseous membrane

Body of tibia

Groove for tendon of tibialis posterior m.

Anterior tibiofibular ligament

Opening for branch of peroneal artery

Posterior tibiofibular ligament

Lateral maleolus

Medial maleolus

Lateral maleolus

Talus

Groove for peroneal tendons

A Anterior

B Posterior

Fig. 7.6: Little motion occurs at the proximal tibiofibular joint, but the distal tibiofibular joint forms the mortise for the talocrural joint. The interosseus membrane joins the full lengths of the tibia and fibula.

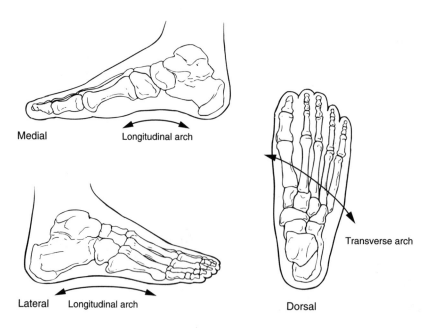

Medial

Longitudinal arch

Lateral

Longitudinal arch

Transverse arch

Dorsal

Fig. 7.7: The arches of the foot.

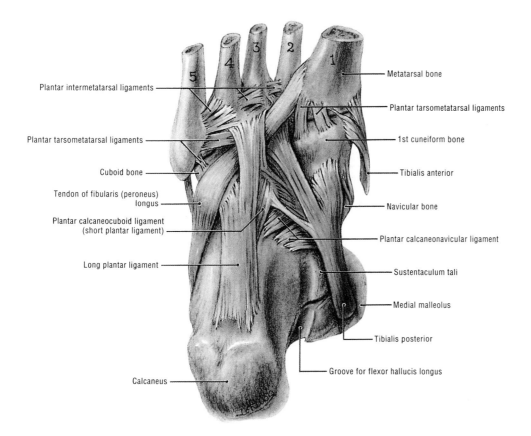

Plantar intermetatarsal ligaments

Plantar tarsometatarsal ligaments

Cuboid bone

Tendon of fibularis (peroneus) longus

Plantar calcaneocuboid ligament (short plantar ligament)

Long plantar ligament

Calcaneus

Metatarsal bone

Plantar tarsometatarsal ligaments

1st cuneiform bone

Tibialis anterior

Navicular bone

Plantar calcaneonavicular ligament

Sustentaculum tali

Medial malleolus

Tibialis posterior

Groove for flexor hallucis longus

Fig. 7.8: The medial longitudinal arch is supported by the spring ligament, short plantar ligament, long plantar ligament, plantar aponeurosis, and the tibialis posterior tendon.

supporter of the medial longitudinal arch, stretching from the sustentaculum tali on the calcaneus to the inferior navicular. The long plantar ligament is the primary support for the lateral longitudinal arch and calcaneocuboid joint. The short plantar ligament assists with these functions. When muscle tension is present, the muscles of the foot, particularly the tibialis posterior, also contribute support to the arches and joints as they cross them.

The **plantar fascia**, or plantar aponeurosis, is a specialized thick interconnected band of fascia that covers the plantar surface of the foot, providing support for the longitudinal arch (**Figure 7-9**). It extends from the posterior medial calcaneus to the proximal phalanx of each toe where it attaches with deep transverse metatarsal ligaments. During the weight-bearing phase of the gait cycle the plantar fascia functions like a spring to store mechanical energy which is then released to help the foot push off from the surface. The plantar fascia may be elongated by stretching the Achilles tendon, because both structures attach to the calcaneus.

Muscles of the Lower Leg and Foot

Thick sheaths of fascia divide the muscles of the leg into four compartments—the anterior, deep and superficial posterior, and lateral compartments (**Figure 7-10**). The anterior compartment contains the tibialis anterior, extensor digitorum longus, extensor hallucis longus, and peroneus tertius (**Figure 7-11**). These muscles can easily be remembered by using the mnemonic Tom, Dick, and Harry too. Muscles in the deep posterior compartment can also be remembered by the Tom, Dick, and Harry mnemonic, and include the tibialis posterior, flexor digitorum longus, and flexor hallucis longus (**Figure 7-12**). The superficial posterior compartment contains the gastrocnemius, soleus and plantaris (**Figure 7-13**). The lateral compartment contains the peroneus longus and peroneus brevis (**Figure 7-14**).

The foot contains both intrinsic and extrinsic muscles (**Figure 7-15**). Intrinsic muscles have both attachments of the muscles contained within the foot while extrinsic muscles have one attachment outside the

Plantar fascia
Specialized band of fascia that covers the plantar surface of the foot and helps support the longitudinal arch

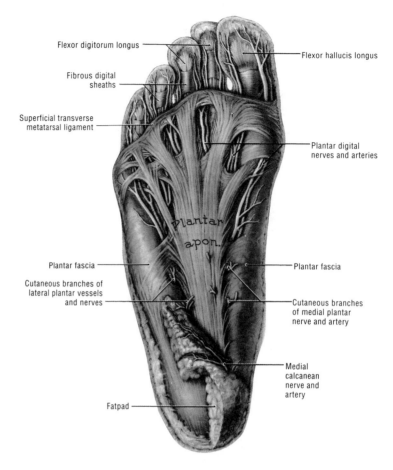

Flexor digitorum longus

Flexor hallucis longus

Fibrous digital sheaths

Superficial transverse metatarsal ligament

Plantar digital nerves and arteries

Plantar apon.

Plantar fascia

Plantar fascia

Cutaneous branches of lateral plantar vessels and nerves

Cutaneous branches of medial plantar nerve and artery

Medial calcanean nerve and artery

Fatpad

Fig. 7.9: The plantar fascia stores mechanical energy each time the foot deforms during the weight-bearing phase of the gait cycle.

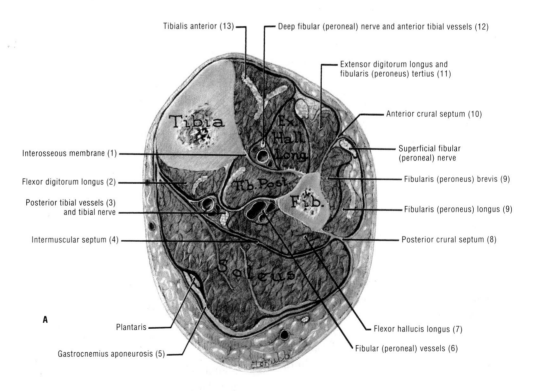

Tibialis anterior (13)

Deep fibular (peroneal) nerve and anterior tibial vessels (12)

Extensor digitorum longus and fibularis (peroneus) tertius (11)

Anterior crural septum (10)

Tibia

Ex. Hall. Long.

Interosseous membrane (1)

Superficial fibular (peroneal) nerve

Flexor digitorum longus (2)

Tb. Post.

Fib.

Fibularis (peroneus) brevis (9)

Posterior tibial vessels (3) and tibial nerve

Fibularis (peroneus) longus (9)

Intermuscular septum (4)

Posterior crural septum (8)

Soleus

A

Plantaris

Flexor hallucis longus (7)

Gastrocnemius aponeurosis (5)

Fibular (peroneal) vessels (6)

Fig. 7.10: The muscles of the leg lie in anterior, deep posterior, superficial posterior, and lateral compartments.

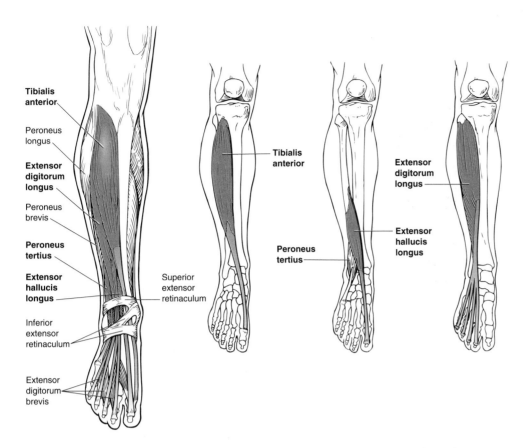

Fig. 7.11: The anterior compartment of the leg contains the tibialis anterior, extensor digitorum longus, extensor hallucis longus, and peroneus tertius.

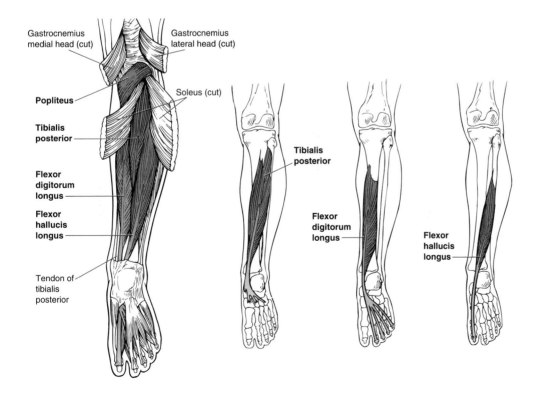

Fig. 7.12: The muscles in the deep posterior compartment pass behind the medial malleolus to enter the foot. Using the **T**om, **D**ick, **an**d **H**arry mnemonic, the structures pass anterior to posterior in this order: **t**ibialis posterior, flexor **d**igitorum longus, tibialis posterior **a**rtery, tibial **n**erve, and flexor **h**allucis longus.

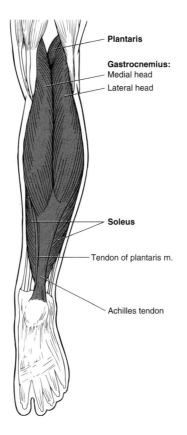

Fig. 7.13: The superficial compartment is composed of the gastrocnemius and soleus. They are collectively called the triceps surae and attach to the calcaneus via the Achilles tendon.

foot. The attachments and primary actions of the major extrinsic muscles of the foot, ankle, and lower leg are summarized in **Table 7-1**.

Nerves of the Foot, Ankle, and Lower Leg

The sciatic nerve and its branches provide primary innervation for the foot, ankle, and lower leg (**Figure 7-16**). Traveling down the posterior aspect of the leg from the lumbosacral spine, the sciatic nerve branches into smaller nerves just proximal to the popliteal fossa. The major branch is the tibial nerve that innervates the posterior aspect of the leg and the common peroneal nerve that spawns the deep and superficial peroneal nerves.

The tibial nerve (L_4-S_3) passes through the popliteal fossa and down the leg between the superficial and deep muscles in the posterior compartment of the leg. It continues medially behind the medial malleolus with the posterior tibial artery to become the medial and lateral plantar nerves. The saphenous nerve (L_2-L_4), which branches from the femoral nerve, supplies cutaneous innervation to the medial aspect of the ankle.

The common peroneal nerve passes laterally around the neck of the fibula to the anterolateral leg where it splits into the deep

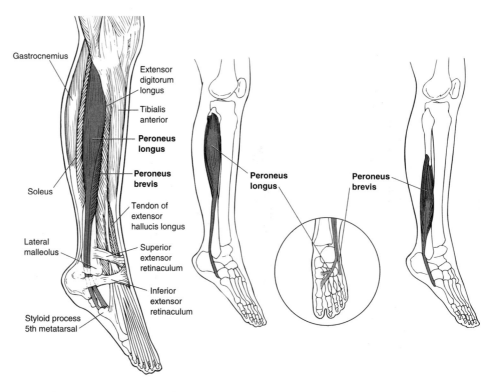

Fig. 7.14: The lateral compartment of the leg contains the peroneus brevis and peroneus longus. Note that the peroneus tertius is an extension of the extensor digitorum longus and is in the anterior compartment.

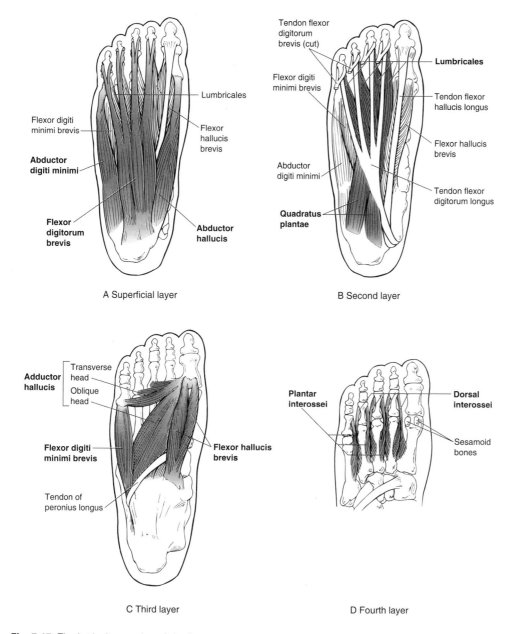

Flexor digiti minimi brevis

Abductor digiti minimi

Flexor digitorum brevis

Lumbricales

Flexor hallucis brevis

Abductor hallucis

A Superficial layer

Tendon flexor digitorum brevis (cut)

Flexor digiti minimi brevis

Abductor digiti minimi

Quadratus plantae

Lumbricales

Tendon flexor hallucis longus

Flexor hallucis brevis

Tendon flexor digitorum longus

B Second layer

Adductor hallucis

Transverse head

Oblique head

Flexor digiti minimi brevis

Tendon of peronius longus

Flexor hallucis brevis

C Third layer

Plantar interossei

Dorsal interossei

Sesamoid bones

D Fourth layer

Fig. 7.15: The intrinsic muscles of the foot.

and superficial peroneal nerves. The deep peroneal nerve (L_4-S_1) innervates the anterior compartment containing the ankle dorsiflexors and toe extensors, then courses over the dorsum of the foot to innervate the skin between the first and second toes. The superficial peroneal nerve (L_5-S_2) innervates the lateral compartment containing the primary evertor muscles and provides cutaneous innervation to the second through fourth toes. The sural nerve (L_4-S_2), a branch from both the common peroneal and tibial nerves, supplies cutaneous innervation to the lateral aspect of the foot. Given the extensiveness of the sciatic nerve supply to the lower extrem-

ity, it is no surprise that impingement of the sciatic nerve by a herniated disc in the lumbosacral region often results in pain, numbness and/or impaired function in the foot and ankle region.

Blood Vessels of the Foot, Ankle, and Lower Leg

The blood supply to the foot, ankle, and lower leg enters the lower extremity as the femoral artery (**Figure 7-17**). The femoral artery becomes the popliteal artery proximal and posterior to the knee, then branches into the anterior and posterior tibial arteries just

Table 7–1. Major Muscles of the Foot and Leg.

Muscle	Proximal Attachment	Distal Attachment	Primary Action(s)	Nerve Innervation
Anterior Compartment				
Tibialis anterior	Upper two-thirds lateral tibia and interosseus membrane	Medial surface of first cuneiform and first metatarsal	Dorsiflexion Inversion	Deep peroneal (L_4, L_5)
Extensor digitorum longus	Upper three-fourths anterior fibula and interosseus membrane	Second and third phalanges of 4 lesser toes	Toe extension Dorsiflexion	Deep peroneal (L_5, S_1)
Extensor hallucis longus	Middle anterior fibula and interosseus membrane	Dorsal surface of distal phalanx of great toe	Extension of great toe	Deep peroneal (L_5, S_1)
Peroneus tertius	Distal third of anterior fibula and interosseus membrane	Dorsal surface styloid process, fifth metatarsal	Eversion Dorsiflexion	Deep peroneal (L_5, S_1)
Lateral Compartment				
Peroneus longus	Proximal two-thirds lateral fibula	Plantar surface of first cuneiform and first metatarsal	Eversion Plantar flexion	Superficial peroneal $(L_5–S_2)$
Peroneus brevis	Distal two-thirds fibula	Lateral side of styloid process, fifth metatarsal	Eversion Plantar flexion	Superficial peroneal $(L_5–S_2)$
Posterior Deep Compartment				
Flexor digitorum longus	Posterior tibia	Distal phalanx of 4 lesser toes	Toe flexion Plantar flexion	Tibial (S_2, S_3)
Flexor hallucis longus	Distal two-thirds posterior fibula	Distal phalanx of the great toe	Flexion of the great toe Plantar flexion	Tibial (S_2, S_3)
Tibialis posterior	Upper two-thirds tibia, fibula and interosseus membrane	Cuboid, navicular, cuneiforms and 2 to 4 metatarsals	Inversion Plantar flexion	Tibial (L_4, L_5)
Popliteus	Lateral condyle of femur	Proximal portion of posterior tibia	Knee flexion Medial rotation of flexed leg	Tibial $(L_4–S_1)$
Posterior Superficial Compartment				
Gastrocnemius	Posterior medial and lateral condyles of the femur	Calcaneal tuberosity via Achilles tendon	Plantar flexion Knee flexion	Tibial (S_1, S_2)
Soleus	Posterior proximal fibula and middle tibia	Calcaneal tuberosity via Achilles tendon	Plantar flexion	Tibial (S_1, S_2)
Plantaris	Posterior femur above lateral condyle	Calcaneal tuberosity by Achilles tendon	Plantar flexion Knee flexion	Tibial (S_1, S_2)

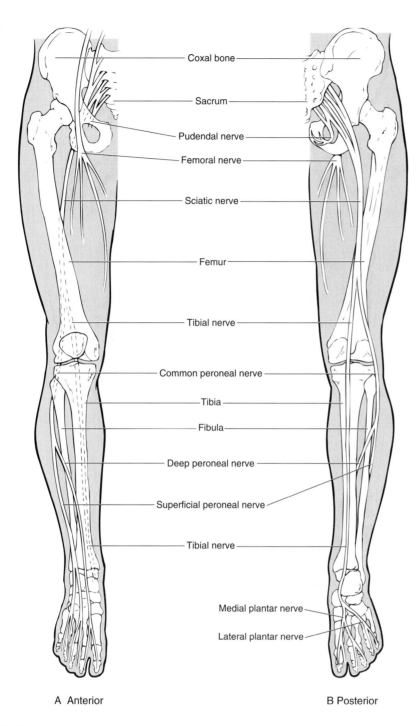

Coxal bone
Sacrum
Pudendal nerve
Femoral nerve
Sciatic nerve
Femur
Tibial nerve
Common peroneal nerve
Tibia
Fibula
Deep peroneal nerve
Superficial peroneal nerve
Tibial nerve
Medial plantar nerve
Lateral plantar nerve

A Anterior

B Posterior

Fig. 7.16: Motor function to the lower leg is supplied by the sciatic nerve (L_4, L_5, S_1). Sensory innervation is supplied by the sciatic nerve and saphenous branch of the femoral nerve (L_2, L_3, L_4).

distal to the knee. The anterior tibial artery becomes the dorsalis pedis artery to supply the dorsum of the foot. The posterior tibial artery gives off several branches that supply the posterior and lateral compartments, and the plantar region of the foot.

Did you determine which structures may be causing the pain on the plantar aspect of the midfoot? If you determined the navicular, medial and middle cuneiforms, medial longitudinal arch and associated ligaments, or the tibialis posterior or toe flexors, you are correct.

Pulses can be taken at the dorsum of the foot (dorsalis pedis) and behind the medial malleolus (tibialis posterior)

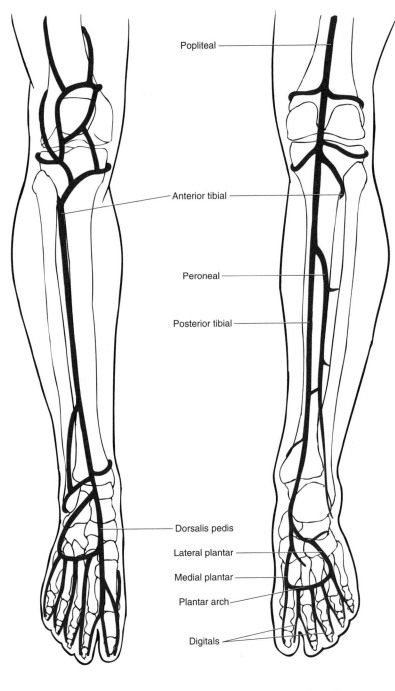

Popliteal

Anterior tibial

Peroneal

Posterior tibial

Dorsalis pedis

Lateral plantar

Medial plantar

Plantar arch

Digitals

A Anterior view

B Posterior view

Fig. 7.17: The blood supply to the leg, ankle, and foot region. The dorsalis pedis artery is easily palpated in the midfoot region between the second and third tendons of the extensor digitorum longus.

KINEMATICS OF THE FOOT, ANKLE, AND LOWER LEG

Many styles of running shoes are designed to control pronation and supination of the foot. At which joints do these motions occur?

Kinematics is the study of spatial and temporal aspects of motion, which translates to movement form or technique. Evaluation of the kinematics of a particular movement can provide information about timing and sequencing of movement, which can then yield important clues for injury prevention. This section describes the kinematics of the foot, ankle, and lower leg, and identifies muscles responsible for specific movements.

Kinematics
Study of the spatial and temporal aspects of movement

The Gait Cycle

Despite variation in individual gait patterns, enough commonality exists in human gaits that one can describe the typical gait cycle (**Figure 7-18**). The gait cycle begins with a period of single leg support in which body weight is supported by one leg while the other leg swings forward. The swing phase can be divided into the initial swing, midswing, and terminal swing. The period of double support begins with the contact of the swing leg with the ground or floor. As body weight transfers from the support leg to the swing leg, the swing leg undergoes a loading response and becomes the new support leg. A new period of single support then begins as the swing leg loses ground contact. The time through which body weight is balanced over the support leg is referred to as midstance. As the body's center of gravity shifts forward, the terminal stance phase of the support leg coincides with the terminal swing phase of the opposite leg.

The gait cycle requires a set of coordinated, sequential joint actions of the lower extremity. Many of these specific motions are described later in the chapter.

Toe Flexion and Extension

Several muscles contribute to flexion of the second through fifth toes. These include the flexor digitorum longus, flexor digitorum brevis, quadratus plantae, lumbricals, and interossei. The flexor hallucis longus and brevis produce flexion of the hallux. Conversely, the extensor hallucis longus, extensor digitorum longus, and extensor digitorum brevis are responsible for extension and overextension of the toes.

Dorsiflexion and Plantar Flexion

Motion at the ankle occurs primarily in the sagittal plane, with ankle flexion and extension being termed dorsiflexion and plantar flexion, respectively (**Figure 7-19**). The medial and lateral malleoli serve as pulleys to channel the tendons of the leg muscles either posterior or anterior to the axis of rotation, thereby enabling their contributions to either dorsiflexion or plantar flexion. Muscles with tendons passing anterior to the malleoli, such as the tibialis anterior, extensor digitorum longus, and peroneus tertius, are dorsiflexors. Those with tendinous attachments running posterior to the malleoli, such as the soleus, gastrocnemius, plantaris, peroneal longus and brevis, tibialis posterior, and toe flexors contribute to plantar flexion.

Inversion and Eversion

Rotations of the foot in the medial and lateral directions are termed inversion and eversion, respectively (**Figure 7-19**). These movements occur primarily at the subtalar joint, with secondary contributions from gliding movements at the intertarsal and tarsometatarsal joints. The tibialis posterior and tibialis anterior are the major inverters. Peroneus longus and peroneus brevis, with tendons passing behind the lateral malleolus, are primarily responsible for eversion, with assistance provided by the peroneus tertius.

Pronation and Supination

The lower extremity moves through a cyclical sequence of movements during gait. Among these, the action at the subtalar joint during weight bearing has the most significant implications for lower extremity injury potential. During heel contact with the support surface, the hindfoot is typically somewhat inverted. As the foot rolls forward and the forefoot initially contacts the ground, the foot is plantar flexed. This combination of calcaneal inversion, foot adduction, and plantar flexion, all at

> Muscles with tendons that pass anterior to the malleoli are dorsiflexors, and tendons that pass posterior are plantar flexors

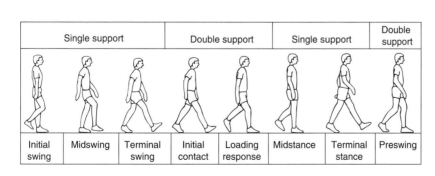

Fig. 7.18: The gait cycle consists of alternating periods of single leg support and double leg support.

Single support			Double support		Single support		Double support
Initial swing	Midswing	Terminal swing	Initial contact	Loading response	Midstance	Terminal stance	Preswing

Supination
Combined motions of calcaneal inversion, foot adduction, and plantar flexion

Pronation
Combined motions of calcaneal eversion, foot abduction, and dorsiflexion

Pes planus
Flat feet

Excessive pronation can result in increased stress within the Achilles tendon

Kinetics
Study of the forces causing, and resulting from, motion

Bones of the lower extremity are subject to tension, compression, bending, and torsion during training

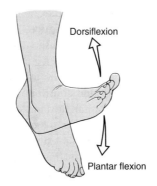

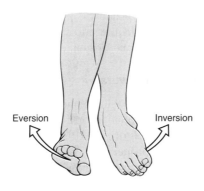

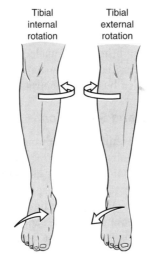

Fig. 7.19: Motions of the leg and ankle. Supination of the subtalar joint results in external rotation of the tibia. Pronation is linked with internal rotation of the tibia.

the subtalar joint, is known as **supination**. During weight bearing at midstance, calcaneal eversion and foot abduction tend to occur, as the foot moves into dorsiflexion. These movements are known collectively as **pronation**. Supination of the subtalar joint also results in external rotation of the tibia, with pronation linked to internal tibial rotation (**Figure 7-19**) (4).

Although a normal amount of pronation is useful in reducing the peak forces sustained during impact, studies have linked excessive pronation and/or prolonged pronation to running-related injuries of the lower extremity (5,6). Normal walking gait typically involves about 6 to 8° pronation, although individuals with **pes planus** (flat feet) may undergo as much as 10 to 12° pronation (7). Because pronation also causes a compensatory inward rotation of the tibia, excessive pronation can result in increased stress within the plantar fascia and Achilles tendon.

Prolonged pronation of the subtalar joint during the support phase of running results in a loose foot with limited ability to provide propulsion during push-off. Prolonged pronation has also been associated with several overuse injuries to the medial side of the foot and lower leg, including stress fractures to the second metatarsal, irritation of the sesamoid bones, plantar fasciitis, Achilles tendinitis, and medial tibial stress syndrome.

Pronation and supination occur at the subtalar joint. However, combined action of all the major joints of the foot are required for smooth, coordinated locomotion.

KINETICS OF THE FOOT, ANKLE, AND LOWER LEG

Stress fractures are common in the foot and lower leg. What factors other than excessive or prolonged pronation can predispose an individual to stress fractures of the lower extremity?

Kinetics is the study of forces associated with motion. Because it is ultimately force that causes injury, understanding the kinetic aspects of foot, ankle, and lower leg function is an important foundation for understanding injury mechanisms.

Forces Commonly Sustained by the Foot, Ankle, and Lower Leg

During training the bones of the lower extremity are subjected to a complex array of loading patterns, including tension, compression, bending, and torsion (8). During running the foot sustains impact forces that can reach two to three times body weight, with the magnitudes of the forces increasing with gait speed (2,9). However, researchers have estimated strength of lower extremity bones to be two to four times that necessary to withstand the maximum stresses normally sustained during running (10,11).

Because repeated impact forces sustained during overtraining can produce stress fractures in the bones of the lower extremity, researchers have studied the factors associated with stress fracture incidence. In a study of infantry recruits, investigators found that thicker bones are generally more resistant to injury (12). Women, who tend to have smaller bones than men, have also been found to incur more stress fractures than men, particularly in the tibia and metatarsals. Stress fractures are also common in runners, ballerinas, and gymnasts, and may be related to decreased bone mineral density (**osteopenia**) secondary to **oligomenorrhea** (13-15).

Foot Deformation during Gait

The structures of the foot are anatomically linked so the load is evenly distributed over the foot during weight bearing. Approximately 50% of body weight is distributed through the subtalar joint to the calcaneus with the remaining 50% channeled through the transverse tarsal joints to the forefoot (2).

If the foot were a more rigid structure, however, each impact with the support surface would generate extremely large forces of short duration through the skeletal system. Because the foot is composed of numerous bones connected by flexible ligaments and restrained by flexible tendons, it deforms with each ground contact, thereby absorbing much of the shock and transmitting a much smaller force of longer duration up through the skeletal system (16).

The process of foot deformation during weight bearing results in the storage of mechanical energy in the stretched tendons, ligaments, and plantar fascia. As the tibia rotates forward over the talus during gait, additional energy is stored in the gastrocnemius and soleus as they develop eccentric tension. During the push-off phase, the stored energy in all of these elastic structures is released, contributing to the force of push-off, and actually reducing the metabolic energy cost of walking or running (17).

Osteopenia secondary to menstrual dysfunction can predispose female sport participants to stress fractures.

PREVENTION OF FOOT, ANKLE, AND LOWER LEG INJURIES

What exercises should be included in a preseason program to reduce the risk of injury to the foot, ankle, and lower leg?

Preventing injuries should be a priority for all sport participants. Several steps can reduce the incidence or severity of injury, and include the use of appropriate protective equipment, footwear, and regular physical conditioning including flexibility and strengthening exercises.

Protective Equipment

Chapter 6 discussed the use of protective braces and equipment for the foot, ankle, and lower leg. Specific foot conditions can be padded and supported with a variety of products including innersoles, semirigid orthotics, rigid orthotics, antishock heel lifts, heel cups, or commercially available pads and devices. Adhesive tape, or an ankle lace-up brace, semirigid orthosis, or air bladder design brace can be used to provide additional stabilization for the ankle joint. Shin pads for the anterior tibial area protect this highly vulnerable region against high velocity-low mass projectiles, such as a ball, bat, stick, or kick from a foot. In addition to commercially available pads and devices, adhesive felt (moleskin), felt, and foam can also be cut to construct similar pads to protect specific areas.

Physical Conditioning

Physical conditioning and strengthening of the body is one of the strongest defenses against injury. The foot and lower leg, however, are often neglected. A flexibility program should be completed prior to any sport participation. A tight Achilles tendon has been shown to predispose an individual to plantar fasciitis, Achilles tendinitis, and lateral ankle sprains. Strengthening exercises for the intrinsic and extrinsic muscles of the region should also be included. For example, to build strength in the foot, pick up marbles or dice with the toes and place them in a container close to the foot. Place a tennis ball between the soles of the feet and roll the ball back and forth from the heel to the forefoot. To increase strength in the lower leg muscles, secure a weight or elastic tubing around the forefoot and move through the ranges of motion doing three sets of 10 to 15 repetitions. Bilateral toe raises and heel raises may also be incorporated. **Field Strategy 7-1** demonstrates several exercises that can be used to prevent injuries to the foot, ankle, and lower leg.

Osteopenia
Pathological condition of reduced bone mineral density

Oligomenorrhea
Menstruation involving scant blood loss

Half of the body's weight is supported by the two calcanei with the remaining half supported by the fore foot

The foot deforms during weight bearing, thereby absorbing a smaller force of longer duration than if it were rigid

Foot deformation during weight bearing causes storage of mechanical energy in the stretched tendons, ligaments, and plantar fascia

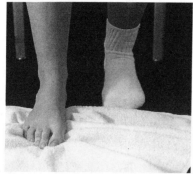

A-3

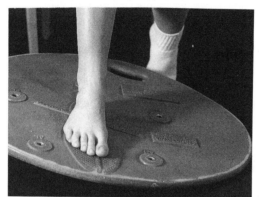

A-7

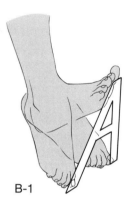

B-1

A.   Foot Intrinsic Muscle Exercises.
  1.   Plantar fascia stretch. Place a towel around the toes and slowly over-extend them. Combine with dorsiflexion of the ankle to stretch the Achilles tendon also.
  2.   Towel crunches. Place a towel between the plantar surfaces of the toes and feet. Push the toes and feet together, crunching the towel between the toes.
  3.   Toe curls. With the foot resting on a towel, slowly curl the toes under bunching the towel beneath the foot. Variation: use two feet. Place a book or small weight on the towel for added resistance.
  4.   Picking up objects. Pick up small objects, such as marbles or dice with the toes and place in a nearby container, or use therapeutic putty to work the toe flexors.
  5.   Shin curls. Slide the plantar surface of the foot up the opposite shin moving distal to proximal.
  6.   Unilateral balance activities. Stand on uneven surfaces with the eyes first open, then closed.
  7.   BAPS board. Seated position: roll the board slowly clockwise, then counterclockwise 20 times.

B.   Ankle/Lower Leg Muscle Exercises.
  1.   Ankle alphabet. Using the ankle and foot only, trace the letters of the alphabet from A to Z; 3 times with capital letters, and 3 times with lowercase.
  2.   Triceps surae stretch. Keeping the back leg straight and heel on the floor, lean against a wall until tension is felt in the calf muscles (a). To isolate the soleus, bend both knees (b).
  3.   Plantar fascia and triceps surae stretch. Standing with the ball of the foot on a stair step, allow body weight to drop the heels below the step until tension is felt in the arch and calf muscles. Combine with toe raises. Variation: use a tilt board. In both exercises, point the toes outward, straight ahead, and inward to stretch the various fibers of the Achilles tendon.
  4.   Theraband or surgical tubing exercises. Secure the Theraband or tubing around a table leg and do resisted dorsiflexion, plantar flexion, inversion, and eversion.

(continued)

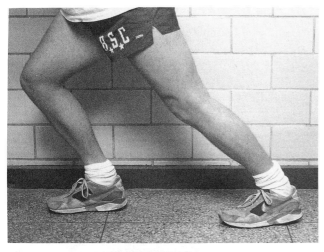

B-2-a

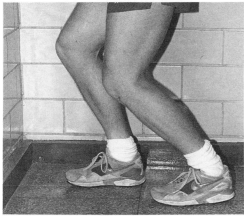

B-2-b

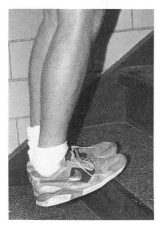

B-3

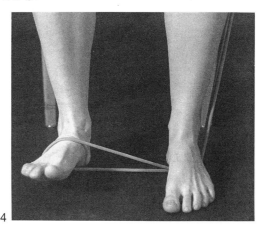

B-4

5. Unilateral balance exercises. Balance on the opposite leg while doing theraband exercises in all directions.

6. BAPS board. Standing position: balance on the involved foot and repeat the process. Additional challenges, such as using no support, or dribbling with a basketball while balancing, can be added.

Footwear

The demands of a particular sport require adaptations in shoe design and selection. Depending on the playing surface, a cleated shoe, or a multicleated design may be necessary. In Chapter 6, shoe selection and guidelines for fitting shoes are discussed in detail. See Field Strategy 6-4 for review.

Strengthening exercises for the intrinsic and extrinsic muscles of the foot and lower leg should be included in a regular preventive program, and should be supplemented by an inclusive self-stretching flexibility program.

TOE AND FOOT CONDITIONS

A football lineman has a throbbing pain on the plantar side of the great toe on the right foot. The pain increases significantly every time the player pushes off the right foot to block his opponent. Think for a minute or two about what may have caused this condition and how you are going to handle this injury.

Many individuals are at risk for toe and foot problems because of a leg length discrepancy, postural deviation, muscle dysfunction (such as muscle imbalance), or a malalignment syndrome (pes cavus, pes planus, pes equinus, hammer or claw toes) (**Figure 7-20**). The resulting strain may lead to turf toe, ingrown toenails, hammer and claw toes, corns, calluses, plantar's neuroma (Morton's neuroma), bunions, Freiberg's disease, or bursitis. Athlete's foot and verrucae plantaris (plantar's warts) may also plague the sport participant. Although many are minor conditions and may even be asymptomatic, each condition can become painful and disabling.

Turf Toe

Turf toe primarily affects football, baseball, field hockey, lacrosse, and soccer players. The condition is caused by jamming the great toe into the end of the shoe, or hyperextending the MTP joint of the great toe. It is related to artificial turf, lightweight shoes that are too flexible, and positions that require forced hyperextension of the toes, as in football linebackers and offensive linemen (18). Hyperextension of the great toe causes the sesamoids to be drawn forward to bear weight under the first metatarsal head. Repetitive overload leads to injury, particularly when associated with a valgus stress. The individual will have pain, tenderness, and swelling on the plantar aspect of the MTP joint of the great toe. Extension of the great toe will be exquisitely painful. Because the sesamoid bones are located in the tendons of the flexor hallucis brevis, this condition is sometimes associated with inflammation or fracture of the sesamoid bones. Initial treatment involves ice therapy, NSAIDs, rest and protection from excessive motion. Taping to limit motion at the MTP joint, a metatarsal pad to lower stress on the first metatarsal, or use of a stiff soled shoe may be helpful (18,19).

Ingrown Toenail

An ingrown toenail is common, yet preventable with proper hygiene and nail care. Improper cutting of the nail, improper shoe size, or constant sliding of the foot inside the shoe traumatizes the nail, causing its edge to grow into the lateral nail fold and surrounding skin. The nail margin reddens and becomes very painful. If a fungal/bacterial infection is present, the condition is called **paronychia**. Two methods to treat this condition are discussed in **Field Strategy 7-2**.

Hammer and Claw Toes

Hammer and claw toes are often congenital, but can develop because of improperly fitted shoes, contractures of the intrinsic or extrinsic muscles of the foot, or malalignment of bony

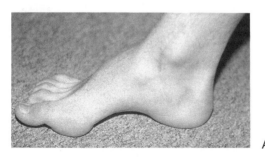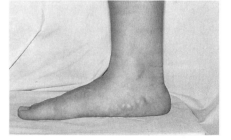

Fig. 7.20: Common foot deformities. (A) Pes cavus. (B) Pes planus.

Field Strategy 7–2. Management of an Ingrown Toenail.

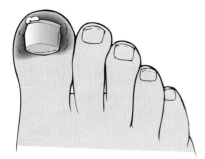

A

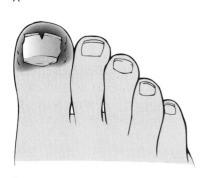

B

Prevention

- Cut toenails straight across to prevent the edges from growing under the skin on the side of the nail
- Allow the toenail to be long enough to extend beyond the underlying skin, but short enough so as not to push into the toe box of the shoe
- Wear properly fitted shoes and socks

Management—Method 1

- Soak the involved toe in hot water (108° to 116°) until the nail bed is soft (usually 10 to 15 minutes)
- Lift the edge of the nail and place a small piece of cotton or tissue under the nail to elevate the nail out of the skinfold (Figure A)
- Apply antiseptic to the area and cover with a sterile dressing
- Repeat the procedure daily, keeping the area clean and dry
- If a purulent infection is present, refer to a physician for antibiotics and drainage of the infection

Management—Method 2

- Soak the toe as above, and cut a V in the center of the nail (Figure B)
- As the nail grows, its edges will pull toward the center, drawing the nail edges from under the skin
- Apply an antiseptic, cover with a sterile dressing, and keep the area clean and dry
- If a purulent infection is present, refer to a physician for antibiotics and drainage of the infection

structures. **Hammer toe** is a flexion deformity of the PIP joint (**Figure 7-21A**). **Claw toe** involves hyperextension of the MTP joint and hyperflexion of the DIP and PIP joints (**Figure 7-21B**). Both can lead to painful callus formation on the dorsum of the IP joint from pressure against the shoe, and under the metatarsal head, particularly the second toe, due to retrograde pressure on the long toe. These conditions are difficult to treat conservatively. A metatarsal pad may assist in controlling symptoms, but surgical resection of the head of the proximal phalanx is often necessary to treat the condition.

Calluses and Corns

Calluses and corns are caused by excessive localized pressure or friction against the foot, such as with improperly fitted shoes, constant sliding of the foot inside a shoe, or with con-

ditions such as hammer toe or claw toe. The thickened skin overlying bony prominences can lead to pain and discomfort.

A small doughnut pad can be used to relieve pressure from corns found between toes. A weak **keratolytic agent**, such as 40 percent salicylic acid in liquid form, can be applied daily. Removal of the dead, macerated tissue can reduce the problem. Corns on top of the toes are often the result of hammer toes. Padding the area with a doughnut pad may be insufficient to relieve pain. The individual may eventually need surgical intervention to correct the toe deformity.

Calluses on the plantar aspect of the foot are treated with a felt or commercial metatarsal pad to spread the metatarsal heads and relieve some pressure, as well as elevate the head to partially correct claw toes. Proper placement of the pad should be proximal to

Hammer toe
A flexion deformity of the distal interphalangeal (DIP) joint of the toes

Claw toe
A toe deformity characterized by hyperextension of the metatarsophalangeal (MTP) joint and hyperflexion of the interphalangeal (IP) joints

Calluses and corns are caused by excessive localized pressure against the foot and toes from improperly fitted shoes, constant sliding of the foot inside a shoe, or with certain toe conditions

Keratolytic agent
An agent that promotes softening and dissolution, or peeling of the horny layer of skin

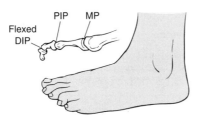

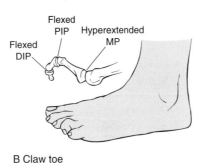

Fig. 7.21: Toe deformities. (A) A hammer toe is a flexion deformity of the PIP joint. (B) A claw toe invovles hyperextension of the MP joint and hyperflexion of the DIP and PIP joints.

Tinea pedis
A common fungal infection found between the toes characterized by small vesicles, itching, and scaling

Verrucae plantaris
Plantar warts

Stratum corneum
The outermost layer of the epidermis; horny layer of dead cells

the head. Experiment with pad placement so it does not irritate the condition. Regular debridement with a callus board or callus shaver can help keep calluses at a minimum. If you run your finger along the callus and feel an edge, the callus is too thick and needs to be reduced. A large callus can become detached from the underlying skin layer tearing small capillaries, which leads to blood under the callus. Do not drain the blood, as it opens an avenue for infection. Soak the foot in ice water, apply a compression pad over the area, and place the individual on crutches to avoid bearing weight on the affected foot. Keep the foot elevated above the heart whenever possible to assist in reabsorption of the blood and fluid. If drainage is necessary, refer to a physician.

Athlete's Foot

Athlete's foot is a common tinea fungal infection known as **tinea pedis**. It can spread in the locker room during casual handling of contaminated socks, or can be picked up by another player on the floor or shower stall. It is, however, based on individual susceptibility and may not affect certain people. The condition is characterized by extreme itching on the sole of the foot and between the toes. The individual may have dry or vesicular lesions that exude a yellowish serum. Scratching the area will lead to scaling, peeling, and cracking fissures in the skin, particularly between the toes. **Field Strategy 7-3** summarizes the prevention and management of athlete's foot.

Verrucae Plantaris

Verrucae plantaris (plantar warts) is a condition found on the plantar aspect of the foot. These warts grow into the thick **stratum corneum** of the foot and have tiny, dark red or black dots within each one that represent capillaries penetrated by the root of the wart. Recurrences are frequent, and no single method of treatment is effective for all

---

 Field Strategy 7–3. Management of Athlete's Foot.

Prevention

- Shower after every practice and competition
- Always dry feet thoroughly after every shower, especially between toes
- Apply absorbant powder, such as Desenex and Tinactin to the shoes, socks and feet, especially between toes
- Change socks daily and allow wet shoes to dry thoroughly before wearing them
- Wear nonocclusive street shoes
- Clean and disinfect the floors in the shower room, dressing room, and training room daily

Management

- Apply topical antifungal agents, such as Micatin, Tinactin, Lotrimin, and Halotex twice daily for one month
- In resistant infections, oral griseofulvin can be used for 4 to 8 weeks
- Follow proper foot hygiene as listed above

lesions. During the competitive season a doughnut pad can be worn to alleviate some of the pressure on the area. After the season, under the direction of a physician, treatment may involve chemical therapy including salicylic acid pads applied every few days following bathing, injections or applications of antimetabolites including intralesional bleomycin or 5-fluorouracil (5-FU) to destroy the wart, cryosurgery (liquid nitrogen), electrosurgery, scalpel excision, or carbon dioxide laser excision (20).

Metatarsalgia

General discomfort around the metatarsal-sheads is called **metatarsalgia**, or Morton's metatarsalgia. Constant overloading of the transverse ligaments lead to callus formation over the middle three metatarsal heads, particularly the second metatarsal head. Intrinsic factors originating from within the body, such as excessive body weight, valgus heel, hammer toes, pes planus, or pes cavus can contribute to excessive pressure on the forefoot. Extrinsic factors external to the body, such as a narrow toe box, landing poorly from a height, repetitive jumping, excessive training, or a running style that puts undue pressure on the forefoot can also contribute to the condition. Although often related to sport participation, age, arthritic disease, gout, diabetes, circulatory disease, and some neurological conditions can also predispose an individual to metatarsal pain (18). Treatment involves reducing the load on the metatarsal heads through activity modification, footwear examination, metatarsal pads or bars, and strengthening the intrinsic muscles of the foot.

Plantar's Neuroma (Interdigital Neuroma)

Plantar's neuroma is a static condition of the foot characterized by localized pain primarily in the second and third metatarsal space that often radiates into the respective toes (**Figure 7-22**). At the metatarsal heads the medial and lateral plantar nerves are compressed between the heads by tight fitting shoes, or a pronated foot. This leads to a painful irritation of the nerves, or **neuritis**. Pain is relieved when barefoot, but increases with tight shoes, deep palpation between the distal metatarsal heads, and during extension of the appropriate MTP and IP joints. Conservative management involves a wider shoe with a low heel and

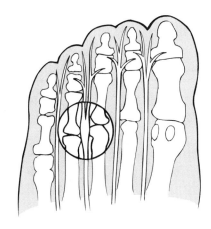

Fig. 7.22: Plantar's neuroma (Morton's neuroma) is caused by pinching the interdigital nerve between the metatarsal heads. While weight bearing in shoes, the individual will have an agonizing pain on the lateral side of the foot, but will be relieved when going barefoot.

appropriate arch padding, but local corticosteroid injections or surgical incision may be necessary to remedy the situation (18).

Bunions (Hallux Valgus)

Bunions are typically found on the medial aspect of the MTP joint of the great toe, but can occur on the lateral aspect of the fifth toe, called a bunionette or tailor's bunion. Pronation of the foot, prolonged pronation during gait, contractures of the Achilles tendon, arthritis, and generalized ligamentous laxity between the first and second metatarsal heads produce a thickening on the medial side of the first metatarsal head as it is constantly rubbed against the inside of the shoe. As the condition worsens, the great toe may shift laterally and overlap the second toe, leading to a rigid nonfunctional hallux valgus deformity (**Figure 7-23**) (18). This condition is exacerbated by high heels and pointed shoe toe boxes, factors that account for women having this condition more often than men. Once the deformity occurs, little can be done. Strapping the great toe as closely to proper anatomical position as possible and wearing wider shoes can provide some relief, but surgical correction is indicated in severe cases.

Freiberg's Disease

Freiberg's disease is an overuse injury to the cartilage or subchondral bone of the metatarsal head that leads to **avascular**

Metatarsalgia
A condition involving general discomfort around the metatarsal heads

Neuritis
Inflammation or irritation of a nerve commonly found between the third and fourth metatarsal heads

Bunions typically occur on the medial aspect of the MTP joint of the great toe, but can also occur on the lateral aspect of the fifth toe, called a bunionette

Freiberg's disease
Avascular necrosis that occurs to the second metatarsal head in some adolescents

Avascular necrosis
Death of tissue due to insufficient blood supply

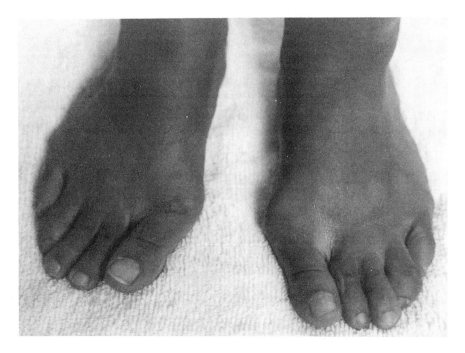

Fig. 7.23: Bunions are generally formed by constantly rubbing the medial aspect of the MTP joint of the great toe against the inside of the shoe. The toe then shifts laterally, forming the hallux valgus deformity.

necrosis. Primarily occurring in the second and third metatarsals, the condition is more often seen in adolescents aged 14 to 18 before closure of the epiphysis. Although not specifically a sport injury, it can lead to diffuse pain in the forefoot region. Early detection is best treated by padding and limiting activity, but often it goes undetected until the condition is so advanced it requires surgical resection of the distal metatarsal head (18).

Bursitis (Pump Bump, Runner's Bump)

External pressure from a constrictive heel cup or excessive pronation can lead to swelling, erythema (redness of the skin) and irritation of the bursa associated with the Achilles tendon. The retrocalcaneal bursa is located between the anterior Achilles tendon insertion and calcaneus **(Figure 7-24)**. Pain is elicited when you reach around the Achilles tendon to palpate the soft tissue just anterior to the tendon. Active plantar flexion during push-off compresses the bursa between the tendon and bone leading to irritation and pain. At times, inflammation may occur in the posterior calcaneal bursa located between the Achilles tendon and overlying skin. Irritation of this bursa is characterized by a slightly thickened, red swollen area. Initial treatment involves ice therapy, NSAIDs, stretching exercises for the Achilles tendon,

> Pain can be palpated in the soft tissue just anterior to the Achilles tendon

shoe modification, or a heel lift to relieve external pressure on the bursa. Occasionally an inflamed bursa can lead to a dramatic large mass referred to as a "pump bump," common in figure skaters and runners, when it is called runner's bump. This bump may be related to an underlying bony spur caused by frequent microtrauma or microavulsions surrounding the distal attachment of the Achilles tendon (18).

Did you determine the football lineman may have a possible turf toe or irritation of the sesamoid bones? If so, you are correct. Ice therapy, taping to limit motion of the great toe, a metatarsal pad, or more rigid shoe may alleviate some of the symptoms.

CONTUSIONS

A soccer player was kicked on the superior lateral leg. Although the initial pain has subsided, the dorsum of the foot feels somewhat numb. How will you handle the immediate problem? What complications might result from this trauma?

Contusions of the foot and leg frequently result from direct trauma, such as dropping a weight on the foot, being stepped on, kicked, or being hit by a speeding ball or implement. Although many of the injuries are minor and easily treated with immediate ice therapy, compression, elevation, and rest,

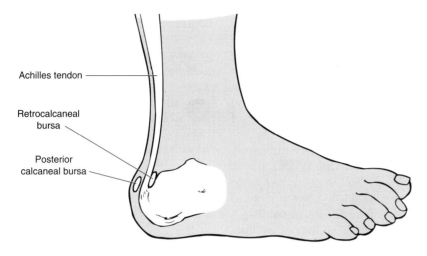

Fig. 7.24: The retrocalcaneal bursa is commonly inflamed when it is pinched between the Achilles tendon and calcaneus during plantar flexion.

Achilles tendon

Retrocalcaneal bursa

Posterior calcaneal bursa

a few injuries can result in complications, such as damage to tendon sheaths leading to tenosynovitis, excessive hemorrhage, periosteal irritation, or nerve damage.

Foot Contusions

Having the midfoot or forefoot stepped on, or having a weight dropped on the foot can be quite painful. A possible fracture to the metatarsals or phalanges should be ruled out, as well as damage to the toe extensor tendons. Inflammation of the synovial sheath surrounding the tendons may lead to tenosynovitis.

With weight bearing, contusions of the plantar aspect of the forefoot may result from a loose cleat or spike irritating the ball of the foot. Repairing and/or replacing the object along with ice therapy to reduce immediate hemorrhage and discomfort is usually sufficient to remedy the situation.

A contusion to the hindfoot, called a "**heel bruise**," can be more serious. Elastic adipose tissue lies between the thick skin and plantar aspect of the calcaneus to cushion and protect the inferior portion of the calcaneus from trauma. It is constantly subjected to extreme stress in running, jumping, and changing directions. Excessive body weight, age, poorly cushioned or worn-out running shoes, increases in training, and hard, uneven training surfaces can predispose an individual to this condition. Walking barefoot is particularly painful. Ice treatments to minimize pain and inflammation, followed by regular use of a heel cup or doughnut pad can minimize the

condition. Despite excellent care, the condition may persist for months.

Lower Leg Contusions

Contusions to the gastrocnemius result in immediate pain, weakness, and partial loss of motion. Hemorrhage and muscle spasm quickly lead to a tender, firm mass that is easily palpable. When applying ice, keep the muscle on static stretch to decrease muscle spasm. If the condition does not improve in 2 to 3 days, ultrasound may be used under the direction of a physician to assist in breaking up the hematoma.

A contusion to the tibia, commonly called a **shin bruise**, may occur in soccer, field hockey, baseball, softball, or football where the lower leg is often subjected to high impact forces. The shin is particularly void of natural subcutaneous fat and is vulnerable to direct blows that irritate the periosteal tissue around the tibia. As such, participants should always wear appropriate shin guards to protect this highly vulnerable area. Although painful, the condition can be managed effectively with ice, compression, elevation, and rest. A doughnut pad over the area and additional shin protection can allow the individual to participate within pain tolerance levels.

A minor blow to the fibular head can lead to contusion of the peroneal nerve. Initially the shock of the blow may send pain shooting down the nerve distribution into the anterolateral leg and foot. Symptoms are usually transient and last only a few seconds or minutes, then should return to normal.

Complications from a leg contusion can include tenosynovitis, excessive hemorrhage, periosteal irritation or nerve damage

Heel bruise
Contusion to the subcutaneous fat pad located over the inferior aspect of the calcaneus

With a heel bruise, walking barefoot is particularly painful

Contusions to the gastrocnemius result in immediate pain, weakness, and partial loss of motion

Shin bruise
A contusion to the tibia, sometimes referred to as tibial periostitis

A minor blow in the area of the fibular head can lead to contusion of the peroneal nerve

Subsequent swelling and edema, however, can result in pressure being placed on the nerve fibers, with numbness, pain, and paresthesia becoming more prolonged. Although rare, swelling or actual hemorrhage within the neural sheath can lead to loss of function to the dorsiflexors of the ankle. Standard acute care will reduce swelling and inflammation. Be careful in applying ice to the area to avoid further damage to the nerve. Increased cold can lead to decreased nerve conduction or cold-induced nerve palsy in the anterior or lateral compartments. If symptoms do not return to normal within a few minutes, refer the individual to a physician for follow-up care.

Acute Compartment Syndrome

An acute compartment syndrome may result from a direct blow to the anterolateral aspect of the leg, a fracture, crushing injury, or circulatory occlusion. The anterior compartment is particularly at risk, as it is bounded by the tibia medially, interosseus membrane posteriorly, fibula laterally, and a tough fascial sheath anteriorly. Hence, the structures within the non-yielding compartment are very vulnerable to increases in internal tissue pressure. An acute anterior compartment syndrome is a medical and surgical emergency. Circulation and tissue function within the closed space are compromised by increased pressure within the compartment.

Signs and symptoms include increasing pain and swelling over the anterior compartment that does not cease with rest. A firm mass, tight skin (because it has been stretched to its limits), loss of sensation between the great toe and second toe on the dorsum of the foot, and diminished pulse at the dorsalis pedis are all late and dangerous signs. However, a normal pulse does not rule out the syndrome. Acute compartment syndrome can produce functional abnormalities within 30 minutes of onset of hemorrhage. Immediate action is necessary, because irreversible damage can occur within 12 to 24 hours (18,21). If numbness in the foot is present, a surgical release of the fascia is indicated to prevent permanent tissue damage.

Immediate care involves ice and total rest. Compression is not recommended because the compartment is already unduly compressed and additional external compression will only hasten the deterioration. Further-

more, the limb must not be elevated, as this decreases arterial pressure and further compromises capillary filling. Referral to a physician for immediate care is absolutely necessary.

After applying standard acute care to the lateral leg, did you determine what complication might occur as a result of the initial trauma? Possible complications might include a contusion to the peroneal nerve or fracture to the fibula.

FOOT AND ANKLE SPRAINS

After going up for a rebound, a basketball player stepped on the foot of an opponent and rolled off the side of the foot, inverting the ankle. Although the player stayed off the ankle and iced it during the night, the ankle appeared swollen and discolored the next morning, and continued to hurt on weight bearing. Think for a minute or two about how you will manage this condition?

Sprains to the foot and ankle region are common in sports, particularly for those individuals who play on badly maintained fields. Uneven terrain, stepping in a hole, or landing on another player's foot and sliding off the side can all be contributing factors to injury for this highly vulnerable area.

Toe and Foot Sprains/Dislocations

Sprains and dislocations to the MP joints and IP joints of the toes may occur by tripping or stubbing the toe. Varus and valgus forces more commonly affect the first and fifth toes, rather than the middle three. Pain, dysfunction, immediate swelling, and if dislocated, gross deformity is clearly evident. Radiographs should be taken to rule out possible fracture, but closed reduction and strapping to the next toe for 10 to 14 days is usually sufficient to remedy the problem.

Midfoot sprains often result from severe dorsiflexion, plantar flexion, or pronation. Although the condition is seen in basketball and soccer players, it is more frequent in activities where the foot is unsupported, such as in gymnastics or dance where slippers are typically worn, or in track athletes who wear running flats. Pain and swelling is deep on the medial aspect of the foot, and weight bearing may be too painful (22).

Depending on the location and severity of pain, adequate strapping, arch supports, and limited weight bearing is warranted during

Immediate action is necessary, because irreversible damage can occur with 12 to 24 hours

Midfoot sprains are more frequently seen in activities where the foot is unsupported

the acute stage. If the condition does not improve, refer the individual to a physician to rule out a possible avulsion fracture at the tarsal joints. Reconditioning exercises should include range of motion and strengthening for the intrinsic muscles of the foot.

Mechanisms of Injury for Ankle Sprains

Ankle sprains are the most common injury in recreational and competitive athletes. They are classified as first-, second-, and third-degree based on the progression of anatomical structures damaged and subsequent disability (**Table 7-2**). In basketball, ankle sprains comprise more than 50 percent of major injuries and in soccer and volleyball, more than 25 percent.

Ankle sprains are generally caused by severe medial (supination or inversion) and lateral (pronation or eversion) rotation motions, and may or may not be coupled with plantar flexion or dorsiflexion. Excessive supination of the foot (adduction, inversion, and plantar flexion) results when the plantar aspect of the foot is turned inward toward the midline of the body, commonly referred to as an inversion ankle sprain. Excessive pronation (abduction, eversion, and dorsiflexion) results when the plantar aspect of the foot is turned laterally, referred to as an eversion ankle sprain.

In many sports, cleated shoes become fixed to the ground whereas the limb continues to rotate around it. In addition, the very nature of changing directions while running places an inordinate amount of strain on the ankle region. For example, when cutting to the left to avoid an opposing player, you decelerate, set the right foot in a position of adduction, inversion, and dorsiflexion, and push-off that foot with plantar flexion at the ankle (**Figure 7-25**). Another method of injury is to step in a hole, step off a curb, or step on an opponent's foot, rolling the foot off the surface.

An eversion sprain may result from lateral rotation stress at the knee coupled with eversion, abduction, and dorsiflexion at the ankle. In more severe cases, the deltoid ligament may avulse a bony fragment from the medial malleolus, rather than rupture. Bone-on-bone shear forces can also lead to malleoli fractures as the talus rocks up into the lateral malleolus. If the force continues, the tibiofibular syndesmosis can be ruptured leading to joint instability (**Figure 7-26**).

Lateral Ankle Sprains

Acute inversion ankle sprains occur during walking, running, or jumping, particularly while changing directions rapidly or when participating on an uneven surface. The medial and lateral malleoli project downward over the talus to form a mortise-tenon joint.

An inversion ankle sprain results from excessive supination of the foot

An eversion ankle sprain results from excessive pronation of the foot

Table 7–2. Mechanisms of Common Ankle Sprains and Resulting Ligament Damage.			
Mechanism	**1st° (Mild)**	**2nd° (Moderate)**	**3rd° (Severe)**
Inversion and plantar flexion	Anterior talofibular stretched	Partial tear of anterior talofibular with calcaneofibular stretched	Rupture of anterior talofibular and calcaneofibular with posterior talofibular and tibiofibular torn (severe)
Inversion	Calcaneofibular stretched	Calcaneofibular torn Anterior talofibular stretched	Rupture of calcaneofibular, anterior talofibular with posterior talofibular stretched
Dorsiflexion	Tibiofibular stretched	Partial tear tibiofibular	Rupture of tibiofibular
Eversion	Deltoid stretched or an avulsion fracture of medial malleolus	Partial tear of deltoid and tibiofibular	Rupture of deltoid, interosseous membrane with possible fibular fracture above syndesmosis

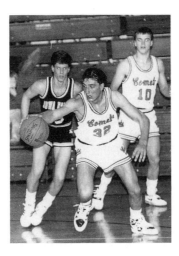

Fig. 7.25: Cutting to avoid an oncoming opponent places the foot in a position of inversion, internal rotation, and dorsiflexion leading to a tremendous strain on the lateral ankle region.

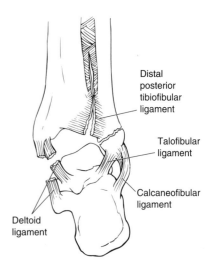

Fig. 7.26: As the talus rocks under the lateral malleolus during eversion, a fracture and tearing of the tibiofibular syndesmosis can occur leading to total joint instability.

The lateral malleolus projects farther downward than the medial, thus limiting lateral talar shifts. As stress is initially applied to the ankle during plantar flexion and inversion, the anterior talofibular ligament first stretches. If the strain continues, the ankle loses ligamentous stability in its neutral position. The medial malleolus acts as a fulcrum to further the inversion, and stretches or ruptures the calcaneofibular ligament (**Figure 7-27**). The overlying inner wall of the peroneal tendon sheath lies adjacent to the calcaneofibular ligament and can absorb some strain to prevent this ligament from being injured. If the peroneal muscles are weak, however, they are unable to help stabilize the joint leading to tearing of the calcaneofibular ligament. With severe injuries, the posterior talofibular ligament is also involved. As the ankle joint becomes unstable the talus can pinch the deltoid ligament against the medial malleolus leading to injury on both sides of the ankle joint.

The individual will usually report a cracking or tearing sound at the time of injury. Swelling and tenderness will be localized over the anterior talofibular ligament and may extend over the calcaneofibular ligament. If no fracture is involved, bony tenderness will only be found at the ligamentous attachments. Swelling and ecchymosis will be rapid and diffuse. Immediate assessment should distinguish between first-, second-, and third-degree sprains. Once swelling has moved into the area, stress testing of the ligamentous structures will be painful and assessment difficult.

> If the peroneal muscles are weak, they are unable to help stabilize the joint leading to tearing of the calcaneofibular ligament

> If no fractures are involved, bony tenderness will only be found at the ligamentous attachments

After assessment for possible fracture and ligamentous damage, initial treatment should consist of ice therapy, compression (with or without a horseshoe pad), elevation, and restricted activity. Radiographs can determine damage to the syndesmosis or detect an osteochondral fracture to the dome of the talus. If the individual is unable to bear weight, crutches should be used. **Field Strategy 7-4** summarizes signs, symptoms, and treatment of lateral ankle sprains.

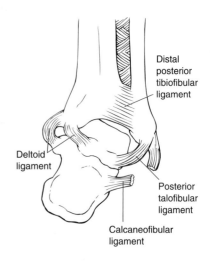

Fig. 7.27: During inversion, the medial malleolus acts as a fulcrum to further invert the talus, leading to stretching or tearing of the calcaneofibular ligament.

Field Strategy 7–4. Management of a Lateral Ankle Sprain.

	Signs and Symptoms	Treatment
First	Pain and swelling on anterolateral aspect of lateral malleolus Point tenderness over anterior talofibular ligament No laxity with stress tests	Immediate ice therapy with wet wrap compression and elevation 15 to 20 minutes; repeat every hour until swelling is controlled Apply a horseshoe pad or open basket weave with tape and/or elastic wrap to protect area, but instruct the individual to remove the elastic wrap during sleeping If limping, fit with crutches Reassess in the morning and start rehabilitation
Second	Tearing or popping sensation felt on lateral aspect Pain and swelling on anterolateral and inferior aspect of lateral malleolus Painful palpation over anterior talofibular and calcaneofibular ligament. May also be tender over posterior talofibular, deltoid ligament, and anterior capsule area Positive anterior drawer and talar tilt test	Treatment as above If fracture is suspected, refer to physician
Third	Tearing or popping sensation felt on lateral aspect Diffuse swelling over entire lateral aspect with or without anterior swelling Immobilize and apply ice Can be very painful or absent of pain right after injury Also positive anterior drawer and talar tilt test	Suspect possible fracture Fit with crutches and refer to physician (A short walking cast may need to be applied)

Another serious sprain that involves the subtalar joint results from a fall from a height (as in basketball or volleyball). The foot lands in inversion, disrupting the interosseous talocalcaneal and talonavicular ligaments. If the foot lands in dorsiflexion and inversion, the calcaneofibular ligament will also be ruptured (22). When the dislocation occurs, the injury is better known as "basketball foot." Because of the potential for peroneal tendon entrapment and neurovascular damage leading to reduced blood supply to the foot, this dislocation is considered a medical emergency.

Medial Ankle Sprains

Eversion ankle sprains are less common than inversion ankle sprains. This is due to the strong deltoid ligament, and the ankle joint anatomy whereby the lateral malleolus extends more distally than the medial malleolus, thus blocking excessive eversion. However, individuals with pronated or hypermobile feet are at greater risk for eversion injuries. Often the individual will step in a hole, or set the foot in extreme pronation in preparation for push-off to avoid an opponent. The talar dome is wider anteriorly than posteriorly. During dorsiflexion, the talus fits more firmly in the mortise supported by the distal anterior tibiofibular ligament. With excessive dorsiflexion and eversion, the talus is thrust laterally against the longer fibula resulting in either a mild sprain to the deltoid ligament, or if the force is great enough, a lateral malleolar fracture. If the force continues after the fracture occurs,

Individuals with pronated or hypermobile feet are at greater risk for eversion injuries

Bimalleolar fracture
Fractures of both medial and lateral malleolus

In severe injuries passive motion may be pain-free in all motions except dorsiflexion

Tenosynovitis
Inflammation of the inner lining of the tendon sheath caused by friction between the tendon and the sheath

Snowball crepitation
Sound similar to that heard when crunching snow into a snowball indicating presence of tenosynovitis

Muscles cramps are associated with dehydration, electrolyte imbalance, or prolonged muscle fatigue

the deltoid ligament may be ruptured or may remain intact avulsing a small bony fragment from the medial malleolus, leading to a **bimalleolar fracture**. In either case, the distal anterior tibiofibular ligament and interosseus membrane may be torn, leading to total instability of the ankle joint and ultimate degeneration (**Figure 7-28**).

Signs and symptoms depend on the severity of injury. In mild to moderate injuries the individual will often be unable to specifically detail the history of the injury. The individual may report some pain initially at the ankle when it was everted and dorsiflexed, but as the ankle returns to its normal anatomical position the pain often subsides and the individual may continue to play. In attempts to run or put pressure on the area, pain will intensify but the individual may not make the connection between the pain and the earlier injury. Swelling may not be as evident as a lateral sprain because hemorrhage occurs deep in the leg and may not be readily visible. Swelling may occur just posterior to the lateral malleolus, between it and the Achilles tendon. Point tenderness can be elicited over the deltoid and distal anterior tibiofibular ligaments, and the anterior and posterior joint lines. In severe injuries passive motion may be pain-free in all motions except dorsiflexion. With fractures of the malleoli, pain will be evident over the fracture site and will increase with any movement of the mortise. Percussion and heel strike will produce increased pain. Appropriate immobilization

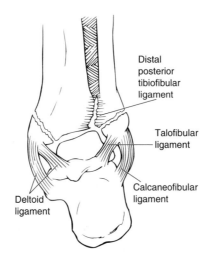

Fig. 7.28: During a severe eversion ankle sprain, the lateral malleolus can fracture, the deltoid ligament can avulse the medial malleolus, and the distal tibiofibular joint can be disrupted.

Distal posterior tibiofibular ligament

Talofibular ligament

Calcaneofibular ligament

Deltoid ligament

with a rigid posterior or vacuum splint, and referral to a physician is warranted because surgical repair is generally indicated when a fracture or ligamentous disruption of the syndesmosis is involved.

After seeing the swollen ankle the next day, did you determine how to manage this condition? After reassessing the ankle for possible fracture, control the inflammatory stage with continued ice therapy, apply a horseshoe pad or open basketweave strapping and an elastic wrap for compression, and fit the individual with crutches. If pain persists, refer the individual to a physician.

ACUTE STRAINS OF THE FOOT AND LOWER LEG

A middle aged tennis player was playing on a cool day when the individual felt a sudden, painful tearing sensation in the calf leading to immediate disability. What factors have contributed to this injury and how will you manage this acute condition?

Foot strains as a result of a direct blow or chronic overuse frequently affect the intrinsic and extrinsic muscles of the foot. **Tenosynovitis** is a condition caused by friction and subsequent irritation between the tendon and its surrounding sheath. The tibialis anterior and extensor tendons of the toes may be injured as a result of shoe laces being too tight or having the feet repeatedly stepped on. Pain, localized edema, inflammation and adhesions may be present. During assessment the involved tendon(s) will have pain on passive stretching, active, and resisted motion. Palpation over the tendon during active motion may reveal a sound similar to that heard when crunching a snowball together, hence the sound is called "**snowball**" crepitation. Treatment involves ice therapy, NSAIDs, and strapping to limit active motion of the tendon. Range of motion and strengthening exercises should be started after acute pain has subsided.

Muscle Cramps

Although the specific nature of cramping is unknown, it is commonly attributed to dehydration, electrolyte imbalance, or prolonged muscle fatigue. For some, acute spasms may awaken them in the night following a day of strenuous exercise. Acute cramps are best treated with ice, pressure, and slow stretch of the muscle as it begins to relax. Prevention of this condition involves an adequate water intake during strenuous activity and a regular stretching program for the gastrocnemius-soleus complex. When participation may extend over two hours in hot weather, increased water intake with a weak electrolyte solution should be consumed during and after strenuous activity.

Peroneal Tendon Strains

Peroneal tendon strains may be acute or chronic. Common mechanisms include exploding off a slightly pronated foot, such as when a football player is in a three-point stance and makes a forward surge; forceful passive dorsiflexion, such as when a skier catches the tip of the ski and falls forward; or by being kicked from behind in the vicinity of the lateral malleolus. The retinaculum that holds the tendons in place on the posterior aspect of the lateral malleolus gives way and the tendons slip forward over the lateral malleolus but usually return spontaneously (**Figure 7-29**). This condition can be overlooked or confused with an ankle sprain because it too, gives a feeling of instability and pain over the lateral malleolus.

A cracking sensation followed by intense pain and an inability to walk will be reported. Swelling and tenderness is localized over the posterior superior aspect of the lateral malleolus, rather than the anterior inferior aspect, as in an inversion ankle sprain. If seen immediately after injury, the dislocated tendons may be palpated when the foot is dorsiflexed

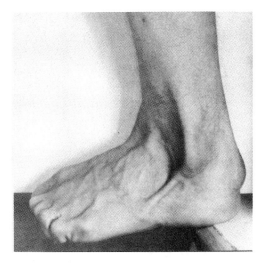

Fig. 7.29: The retinaculum holding the peroneal tendons can be ruptured leading to a foreward subluxation of the tendons over the lateral malleolus.

and everted against resistance. This is obscured with swelling and ecchymosis. Acute injuries may respond to cast immobilization. External padding and strappings may help stabilize the tendons but often surgery is still required (19).

Tibialis Posterior Tendon Strain

Acute strains to the tibialis posterior tendon often occur as it courses behind the medial malleolus. Pain and mild swelling may lead to acute tendinitis and tenosynovitis. If the tendon ruptures, a painful pop can be felt. Point tenderness, swelling, and weakness in plantar flexion will be present. Because the tendon aids in support of the medial longitudinal arch, collapse of the midfoot and hyperpronation may be visible. Treatment will depend on the severity of injury, and may include ice therapy, NSAIDs, restricted activity, and support with tape. In chronic cases involving a partial tear of the tendon, painful, palpable nodular scar tissue may build up in the tendon sheath requiring surgical debridement.

Achilles Tendon Strain

Strains to the distal attachment of the Achilles tendon often result from vigorous jumping, or excessive endurance running. It can be severely incapacitating because each time the calf muscles contract during walking or running, severe pain occurs at the injury site. Occasionally, a chronic strain can lead to calcification in the tendon. Activity modification, NSAIDs, and a heel pad on both feet can relieve some tension, but passive stretching and range of motion exercises should be started immediately.

Achilles Tendon Rupture

Acute rupture of the Achilles tendon is probably the most severe acute muscular problem in the lower leg. It is more commonly seen in individuals 30 to 50 years old (23). The usual mechanism is a push-off of the forefoot while the knee is extending, a common move in many propulsive activities. Tendinous ruptures usually occur 1 to 2 inches proximal to the distal attachment of the tendon on the calcaneus (**Figure 7-30**). The individual hears and feels a characteristic "pop" sensation in the tendon area. Clinical signs and symptoms include a visible defect in the ten-

An individual can dislocate the peroneal tendons by being kicked from behind the lateral malleolus, with forceful passive dorsiflexion, or a forward surge on a slightly pronated foot

If evaluated soon after injury, the dislocated peroneal tendons may be palpated when the foot is dorsiflexed and everted against resistance

Because the tendon aids in support of the medial longitudinal arch, collapse of the midfoot and hyperpronation may be visible

Achilles tendon ruptures are commonly seen in individuals 30 to 50 years old

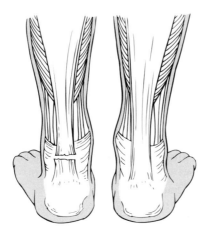

Fig. 7.30: The Achilles tendon is often ruptured 1 to 2 inches proximal to its distal attachment. The individual will hear and feel a characteristic "pop" sensation of being kicked in the tendon.

don, inability to stand on tiptoes or even balance on the affected leg, swelling and bruising around the malleoli, excessive passive dorsiflexion, and a positive Thompson's test (failure of plantar flexion to occur with passive compression of the gastrocnemius on the affected side) (18). Because the peroneal longus, peroneal brevis, and muscles in the deep posterior compartment are still intact, the individual may limp or walk with the foot and leg externally rotated, because this does not require push-off with the superficial calf muscles.

A compression wrap should be applied from the toes to the knee. The leg and foot can be immobilized in a posterior splint and the individual should be referred immediately to an orthopedist. Nonoperative treatment offers excellent functional results for partial tears in older, noncompetitive individuals. In delayed diagnosis or in highly competitive individuals, surgical repair provides better push-off strength and prevents overelongation of the tendon, thus lowering the risk for reinjury (18,24). The course of action depends on the supervising physician, but either way, full range of motion and strength may not be achieved until 6 months after the injury.

Gastrocnemius Muscle Strain

Strains to the medial head of the gastrocnemius are often seen in tennis players over 40, and is sometimes referred to as "tennis leg." The individual experiences a sudden, painful

> The individual will experience a sudden, painful tearing sensation in the calf muscles, particularly when the foot is plantar flexed, then suddenly dorsiflexed.

tearing sensation in the calf muscles, particularly when the foot is plantar flexed, then suddenly dorsiflexed, as in hill climbing or jumping. The disability is immediate with swelling and eccyhmosis progressing down the leg into the foot and ankle. Palpation will reveal minimal swelling in a first degree strain, ranging to a possible defect on the medial head of the gastrocnemius at the musculotendinous junction in a severe strain (**Figure 7-31**). Often however, by the time the individual is seen, swelling obscures this defect. Acute care consists of ice therapy to control inflammation, restricted activity, gentle stretching of the gastocnemius, heel lifts, and a progressive strengthening program. In more severe cases, immobilization and non-weight bearing may be necessary to allow the muscle to fully heal.

Did you determine that the middle aged tennis player had "tennis leg?" Age, physical condition, and cool climate may have contributed to this condition. What suggestions might you make to prevent the injury from recurring?

OVERUSE CONDITIONS

A novice runner has pain along the distal medial tibial border at the start of run-

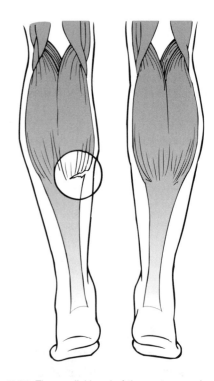

Fig. 7.31: The medial head of the gastrocnemius muscle is commonly strained in individuals over 40 years of age. A defect can often be palpated at the musculotendinous junction.

ning. As activity progresses, the pain diminishes only to recur hours after activity has ended. What factors may have initiated this condition? How will you manage this injury?

The leg is subjected to a number of overuse conditions, many of which are common to specific sports, such as plantar fasciitis in running; Achilles tendinitis in basketball and soccer; medial tibial stress syndrome (shin splints) in football, dance, or running; and exercise-induced compartment compression syndromes in soccer or distance running. Repetitive microscopic injury or overloading of tendinous structures lead to inflammation that overwhelms the tissue's ability to repair itself. Other factors, such as faulty biomechanics, poor cushioning or stiff-soled shoes, or excessive downhill running, also contribute to inflammation of the tendons (25). Many individuals complain of vague leg pain, but will have no history of a specific injury that caused the pain. A common complaint is pain caused by activity.

Plantar Fasciitis

Excessive tightness of the Achilles tendon, excessive or prolonged pronation, or obesity can overload the plantar fascia origin on the calcaneus during weight-bearing activities. Although it can occur in anyone who plays on hard surfaces, it is the most common hind foot problem in runners (26). The individual will complain of pain upon arising in the morning that diminishes within 5 to 10 minutes, but builds throughout the day. Pain and stiffness on weight bearing are related to muscle spasm and splinting of the fascia secondary to inflammation. Hence, normal muscle length is not easily attained and leads to additional pain and irritation (26). Point tenderness is elicited over the medial tubercle of the calcaneus and increases with forefoot dorsiflexion and toe extension (19,20). Therapeutic modalities used to alleviate symptoms may include ice, deep friction massage, ultrasound, and electrical muscle stimulation (26). Achilles tendon stretching exercises, stretching of the toe flexor tendons, strengthening of the intrinsic muscles, NSAIDs, a heel lift or doughnut pad may also be helpful. A moleskin plantar fascia strap or figure-eight strapping are effective means of support. However, circular strips of tape around the foot are contraindicated because they may overstretch the fascia and prolong recovery. **Field Strategy 7-5** highlights the management of plantar fasciitis.

A common complaint with overuse injuries is pain brought on by activity

Point tenderness is elicited over the medial tubercle of the calcaneus and increases with forefoot dorsiflexion and toe extension

---

 Field Strategy 7–5. Management of Plantar Fasciitis.

Signs and Symptoms

Pain in the foot upon arising in the morning, particularly in the proximal medial longitudinal arch
Point tenderness can be elicited just over and distal to the medial calcaneal tubercle
Passive extension of the great toe and dorsiflexion of the ankle will increase pain and discomfort
Pain increases with weight bearing
Initial pain is relieved with activity, but returns with rest
As condition worsens, pain during and after activity

Treatment

Ice therapy and NSAIDs
Insert shock-absorbing heel pad or soft plantar arch orthotic
Figure-eight strapping may help

Rehabilitation

Heel cord stretching three times a day in position of toes straight ahead, toes in, and toes out
Gentle isometric contractions for intrinsic muscles of the foot initially
Progress to active range of motion within pain-free ranges, such as toe curls, marble pick-up, towel crunches, and towel curls to fatigue
Strengthen intrinsic and extrinsic muscles of leg
Maintain body fitness and strength, and aerobic fitness with non-weight bearing activities.

Achilles Tendinitis

Jumping and running can cause repetitive overextension and overload of the Achilles tendon. Commonly seen in joggers, runners, ballet dancers, skaters, and soccer and basketball players, Achilles tendinitis is one of the most common overuse problems in sport activity. Risk factors include tight heel cords, foot malalignment deformities, a recent change in shoes or running surface, a sudden increase in distance or intensity during a workout session, or excessive hill climbing (18,23).

Signs and symptoms include a history of pain during and after activity. Pain increases with passive stretching of the tendon into dorsiflexion, and with resisted plantar flexion. Point tenderness can be elicited on the tendon, and diffuse or localized swelling can be seen. Occasionally fine crepitation can be palpated in the middle of the tendon during movement, indicating friction between the tendon and its sheath.

Treatment involves ice therapy, NSAIDs, and activity modification in mild cases. In moderate to severe cases, complete restriction of activity may be necessary for 3 weeks. Active stretching of the Achilles tendon before and after activity along with a full strengthening program for the Achilles tendon including eccentric loading is initiated immediately after acute pain has subsided. Placing heel lifts in the shoe can decrease tension on the tendon temporarily, but correcting biomechanical abnormalities of the foot with orthotics should be a priority.

Occasionally, chronic degenerative changes caused by a long-time partial tear to the tendon can lead to a thickened, fibrotic, and constrictive tendon sheath. This should be referred to a physician. Surgical intervention to excise any degenerative area and stripping the tendon of its thickened mass may be necessary to properly repair the tendon. With stripping of the tendon, a gradual stretching and strengthening program can begin almost immediately with the individual returning to activity in 3 to 6 weeks. If a partial tear is surgically repaired, however, return to full activity will be somewhat longer (21).

Medial Tibial Stress Syndrome (MTSS)

Medial tibial stress syndrome encompasses any pain along the medial tibial border, usually in the distal third, not associated with a stress fracture or compartment syndrome (27). A major contributing factor to the condition involves excessive pronation or prolonged pronation of the foot leading to localized inflammation of the tibialis posterior muscle, a main supporting structure of the medial longitudinal arch. Other contributing factors include recent changes in running distance, speed, form, stretching, footwear, or running surface. Typically seen in runners or jumpers, pain initially is present at the start of activity. As activity progresses, pain diminishes only to recur hours after activity has ceased. In later stages, pain will be present before, during, and after activity, and may restrict performance.

Point tenderness will be elicited in a 3 to 6 cm area along the posterior medial edge of the distal one third of the tibia (27). Pain is aggravated by active plantar flexion and inversion of the ankle indicating strain of the tibialis posterior muscle. Possible stress fractures to the tibia should be ruled out through appropriate radiograph or scanning procedures.

Cryotherapy, NSAIDs, and activity modification, such as nonimpact or low impact activities, relieves initial acute symptoms. Pain-free stretching of both the anterior and posterior musculature will help improve joint mobility, increase muscle and tendon strength and coordination, and aid the musculoskeletal system to adapt to the physical demands of a specific sport (27). Analysis of the individual's running motion, foot alignment, running surface, and footwear may prevent reccurrence. **Field Strategy 7-6** summarizes the classification and management of medial tibial stress syndrome.

Exercise-Induced Compartment Syndrome

A **compartment syndrome** exists when increased intramuscular pressure during exercise impedes blood flow and function of the tissues within that compartment. With activity, blood flow increases to the various compartments which precipitates an increase in volume leading to an increase in pressure within the specific compartment. The anterior and deep posterior compartments are most frequently involved, however, the lateral and superficial posterior compartments may also be affected. Virtually any macrotrauma or microtrauma, including fractures, strains, contusions, and overuse associated with bleeding or edema formation within the com-

Compartment syndrome
Condition where increased intramuscular pressure brought on by activity impedes blood flow and function of tissues within that compartment

Field Strategy 7-6. Management of Medial Tibial Stress Syndrome.

Signs and Symptoms

Initial pain begins at start of activity, then ceases, but recurs hours after activity stops
In late stages, pain is present before, during and after activity
In experienced runners, condition is usually secondary to mechanical abnormalities
Pain along posterior medial border of tibia in a 3 to 6 cm area, usually in distal third
Pain is aggravated by active plantar flexion and inversion of ankle (posterior tibialis muscle)

Treatment

Ice, compression, elevation, NSAIDs, and activity modification
Evaluate and correct any foot malalignment
Keep a watchful eye on condition and determine a possible stress fracture with a tuning fork
If condition does not improve in 2 to 3 days, refer to physician for possible radiograph or bone scan
Conduct a biomechanical assessment of the running motion and correct any technique problems
Change running surface and possibly shoes
Increase flexibility in muscles in anterior and posterior compartment
Increase strength in all muscles of lower leg and foot

partment can lead to a compartment syndrome (28).

Chronic syndromes present as lower leg pain during exercise, and are relieved after rest. Pain often arises at a specific point in the training session, depending on speed and terrain, and does not seem to worsen over time. As swelling continues to expand the fascia to its maximum limit, the increased pressure on the deep neurovascular structures leads to numbness and tingling in the nerve distribution that traverses the particular compartment. The anterior compartment is often affected by skiing and walking, and the posterior compartment by running and jogging (18).

Intermittent excessive pressure within the closed fascial compartment can lead to **chronic exertional compartment syndrome**, which can also reduce blood flow through the compartment (23). Pain is rarely present before activity but pressure and subsequent pain increase with activity. Both pain and pressure cease after activity has ended, only to redevelop within 12 hours after exercise. The individual typically describes a deep throbbing of unyielding pressure. The skin may be shiny and warm. Pain increases with passive stretch of the compartment muscles and weakness is evident in active muscle contraction. In a chronic anterior compartment syndrome, dorsiflexion is limited and weak.

Extrinsic factors such as training patterns, technique, footwear, and running surfaces should be evaluated. Intrinsic factors such as alignment, muscle imbalance, and flexibility

should be assessed. In minor conditions, cryotherapy, NSAIDs and occasionally diuretics may assist the stretching, strengthening, orthotics, and activity modification (18). When high compartment pressures have been confirmed by a physician, however, surgery, called a fasciotomy, is the treatment of choice.

Did you determine the runner may have medial tibial stress syndrome? If so, you are correct. As part of the assessment check foot alignment, gait, and shoes for problems that may have contributed to the condition. Continue to check this individual for a possible stress fracture or compartment syndrome.

FRACTURES

A basketball player is complaining of pain in the forefoot region during sprinting and jumping drills. When you encircle the forefoot and compress the metatarsals, the individual winces in pain, but reports it only hurts "a little." What will your next course of action be?

Fractures in the foot and lower leg region seldom result from a single traumatic episode. Often, repetitive microtraumas lead to apophyseal or stress fractures. Tensile forces associated with severe ankle sprains can lead to avulsion fractures of the fifth metatarsal. Excessive compressive forces coupled with severe twisting can lead to displaced and undisplaced fractures in the foot,

Pain often arises at a specific point in the training session and does not seem to worsen over time

Chronic exertional compartment syndrome
Intermittent excessive pressure that reduces blood flow through a muscular compartment causing pain and possible paresthesis

ankle, or lower leg. A combination of forces can lead to a traumatic fracture-dislocation. In this section apophyseal, avulsion, stress, osteochondral, displaced and undisplaced fractures, and fracture-dislocation will be discussed.

Apophysitis of the Calcaneus (Sever's Disease)

In adolescents aged 10 to 15, a special condition called **Sever's disease**, or calcaneal apophysitis, occurs on the calcaneus where the Achilles tendon attaches. Because the apophyseal plate is vertically oriented, it is particularly susceptible to shearing stresses from the gastrocnemius. Being kicked in the region or an off-balance landing may also precipitate this condition. It is frequently seen in young gymnasts because of repetitive jumping or landing from a height with little or no support provided by the slippers typically worn during exercise (18). The individual will complain of posterior heel pain during activity relieved with rest. Palpable heel pain can be located just below the Achilles tendon attachment. The condition usually resolves itself with closure of the apophysis. Until then, NSAIDs, heel lifts, strapping the foot in slight plantar flexion to relieve some strain on the Achilles tendon, and activity modification will usually relieve symptoms.

Stress Fractures

Stress fractures are often seen in running and jumping, particularly after a significant increase in the training regimen, changing to a less resilient surface, or in individuals who wear shoes that no longer provide adequate padding or support for the foot. Women with **amenorrhea** and oligomenorrhea have a higher incidence of stress fractures of the foot and leg during sport activity (13). The neck of the second metatarsal is the most common location for a stress fracture, although it is also seen on the fourth and fifth metatarsals. Other frequent sites are the sesamoid bones, navicular, calcaneus, fibula, and tibia.

The two sesamoid bones of the great toe are often fractured as a result of constant weight bearing on a hyperextended great toe, or because of prolonged pronation during running. Individuals with a pes cavus or tight plantar fascia are predisposed to this injury because of the large tensile forces placed on the bones (18). Pain and swelling will be pres-

ent in the ball of the foot, and the individual will be unable to roll through the foot to stand on the toes. During hyperextension of the great toe, the sesamoid bones move distally as does the tenderness (**Figure 7-32**). Radiographs may be inconclusive, because it is common for sesamoid bones to be **biparte**.

Stress fractures of the metatarsals usually present with pain on weight bearing, and have swelling and point tenderness over the fracture site. Encircling the forefoot with your hand and squeezing the fingers together produce added discomfort.

Stress fractures to the navicular are common in jumpers, ballet dancers, and equestrians due to the nature of foot positions, motions, and inevitable stresses produced in the midfoot. Often seen in young men, this fracture is difficult to assess. A high degree of suspicion about this condition being present is required when the individual complains of generalized foot pain on the dorsomedial aspect of the midfoot brought on by activity and relieved with rest. In advanced stages, overlying swelling and pain on walking become evident.

Stress fractures to the calcaneus produce significant pain on heel strike. There is often a history of a substantial increase in the individual's activity level, particularly in distance runners. Palpation will reveal maximum pain on the medial and lateral aspects of the plantar-calcaneal tuberosity (19). Squeezing the calcaneus will also produce pain.

Stress fractures to the tibia and fibula result from repetitive stress to the leg leading to muscle fatigue. The resulting loss in shock

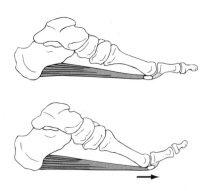

Fig. 7.32: The sesamoid bones are located within the tendons of the flexor hallucis brevis. When the great toe is hyperextended, the bones move distally as does the tenderness. With a fracture, the individual will be unable to roll through the foot to stand on the toes.

absorption increases stress to the bone and periosteum. In the tibia, most stress fractures occur at the junction of the mid and distal thirds, the posterior medial tibial plateau, or just distal to the tibial tuberosity (23). Fibular stress fractures usually occur in the distal metadiaphyseal region.

Symptoms associated with nearly all stress fractures usually begin with mild discomfort during running, but decrease or stop after activity and when non-weight bearing. Localized point tenderness over the fracture site and pain can be elicited with percussion, a tuning fork, or ultrasound. Frequently radiographs are negative early, but periosteal reaction or cortical thickening can be seen two to four weeks later. Bone scans usually reveal the presence of a fracture long before it becomes evident on radiography (**Figure 7-33**). Early treatment involves ice therapy, NSAIDs, activity modification, and correcting any mechanical abnormalities that may have contributed to the condition. Protected weight bearing, a stiff shoe, rigid orthosis, or walking cast may be indicated in fractures to the metatarsals, calcaneus, or tibia. Wearing stiff soled shoes or a heel cup may be helpful with stress fractures to the sesamoid bones and calcaneus, respectively. Most stress fractures heal in 4 to 6 weeks, but can take as long as 12 weeks. The individual should be completely asymptomatic before returning to participation.

Avulsion Fractures

Avulsion fractures may occur at the site of any ligamentous or tendinous attachment. Severe eversion ankle sprains may result in the deltoid ligament avulsing a portion of the distal medial malleolus rather than tearing the ligament. Inversion ankle sprains can provide sufficient overload to cause the peroneus brevis tendon to avulse the base of the fifth metatarsal. If the styloid process is avulsed it is termed a Type 2 fracture (18). Treatment usually involves a short walking cast initially to relieve pain. The individual may progress into a commercial protective device and return to sport participation after being fully reconditioned.

A much more complicated avulsion fracture seen in sprinters and jumpers involves a Type I transverse fracture into the proximal shaft of the fifth metatarsal, called **Jones's fracture (Figure 7-34)**. It is often overlooked in conjunction with a severe ankle sprain. Healing may be delayed, or may result in a **nonunion fracture**. Without wide displacement, a short leg cast and weight bearing as tolerated is employed. Surgery with bone grafting and internal fixation, however, may be necessary with wider displacement (18).

Osteochondral Fracture of the Talus

Severe ankle sprains can impinge the dome of the talus against the malleoli leading to a fracture of the cartilaginous cover. Anterolateral fractures result from forceful inversion of a dorsiflexed ankle. Posteromedial fractures result from forceful inversion of a plantar flexed ankle (**Figure 7-35**) (29). The fragment may remain nondisplaced or may float freely in the joint. **Osteochondritis dissecans** of the talus can develop if the fragment, particularly one of the corners, floats freely in the ankle joint, thus losing its blood supply. Symptoms may be nonspecific, and include a deep, aching pain aggravated by activity, ankle swelling, stiffness, occasional crepitus, clicking, locking, or a catching sensation (18,29). Passive plantar flexion and palpation of the anterolateral and posteromedial corner of the talus will elicit point tenderness. A palpable lesion or crepitus may also be palpated on the corners. If pain and joint effusion per-

Jones's fracture
A transverse stress fracture of the proximal shaft of the fifth metatarsal

Nonunion fracture
A fracture where healing is delayed or the bone fails to unite at all

Osteochondritis dissecans
Inflammation of both bone and cartilage that can split the pieces into the joint, and result in loss of blood supply to the fragments

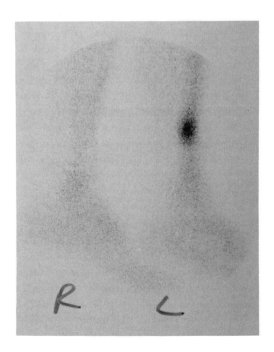

Fig. 7.33: Bone scans detect stress fractures long before the fractures become apparent on x-rays.

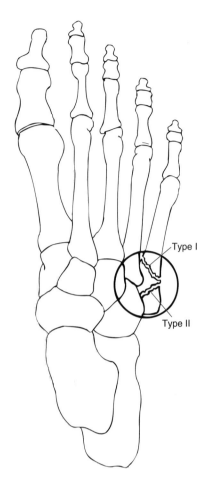

Fig. 7.34: A Type I transverse fracture into the proximal shaft of the 5th metatarsal is often overlooked in an inversion ankle sprain, resulting in a nonunion fracture. A Type II fracture invovles the styloid process of the 5th metatarsal.

sist after a inversion ankle sprain or ankle fracture, or if symptoms return after an asymptomatic period, suspect a more serious underlying condition. Decreased activity, limited weight bearing, and/or immobilization, and NSAIDs are used to treat undisplaced fractures. In displaced fractures, treatment may involve immobilization for 4 to 6 weeks, surgical excision, or internal fixation.

Displaced and Undisplaced Fractures

Displaced and undisplaced fractures result from direct compression in acute trauma (e.g., falling from a height or being stepped on), or from combined compression and shearing forces, such as during a severe twisting action. Because of the proximity of major blood vessels and nerves, many displaced and undisplaced fractures necessitate immediate

immobilization and referral to the nearest trauma center.

Phalangeal fractures are commonly caused by crushing injury or jamming the toe into an immovable object. With the exception of a fracture to the great toe, most are minor injuries. Swelling, ecchymosis, and pain are primary symptoms. Although tenderness may persist for several weeks, two to three weeks of limited weight bearing is usually sufficient to allow for good healing. If the bony fragment is nondisplaced, padding, splinting, and wearing a shoe with a wide toe box may help. If the great toe is fractured, wearing a stiff shoe is helpful, however, if displaced, casting for a few days may be necessary.

Fractures to the metatarsals produce palpable pain directly over the area and/or compression along the long axis of the bone. Ordinarily there is little displacement of the bone ends and a short slipper cast is sufficient for immobilization.

The lateral process of the talus can be fractured by a traumatic ankle sprain leading to swelling, ecchymosis, and point tenderness just anterior and inferior to the tip of the lateral malleolus. Major symptoms include persistent ankle pain, swelling, and an inability to stand or walk for long periods.

Posterior fractures to the talus are seen in individuals aged 15 to 30, particularly in those sports requiring forced plantar flexion of the foot, such as ballet or soccer, and may be either acute or stress-related (18). Posterior pain is present when jumping, running, or kicking with the instep of the foot, and is increased on forced plantar flexion and resisted great toe flexion stemming from the close proximity of the flexor hallucis longus tendon to the fractured process. Fractures to the neck of the talus can occur with a forceful dorsiflexion injury. Because the blood supply to the talus may be lost with this type of injury, immediate immobilization and referral to a physician is necessary.

Traumatic fractures to the calcaneus are rare and considered an orthopedic emergency. Occasionally fractures will occur to the anterior process by either forceful plantar flexion and adduction, or compression. Intense pain can be palpated directly over the process, located just distal to the sinus tarsi (30).

On inversion sprains, the medial malleolus is typically fractured at the level of the talar dome, or may occur as a spiral fracture at the distal tibial metaphysis. Eversion and dorsiflexion injuries lead to spiral or comminuted

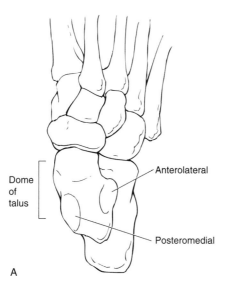

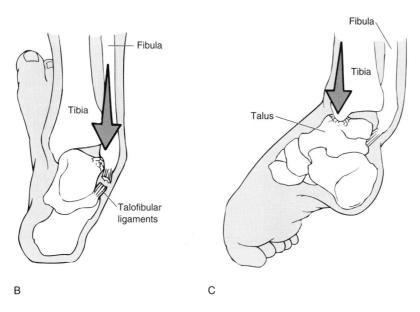

Fig. 7.35: (A) A severe ankle injury that can fracture a portion of the cartilaginous cover on the dome of the talus is called an osteochondral fracture. (B) Forceful inversion of a dorsiflexed ankle can produce damage to the anterolateral talar dome. (C) Forceful inversion of a plantar flexed ankle can produce damage to the posteromedial aspect of the dome.

fractures of the lateral malleolus (21). With lateral malleolar fractures, the risks are high for a bimalleolar fracture due to the deltoid ligament avulsing the medial malleolus. Often a "crack" will be heard and the individual is unable to bear weight on the injured extremity because of intense pain. Palpation elicits pain and crepitus over the involved bone. Deformity may or may not be present. Immediately check circulation, sensation, and motor function of the foot. Nondisplaced fractures are treated conservatively with cast immobilization for four to six weeks followed by a functional brace until completely healed (23). Displaced fractures involving joint sta-

bility require surgical intervention with open reduction and internal fixation. Healing after surgery usually takes two to three months or longer, followed by extensive rehabilitation.

Fractures to the fibula usually occur at midshaft as a result of a blow to the lateral aspect of the calf. Because the fibula is a non-weight-bearing bone, the individual may not even be aware of the fracture, and may walk or even run off the field. Pain is not a good indicator, as the condition may be confused with a deep contusion. Treatment for fractures in the distal third of the fibula involve a short leg walking cast for four to six weeks, but fractures to the midshaft and upper por-

On inversion sprains, the medial malleolus is typically fractured at the level of the talar dome

With a fibular fracture, the individual may not even be aware of the fracture and may walk or even run off the field

tions may be treated with a simple compressive dressing and crutches (21).

Tibial fractures usually result from direct or indirect compression and bending of the bones during sport participation. Most traumatic tibial fractures occur either below the tibial plateau or more commonly, above the malleolus. Any acute fracture to the tibia must be assessed to determine if it is open, and if so, appropriate covering of the area with a sterile dressing is indicated to prevent infection and potential loss of blood. Gross deformity, gross bone motion at the suspected fracture site, crepitus, immediate swelling, extreme pain, or pain with motion should signal immediate action. The neurovascular integrity must be assessed before and after immobilization by taking a distal pulse at the posterior tibial artery, dorsalis pedis artery, or blanching the toe nails to determine capillary refill. Because shock is possible, an ambulance should be summoned to immobilize and transport the individual to the nearest medical facility.

Fracture-Dislocations

Fracture-dislocations usually result from landing from a height with the foot in excessive eversion or inversion, or being kicked from behind while the foot is firmly planted on the ground. The foot will typically be displaced laterally at a gross angle to the lower leg, and extreme pain will be present. This position can compromise the posterior tibial artery and nerve. The shoe and sock should be cut away from the foot. Note the skin color of the foot and toes. Feel the toes for warmth, and blanch the toe nails to determine capillary refill. Stroke the pulp of your finger across the top of the distal metatarsal heads, and ask the individual if they can feel your finger. Repeat with the finger nail. Summon EMS! The foot and ankle should be immobilized by the ambulance attendants in the position found and the individual transported immediately to the nearest medical facility.

Did you determine the basketball player had a possible stress fracture of the metatarsals due to repetitive overloading of the region? If so, you are correct. This individual should be referred to a physician for further assessment and treatment.

ASSESSMENT OF THE FOOT, ANKLE, AND LOWER LEG

An individual is complaining about vague pain on the dorsum of the foot

brought on by activity. Can you limit the assessment to only the foot or should you assess the entire lower leg? How will you proceed?

Although pain, discomfort, or weakness may occur at a specific site, the lower extremities work as a unit to provide a foundation of support for the upright body, propulsion through space, absorption of shock, and adaptation to varying terrains. As such, assessment must include the entire lower extremity to evaluate how the body segments work together to provide motion. Always enter the assessment with an open mind because pain may be referred to the foot, ankle, and lower leg from conditions in the lumbar spine, sacrum, hip or knee. Keep this in mind as you progress through the assessment.

HISTORY

What information do you need from the individual complaining of vague pain on the dorsum of the foot? How will you phrase the questions to identify the main components of the primary complaint?

Many conditions in the foot, ankle, and lower leg are related to family history, congenital deformities, poor technique, and recent changes in training programs, surfaces, or foot attire. In addition to general questions discussed in Chapter 4, specific questions related to the foot, ankle, and lower leg are listed in **Field Strategy 7-7**.

You have learned from the individual that pain on the dorsum of the foot started two weeks ago and generally intensifies during physical activity. Recently while playing tennis, pain was so intense the individual had to stop and remove the tennis shoes because the laces were irritating the top of the foot. Nothing like this has ever happened before, nor does the individual recall any member of the family having a similar experience.

OBSERVATION AND INSPECTION

Think for a minute or two about the position(s) in which you want to observe this individual. Would a posture and gait analysis help? Why? What specific malalignment conditions might contribute to pain in the foot, ankle, or leg?

Both lower legs should be clearly visible to denote symmetry, any congenital deformity, swelling, discoloration, hypertrophy, muscular atrophy, or previous surgical incisions. The individual should wear running shorts to

A fracture-dislocation at the ankle can compromise the posterior tibial artery and nerve

Field Strategy 7–7. Developing a History of the Injury.

Current Injury Status

1. What are your normal activities? Do you stand, sit, or walk on uneven surfaces for long periods? Have you recently increased your training intensity or duration? What types of surfaces give you the most problem? What type of shoe do you wear when the pain sets in? (Check the height of the heel, wear pattern on bottom, and internal arch and heel padding)

2. Where is the pain (or weakness) located? Can you point to the most uncomfortable area? On a scale of 1 to 10 with 10 being very severe, how would you rate the pain (weakness)? What type of pain is it? (dull ache, throbbing, sharp, intermittent, "red-hot" or burning)?

3. Did the pain come on gradually (overuse problem) or suddenly (acute problem)? How long has it been a problem? Was the pain greatest when the injury first occurred or did it get worse the second or third day? What has been done for the condition?

4. If an acute problem, identify the mechanism of injury. Ask: What were you doing at the time of the injury? How did the injury occur? If the injury came on gradually ask: What different activities have you been doing in the last week? (Look for changes in frequency, duration, intensity, type, or method)

5. Did you hear any sounds during the incident? Any snaps, pops, or cracks? Has the joint ever locked on you (indicating a possible talar dome lesion)? Did you notice any swelling or discoloration at the time of the injury? How soon did it occur? What did you do for it?

6. What actions or motions bring on the pain? Is it worse in the morning, during activity, after activity, or at night? When the pain sets in, how long does it last? Has there been any improvement in the condition?

7. Are there certain activities you are unable to perform because of the pain? Which ones? How old are you? Which foot is dominant?

Past Injury Status

1. Have you ever injured your leg before? When? How did that occur? Who evaluated and cared for the injury? What was the diagnosis? What was done at the time of injury? What have you done since then to strengthen the area? Did you have any difficulty returning to your full functional status?

2. Have you had any medical problems recently? (Look for problems that may refer pain to the area from the lumbar spine, hip, or knee). Are you on any medication? Do you have any musculoskeletal problems elsewhere in the body? (These may result in changes in gait or technique that transfers abnormal forces to structures in the involved limb)

allow full view of the lower extremity. Ask them to bring along the shoes they normally wear when pain is present. Inspect the sole, heel box, toe box, and general condition of the shoes for unusual wear, thus indicating a biomechanical abnormality.

In an ambulatory patient, begin observations by completing a postural exam. At the foot, note the presence, or lack, of an arch on weight bearing and non-weight bearing. A supple, or flexible, flat foot appears flattened when weight bearing but produces an obvious arch when non-weight bearing. In contrast, a rigid flat foot appears flattened on weight bearing and non-weight bearing. Specific areas to focus on in the lower extremity are summarized in **Field Strategy 7-8**. Next, place the individual prone on a table with the knee extended and the feet over the end of the table. Observe the relationship of the rearfoot to forefoot alignment. After completing a static exam observe the individual walking barefoot from anterior, posterior, and lateral views. Note any abnormalities in gait, favoring one limb, heel-toe floor contact, and heel alignment. Have the individual put on shoes and any orthoses, and repeat the gait analysis to get a better perspective of the wear pattern. Inspect the injury site for obvious deformities, discoloration, edema, scars that might indicate previous surgery, and note the general condition of the skin. Remember to compare the affected limb with the unaffected limb.

The individual has bilateral low arches and the calcaneus appears to evert

A supple flatfoot appears to have an arch when non-weight bearing, however, a rigid flatfoot is flat on weight bearing and non-weight bearing

Anterior View

- The iliac crests should be level with equal space between the arms and waist. Both thighs should look the same. Check for hypertrophy or atrophy. The patellas should be at the same height and face straight forward
- The legs should be straight. The knees may be in genu valgum (knock kneed) or genu varum (bow legged)
- The medial and lateral malleoli should be level as compared to the opposite foot. Is there swelling in the ankle joint?
- Both feet should be angled equally. Tibial torsion may result in the foot either pointing inward ("pigeon toes"), or pointing slightly lateral. Check for supination or pronation of the feet. Both feet should have visible equal arches. Note any pes cavus (high arch) or pes planus (flat foot). Are the feet splayed (widening of the forefoot)? Are the toes straight and parallel? Do the nails appear normal?
- Check the skin for normal contours, discolored lesions, exostosis or other bumps, corns, calluses, and scars indicating a previous injury or surgery. Note any signs of circulatory impairment or varicose veins

Posterior View

- The gluteal folds and knee folds should be level. The hamstrings and calf muscles should have equal bulk
- The Achilles tendons should go straight down to the calcaneus. If they appear to angle out, excessive pronation may be present. The heels should appear to be straight with equal shape and position
- The lateral malleoli should extend slightly more distal than the medial malleoli, and the medial malleoli will be slightly more anterior than the lateral malleoli

Side View

- The knees should be slightly flexed (0 to 5°)
- The lateral malleolus should be slightly posterior to the center of the knee

Non-Weight Bearing View

- Check for abnormal calluses, plantar warts, arches and scars on the plantar side of the foot

slightly. With the exception of prolonged pronation on the right foot, gait appears normal. The dorsa of both feet are red and swollen.

PALPATIONS

With pain centered on the dorsum, think for a minute where you should begin to palpate the various structures. During palpations, what factors are you looking for?

Bilateral palpations can determine temperature, swelling, point tenderness, crepitus, deformity, muscle spasm, and cutaneous sensation. Vascular pulses can be taken at the posterior tibial artery behind the medial malleolus and at the dorsalis pedis artery on the dorsum of the foot. Proceed proximal to distal, but palpate the most painful areas last. Allow the individual to sit on a table so you can perform bilateral palpations.

Anterior and Medial Palpations

1. Shaft of the tibia
2. Medial malleolus
3. Posterior tibial artery
4. Tibialis posterior, flexor digitorum longus, and flexor hallucis longus muscles and tendons
5. Deltoid ligament
6. Sustentaculum tali
7. Talar dome and neck (plantar flexion will expose this area)
8. Joint capsule
9. Tibialis anterior, extensor hallucis longus, extensor digitorum longus muscles and tendons, and dorsalis pedis artery
10. Navicular bone and tubercle of the navicular
11. Medial, middle, and lateral cuneiforms

12. Calcaneonavicular ligament (spring ligament)
13. Medial calcaneus
14. Plantar fascia
15. Head of first metatarsal, sesamoid bones, great toe
16. Second metatarsal and second toe

Anterior and Lateral Palpations

1. Head of the fibula, peroneal longus and brevis
2. Distal tibiofibular joint and ligament
3. Lateral malleolus
4. Anterior and posterior talofibular ligaments, calcaneofibular ligament, peroneal tubercle, and peroneal tendons
5. Sinus tarsi
6. Joint capsule
7. Cuboid bone
8. Styloid process of the fifth metatarsal, shafts of the third, fourth, and fifth metatarsals
9. Third through fifth toes

Posterior Palpations

1. Triceps surae and Achilles tendon
2. Calcaneus and retrocalcaneal bursa
3. Posterior aspect of heel pad and calcaneus

If a fracture is suspected, perform percussion, compression, and distraction prior to any movement of the limb. These tests should be completed before a postural or gait analysis. Depending on the site, techniques listed in **Field Strategy 7-9** may be helpful. If a fracture is suspected, check sensation and circulation distal to the fracture site. Immobilize the area and refer to a physician for follow up care.

You found increased pain and warmth on palpation of the toe extensor tendons over the proximal shafts of the second, third, and fourth metatarsals. Localized swelling and a slight increase in skin temperature is also present in the region.

SPECIAL TESTS

Pain and swelling are localized over the proximal forefoot with specific pain increasing with palpation of the toe extensor tendons. What special tests can be performed to determine if the injury is muscular, bony, or ligamentous?

Special tests should be performed in a comfortable position with the individual lying on a table with feet hanging over the end or with the individual sitting. Bilateral comparison is used to assess normal level of function.

Active Movements

Active movements are best performed with the individual sitting on a table with the leg flexed over the end of the table. Stabilize the thigh and knee. Perform those actions causing pain last to prevent any painful symptoms from overflowing into the next movement. The following motions should be performed weight bearing and non-weight bearing.

1. Dorsiflexion of the ankle (20°)
2. Plantar flexion of the ankle (30 to 50°)
3. Pronation (15 to 30°)
4. Supination (45 to 60°)
5. Toe extension

 Field Strategy 7–9. Determine a Possible Fracture in the Foot and Lower Leg.

- Percussion, or tapping, on the head of the fibula or tibial shaft can be used to detect a fracture of the malleolus.
- Strike the bottom of the heel with the palm to drive the talus into the mortise. Increased pain may indicate an osteochondral fracture, malleolar fracture, or increased mortise spread.
- Compress the tibia and fibula together just distal to the knee. This causes the distal malleoli to distract. Increased pain distally may indicate a fracture.
- Encircle the mid foot with the hand and slowly squeeze the metatarsal heads. Increased pain may indicate a tarsal or metatarsal fracture.
- Place a vibrating tuning fork near the suspected fracture site. Increased localized pain is a positive sign.
- Tap or compress the ends of the toes and metatarsals along the long axis of the bone. Follow this with distraction along the long axis. If a fracture is present percussion and compression should increase pain, but distraction should decrease pain.

6. Toe flexion
7. Toe abduction and adduction

Passive Range of Motion

If the individual is able to perform full range of motion during active movements, apply gentle pressure at the extremes of motion to determine end feel. The end feel for dorsiflexion, plantar flexion, pronation, supination, toe flexion and extension is tissue stretch. If the individual is unable to perform full active movements, passive movement should then be performed to determine available range of motion and end feel. **Figure 7-36** demonstrates proper positioning for goniometry measurement at the ankle.

Resisted Muscle Testing

Stabilize the thigh and perform all resisted muscle testing throughout the full range of motion. As always, painful motions should be delayed until last. **Figure 7-37** demonstrates motions that should be tested (myotomes are listed in parentheses):

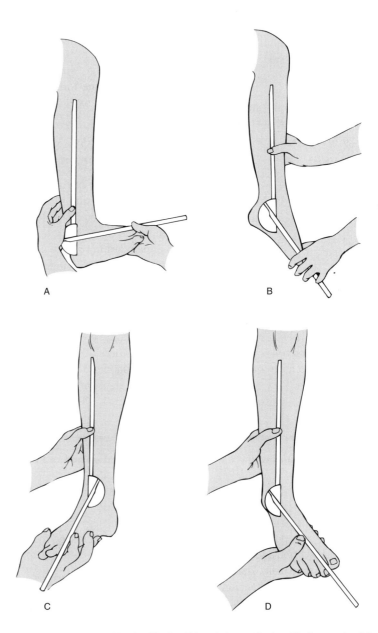

Fig. 7.36: Goniometry measurement. Ankle dorsiflexion (A) and plantar flexion (B). Center the fulcrum over the lateral malleolus. Align the proximal arm along the fibula using the head of the fibula for reference. Align the distal arm parallel to the midline of the 5th metatarsal. Pronation (C) and supination (D). Center the fulcrum over the anterior ankle midway between the malleoli. Align the proximal arm with the midline of the crest of the tibia. Align the distal arm with the midline of the 2nd metatarsal.

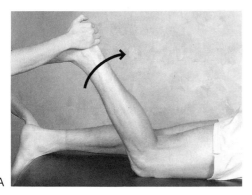

A

Fig. 7.37: Resisted manual muscle testing. (A) Knee flexion.

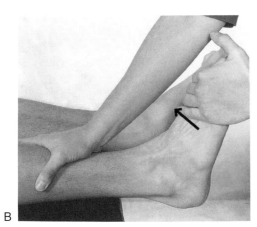

B

Dorsiflexion.

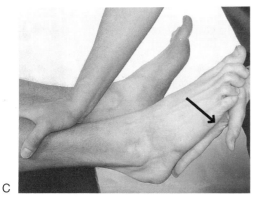

C

Plantar flexion.

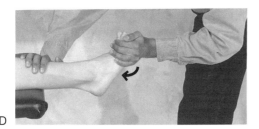

D

Pronation

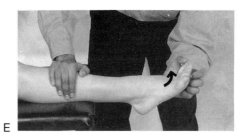

E

Supination.

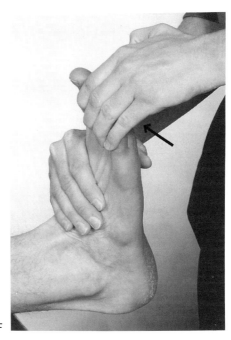

F

Toe extension.

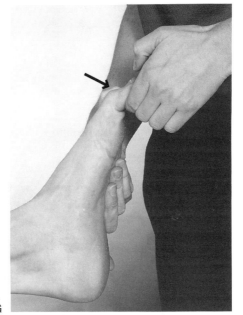

G

Toe flexion.

1. Knee flexion (**S₁ and S₂**)
2. Dorsiflexion (**L₄**)
3. Plantar flexion (**S₁**)
4. Pronation
5. Supination
6. Toe extension (**L₅**)
7. Toe flexion

Neurological Assessment

Assess neurological integrity with isometric muscle testing of the myotomes, reflex testing, and sensation in the segmental dermatomes and peripheral nerve cutaneous patterns.

Myotomes

Isometric muscle testing should be performed in the following motions to test specific segmental myotomes: knee extension (L_3); ankle dorsiflexion (L_4); toe extension (L_5); and ankle plantar flexion, foot eversion, or hip extension (S_1).

Reflexes

Reflexes in the lower leg region include the patella (L_3, L_4) and Achilles tendon reflex (S_1). To test the patellar reflex, flex the knee at 90° (seated), and strike the tendon with the flat end of the reflex hammer using a crisp wrist-flexion action (**Figure 7-38A**). A normal reflex exhibits a slight jerking motion in extension. To test the Achilles tendon reflex, slightly dorsiflex the ankle to place the tendon on stretch, and tap the tendon with the flat end of the reflex hammer (**Figure 7-38B**). An alternative position is to have the individual lie prone on a table, or place the knee on a chair with the foot extended beyond the edge (**Figure 7-38C**). A normal reflex should elicit a slight plantar flexion jerk.

Cutaneous Patterns

In testing cutaneous sensation, run sharp and dull objects over the skin, i.e., blunt tip of taping scissors and the flat edge of taping scissors. With their eyes closed or looking away, ask the individual if they can distinguish sharp and dull. The segmental nerve dermatome patterns for the foot and lower leg are demonstrated in **Figure 7-39**. The peripheral nerve cutaneous distribution patterns are demonstrated in **Figure 7-40**.

Stress and Functional Tests

From information gathered during the history, observation, inspection, and palpation,

> To isolate the anterior talofibular ligament, apply a forward motion in slight plantar flexion and inversion

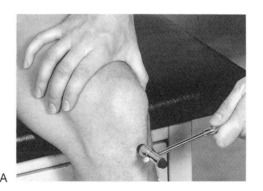

A

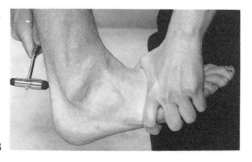

B

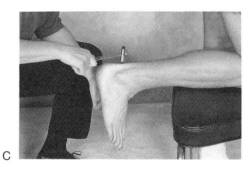

C

Fig. 7.38: Reflex testing. (A) The patellar reflex. (B) The Achilles reflex. (C) Alternative position for the Achilles reflex.

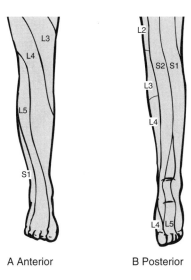

A Anterior   B Posterior

Fig. 7.39: Dermatomes for the lower leg, ankle, and foot.

determine which tests most effectively assess the condition. Only those tests deemed relevant should be used.

*Thompson's Test for
Achilles Tendon Rupture*

With the individual prone on a table squeeze the calf muscles. A normal response elicits slight plantar flexion. Always compare the amount of motion to the uninjured side, however, as some plantar flexion may occur if the plantaris muscle is intact. A positive test, indicating a rupture of the Achilles tendon, is indicated by the absence of plantar flexion (**Figure 7-41**).

Anterior Drawer Test

This test can assess collateral ligament integrity of the ankle. Place the individual supine and extend the foot beyond the table.

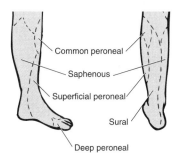

Common peroneal
Saphenous
Superficial peroneal
Sural
Deep peroneal

Fig. 7.40: Peripheral nerve distribution in the lower leg, ankle, and foot.

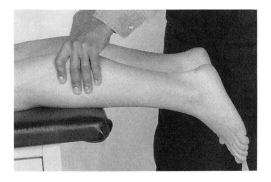

Fig. 7.41: To perform the Thompson test, do passive compression of the calf muscles. This should produce slight plantar flexion at the ankle. If no plantar flexion occurs, suspect a possible rupture of the gastrocnemius-soleus complex or the Achilles tendon.

Stabilize the tibia and fibula in one hand and cup the individual's heel in the other hand. To test both the anterior talofibular ligament and deltoid ligament, apply a straight anterior movement with slight dorsiflexion (**Figure 7-42A**). If the entire dome of the talus shifts equally forward, it indicates both medial and lateral ligament damage. To isolate the anterior talofibular ligament and anterolateral capsule, apply a straight anterior movement with slight plantar flexion and inversion. A positive test will result in the lateral side of the talus shifting forward, indicating anterolateral rotary instability.

Talar Tilt

The calcaneofibular and deltoid ligaments are tested in the same position described for the anterior drawer test. Maintain the calcaneus in normal anatomic position (90° flexion). The talus is then slowly rocked between inversion and eversion (**Figure 7-42B**). Inversion tests the calcaneofibular ligament; eversion the deltoid ligament.

Functional Tests

Functional tests should be performed pain-free before clearing any individual for re-entry into competition. These may include any or all of the following:

1. Squatting with both heels maintained on the floor
2. Going up on the toes at least 20 times without pain
3. Walking on the toes for 20 to 30 feet
4. Balancing on one foot at a time

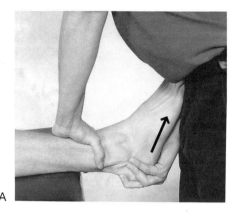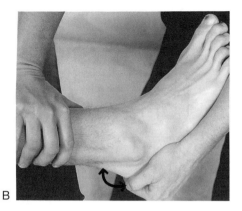

Fig. 7.42: Stress tests for the ankle collateral ligaments. (A) Anterior drawer test. (B) Talar tilt test.

The rehabilitation program should restore motion and proprioception, maintain cardiovascular fitness, and improve muscular strength, endurance, and power predominantly through closed chain exercises

5. Running straight ahead, stopping, and running backwards
6. Running figure-8s with large circles slowly decreasing in size
7. Running at an angle sideways and making V-cuts
8. Jumping rope for at least 1 minute
9. Jumping straight up and going to a 90° squat

These activities are examples that can be used to test the integrity of injured anatomical structures. All should be performed pain-free and without a limp or antalgic gait.

Increased pain occurred on toe extension of the middle three toes and on dorsiflexion. While palpating the tendons you felt slight snowball crepitation during resisted motion. All other tests were negative. What condition may be present here? How will you treat it?

REHABILITATION

A basketball player is recovering from a mild second degree inversion ankle sprain. After controlling acute swelling and inflammation, what exercises should be included in the rehabilitation program?

Rehabilitation exercises for the foot, ankle, and lower leg can be initiated during the acute inflammatory phase so long as the condition is not further irritated. For example, while icing an ankle, the gastrocnemius and soleus can be passively stretched, or strengthening exercises for the foot intrinsic muscles can be started. Pain and swelling dictate the amount of exercise tolerated, and may necessitate restricted weight bearing. The rehabilitation program should restore motion and proprioception, maintain cardiovascular fitness, and improve

muscular strength, endurance, and power predominantly through closed chain exercises.

Restoration of Motion

Field Strategy 7-1 introduced several range of motion exercises that can be performed non-weight bearing. For example, towel pulls stretching the Achilles tendon, writing the alphabet in large circles, picking up objects in the toes and combining the action with shin curls, and use of a BAPS board can all be done in a seated position. As pain subsides and weight bearing is initiated, Achilles tendon stretches, toe raises, balance exercises, and use of the BAPS board can be completed in a standing position.

Restoration of Proprioception and Balance

Proprioception and balance must be regained to allow safe return to sport participation. Early exercises may include shifting one's weight while on crutches, doing bilateral mini-isquats, or using a BAPS board in a seated position. As balance improves, BAPS board exercises can progress to partial weight bearing while supported by a table, to full weight bearing exercises, or the KAT 1000 may be used (**Figure 5-9A**). Running in place on a minitrampoline or use of a slide board are also closed chain exercises that improve proprioception and balance.

Muscular Strength, Endurance, and Power

Early emphasis is placed on strengthening the foot's intrinsic muscles. Towel crunches were demonstrated in **Field Strategy 7-1** . As the condition allows, toe raises and Theraband or surgical tubing exercises are added. Use of a multi-axial ankle machine, toe raises with weights, squats and lunges, and isokinetic exercises will continue to strengthen the lower leg musculature. In later stages, jogging, running side to side, and multiangle plyometrics can assist the individual in returning gradually to sport participation.

Cardiovascular Fitness

Maintenance of cardiovascular fitness can begin immediately after injury with use of an upper body ergometer (UBE) or hydrotherapeutic exercise. Running in deep water and performing sport-specific exercises can provide mild resistance in a non-weight bearing medium. When range of motion is adequate, a stationary bicycle may be used. Light jogging, running backwards, and running side-to-side should increase in intensity and duration to facilitate return to activity. **Field Strategy 7-10** lists several rehabilitation exercises that may be incorporated in a complete program for the lower leg.

 Field Strategy 7–10. Rehabilitation Exercises for the Lower Leg.

A. Phase one. Control inflammation. Minimize inversion and eversion exercises to allow for healing. Dorsiflexion and plantar flexion should be performed within the limits of pain. Exercises should be combined with ice therapy or electrical stimulation with elevation. Use those exercises listed in Field strategy 7–1 as tolerated
  1. Plantar fascia stretch
  2. Towel crunches
  3. Toe curls
  4. Picking up objects
  5. BAPS board in seated position
  6. Triceps surae stretch, non-weight bearing
  7. Pool therapy or upper body ergometer (UBE) exercises for cardiovascular fitness
B. Phase two. As pain and tenderness subside, initiate inversion and eversion range of motion. Initiate strengthening exercises as tolerated. Include:
  1. Shin curls
  2. Ankle alphabet
  3. Triceps surae stretch, standing position
  4. Toe raises
  5. Theraband or surgical tubing exercises in dorsiflexion, plantar flexion, inversion and eversion
  6. Unilateral balance-BAPS board activities with support
  7. Pool therapy, UBE, and stationary bike (if tolerated) for cardiovascular fitness
C. Phase three
  1. Toe raises with weights
  2. Multiaxial ankle machine
  3. Squats and lunges
  4. Balance exercises with challenges, such as dribbling while balancing on one leg, doing Theraband exercises while balancing on one leg, or balancing on an even surface
  5. Straight ahead jogging if able to walk without a limp
D. Phase four. (Use external support for the ankle as needed)
  1. Isokinetic exercises to work functional speeds
  2. Multiangle plyometrics including single and double limb jumping; front to front, side to side, and diagonals
  3. Side to side running
  4. Running backwards
  5. Jumping for height and distance (long jump)
  6. Slide board
  7. Gradual return to sport activity with protection

In addition to exercises, it is suggested the individual be assessed for biomechanical anomalies, and that appropriate orthotics be fabricated to correct any malalignment. With ankle injuries, it may be necessary to provide external support to the ankle region. After the rehabilitation program is completed, and the individual is cleared for full participation, a proper maintenance program of stretching and strengthening exercises should be provided.

The basketball player can strengthen the intrinsic muscles of the foot and maintain plantar flexion and dorsiflexion at the ankle in the early stages of rehabilitation. If the condition is irritated, however, adjustments must be made in the intensity of exercise. As the condition improves, surgical tubing exercises and closed chain exercises are used to improve strength, endurance, power, balance, and proprioception. A UBE or hydrotherapeutic exercises can maintain cardiovascular fitness until the condition allows for light jogging and more intense weight bearing activities.

SUMMARY

The foot, ankle, and lower leg are highly susceptible to injury during sport participation. Tremendous stress is placed on the region in walking and running on uneven surfaces, stopping and starting to change direction rapidly, and jumping from heights. Congenital abnormalities, muscle imbalance, muscle dysfunction, and postural deviations can also predispose an individual to chronic injuries. Because of this, a systematic, thorough assessment must be completed for all lower leg injuries as summarized in **Field Strategy 7-11**.

Throughout the assessment remember that pain may be referred from the lumbar spine, hip, or knee. If a significant finding is assessed, immediately refer the individual to a physician for further evaluation. Conditions that warrant special attention include: obvious deformity suggesting a dislocation or fracture; significant loss of motion or weakness in a myotome; excessive joint swelling; possible epiphyseal or apophyseal injuries; abnormal or absent reflexes; abnormal sensations in either the segmental dermatomes or peripheral cutaneous patterns; absent or weak pulse; gross joint instability; or any unexplained pain. The final rule of thumb is always "when in doubt, refer!"

 Field Strategy 7–11. Foot, Ankle, and Lower Leg Evaluation.

History

Primary complaint including:
    Description and mechanism of current injury
    Onset of symptoms
Pain perception and discomfort
Disability and functional impairments from the injury
Previous injuries to the area
Family history

Observation and Inspection

Postural assessment
    Gait analysis
    Inspection of injured area for:

Muscle symmetry	Hypertrophy or muscle atrophy
Swelling	Visible congenital deformity
Discoloration	Surgical incisions or scars

Palpation

Bony structures to determine possible fracture
Soft tissue structures to determine:

Temperature	Crepitus
Swelling	Muscle spasm
Point tenderness	Cutaneous sensation
Deformity	Vascular pulses

Special Tests

Active movements
Passive range of motion
Resisted muscle testing
Neurologic testing
Stress and functional tests
    Thompson's test for Achilles tendon rupture
    Anterior drawer test
    Talar tilt
    Functional tests

Should you decide to refer the individual to a physician, remove the individual from activity and immobilize the limb in a comfortable position. Immobilization may consist of simple strapping to support the area, or use of a posterior splint, vacuum splint, or any commercial splints available to pad and protect the injured area. If necessary, fit the individual with crutches. Apply ice, compression, and elevation when appropriate to control inflammation and swelling, and transport the individual appropriately.

Functional tests should be performed pain-free without limp or antalgic gait before clearing any individual for re-entry into competition. In addition, the individual should have bilaterally equal range of motion, strength, proprioception, and a high cardiovascular fitness level before being allowed to return to activity. When necessary, protective equipment or braces should be used to prevent reinjury.

REFERENCES

1. Johnson, RE, and Rust, RJ. 1985. Sports related injury: An anatomic approach, part 2, Minn Med, 68(11):829–831.

2. Norkin, CC, and Levangie, PK. *Joint structure and function: A comprehensive analysis.* Philadelphia: FA Davis, 1992.

3. Engsberg, JR. 1987. A biomechanical analysis of the talocalcaneal joint—in vitro. J Biomech, 20(4):429–442.

4. Edington, CJ, Frederick, EC, and Cavanagh, PR. "Rearfoot motion in distance running." In *Biomechanics of distance running*, edited by PR Cavanagh. Champaign, IL: Human Kinetics, 1990.

5. Frederick, EC. 1986. Kinematically mediated effects of sport shoe design: A review. J Sport Sci, 4(3):169–184.

6. Nigg, BM, and Bahlsen, HA. 1988. Influence of heel flare and midsole construction on pronation, supination and impact forces for heel-toe running. Int J Sport Biomech, 4(3):205–219.

7. Renstrom, P, and Johnson, RJ. 1985. Overuse injuries in sports: A review. Sports Med, 2(5):316–333.

8. Lovejoy, CO, Burstein, AH, and Heiple, KC. 1976. The biomechanical analysis of bone strength: A method and its application to platycnemia. Am J Phys Anthrop, 44(3):489–505.

9. Hamill, J, Bates, BT, Knutzen, KM, and Sawhill, JA. 1983. Variations in ground reaction force parameters at different speeds. Hum Mvt Sci, 2:47–56.

10. Rubin, CT. 1984. Skeletal strain and the functional significance of bone architecture. Calcif Tissue Int, 36 (S1):S11–18.

11. Frost, HM. 1988. Vital biomechanics: proposed general concepts for skeletal adaptations to mechanical usage. Calcif Tissue Int, 42(3):145–156.

12. Milgrom, C, Giladi, M, Simkin, A, Rand, N, Kedem, R, Kashtan, H, Stein, M, and Gomori, M. 1989. The area moment of inertia of the tibia: A risk factor for stress fractures. J Biomech, 22(11/12): 1243–1248.

13. Lloyd, T, Triantafyllow, SJ, Baker, ER, Houts, PS, Whiteside, JA, Kalenak, A, and Stumpf, PG. 1986. Women athletes with menstrual irregularity have increased musculoskeletal injuries. Med Sci Sports and Exer, 18(4):374–379.

14. Warren, MP, Brooks-Gunn, J, Hamilton, LH, Warren, LF, and Hamilton, WG. 1986. Scoliosis and fractures in young ballet dancers: Relation to delayed menarche and secondary amenorrhea. N Engl J Med, 314(21):1348–1353.

15. Lloyd, T, Meyers, C, Buchanan, JR, and Demers, LM. 1988. Collegiate women athletes with menstrual irregularity have increased musculoskeletal injuries. Obstet and Gyn, 72(4):639–642.

16. Salathe, EP, Jr, Arangio, GA, and Salathe, EP. 1990. The foot as a shock absorber, J Biomech. 23(7):655–659.

17. Winter, DA. 1983. Moments of force and mechanical power in jogging. J Biomech, 16(1):191–97.

18. Reid, DC. *Sports injury assessment and rehabilitation.* New York: Churchill Livingstone, 1992.

19. Hunter, SC, Cappiello, WL, Hess, GP, and Joyce, D. "Foot problems." In *The team physician's handbook*, edited by MB Mellion, WM Walsh, and GL Shelton. Philadelphia: Hanley & Belfus, 1990.

20. Ransey, ML. 1992. Plantar warts: Choosing treatment for active patients. Phys Sportsmed, 20(11):69–88.

21. American Academy of Orthopaedic Surgeons. *Athletic training and sports medicine.* Park Ridge, IL: American Academy of Orthopaedic Surgeons, 1991.

22. Irvine, WO. Feet under force: Treating sprains and strains. Phys Sportsmed. 20(9):137–144.

23. Brown, DE. "Ankle and leg injuries." In *The team physician's handbook*, edited by MB Mellion, WM Walsh, and GL Shelton. Philadelphia: Hanley & Belfus, 1990.

24. Wills, CA, Washburn, S, Caiozzo, V, Prietoo, CA. 1986. Achilles tendon rupture: A review of the literature comparing surgical versus non-surgical treatment. Clin Orthop, 207:156–163.

25. Herring, SA, and Nilson, KL. "Introduction to overuse injuries." In *Clinics in sports medicine*, edited by LY Hunter Griffin, vol. 6, no. 2. Philadelphia: WB Saunders, 1987.

26. Middleton, JA, and Kolodin, EL. 1992. Plantar fasciitis—Heel pain in athletes. J Ath Train, 27(1):70–75.

27. Fick, DS, Albright, JP, and Murray, BP. 1992. Relieving painful 'shin splints.' Phys Sportsmed, 20(12):105–113.

28. Allen, MJ. 1990. Compartment syndromes of the lower limb. J R Coll Surg Edinb, 35(6 Suppl):S33-6.

29. Shea, MP, and Manoli, A. 1993. "Recognizing talar dome lesions." Phys Sportsmed, 21(3):109–121.

30. Davis, AW, and Alexander, IJ. "Problematic fractures and dislocations in the foot and ankle of athletes." In *Clinics in sports medicine*, edited by JT Watson and JA Bergfeld, vol. 9, no. 1. Philadelphia: WB Saunders, 1990.

Chapter 8

The Knee

After you have completed this chapter, you should be able to:

■ Locate the important bony and soft tissue structures of the knee region

■ Describe the motions of the knee and identify the muscles that produce them

■ Explain what forces produce the loading patterns responsible for common injuries at the knee

■ Identify basic principles in the prevention of knee injuries

■ Recognize and manage specific injuries at the knee

■ Demonstrate a thorough assessment of the knee and patellofemoral joint

■ Demonstrate general rehabilitation exercises for the region

The knee is a large, complex joint frequently injured during sport participation. During walking and running, the knee moves through a considerable range of motion while bearing loads equivalent to three to four times body weight. The knee is also positioned between the two longest bones in the body, the femur and tibia, creating the potential for large, injurious torques at the joint. These factors, coupled with minimal bony stability, make the knee susceptible to injury, particularly during participation in field and/or contact sports.

This chapter begins with a review of the anatomy of the knee, and discusses its kinematics and kinetics. General principles to prevent injuries will then be followed by discussion of common injuries to the knee complex. Finally, a step-by-step injury assessment of the region is presented, and examples of rehabilitative exercises will be provided.

ANATOMY REVIEW OF THE KNEE

❓ *A female runner is complaining of pain on the lateral side of her left knee just above the joint line. The pain is more noticeable when she runs on city streets facing traffic. What structures might be inflamed in this region?*

The knee is a large synovial joint including three articulations within the joint capsule. The weight-bearing joints are the two condylar articulations of the tibiofemoral joint, with the third articulation being the patellofemoral joint. The soft tissue connections of

the proximal tibiofibular joint also exert a minor influence on knee motion (1).

Tibiofemoral Joint

The distal femur and proximal tibia terminate in medial and lateral condyles that articulate to form two side-by-side condyloid joints known collectively as the **tibiofemoral joint**, **(Figure 8-1)**. These joints function together primarily as a modified hinge joint because of the restricting ligaments, with some lateral and rotational motions allowed. Because the medial and lateral condyles of the femur differ somewhat in size, shape, and orientation, the tibia rotates laterally on the femur during the last few degrees of extension to produce "locking" of the knee. This phenomenon, known as the **"screwing-home" mechanism**, brings the knee into the close packed (most stable) position of full extension.

Menisci

The **menisci**, also known as semilunar cartilages because of their half-moon shapes, are discs of fibrocartilage firmly attached to the superior plateaus of the tibia by the coronary ligaments and joint capsule (2). They are also joined to each other by the transverse ligament. The menisci are thicker along the lateral margin and thinner on the medial margin, serving to deepen the concavities of the tibial plateaus. The medial meniscus is semicircular, whereas the lateral meniscus is somewhat more circular **(Figure 8-1)**. The

Tibofemoral joint
Dual condyloid joints between the tibial and femoral condyles that function primarily as a modified hinge joint

Screwing home mechanism
Rotation of the tibia on the femur during extension that produces an anatomical "locking" of the knee

Menisci
Fibrocartilaginous discs within the knee that reduce joint stress

The menisci are attached to the tibia by the coronary ligaments and joint capsule, and to each other by the transverse ligament

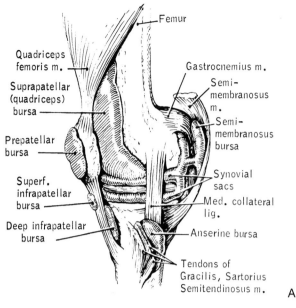

Femur

Quadriceps
femoris m.

Suprapatellar
(quadriceps)
bursa

Prepatellar
bursa

Superf.
infrapatellar
bursa

Deep infrapatellar
bursa

Gastrocnemius m.

Semi-
membranosus
m.

Semi-
membranosus
bursa

Synovial
sacs

Med. collateral
lig.

Anserine bursa

Tendons of
Gracilis, Sartorius
Semitendinosus m.

A

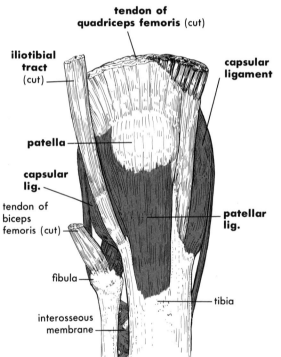

tendon of
quadriceps femoris (cut)

iliotibial
tract
(cut)

capsular
ligament

patella

capsular
lig.

tendon of
biceps
femoris (cut)

patellar
lig.

fibula

tibia

interosseous
membrane

B

Fig. 8.1: The knee. (A) Bursae of the knee. (B) Ligaments of the knee (anterior view). (C) Ligaments of the knee (posterior view—superficial and deep structures). (D) Superior surface of tibia with menisci and associated structures.

The ends of the menisci, called the horns, are attached to the intercondylar tubercles

The largest bursa of the body is the suprapatellar located between the femur and quadriceps femoris muscle tendon

inner edges of both menisci are unattached to the bone, but the two ends of the menisci, known as the anterior and posterior horns, are attached to the intercondylar tubercles. The medial meniscus is also attached to the deep medial collateral ligament and fibers from the semimembranosus muscle. It is injured much more frequently than the lateral meniscus. This is partly due to the medial meniscus being more securely attached to the tibia, and therefore less mobile. The lateral meniscus is a more freely moveable structure. In addition

to its attachments to the joint capsule, intercondylar tubercles, and transverse ligament, the lateral meniscus is attached to the posterior cruciate ligament through the meniscofemoral ligament (Wrisberg's Ligament) and popliteus muscle (3).

Joint Capsule and Bursae

The thin articular capsule at the knee is large and lax, encompassing both the tibiofemoral and patellofemoral joints (**Figure 8-1**). Anteriorly it extends about 2.5 centimeters above

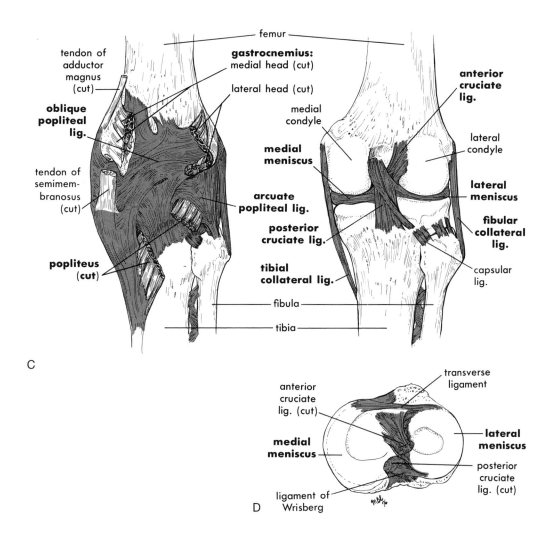

femur

tendon of
adductor
magnus
(cut)

gastrocnemius:
medial head (cut)

lateral head (cut)

**oblique
popliteal
lig.**

medial
condyle

**medial
meniscus**

tendon of
semimem-
branosus
(cut)

**arcuate
popliteal lig.**

**posterior
cruciate lig.**

**popliteus
(cut)**

**tibial
collateral lig.**

fibula

tibia

**anterior
cruciate
lig.**

lateral
condyle

**lateral
meniscus**

**fibular
collateral
lig.**

capsular
lig.

C

anterior
cruciate
lig. (cut)

transverse
ligament

**medial
meniscus**

**lateral
meniscus**

posterior
cruciate
lig. (cut)

ligament of
Wrisberg

D

the patella to attach along the edges of the superior patellar surface. The deep bursa formed by this capsule above the patella, the suprapatellar bursa, is the largest in the body. It lies between the femur and quadriceps femoris tendon, and functions to reduce friction between the two structures. Posteriorly, two other bursae communicate with the joint capsule, the subpopliteal and semimembranosus bursae. The subpopliteal bursa lies between the lateral condyle of the femur and popliteal muscle. The semimembranosus bursa lies between the medial head of the gastrocnemius and semimembranosus tendons.

During flexion and extension the synovial fluid moves throughout the bursal recesses to lubricate the articular surfaces. In extension, the gastrocnemius and subpopliteal bursae are compressed, driving the synovial fluid anteriorly. In flexion, the suprapatellar bursa is compressed, forcing fluid posteriorly (2). When the knee is in a semiflexed, or open packed position, the synovial fluid is under the least amount of pressure. This position

provides relief of pain caused by swelling in the joint capsule and surrounding bursae.

Three other key bursae associated with the knee, but not contained in the joint capsule, are the prepatellar, superficial infrapatellar, and deep infrapatellar bursae. The prepatellar bursa is located between the skin and anterior surface of the patella, allowing free movement of the skin over the patella during flexion and extension. The superficial infrapatellar bursa is located between the skin and patellar tendon. Inflammation of this bursa due to excessive kneeling is sometimes referred to as "housemaid's knee." The deep infrapatellar bursa is located between the tibial tuberosity and the patellar tendon, and is separated from the joint cavity by the infrapatellar fat pad. This bursa reduces friction between the ligament and the bony tuberosity.

Ligaments of the Knee

Because the shallow articular surfaces of the tibiofemoral joint contribute little to knee

During motion at the knee the synovial fluid moves throughout the synovial cavity to lubricate the articular surfaces

stability, the stabilizing role of the ligaments crossing the knee is of great significance. Two major ligaments of the knee are the anterior and posterior **cruciate ligaments (Figure 8-1)**. The name *cruciate* is derived from the fact that these ligaments cross each other, with *anterior* and *posterior* referring to their respective tibial attachments. These ligaments are termed **intracapsular** because they are located within the articular capsule, and **extrasynovial** because they lie outside the synovial cavity. The anterior cruciate ligament stretches from the anterior aspect of the intercondyloid fossa of the tibia just medial and posterior to the anterior tibial spine in a superior, posterior direction to the posterior medial surface of the lateral condyle of the femur. The shorter and stronger posterior cruciate ligament runs from the posterior aspect of the tibial intercondyloid fossa in a superior, anterior direction to the lateral anterior medial condyle of the femur. These ligaments restrict the forward and backward sliding of the femur on the tibial plateaus during knee flexion and extension, and also serve to limit knee hyperextension. The anterior cruciate is considered to be the weaker of the two ligaments, and is frequently subject to deceleration injuries.

The medial and lateral **collateral ligaments** are referred to respectively as the tibial and fibular collateral ligaments after their distal attachments. Fibers of the medial collateral ligament merge with the joint capsule and medial meniscus to connect the medial epicondyle of the femur to the medial tibia. It attaches just below the pes anserinus, the common attachment of the semitendinosus, semimembranosus, and gracilis to the tibia, thereby positioning the ligament to resist medially directed shear (valgus) and rotational forces acting on the knee. The lateral collateral ligament connects the lateral epicondyle of the femur to the head of the fibula, contributing to lateral stability of the knee. The ligament is separated from the lateral meniscus by a small fat pad (4).

Other Structures Stabilizing the Knee

Several other structures also contribute to knee integrity. Posteriorly, the oblique popliteal ligament forms an extension of the semimembranosus tendon, and the arcuate popliteal ligament connects the lateral condyle of the femur to the head of the fibula.

Although the knee is only partially surrounded by a joint capsule, the capsule is reinforced by several tendons and ligaments, including the expanded tendons of the quadriceps, the tendon of the semimembranosus, and the oblique popliteal ligament. Laterally, the iliotibial tract, a broad, thickened band of the fascia lata extends from the tensor fascia lata over the lateral epicondyle of the femur to Gerdy's tubercle on the lateral tibial plateau. This resisting band has been hypothesized to function as an anterolateral ligament of the knee (5). **Table 8-1** lists the structures providing stability to the knee.

Patellofemoral Joint

The patella is a triangular bone commonly known as the kneecap. It articulates with the patellofemoral groove between the femoral condyles to form the **patellofemoral joint** **(Figure 8-1)**. The posterior surface of the patella is covered with articular cartilage, with a central vertical ridge separating the medial and lateral regions.

The **Q-angle** is formed between the line of resultant force produced by the quadriceps muscles and the line of the patellar tendon **(Figure 8-2)**. The normal Q-angle ranges from approximately 13° in males to approximately 18° in females when the knee is extended. A Q-angle less than 13° or greater than 18° is considered abnormal, and can predispose the sport participant to patellar injuries or degeneration (6).

In the sagittal plane, the patella serves to increase the angle of pull of the patellar tendon on the tibia, thereby improving the mechanical advantage of the quadriceps muscles for producing knee extension. The patella also provides some protection for the anterior aspect of the knee.

Muscles Crossing the Knee

The muscles of the knee develop tension to produce motion at the knee and also contribute to the knee's stability. The attachments and primary actions of the muscles crossing the knee are summarized in **Table 8-2**.

Nerves of the Knee

The tibial nerve (L_4, L_5, S_1-S_3) is the largest and most medial continuation of the sciatic nerve. It innervates all of the muscles in the hamstring group except the short head of the

Table 8–1. Structures Contributing to the Stability of the Knee.

Direction of Stability	Ligaments (Static)	Muscles and Tendons (Dynamic)
Medial	Medial collateral ligament Meniscofemoral ligament Coronary ligaments Posterior cruciate ligament	Pes anserinus Semimembranosus
Lateral	Lateral collateral ligament Meniscofemoral ligament Coronary ligaments Anterior and posterior cruciate ligament Arcuate ligament	Popliteus Biceps femoris Iliotibial band
Anterior	Anterior cruciate ligament Medial and lateral collateral ligament	Extensor retinaculum Patella
Posterior	Posterior cruciate ligament Oblique popliteal ligament Arcuate ligament	Biceps femoris Gastrocnemius Semimembranosus Popliteus
Anteromedial and anterolateral	Medial collateral ligament Anterior cruciate ligament Oblique popliteal ligament Meniscofemoral ligament Coronary ligaments	

biceps femoris, and also supplies all muscles in the calf of the leg (**Figure 8-3**).

The common peroneal nerve (L_4, L_5, S_1, S_2) is the lateral terminal branch of the sciatic nerve. It innervates the short head of the biceps femoris in the thigh, then passes through the popliteal fossa to wind laterally along the subcutaneous surface to just below the proximal head of the fibula, where it can be easily damaged. As it passes between the fibula and the peroneus longus muscle it subdivides into the superficial and deep peroneal nerves. An articular branch to the knee may arise from either the deep peroneal nerve or from both deep and superficial peroneal nerves as a terminal branch of the common peroneal nerve (7).

The femoral nerve (L_2-L_4) courses down the anterior aspect of the thigh adjacent to the femoral artery to supply the quadriceps group. The L_2 and L_3 branches of the femoral nerve also innervate the sartorius.

Blood Vessels of the Knee

Just proximal to the knee, the main branch of the femoral artery becomes the popliteal artery. The popliteal artery courses through the popliteal fossa and then branches, forming the medial and lateral superior genicular,

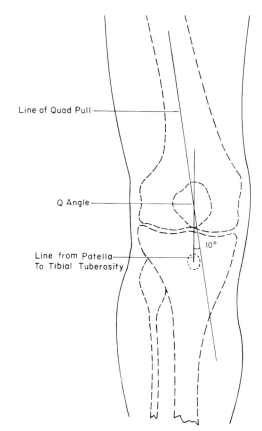

Line of Quad Pull

Q Angle

Line from Patella To Tibial Tuberosity

10°

Fig. 8.2: The Q-angle is formed between the line of quadriceps pull and the imaginary line connecting the center of the patella to the center of the tibial tuberosity.

The tibial nerve innervates all muscles in the hamstring group except the short head of the biceps femoris

The genicular arteries are branches of the popliteal artery that supply the knee with nourishment

Table 8–2. Muscles Acting on the Knee.

Muscle	Proximal Attachment	Distal Attachment	Primary Action(s)	Nerve Innervation
Rectus femoris	Anterior inferior iliac spine (AIIS)	Patella	Extension	Femoral (L_2,L_3,L_4)
Vastus lateralis	Greater trochanter and lateral linea aspera	Patella	Extension	Femoral (L_2,L_3,L_4)
Vastus intermedius	Anterior femur	Patella	Extension	Femoral (L_2,L_3,L_4)
Vastus medialis	Medial linea aspera	Patella	Extension	Femoral (L_2,L_3,L_4)
Semitendinosus	Ischial tuberosity	Proximal, medial tibia at pes	Knee flexion and medial rotation	Sciatic (L_5,S_1,S_2)
Semimembranosus	Ischial tuberosity	Proximal, medial tibia	Knee flexion and medial rotation	Sciatic (L_5,S_1,S_2)
Biceps femoris	*Long head:* ischial tuberosity. *Short head:* lateral linea aspera	Fibular head and lateral condyle of tibia	Knee flexion and lateral rotation	Sciatic (L_5,S_1,S_2)
Sartorius	Anterior superior iliac spine (ASIS)	Proximal medial tibia at pes	Knee flexion and medial rotation	Femoral (L_2,L_3)
Gracilis	Symphysis pubis and the pubic arch	Proximal medial tibia at pes	Knee flexion and medial rotation	Obturator (L_2,L_3)
Popliteus	Lateral condyle of the femur	Posterior, medial tibia	Medial rotation Knee flexion	Tibial (L_4,L_5)
Gastrocnemius	Posterior medial and lateral femoral condyles	Calcaneus, via the Achilles tendon	Knee flexion	Tibial (S_1,S_2)
Plantaris	Posterior femur above lateral condyle	Calcaneus	Knee flexion	Tibial (S_1,S_2)

the middle genicular, and the medial and lateral inferior genicular arteries that supply the knee **(Figure 8-4)**. The superior and inferior genicular arteries intertwine with each other about the knee.

💡 *The structure most likely to be irritated on the lateral superior aspect of a runner's knee is the iliotibial tract, which is subjected to friction against the local surrounding structures by running.*

KINEMATICS AND MAJOR MUSCLE ACTIONS OF THE KNEE

❓ *Why does the rotational capability of the knee vary throughout the range of flexion/extension? What anatomical features are responsible for this phenomenon?*

The knee functions primarily as a hinge joint. However, the different shapes of the femoral condyles serve to complicate joint function.

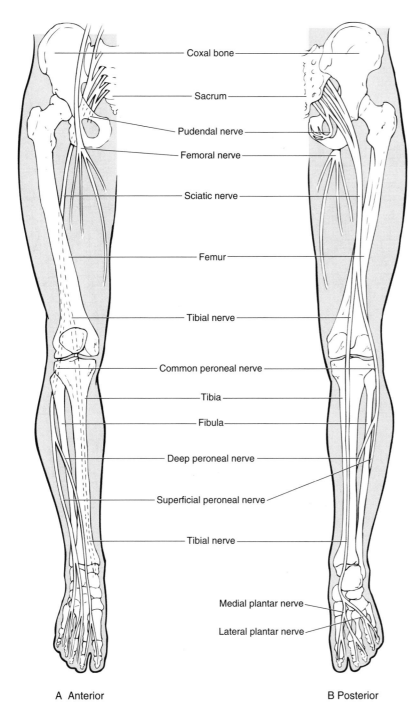

Fig. 8.3: The innervation of the knee.

Coxal bone	
Sacrum	
Pudendal nerve	
Femoral nerve	
Sciatic nerve	
Femur	
Tibial nerve	
Common peroneal nerve	
Tibia	
Fibula	
Deep peroneal nerve	
Superficial peroneal nerve	
Tibial nerve	
Medial plantar nerve	
Lateral plantar nerve	

A Anterior   B Posterior

Flexion and Extension

The primary motions permitted at the tibiofemoral joint are flexion and extension. In full extension, the joint's close packed position, maximal bony contact occurs between the femur and tibia, resulting in the joint being anatomically "locked." This occurs because the articulating surface of the medial condyle of the femur is longer than that of the

lateral condyle in this locked position, rendering motion almost completely impossible (2). For flexion to be initiated from a position of full extension, the knee must first be "unlocked." The role of locksmith is provided by the popliteus, which acts to laterally rotate the femur with respect to the tibia, thereby freeing the joint for motion.

Once the knee is unlocked from full extension, bony contact is diminished and motion

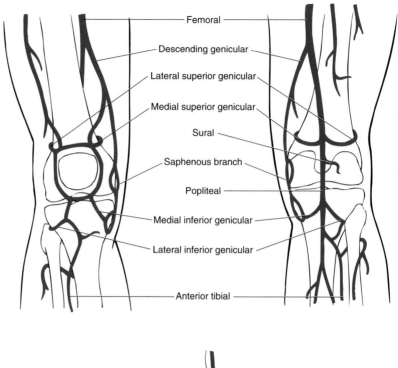

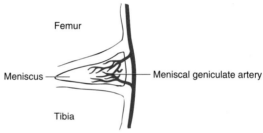

Fig. 8.4: Collateral circulation around the knee.

in the transverse and frontal planes becomes freer. As the knee moves into flexion, the femur slides anteriorly on the tibia, and during extension, the reverse occurs, with the femur sliding posteriorly on the tibia.

Rotation and Passive Abduction and Adduction

Rotational capability of the tibia with respect to the femur is maximal at approximately 90° of knee flexion. A few degrees of passive abduction and adduction are also permitted when the joint is positioned in the vicinity of 30° of flexion (7).

Knee Motion During Gait

During midstance of normal gait the knee is flexed to about 20°, internally rotated approximately 5°, and slightly abducted. Knee motion during the swing phase includes

around 70° of flexion, 15° of external rotation, and 5° of adduction (8).

Patellofemoral Joint Motion

During flexion/extension movements the patella glides superiorly and inferiorly against the distal end of the femur in a primarily vertical direction with an excursion of as much as 8 cm (1). The patella also undergoes medial and lateral displacement as the tibia is rotated laterally and medially, respectively.

Tracking of the patella against the femur is dependent on the direction of the net force produced by the attached quadriceps. The vastus lateralis tends to pull the patella laterally in the direction of the muscle's action line, parallel to the femoral shaft. The iliotibial tract and lateral extensor retinaculum also exert a lateral force on the patella. Although there is considerable debate as to the role of the vastus medialis oblique, it seems to

Rotation of the tibia is maximal at about 90° of knee flexion

oppose the lateral pull of the vastus lateralis, thereby keeping the patella centered in the patellofemoral groove. If the magnitude of the force produced by the vastus lateralis exceeds that produced by the vastus medialis oblique, the patella is pulled laterally out of its groove during tracking. Mistracking of the patella during knee flexion/extension can be extremely painful and requires medical attention.

Rotational capabilities at the knee vary throughout the range of motion depending on where the femoral condyles are in relation to the tibia. Rotation is maximal at about 90° of knee flexion.

KINETICS OF THE KNEE

Why are deep knee bends contraindicated? What structures are placed in danger by such activities?

Because the knee is positioned between the body's two longest bony levers, (the femur and the tibia), the potential for torque and force development at the knee is great. The key role played by the knee during weight bearing also makes the knee subject to large forces during the gait cycle.

Forces at the Tibiofemoral Joints

Both compression and shear forces are created at the tibiofemoral joints during daily activities. Weight bearing and tension development in the muscles crossing the knee contribute to these forces, with compression dominating when the knee is fully extended. As knee flexion occurs and the angle at the joint increases to 90°, the shear component of joint force produced by weight bearing increases. Shear at the knee, which causes a tendency for the femur to displace anteriorly on the tibial plateaus, must be resisted by the ligaments and other supportive structures crossing the knee. Because these structures can be stretched or even ruptured under such stress, activities like deep knee bends and full squats that require load bearing during extreme knee flexion are not recommended.

Compressive force at the tibiofemoral joint has been reported to be slightly greater than three times body weight during the stance phase of gait, increasing to around four times body weight during stair climbing (9). During sport participation, knee forces are undoubtedly greater, although quantita-

tive estimates are lacking. It has also been found that tension in the knee extensors increases lateral stability of the knee, with tension in the knee flexors contributing to medial stability (10).

The menisci assist with force absorption at the knee, bearing as much as an estimated 45% of the total load (11). The medial two-thirds of each meniscus has an internal structure particularly well-suited to resisting compression (2). The menisci also serve to distribute force from the femur over a broader area, thus reducing the magnitude of joint stress. Tibiofemoral joint stress is an estimated three times higher during weight-bearing when the menisci have been removed (12). Because the menisci also serve to protect the articulating bone surfaces from wear, knees that have undergone complete or partial meniscectomies may still function adequately, but are more likely to develop degenerative conditions.

Forces at the Patellofemoral Joint

Compressive force at the patellofemoral joint has been found to be half the body weight during normal walking gait, increasing up to over three times body weight during stair climbing. The squat exercise, known for being particularly stressful to the knee complex, produces a patellofemoral joint reaction force about 7.6× body weight (13). Given the small contact area between the articulating bone surfaces, the transmitted stress at the patellofemoral joint during such maneuvers is high.

Activities, such as deep knee bends, create large shear forces at the knee, causing a tendency for the femur to displace anteriorly on the tibial plateaus. This tendency must be resisted by the ligaments and other supportive structures crossing the knee, which can be stretched or ruptured under high levels of stress.

PREVENTION OF KNEE INJURIES

What exercises should be included in a preseason conditioning program for the knee? Does gender affect the potential for knee or patellofemoral injuries?

Because the knee is positioned between the body's two longest levers, (the femur and tibia), the potential for torque and force development at the knee is enormous. Prevention of injuries must focus on a well-

Compressive force at the tibiofemoral joint is 4× body weight during walking and 4× body weight during stair climbing

The menisci assist with force absorption at the knee, bearing as much as 45% of the total load

Tibiofemoral joint stress is 3× higher during weight bearing with the menisci removed

rounded physical conditioning program. Many of the muscles that move the knee have their proximal attachments in the hip and thigh region. Therefore, preventative exercises for these muscles will contribute to the prevention of injuries at the hip, as well as the knee. Although much debate continues as to the effectiveness of prophylactic knee braces (See Chapter 6), recent rule changes and improved shoe design have contributed more to a reduction of injuries at the knee.

Physical Conditioning

The development of a well-rounded physical conditioning program is the key to injury prevention. Exercises should include flexibility, muscular strength, endurance, and power, as well as speed, agility, balance, and cardiovascular fitness. Stretching exercises should focus on the quadriceps, hamstrings, gastrocnemius, iliotibial tract, and adductors. Because many of these muscles contribute to knee stability, strengthening programs should also focus on these muscle groups. Specific exercises to prevent injury to the musculature are provided in **Field Strategy 8-1**. Many of these exercises can be supplemented with tubing to add resistance to the exercise.

Rule Changes

Rule changes in contact sports, particularly football, have reduced injuries to the knee region. Modifications in acceptable techniques that prohibit tackling at or below the knee, or tackling from behind have reduced traumatic injuries. Proper training methods on correct technique should continue throughout the season to ensure compliance with specific rules designed to prevent injury.

Shoe Design

In Chapter 6, changes in shoe design were discussed. In football, a cleated shoe with a higher number of shorter, broader cleats can prevent the foot from becoming fixed to the ground. The length of the cleats still allows for good traction on running and cutting maneuvers. Other sports, particularly those played on artificial turf surfaces, use the multi-cleated soccer style shoe. These cleat designs can be seen in Chapter 6.

Flexibility, muscular strength, endurance, and power exercises should be included in a physical conditioning program to prevent knee injury. *In addition, agility, speed, balance, and cardiovascular fitness exercises should also be included. Women, because of their wider hips and larger Q-angle, may be at a greater risk for knee or patellofemoral injuries.*

CONTUSIONS

A soccer player was kicked on the anterolateral side of the proximal tibia. Mild swelling and discoloration, but no apparent loss in function or excessive pain, were present. What complications or other problems should be ruled out before the individual returns to play? How will you manage this injury?

Contusions resulting from compressive forces (i.e., a kick or falling on the knee) are common injuries at the knee. General signs and symptoms include localized tenderness, pain, swelling, and ecchymosis. If swelling is extensive, other injuries may be obscured. For example, being kicked on the medial aspect of the tibia may appear as a contusion, when in fact the impact may have caused an avulsion fracture of the medial collateral ligament or an epiphyseal injury in an adolescent. Extreme point tenderness and positive findings on any of the special tests should indicate a more serious injury is present, and referral to a physician is indicated.

Fat Pad Contusion

The infrapatellar fat pad may become entrapped between the femur and tibia, or inflamed during arthroscopy leading to a tender, puffy fat pad contusion. Signs and symptoms include locking, catching, giving way, palpable pain on either side of the patellar tendon, and extreme pain on forced extension. After a full assessment to rule out fracture and major ligament damage, initial treatment includes ice, compression, elevation, rest, and NSAIDs. Sport activity is usually not limited. However, the area should be protected to prevent further insult.

Peroneal Nerve Contusion

The common peroneal nerve leaves the popliteal space, and winds around the fibular neck to supply motor and sensory function to the anterior and lateral compartments of the lower leg (**Figure 8-5**). A kick or blow to the posterolateral aspect of the knee can contuse this nerve leading to temporary or permanent

A kick to the posterolateral aspect of the knee can contuse the peroneal nerve leading to temporary or permanent paralysis

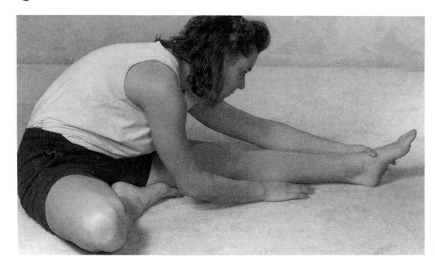

1

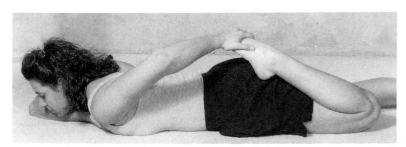

2

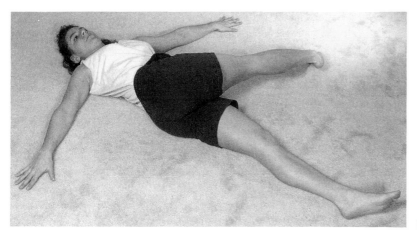

3

1. Hamstrings stretch, seated position. Place the leg to be stretched, straight out with the opposite foot tucked toward the groin. Reach toward the toes until a stretch is felt
2. Quadriceps stretch, prone position. Push the heel toward the buttocks, then raise the knee off the floor until tension is felt.
3. Iliotibial band stretch, supine position. With the trunk stabilized, adduct the leg to be stretched over the other leg and allow gravity to passively stretch the iliotibial band

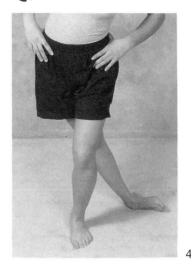

4

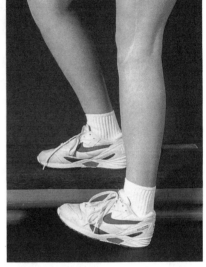

5a

5b

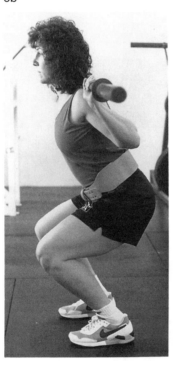

5c

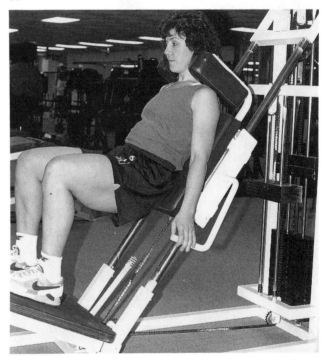

4. Iliotibial band stretch, standing position. Cross the limb to be stretched behind the other, extending and adducting the hip as far as possible
5. Closed chain exercises
    a. Step ups, step downs, and lateral step ups
    b. Squats. (Never below 85 to 90°)
    c. Leg press
    d. Lunges
6. Open chain exercises
    a. Knee extension. (quadriceps)
    b. Knee flexion. (hamstrings)

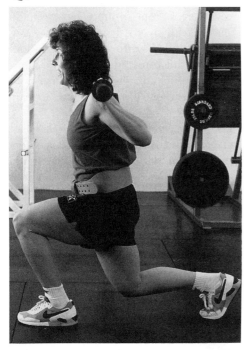

5d

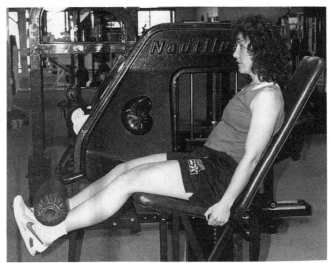

6a

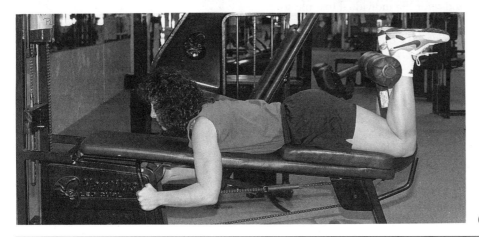

6b

Neoplasm
Tumor that can be benign or malignant

Acute traumatic bursitis leads to a grossly distended, warm bursa filled with bloody effusion

Pyarthrosis
Suppurative pus within a joint cavity

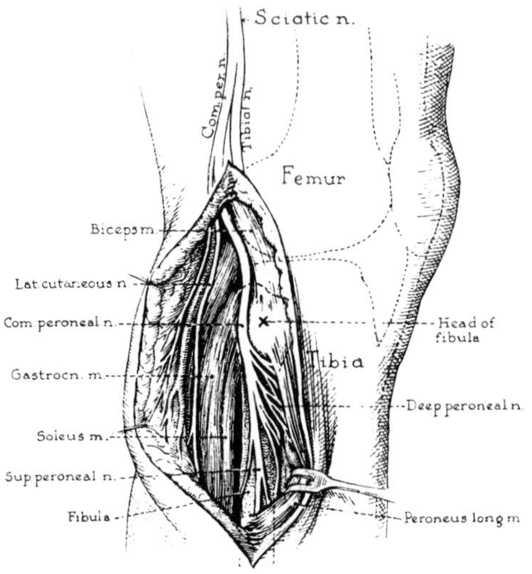

Fig. 8.5: Getting kicked on the posterolateral aspect of the knee can contuse the peroneal nerve as it winds around the neck of the fibula. This may lead to temporary or permanent paralysis of the foot.

paralysis. In mild contusions, an immediate "shocking feeling" of pain may radiate down the lateral aspect of the leg and foot. If the actual nerve is not damaged, tingling and numbness may persist for several minutes. In severe cases where the nerve may be crushed, initial pain is not immediately followed by tingling or numbness. Rather, as swelling increases within the nerve sheath, muscle weakness in dorsiflexion or eversion, and loss of sensation on the dorsum of the foot, particularly between the great and second toes, may progressively occur days or weeks later. Treatment involves standard acute care for contusions. If the condition does not rapidly improve, however, carefully monitor any sensory changes or motor weakness as previously indicated, and refer the individual to a physician at the first sign of any change.

Did you rule out a fracture of the head of the fibula and proximal tibia? Did you assess muscle weakness in dorsiflexion and eversion, and check cutaneous sensation on the dorsum of the foot? If the condition does not improve after standard acute care, refer the individual to a physician.

BURSITIS

A wrestler has an aching, warm, swollen knee. An outline of the patella is not visible. Is the swelling intra-articular or extra-articular? How are you going to handle this injury?

Bursitis may be caused by direct trauma, infections, metabolic abnormalities, rheumatic afflictions, and **neoplasms** (14). Compressive forces from a direct blow can be associated with a grossly distended, warm bursal sac filled with bloody effusion. Repeated insult can lead to the more common chronic bursitis. Here, the bursal wall thickens and when filled with fluid, appears distended.

Abrasions or penetrating injuries can lead to infected bursitis caused by bacteria entering the broken skin. This condition differs from acute bursitis because of the localized intense redness, increased pain, enlarged regional lymph nodes, spreading cellulitis, and subsequent fever and malaise (15). If infection is suspected, immediate referral to a physician is warranted for proper cleansing, irrigation, and closure (often with a drain). The infection can enter the lymph system causing **pyarthrosis** at the knee.

Prepatellar Bursitis

The prepatellar bursa lies between the skin and anterior surface of the patella. Because of its location, it is the most commonly injured bursa by compressive forces (**Figure 8-6**). Swelling may occur immediately or over a 24 hour period obscuring the visible outline of the patella. Occasionally the swelling may be

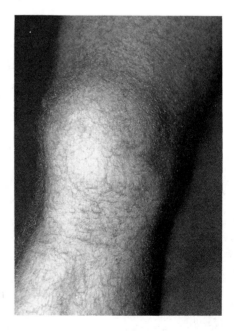

Fig. 8.6: The prepatellar bursa is commonly injured by compression from a direct blow or during a fall on a flexed knee.

mixed with blood, constituting a hemobursa. Direct pressure over the bursa and passive flexion of the knee leads to considerable pain. With chronic prepatellar bursitis, the condition may remain asymptomatic, except for mild discomfort when firm pressure is applied directly over the bursa.

Deep Infrapatellar Bursitis

The deep infrapatellar bursa lies posterior to the patellar tendon, and anterior and distal to the infrapatellar fat pad and tibia. It does not normally communicate with the knee joint. The cause of damage to this bursa is different than the prepatellar bursa, because the infrapatellar bursa is well protected from direct blows. Inflammation of this bursa is usually caused by overuse and subsequent friction between the patellar tendon and structures behind it (fat pad and tibia). Because this bursa lies posterior to the patellar tendon, inflammation of the bursa is often confused with Osgood-Schlatter's disease in adolescents, and patellar tendinitis in older individuals. Careful palpation and noting the specific area of tenderness determines which condition is present.

Pes Anserine Bursitis

The pes anserine bursa lies between the pes anserinus tendons (gracilis, sartorius, and semitendinous) and medial collateral ligament on the anteromedial aspect of the proximal tibia. Inflammation typically develops from friction but may occur from direct trauma. It is often seen in runners, cyclists, and swimmers who are subjected to excessive valgus stress at the knee. Initial symptoms include point tenderness beneath the pes tendons (usually 2 cm below the joint line), localized swelling, pain aggravated by flexion of the knee, and crepitation.

Baker's Cyst

The term Baker's cyst identifies almost any synovial herniation of the posterior joint capsule or bursitis on the posterior aspect of the knee. With no obstruction posteriorly, internal derangement injuries (i.e., meniscal problems, cruciate ligament tears, or arthritis) commonly lead to joint effusion expanding into the bursa sac. The semimembranosus bursa is most commonly involved, as it often communicates with the joint capsule. A soft tumorous mass can be palpated in the medial popliteal space and may or may not be painful. A Baker's cyst does not pose a serious problem, although it may be bothersome during full flexion or extension of the knee.

Treatment of Bursitis

Treatment consists of ice therapy, a compressive wrap, NSAIDs, avoiding activities that irritate the condition, or total rest until acute symptoms subside. A protective foam, or doughnut pad may protect the area from further insult. If the skin is broken during the initial injury, there is a risk of infection. As such, the physician may culture any aspirated fluid to detect bacteria with subsequent medication prescribed. Corticosteroid injections may be administered by the physician when other means of treatment have been ineffective in decreasing inflammation. Because these injections can weaken surrounding tendons or ligaments, they should not be injected close to these structures.

💡 *Did you determine the wrestler had an acute prepatellar bursitis injury with extra-articular swelling? After initial acute care, refer the individual to a physician for possible aspiration and culture work to rule out an infected bursa.*

LIGAMENTOUS INJURIES

❓ *A basketball player decelerated, set the left foot, then forcefully pushed off the left leg to perform a right-handed lay up shot. However, the player suddenly fell to the floor grasping the left knee. The individual reported a popping sensation and feeling of giving way in the knee. There is extreme pain on the anteromedial joint line. What structures might have been damaged? What is your course of action?*

Knee joint stability depends primarily on a static passive system of support from its ligaments and capsular structures, rather than from an active dynamic system from the surrounding muscles. Bones and menisci provide some additional stability via their shape and inherent stability when two adjoining structures are in a close packed position. The American Academy of Orthopaedic Surgeons (AAOS) classifies ligamentous injuries at the knee according to the functional disruption of a specific ligament, the amount of laxity, and direction of laxity. The amount and direction

> Deep infrapatellar bursitis is caused by overuse and subsequent friction between the patellar tendon and fat pad on the tibia

> Knee stability is dependent on static support from its ligaments and capsular structures

Table 8–3. Classification of Ligament Injury.

Degree	Straight laxity	Rotary laxity
First degree	Mild (less than 5 mm distraction)	Mild
Second degree	Moderate (5 to 10 mm distraction)	Moderate
Third degree	Severe (over 10 mm distraction)	Severe

Valgus laxity
An opening on the medial side of a joint caused by the distal segment moving laterally

Varus laxity
An opening on the lateral side of a joint caused by the distal segment moving medially

of laxity gives a clearer understanding of the true severity of injury (**Table 8-3**). The direction of laxity divides injuries into four straight laxities and four rotatory laxities (**Table 8-4**). Knowing the knee position at impact and the direction the tibia displaces or rotates denotes the damaged structures. **Table 8-5** lists the signs and symptom in the various stages of ligament failure.

Unidirectional Instabilities

In straight medial laxity, or **valgus laxity**, lateral forces cause tension on the medial aspect of the knee, potentially damaging the tibial (medial) collateral ligament, posterior oblique ligament, and posteromedial capsular ligaments (**Figure 8-7**). A first degree sprain of the tibial collateral ligament is characterized by mild pain on the medial joint line, little to no joint effusion, full range of motion although somewhat uncomfortable, and a stable joint when doing the valgus stress test. A positive valgus test in 30° of flexion (See **Figure 8-31A**) indicates at least a second degree injury to the middle third of the capsular ligament and tibial collateral ligament. The individual may be unable to fully extend the leg, and will often walk on the ball of the foot, unable to keep the heel flat on the ground.

Straight lateral laxity, or **varus laxity**, results from medial forces that produce tension on the lateral aspect of the knee damaging the fibular collateral ligament, lateral capsular ligaments, and joint structures (**Figure 8-8**). This isolated injury is rare because the biceps femoris, iliotibial tract, and popliteus provide a strong stabilizing effect. In wrestling, however, the opponent is often between the individual's legs and is able to deliver an excessive varus force that can lead to injury. Damage to the fibular collateral ligament follows general signs and symptoms associated with a tibial collateral sprain. Occasionally, the individual may hear or feel a "pop" accompanied with sharp lateral pain. Swelling will be minimal because the ligament is not attached to the joint capsule. Instability will be subtle because other structures are intact, but a positive varus test in 30° of flexion should confirm damage to the ligament (See **Figure 8-31B**). If tenderness is detected on the head of the fibula, a possible avulsion fracture may be involved.

With straight anterior laxity, or true anterior instability, there is a straight anterior displacement of the tibia on the femur. This cannot occur unless the anterior cruciate is damaged, as it provides nearly 87% of the

Table 8–4. Classification of Knee Instability and Structures Injured.

Classification of laxity	Primary ligament or joint structure injured
Straight medial (valgus)	Tibial collateral, posterior oblique, posteromedial capsule
Straight lateral (varus)	Fibular collateral, posterolateral capsule, popliteus
Straight anterior	Anterior cruciate ligament
Straight posterior	Posterior cruciate ligament
Anteromedial (anterior external rotation)	Tibial collateral, medial meniscus, anterior cruciate
Anterolateral (anterior internal rotation)	Anterior cruciate, iliotibial band, anterior and middle lateral capsule
Posteromedial (posterior internal rotation)	Tibial collateral, posterior cruciate, posterior oblique, posteromedial capsule
Posterolateral (posterior external rotation)	Posterior cruciate, fibular collateral, popliteus, posterolateral capsule

Table 8–5. Signs and Symptoms of Ligament Failure.

Minimal ligament failure (less than 5mm distraction)

Less than one third of the fibers are torn
Mild swelling is localized over the injury site
With the medial collateral ligament, pain is typically in the proximal 1 to 2 inches
Active and passive range of motion will be normal
Muscular strength will be normal or slightly decreased
No joint laxity is apparent during stress test
Definite end feel is present

Partial ligament failure (5 to 10 mm distraction)

One third to two thirds of the ligament has been damaged with microtears present
More localized swelling and joint effusion may be due to deep capsular tears, meniscal
  damage, or cruciate ligament damage
Pain is usually sharp and may be transient or lasting
Individual may complain of instability and an inability to walk with the heel on the ground
Range of motion is decreased initially by pain and hamstring muscle spasm; later by soft tissue
  swelling or effusion
Inability to fully extend the knee actively
Visible translation of the tibia during stress tests

Complete ligament failure (over 10 mm distraction)

Over two thirds of the ligament has been ruptured
Swelling is diffuse indicating severe capsular tear and damage to intracapsular structures
Pain is initially sharp and often disappears within a minute
Individual is aware of the feeling of instability or the knee giving way
Significant loss of range of motion
Visible distraction over 10 mm during stress testing that may appear as a subluxation

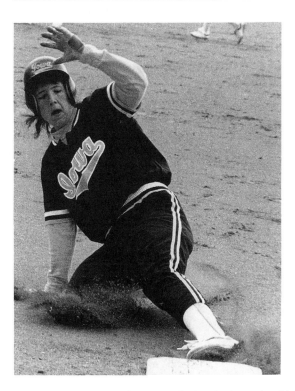

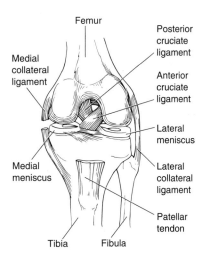

Fig. 8.7: When a valgus force is applied to the knee, the tibial collateral ligament and medial capsular ligaments, are damaged leading to valgus laxity.

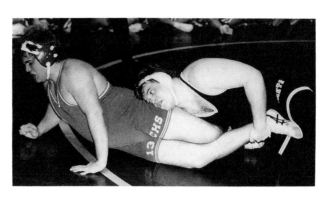

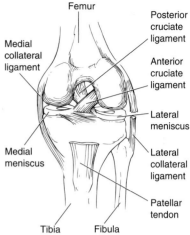

Femur
Posterior cruciate ligament
Medial collateral ligament
Anterior cruciate ligament
Lateral meniscus
Medial meniscus
Lateral collateral ligament
Patellar tendon
Tibia   Fibula

Fig. 8.8: In wrestling, the opponent is often between the athlete's legs and is able to deliver an isolated varus force damaging the fibular collateral ligament leading to varus laxity.

> Damage to the anterior cruciate ligament commonly occurs during a cutting maneuver, sudden deceleration, or landing in an off-balance position after a jump

resisting force to anterior movement (15). Isolated anterior laxity is rare. Instead, an anteromedial or anterolateral laxity usually occurs, and is determined with the Lachman test (See **Figure 8-32A**). Damage to the anterior cruciate ligament is typically seen in running/jumping sports, such as football, basketball, soccer, and gymnastics. It commonly occurs during a cutting or turning maneuver, landing in an off-balance position after a jump, or during sudden deceleration (**Figure 8-9**). It is also common in skiing if the tip of the ski catches in the snow and throws the skier forward. Pain can range from minimal and transient to severe and lasting, and may be described as being located deep in the knee, but is more often felt anterior on either side of the patellar tendon or laterally on the joint line. Joint effusion may not initially be present but appears one to two hours after injury even if acute care protocol is followed. Largely bloody joint effusion is clearly evident 24 hours post injury. With a significant ligament tear, a characteristic "pop" or "snap" is heard and the unstable knee immediately causes the individual to fall. Weight bearing

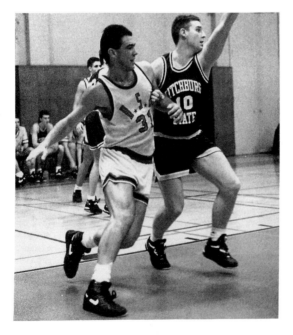

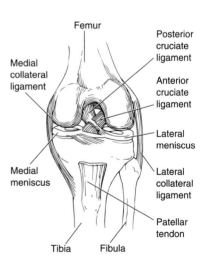

Femur
Posterior cruciate ligament
Medial collateral ligament
Anterior cruciate ligament
Lateral meniscus
Medial meniscus
Lateral collateral ligament
Patellar tendon
Tibia   Fibula

Fig. 8.9: When changing directions during deceleration, as in basketball, the anterior cruciate ligament can be damaged.

leads to a feeling of the knee giving way or "just not feeling right". The high incidence of damage to other internal structures necessitates immediate referral to a physician.

In straight posterior laxity, the tibia is displaced posteriorly in a neutral position without rotation. Again, the posterior cruciate provides nearly all resistance to prevent this motion. Hyperextension is the most common mechanism, although the ligament can also be damaged when the knee is flexed at 90° and the upper tibia is driven posteriorly, such as in an automobile accident when the person's knee is driven into the dashboard of a car, or when a hockey player collides with the boards (**Figure 8-10**). In milder cases, intense pain and a sense of stretching are felt in the posterior aspect of the knee. In a total rupture, a characteristic "pop" or "snap" is felt and heard. Effusion and hemarthrosis occur rapidly and the individual is acutely aware of swelling. Knee extension is limited because of the effusion, stretching of the posterior capsule, and gastrocnemius. A positive gravity drawer test (posterior sag sign) confirms damage to the posterior cruciate ligament (See **Figure 8-32B**).

Multidirectional Instabilities

Anteromedial instability results from anterior external rotation of the medial tibia condyle on the femur leading to damage of the medial ligaments (superficial tibial collateral, posterior and medial capsular ligaments), medial meniscus, and anterior cruciate (**Figure 8-11**). Although referred to as the "unhappy triad," the tibial collateral ligament is the primary lig-

amentous restraint to this motion. The anterior cruciate may be partially intact, and if so, anterior tibial displacement is minimal.

Anterolateral instability is characteristic of an anterior internal subluxation of the lateral tibial condyle on the femur. The anterior cruciate ligament is the primary structure damaged by this instability, but the iliotibial tract and lateral capsule can also be damaged. It is typically caused by a sudden deceleration and cutting maneuver, and is the most frequent rotatory instability at the knee (**Figure 8-12**).

In posterolateral instability, the lateral tibial plateau rotates posteriorly. This is often caused by a sudden anteromedial force that brings the knee joint from near full extension into full extension or hyperextension, resulting in rupture to the posterolateral structures. These structures include the arcuate ligament, popliteal tendon, posterolateral capsule, and fibular collateral ligament (**Figure 8-13A**).

In posteromedial rotatory instability, the medial tibial plateau shifts posteriorly on the femur and gives a medial opening. This is a severe injury and is indicative of damage to the superficial tibial collateral ligament, the medial capsule, and both cruciate ligaments (**Figure 8-13B**).

Management of Ligament Injuries

Injuries involving minimal ligament failure are managed conservatively with ice application, compression, elevation, and protected rest until acute symptoms subside. A compression wrap, consisting of an inverted horseshoe around the patella secured by an elastic wrap

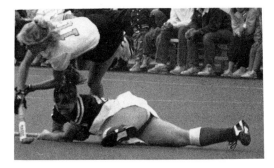

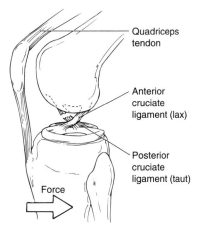

Quadriceps tendon

Anterior cruciate ligament (lax)

Posterior cruciate ligament (taut)

Force

Fig. 8.10: During hyperextension of the knee or when the knee is flexed and the tibia is driven posterior, the posterior cruciate ligament can be damaged.

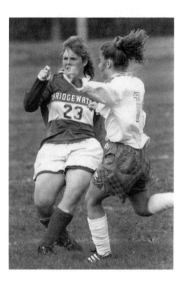

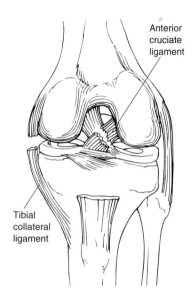

Fig. 8.11: When a valgus stress is applied to a fixed foot with the tibia externally rotated, the tibial collateral ligament, anterior cruciate ligament, and medial meniscus can be damaged leading to anteromedial instability, more commonly called an "unhappy triad."

can be used with a knee immobilizer to reduce swelling. Modalities and NSAIDs are used to reduce pain and inflammation.

In a moderate injury with partial ligament failure, ice, compression, elevation, and protected rest should be continued for 24 to 72 hours. Crutches are used until the individual walks without a limp. Progression to partial weight bearing with heel-to-toe gait can begin as tolerated. Rehabilitation should be initiated as soon as acute symptoms subside. Range of motion exercises should include assisted knee flexion and knee extension. Isometric exercises of the quadriceps and

straight leg raises in all directions should progress to resisted exercises throughout the full range of motion. Closed chain strengthening exercises and maintenance of range of motion can be supplemented by cardiovascular exercises as tolerated. In ligament injuries where isolated complete ligament failure has occurred, or when more than one major ligament is involved, referral to an orthopedist is warranted for possible surgical repair. **Field Strategy 8-2** lists management and rehabilitation of a mild anterior cruciate injury.

The basketball player reported a popping sensation and buckling of the knee after

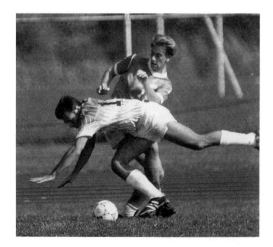

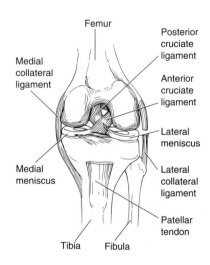

Fig. 8.12: Sudden deceleration and cutting actions lead to injury to the anterior cruciate ligament, lateral capsule, and iliotibial band leading to anterolateral instability.

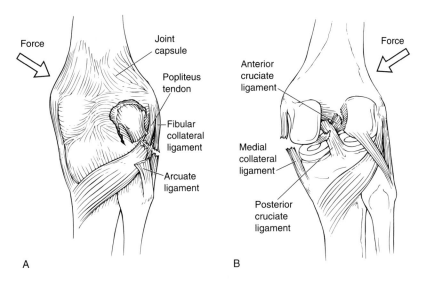

Fig. 8.13: (A) A sudden anteromedial force can bring a nearly extended knee joint into full extension or hyperextension causing posterolateral instability with damage to the arcuate ligament, popliteal tendon, posterolateral capsule, and fibular collateral ligament. (B) Posteromedial instability involves a sudden anterolateral force that damages the tibial collateral ligament, the joint capsule, and both cruciate ligaments.

deceleration. Did you suspect a possible anterior cruciate injury? If so, you are correct. Because anterior cruciate injuries seldom occur as an isolated injury, always assess the collateral ligaments and associated joint structures.

MENISCAL INJURIES

❓ *A softball catcher complains of mild swelling and posteromedial joint line tenderness. Although the pain has been persistent over the past several weeks, it now hurts to remain in a prolonged squatting position. What may be occurring? How will you manage this injury?*

Menisci become stiffer and less resilient with age, and are injured in similar manners as ligamentous structures. In addition to compression and tensile forces, shearing forces caused when the femur rotates on a fixed tibia trap the posterior horns of both menisci leading to some tearing. Tears are classified according to age, location, or axis of orientation, and include longitudinal, bucket-handle, horizontal, and parrot-beak (**Figure 8-14**) (14). Peak incidence of injuries has been found to occur in men between the ages of 21 and 40, and in girls and women between the ages of 11 and 20, and again between 61 and 70 (16). Medial meniscus damage is more common than lateral meniscus damage.

Longitudinal tears result from a twisting motion when the foot is fixed and knee flexed. This action produces compression and torsion on the posterior peripheral attachment. The tear can be partial, affecting only the peripheral segment of the meniscus, or complete, involving the substance of the meniscus itself. A "**bucket-handle**" tear occurs when an entire longitudinal segment is displaced medially toward the center of the tibia. This tear can lead to locking of the knee at about 10° flexion. However, a fixed locked position occurs in only 40% of complete meniscal tears (15).

Horizontal cleavage tears result from degeneration and often affect the posterior medial portion of the meniscus. With age, shearing forces from rotational motions tear the inner substance of the meniscus. If detached, momentary locking, associated pain, and instability may occur. A **parrot-beak** tear is seen in adolescents with a history of previous trauma or some cystic pathology that makes the meniscus more fixed at its periphery. Two tears commonly occur in the middle segment of the lateral meniscus leading to the characteristic shape of a parrot's beak.

Meniscal injuries are difficult to assess because of the limited sensory nerve supply. A chronic degenerative meniscal tear often results from multiple episodes of minimal trauma leading to almost no pain, disability, or swelling. Chronic tears in the absence of degeneration have point tenderness only over

Menisci become stiffer and less resilient with age

Bucket-handle tear
Longitudinal meniscal tear of the central segment that can displace into the joint leading to locking of the knee

Parrot-beak tear
Horizontal meniscal tear typically in the middle segment of the lateral meniscus

Chronic degenerative meniscal tears may have no pain, disability, or swelling

Field Strategy 8–2. Management of an Anterior Cruciate Injury.

Phase 1

PRICE

Ice, elevation, compression wrap and rest with a knee immobilizer to reduce swelling. Use crutches if the individual cannot bear weight without pain

Range of motion exercises within pain free limits.

Heel slides

Prone knee flexion assisted with the opposite leg

Passive knee extension in a supine or seated position

Strengthening exercises

Bent leg raises in all directions

Multiangle isometric exercises for the quadriceps, hamstrings, and hip adductors

Phase 2

Range of Motion.

Continue exercises to regain full range of motion

Unilateral balance activities.

See Field Strategy 7–1, and progress as tolerated

Strengthening exercises.

Do slow, controlled, eccentric closed chain exercises, such as two legged squats to 60°, step ups, step downs, and lateral step ups.

Calf raises (seated position) can progress to standing position when pain free

Straight leg raises in all directions with tubing added as tolerated

Cardiovascular fitness exercises may include the UBE and unilateral leg cycling

Phase 3

Range of Motion.

Maintain full range of motion and flexibility in the lower extremity

Strengthening

Hip leg press and squats

Toe raises with weights

Lunges

Isokinetic open and closed chain exercises

Cardiovascular fitness

Bilateral minimal tension cycling if 100 to 115° of knee flexion is present. Avoid full knee extension

Pool running, swimming with a flutter kick, jogging in place on a trampoline, and power walking

Phase 4

Balance and proprioception.

Continue exercises given above

Functional activities

Running drills, e.g., circles, figure-8s, cross over steps (kariocas), jumping with double limb/single limb progressing from standing in place, front to back, to diagonals

Multidirectional high speed balance drills are added after the individual can run 2 to 3 miles

Jumping, bounding, and skipping (plyometrics)

Slide board

the site of the lesion. Because the meniscal periphery is attached to the synovial lining, tensile forces may cause synovial inflammation and slight joint effusion. Pain will occur on rotation and extreme flexion of the knee. The individual may experience a popping, grinding, or clicking sensation that can lead to the knee buckling or giving way causing the

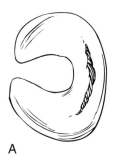 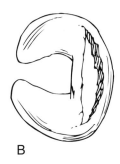 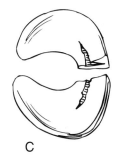 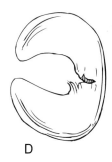

Fig. 8.14: Mensical tears. (A) Longitudinal. (B) Bucket-handle. (C) Horizontal. (D) Parrot-beak.

individual to stumble or fall. Traumatic meniscal tears usually occur in conjunction with other knee injuries and produce severe pain, disability, and swelling.

Special tests used to identify possible meniscal injuries include McMurray's test, the cross-over test, and Apley's compression test (See the Assessment section later in this chapter.). In addition, the inability of the individual to perform a deep squat or do a duck walk may also indicate meniscal injury.

Initial treatment depends on the extent of damage. Mild cases of pain and swelling can be managed with standard acute care—ice, compression, elevation, protected rest, and crutches as needed. Isometric strengthening exercises can be initiated when swelling has subsided. If joint effusion is extensive, aspiration of the fluid by a physician may be necessary. **Field Strategy 8-3** summarizes the initial management and suggested rehabilitation exercises for a meniscal injury.

If the knee is locked and cannot be spontaneously reduced, surgical intervention is needed. Recent studies of the function, biomechanics, and blood supply to the menisci have shown a partial meniscectomy preferable to total, and that certain peripheral meniscal tears can be surgically repaired through arthroscopy, avoiding excision (15,16). Total meniscectomy increases rotary instability and can lead to arthritis. Bucket-handle tear segments can also be surgically excised without removing the total meniscus, although regeneration of the centrally displaced portion will not occur.

In the softball catcher, did you suspect a possible chronic meniscal tear aggravated when the knee is fully flexed? If so, you are correct. This individual should be referred to a physician.

PATELLAR AND RELATED INJURIES

A female rower is complaining of a deep, aching pain in the knee during activity. Slight joint effusion is present. Palpable pain is elicited over the lateral patellar border. Intense pain is felt when the patella is pushed downward into the patellofemoral groove. What factors may contribute to this condition? What long-term management should be considered after acute symptoms have subsided?

The patellofemoral joint is the region most commonly associated with anterior knee pain. Patellar tracking disorders and instability within the joint, along with obesity, direct trauma, and repetitive motions all contribute to a variety of injuries. The quadriceps mechanism, more accurately called the **extensor mechanism**, is composed of dynamic and static stabilizers that combine rolling and gliding motions to place the femur and patella in specific positions to effect deceleration of the patellofemoral articulation in providing stability and function at the knee **(Figure 8-15)** (17). The medial patellar retinacula is an extension of the vastus medialis oblique, or VMO, and is the dynamic medial stabilizer that resists lateral displacement of the patella. Atrophy of this muscle is nearly always evident in patellofemoral dysfunction. Both medial and lateral retinacula assist in knee extension even though the patellar tendon may be ruptured.

Deficiencies in stabilization of the extensor mechanism can be due to several abnormalities of the patellofemoral region and may include (15,18):

1. Patellar instability due to an abnormally shaped medial patellar facet, shallow trochlear groove, variable length and width of the patellar tendon, and patella alta (high riding patella)

Partial meniscectomies are preferable to total meniscectomies

Extensor mechanism
Complex interaction of muscles, ligaments, and tendons that stabilize and provide motion at the patellofemoral joint

The VMO is the dynamic medial stabilizer that resists lateral displacement of the patella

Field Strategy 8–3. Management of a Partial Menisectomy

Phase 1

PRICE
  Ice, elevation, compression, and bracing to reduce swelling. Use crutches if needed.
Range of motion exercises within pain free limits
  Heel slides
  Supine wall slides
  Prone knee flexion assisted with the opposite leg
  Passive knee extension in a supine or seated position

Phase 2

Range of Motion
  Continue exercises as tolerated
Unilateral balance activities
  See Field Strategy 7–1
Strengthening exercises including:
  Multiangle isometric exercises for the quadriceps, hamstrings, and hip adductors
  Straight leg raises in all directions. Add tubing or ankle weights in later stages
  Short arc quadriceps extension exercises. Place a pillow or bolster under the knee to support
  the knee at 45° flexion. Extend the knee and hold for 10 seconds. Add ankle weights to
  increase resistance
  Toe raises from a seated position can progress to standing position when pain free
  Straight leg raises in all directions with tubing added as tolerated
Cardiovascular fitness. UBE, and stationary cycling with bilateral minimal tension if 115 to 120° of
knee flexion is present. Avoid full knee extension.

Phase 3

Range of Motion. Maintain full range of motion and flexibility in the lower extremity
Strengthening
  Hip leg press and squats
  Toe raises with weights
  Lunges
  Isokinetic open and closed chain exercises
Cardiovascular fitness
  Pool running, swimming with a flutter kick, jogging in place on a trampoline, and power
  walking

Phase 4, Return to Activity

Maintain range of motion, flexibility, strength, and balance
Functional activities. Same as those listed in Field Strategy 8–2

2. Weakness in the supporting muscles and guiding mechanisms, such as a weak VMO
3. Hypermobility of the patella as a result of muscle atrophy after an injury and tightness of the lateral retinaculum, iliotibial tract, and hamstrings
4. Malalignment of the extremity from structural abnormalities, such as excessive femoral or tibial rotation, genu valgum, congenital genu recurvatum (hyperexten-

sion at the knees), increased Q-angle, and excessive foot pronation
5. Plica syndromes and repetitive minor trauma

Each condition can be counterbalanced in a healthy knee by the triangular shape of the patella, depth of the patellofemoral groove, and limiting action of the static ligamentous structures. Failure of medial structures to restrain the patella in a balanced position, and/or the presence of bony anomalies can

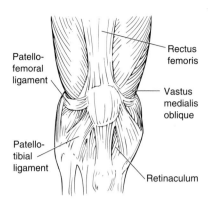

Fig. 8.15: The extensor mechanism is composed of dynamic and static stabilizers. Working together, they combine rolling and gliding motions to place the femur and patella in specific positions to effect the deceleration mechanism of the patellofemoral articulation to provide stability and function at the knee. Oblique condensations of the retinacula produce the patellofemoral ligament and medial and lateral patellotibial ligaments.

result in lateral tilting or lateral excursion of the patella which leads to patellofemoral **arthralgia**, or severe joint pain. This pain may be due to patellofemoral stress syndrome, chondromalacia patellae, or patellar subluxation or dislocation. Other patellar injuries include patella plica syndrome, patellar tendinitis, Osgood-Schlatter disease, and extensor tendon ruptures.

Patellofemoral Stress Syndrome

Patellofemoral stress syndrome, also called lateral patellar compression syndrome, occurs when either the VMO is weak or the lateral retinaculum that holds the patella firmly to the femoral condyle is excessively tight. In either case, the end result is lateral excursion of the patella. An excessive Q-angle, more common in women, internal femoral rotation (anteversion), and external tibial torsion can also increase lateral excursion. Hence, patella mobility is decreased and cannot be displaced medially even when muscles are relaxed (19).

Pain may result when a tense lateral retinaculum passes over the trochlear groove, or from increased patellofemoral stresses that are transferred from the articular cartilage to pain fibers in the subchondral bone (20). The individual may report a dull, aching pain in the center of the knee. Point tenderness can be located over the lateral facet of the patella with intense pain and crepitus elicited when

the patella is manually compressed into the patellofemoral groove. Synovial inflammation may also be present.

Treatment involves standard acute care and NSAIDs. The McConnell taping technique utilizes passive taping of the patella to correct patellar position and tracking during knee motion. Other patellofemoral support devices, such as those demonstrated in Chapter 6 are also used to prevent lateral displacement of the patella. Examples of open kinetic chain exercises to correct the problem include isometric hip adduction at 0° extension, or isometric quadriceps contractions in the 60 to 90° arc of motion, or concentric isokinetic exercise at 120°/sec in the 60 to 85° arc of motion (21). Resisted terminal knee extension exercises, straight leg raises in hip flexion and adduction, and quadriceps isometric, isotonic, and high speed isokinetic exercises in a 60 to 90° arc may also be performed. Examples of closed kinetic chain exercises include knee flexion in 30 to 70°, and lateral steps up from 1 to 8" to allow eccentric and concentric movements (21,22). Weight training programs that load the patellofemoral joint, such as bent-knee exercises should be avoided.

Chondromalacia Patellae

Chondromalacia patellae is a true degeneration in the articular cartilage of the patella, which results when compressive forces exceed the normal physical range, or when alterations in patellar excursion produce abnormal shear forces that damage the articular surface. The medial and lateral patellar facets are most commonly involved. The condition is confirmed when pain results from the Clarke's test (See **Figure 8-35B**) and Waldron's test. Chondromalacia has four stages **(Figure 8-16)**:

Stage 1. Articular cartilage shows only softening or blistering
Stage 2. Fissures appear in the cartilage
Stage 3. Fibrillation of the cartilage occurs, causing a "crab-meat" appearance
Stage 4. Full cartilage defects are present and subchondral bone is exposed

Asymtomatic chondromalacia does not require treatment. If the condition becomes symptomatic, follow standard acute care protocol. Most individuals respond well to mild anti-inflammatory medication, quadriceps strengthening, and a hamstring flexibility program. All resisted exercises with knee extension from a fully flexed position,

Arthralgia
Severe joint pain

Patellofemoral stress syndrome
Condition whereby the lateral retinaculum is tight, or the vastus medialis oblique is weak leading to lateral excursion and pressure on the lateral facet of the patella causing a painful condition

Weight training programs that load the patellofemoral joint and bent-knee exercises should be avoided

Chondromalacia patellae
Degenerative condition in the articular cartilage of the patella caused by abnormal compression or shearing forces

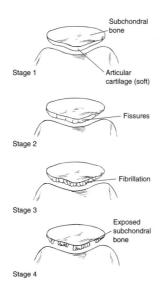

Fig. 8.16: Four stages of chondromalacia patellae. Stage 1 involves softening or blistering of the cartilage. Stage 2 reveals fissures in the cartilage. Stage 3 is reached when fibrillation of the cartilage occurs causing a "crab-meat" appearance. Stage 4 reveals cartilage defects with subchondral bone exposed.

crouches, or deep knee-bends should be avoided, because these positions may aggravate the condition. A knee sleeve with a patellar cutout, as shown in Chapter 6 may be helpful. If this does not reduce the symptoms, surgical intervention may be necessary, such as arthroscopic patellar debridement, lateral retinacular release, extensor mechanism realignment, or elevation of the tibial tubercle to relieve patellar compression forces.

Acute Patellar Subluxation and Dislocation

Subluxation of the patella may result from hypertrophy of the vastus lateralis, presence of patella alta, atrophy of the VMO, increased Q-angle, tight lateral retinaculum, or lateral passive mobility (20,23). Although ligament laxity and internal derangement may have been ruled out in an acute injury, the individual stills complains of pain and a feeling that the leg is giving way. Joint effusion may develop but improves rapidly with the individual resuming activity. Chronic subluxations produce less swelling, pain, and disability.

The condition is verified by observing patellar position during active knee flexion and extension, and with a positive patellar apprehension test (See Assessment section later in this chapter.). An individual with patellofemoral stress syndrome will not be apprehensive about this test, whereas one with patellar pain due to subluxating patella will resist any attempt to displace the patella laterally.

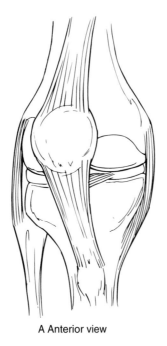

A Anterior view

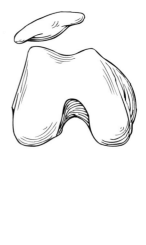

B Skyline view

Fig. 8.17: A dislocated patella often displaces laterally, and is accompanied by an audible pop and violent collapse of the knee following deceleration involving a cutting maneuver.

Dislocation of the patella is an acute, severe injury that commonly occurs during deceleration with a cutting maneuver (**Figure 8-17**). Nearly all medial muscular and retinaculum attachments are torn from the medial aspect of the patella leading to an audible pop and violent collapse of the knee. Many dislocations will spontaneously reduce themselves, leaving a painful, swollen tender knee. Palpate the area to assess any defects in the medial retinaculum and vastus medialis attachment before they are obscured by swelling. Occasionally a fracture of the patella or lateral femoral condyle also occurs, resulting in a loose bony fragment in the joint.

Immediate treatment includes ice, elevation, immobilization, and immediate referral to a physician. After the physician reduces the dislocation, the knee is immobilized for four to six weeks. While immobilized, isometric quadriceps exercises and straight leg raises can be performed. When immobilization is removed, a full rehabilitative program to strengthen the dynamic stabilizers of the patellofemoral joint, particularly the VMO, and a flexibility program for the hamstrings and iliotibial tract should be initiated. A knee sleeve with lateral pad to restrict lateral excursion and activity modification may be helpful. Nearly 80 to 90% of individuals with patellofemoral tracking disorders and instability can improve and return to activity without surgical intervention (20).

Patella Plica Syndrome

The **patella plica** shelf is a fold in the synovial lining of the knee. It is typically crescent shaped and extends from the infrapatellar fat pad medially, loops around the femoral condyle, crosses under the quadriceps tendon in the suprapatellar region, then passes laterally over the lateral femoral condyle to the lateral retinaculum (**Figure 8-18**) (15,16). This tissue can become inflamed and thickened from overuse or trauma as it extends over the medial femoral condyle.

Often pain comes on gradually and is aggravated by quadriceps exercises. In about 25% of the cases, there is a positive "moviegoer's sign", or pain with prolonged sitting. As the individual stands and begins to walk, a sharp pain is felt for 8 to 10 steps, then disappears (15). The pain is due to the plica being maximally stretched and impinged within the

Patella plica
A fold in the synovial lining that may cause medial knee pain without associated trauma

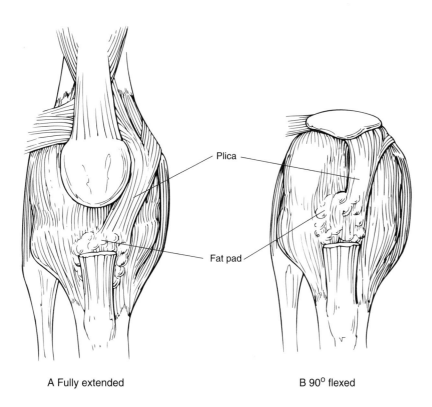

A Fully extended   B 90° flexed

Fig. 8.18: Patella plica is a fold in the synovial lining of the knee joint that can become inflamed and thickened due to trauma as it extends over the femoral condyle, or from microtrauma from overuse.

Plica can lead to a pop or snap as the individual flexes and extends the knee, or pseudolocking may occur, mimicking a torn meniscus

patellofemoral joint. As the articularis genus muscle contracts several times, it elevates the plica enough to prevent further impingement. Occasionally adhesions present in the plica lead to a pop or snap as the individual flexes and extends the knee, or pseudolocking may occur, mimicking a torn meniscus.

Assessment reveals slight joint effusion, palpable pain, and crepitus in the medial and lateral retinacular regions, particularly along the edge of the medial femoral condyle with the knee flexed at 45°. Treatment is symptomatic with ice therapy, NSAIDs, and activity modification. Strengthening exercises for the quadriceps is important, as well as hamstrings stretching. Tight hamstrings can produce higher patellofemoral forces at the knee predisposing an individual to this injury. If the condition warrants, the plica shelf can be removed arthroscopically.

Patellar Tendinitis (Jumper's Knee)

The patellar tendon frequently becomes inflamed and tender from repetitive or eccentric knee extension activities, such as in running and jumping, hence the name "Jumper's Knee." Patellar subluxation or patellofemoral stress syndrome can also overload the patellar tendon. It should be differentiated from tendinitis. Initially, pain after activity is concentrated on the inferior pole of the patella, but also occurs at the insertion of the patellar tendon into the tibial tuberosity **(Figure 8-19)**. As the condition progresses, pain is present at the beginning of activity, then subsides during warm-up, then reappears after activity. In-

creased pain is often reported while ascending and descending stairs or after prolonged sitting. Pain can be elicited during passive knee flexion beyond 120° and during resisted knee extension (24). The fat pad lying beneath the tendon can also become inflamed contributing to the symptoms. Eventually pain is present during and after activity, and can become too severe for the individual to participate. Chronic tendinitis may occasionally lead to cystic changes at the distal pole of the patella, or ectopic calcification and nodule formation in the tendon (25).

Immediate treatment involves ice, compression, elevation, rest, restricted activity, and NSAIDs. Other common modalities in early stages of patellar tendinitis include heat therapy, electrical stimulation, phonophoresis, iontophoresis, and ultrasound (24). Painful activities should be eliminated. Eccentric quadriceps strengthening and a stretching program for the quadriceps, hamstrings, plantar flexors, hip flexors and extensors will assist in absorbing strain. Aquatic therapy is very useful in early stages to reduce gravitational forces. As the patient progresses, changing to a more resilient spring loaded floor may also help. **Field Strategy 8-4** summarizes the management and suggested exercises for patellar tendinitis.

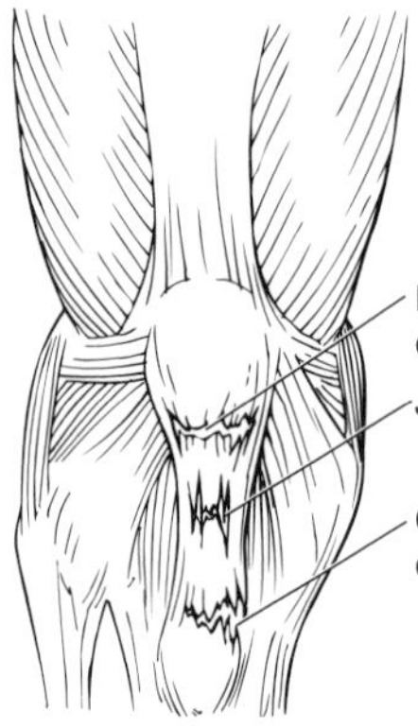

Osgood-Schlatter Disease

Osgood-Schlatter disease is a traction-type injury to the tibial apophysis where the patellar tendon attaches onto the tibial tuberosity. Pain and swelling are evident with activity, but relieved with rest. It is more common in boys between ages 10 and 15. Although it commonly affects only one limb, it can be seen bilaterally in about 25 to 33% of patients (15). In cases of long duration, the tibial tuberosity appears enlarged and prominent. Occasionally cartilage fragments and bony ossicles form in the patellar tendon. Point tenderness can be elicited directly over the tuberosity but range of motion is usually not affected. Pain is present at the extremes of knee extension and forced flexion. Treatment is symptomatic. In most cases, activity is unrestricted unless pain is disabling. The condition rectifies itself with closure of the apophysis.

A similar condition is **Larsen-Johansson disease**, but this occurs at the inferior pole of the patella. Pain, swelling, and tenderness

Osgood-Schlatter disease
Inflammation or partial avulsion of the tibial apophysis due to traction forces

Osgood-Schlatter disease is commoner in boys aged 10 to 15

Larsen-Johansson disease
Inflammation or partial avulsion of the apex of the patella due to traction forces

Fig. 8.19: Patellar conditions may involve Larsen-Johansson disease, patellar tendinitis, or Osgood-Schlatter disease. The location of pain will typically define which problem is present.

Signs and symptoms

Initial pain after activity is concentrated on the inferior pole of the patella or the distal attachment
of the patellar tendon on the tibial tuberosity
As the condition progresses, pain is present at the start of activity, subsides with warm-up, then
reappears after activity
Pain is then present while ascending and descending stairs
Pain occurs on passive knee flexion beyond 120° and during resisted knee extension

Management

After standard acute care to control inflammation and pain, avoid activities that lead to increased
pain
Transverse friction massage for 6 to 8 minutes may help facilitate healing during the acute phase
Initiate early flexibility exercises for the gastrocnemius-soleus complex, quadriceps, and hamstrings
Progressive resistance strengthening exercises may include:
Straight leg raises in all directions
Short-arc knee extension exercises.
One-quarter knee squats.
Eccentric strengthening exercises for the quadriceps and dorsiflexors, such as drop squats
(i.e., landing from a jump). Focus on the deceleration between the upward and downward
phase. Increase deceleration as tolerated by the patient
Heat and ice may be used prior to and after exercise, respectively. Other modalities that may be
effective are electrical stimulation, phonophoresis, iontophoresis, ultrasound, and NSAIDs
Cardiovascular fitness should be maintained with exercises that do not involve powerful knee
extension (i.e., UBE, swimming, stationary bike with minimal tension)
In the later stage, plyometrics may be incorporated (i.e., single leg hop, double leg hop, single leg
vertical jump, and bounding)
A patellofemoral knee sleeve may be applied to reduce mobility of the patellar tendon during activity

result from excessive strain on the patellar tendon. Treatment is similar to that of Osgood-Slatter disease.

Extensor Tendon Rupture

Extensor tendon ruptures can occur at the superior pole of the patella, inferior pole of the patella, tibial tuberosity, or within the patellar tendon itself. Ruptures result from powerful muscle contractions, or in conjunction with severe ligamentous disruption at the knee. The rupture may be partial or total. A partial rupture will produce pain and muscle weakness in knee extension. If a total rupture occurs distal to the patella, assessment will reveal a high riding patella, a palpable defect over the tendon, and an inability to do knee extension. If the quadriceps tendon is ruptured from the superior pole of the patella and the extensor retinaculum is still intact, knee extension is still possible, although it will be weak and painful. Individuals with a history of prior corticosteriod injections, ana-bolic steroid abuse, or use of systemic steroids are at a greater risk for tendon ruptures. Steroid use can cause softening or weakening of collagen fibers in the muscle tendon, predisposing the tendon to premature rupture. Treatment depends on the location and displacement of any bony fragment. In partial ruptures involving a shredded tendon, wiring may be necessary through the patella to relieve tension on the healing tendon. In total ruptures, surgical repair is necessary.

The repetitive motions performed by the female rower, coupled with an increased Q-angle, can lead to stress on the patellofemoral region. The VMO should be strengthened with eccentric and concentric closed chain exercises.

ILIOTIBIAL BAND FRICTION SYNDROME

A female volleyball player is complaining of a mild aching sensation on the lateral side of the knee that increases in intensity throughout practice. Initially it hurt only at the start of practice, but efforts to play through the pain have now led to persistent pain during walking and climbing stairs. How will you handle this situation?

A condition common in runners, cyclists, weight lifters, and volleyball players is iliotibial band friction syndrome. The iliotibial band continues the line of pull from the tensor fascia latae and gluteus maximus muscle. The deep fibers are associated with the lateral intermuscular septum. The distal fibers become thicker at their attachment on Gerdy's tubercle adjacent to the tibial tubercle on the lateral proximal tibia. The band drops posteriorly behind the lateral femoral epicondyle with knee flexion, then snaps forward over the epicondyle during extension (**Figure 8-20**). Weight bearing increases compression and friction forces over the greater trochanter and lateral femoral condyle (26). Individuals with a malalignment problem, such as genu valgum, large Q-angle, excessive foot pronation, or a leg-length discrepancy are predisposed to this injury. Runners who constantly run on the same side of the street may also be prone to this condition. Most streets are crowned for water run off, therefore one leg always runs lower than the other and places considerable strain on lateral joint structures.

Initially, pain is present only while running. As the condition progresses, pain is evident in running uphill and downhill, climbing stairs, and during walking. It is particularly intense on weight bearing from foot strike through midstance. It is during this part of the gait cycle that the iliotibial band is most compressed between the lateral femoral epicondyle and greater trochanter of the femur. Point tenderness is localized over the lateral femoral condyle about 2 to 3 cm above the lateral joint line, and occasionally radiates distally to the tibial attachment or proximally up the thigh (15,26). Positive Ober's and Noble's Compression tests confirm the condition. (See **Figure 8-37.**) **Field Strategy 8-5** lists signs and symptoms, and management of iliotibial band friction syndrome (16).

Because the volleyball player is female, the increased Q angle, coupled with the extensive knee flexion and extension required in the sport can additionally strain the iliotibial band. After controlling inflammation, an extensive flexibility program for the iliotibial band should be initiated.

FRACTURES AND ASSOCIATED INJURIES

A basketball player has had a progressively persistent pain on the proximal tibia since the start of the basketball season, and now reports that it hurts just to walk. Mild swelling is present on the anteromedial aspect of the proximal tibia just below the joint line, but no other obvious signs are present. What might be happening to this player?

Traumatic fractures about the knee area are rare in sports competition unless you include high velocity sports, such as motorcycling and auto racing. These fractures are usually associated with multiple trauma. However, other more common fractures, and associated bony conditions can occur in sport participation.

Avulsion Fractures

Avulsion fractures are caused by compressive forces from direct trauma, excessive tensile forces from an explosive muscular contraction, repetitive overuse, or a tensile force that pulls a ligament from its bony attachment. For example, getting kicked on the lateral aspect of the knee may avulse a portion of the lateral epicondyle, or the tibial tuberosity may be avulsed when the extensor mechanism

Predisposing factors include:
  Malalignment conditions
  Large Q-angle
  Excessive foot pronation
  Leg-length discrepancy

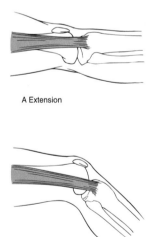

A Extension

B Flexion

Fig. 8.20: The iliotibial band drops posteriorly behind the lateral femoral epicondyle during knee flexion, then snaps forward over the epicondyle during extension. Malalignment problems or constant irritation can inflame the iliotibial band or lead to bursitis.

Field Strategy 8–5. Management of Iliotibial Band Friction Syndrome.

Predisposing factors

Genu varum
Excessive pronation in feet
Leg length discrepancy
Prominent greater trochanter of femur
Training errors, e.g., excessive distance in a single run, increasing mileage too quickly,
  inadequate warm-up, running on the same side of a high-crowned road

Signs and Symptoms

Initially pain comes on after running but does not restrict distance or speed
As condition worsens, pain is present during running and may restrict distance and speed
Pain is especially noticeable during weight-bearing flexion and extension actions at the knee,
  such as in walking down stairs
Eventually pain restricts all running and becomes continuous during activities of daily living
Extreme point tenderness is palpated 2 to 4 cm proximal to the lateral joint line over the lateral
  femoral epicondyle with the leg flexed at 30°
Flexion and extension of the knee may produce a creaking sound
Positive Ober's and Noble's compression tests

Management

Ice, compression, elevation, NSAIDs, and rest until acute symptoms subside
Stretching exercises should include the hip abductors, flexors, and lateral thigh muscles
Foot orthotics may correct some structural problems
Non-weight bearing strengthening exercises, such as leg lifts, and isometric exercises for knee
  flexion, extension, hip abduction, and adduction can be initiated when pain free, followed by
  concentric and eccentric strengthening of the hip and thigh muscles
Hill running should be avoided until asymptomatic
Running or training should be modified to the point of little or minimal pain with a graduated
  schedule of activity planned. Cardiovascular fitness can be maintained with swimming
Ice massage before and after running may be helpful
Steroid injections may be used in resistant cases
Full return to participation should be gauged on painless completion of all functional tests.

pulls a fragment away. The individual has localized pain and tenderness over the bony site. In some instances, a fragment may be palpated. If a musculotendinous unit is involved, muscle function will be limited. When the anterior cruciate is involved, the bony fragment may lodge in the joint causing the knee to "lock".

Epiphyseal and Apophyseal Fractures

Adolescents in contact sports are particularly susceptible to epiphyseal fractures in the knee region. Nearly 65% of the lower extremity longitudinal growth occurs at the knee: 40% at the distal femoral epiphysis and 25% at the proximal tibial epiphysis (14). A shearing force across the cartilaginous growth plate may lead to a disruption of growth and a shortened limb.

The tibial tuberosity is a common site for apophyseal fractures in boys, and may occur as a result of Osgood-Schlatter's disease. These fractures usually result from forced flexion of the knee against a straining quadriceps contraction, or a violent quadriceps contraction against a fixed foot (27-29). These injuries are commonly seen in jumping activities like basketball, long jump, high jump, or hurdling. The individual will have pain, swelling, and tenderness directly over the tuberosity. When a small fragment of the tuberosity avulses, knee extension will be painful and weak. With larger fractures involving extensive retinacular damage, knee extension will be impossible. Displaced frag-

Nearly 65% of the longitudinal growth of the lower extremity occurs at the knee

ments will need open reduction and internal fixation.

Fractures to the proximal tibial epiphysis and distal femoral epiphysis are more serious because of possible arterial damage to the growth plate of each bone. These fractures often occur when a varus or valgus stress is applied on a fixed weight-bearing foot. Undisplaced fractures are usually treated with closed reduction and casting, and will have fairly good resolution, although it may take weeks for resolution to occur (27). More serious fractures will require internal fixation and may result in angular or leg-length discrepancy.

Stress Fractures

The femoral supracondylar region, medial tibial plateau, and tibia tuberosity are common regions for stress fractures. These fractures result from repetitive overload of the bone due to unusual changes in training intensity, duration, frequency, running surface, or unevenly worn shoes (30). The individual will complain of localized pain before and after activity that is relieved with rest and nonweight bearing. In a stress fracture of the medial tibial plateau, pain runs along the anteromedial aspect of the proximal tibia just below the joint line. Localized tenderness and edema will be present but initial radiographs

of the stress fracture may be negative. As the condition progresses, pain becomes more persistent. Follow-up radiographs 3 weeks post injury may then show periosteal new bone development. Early bone scans are highly recommended. Treatment may involve rest, crutches, or casting.

Chondral and Osteochondral Fractures

A **chondral fracture** is a fracture involving the articular cartilage at a joint. An **osteochondral fracture** involves the articular cartilage and underlying bone **(Figure 8-21)**. These fractures result from compression from a direct blow to the knee causing shearing or forceful rotation. A considerable amount of articular surface on the involved bone can be damaged.

The individual will usually feel a painful "snap" and report considerable pain and swelling within the first few hours after injury. Displaced fractures can cause locking of the joint and produce crepitation during range of motion. Aspiration of the joint often yields bloody fluid containing fat. MRIs may be indicated because some fractures may not appear on standard radiographs. Small fragments can be removed during arthroscopic surgery. Internal fixation is necessary with larger fragments. Following surgery, range of motion exercises are performed to improve

With a stress fracture of the medial tibial plateau, pain occurs on the anteromedial aspect of the proximal tibia just below the joint line

Chondral fracture
Fracture involving the articular cartilage at a joint

Osteochondral fracture
Fracture involved the articular cartilage and underlying bone

The individual will feel a painful "snap" and have considerable pain and swelling within the first few hours of the injury

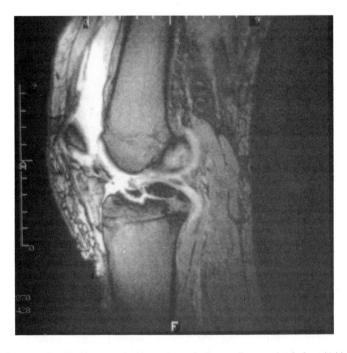

Fig. 8.21: This traumatic osteochondral fracture involves the articular cartilage and subchondral bone on the medial epicondyle of the tibia.

articular cartilage nutrition, limit joint adhesions, and prevent muscular atrophy.

Osteochondritis Dissecans

Osteochondritis dissecans occurs when a fragment of bone adjacent to the articular surface of a joint is deprived of its blood supply leading to avascular necrosis. Although found in several joints, it is typically associated with the knee, particularly in males ages 10 to 20 (**Figure 8-22**). The avascular bone fragment may displace and form a loose body within the knee joint leaving a defect in the articular cartilage (31). Causes include direct and indirect trauma, skeletal abnormalities associated with endocrine dysfunction, a prominent tibial spine that impacts the medial femoral condyle, and generalized ligamentous laxity (15). Common sites include the lateral portion of the medial femoral condyle, lateral femoral condyle, femoral groove, and patella (31).

The most common symptom is an aching, diffuse pain and/or swelling with activity. If the site of the lesion is on the lateral aspect of the medial femoral condyle, pain can be elicited when the knee is acutely flexed, and during resisted knee extension with the tibia internally rotated (15). If the bony fragment has displaced and is free floating within the joint, the knee may momentarily lock. A positive diagnosis is made from a radiograph.

Treatment depends on the age of the individual, size and location of the lesion, as well as the radiographic appearance of the fragment and articular cartilage. If the fragment has not separated, a soft knee immobilizer with restricted activity for four to six weeks may be indicated. If the fragment is separated, or is a chronic lesion, internal fixation or removal of the fragment is indicated. Older individuals do not heal as well because degenerative joint changes may have already developed within the joint. Rehabilitation should include regaining range of motion, quadriceps strength, muscle power, balance, and cardiovascular fitness.

Displaced and Undisplaced Femoral Fractures

Distal femoral fractures result from axial loading or rotational forces with added valgus or varus stress, and tend to angulate and displace posteriorly. The adductor muscles contract to rotate and shorten the femoral shaft giving a characteristic posture (**Figure 8-23**). This can be serious if the neurovascular structures are damaged by bony fragments. If

Osteochondritis dissecans
Localized area of avascular necrosis resulting from complete or incomplete separation of joint cartilage and subchondral bone

---

Common sites include the lateral portion of the medial femoral condyle, lateral femoral condyle, femoral groove, and patella

---

Distal femoral fractures result from axial loading or rotational forces with added valgus or varus stress, and tend to angulate and displace posteriorly

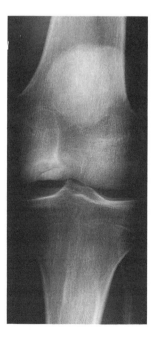

Fig. 8.22: Osteochondritis dissecans occurs when a fragment of bone adjacent to the articular surface of a joint is deprived of its blood supply leading to avascular necrosis. In this patient, a portion of the medial epicondyle of the femur is damaged.

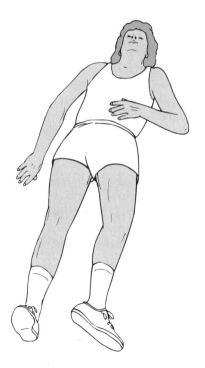

Fig. 8.23: In a fractured femur the adductor muscles contract, leading to internal rotation of the femur and a shortened appearance of the leg.

the femoral artery is ruptured, more than a liter of blood can be lost into the soft tissue leading to shock. Although uncommon in sport because of the extreme force needed to fracture this area, older individuals with osteoporosis who fall on a flexed knee may fracture this region (14).

Severe pain, swelling, deformity, and crepitus at the fracture site will be evident in the distal thigh. In addition, intercondylar fractures are often associated with crepitus on passive knee flexion and diffuse knee effusion that accumulates several hours after injury. Condylar fractures, although not as common as supracondylar or intercondylar, produce a large **hemarthrosis** within one to two hours after injury leaving a tense, inflamed knee.

Femoral fractures can be life threatening because of the blood loss and subsequent shock. EMS should be summoned to properly immobilize the limb in a traction splint (see Figure 3-5), and transported to the nearest medical center.

Patellar Fractures

Patellar fractures account for about 1% of all skeletal injuries and may occur at any age (14). Compression forces from a direct blow or tensile forces when an eccentric contraction of the quadriceps overloads the intrinsic tensile strength of the bone, such as in jumping activities, are common mechanisms. Patella fractures may be transverse, stellate or comminuted, or longitudinal, and may involve tears in the surrounding retinacular tissue. Stress fractures are rare and typically involve the inferior pole of the patella. A bipartite patella, although not a fracture, is present in 1 to 6% of adolescents, and is nine times more common in males (14). It is typically seen on the superior lateral corner of the patella and will have rounded edges rather than sharp edges. The individual will lack point tenderness over the area and can maintain knee extension, differentiating itself from a true fracture.

A patella fracture will produce diffuse extra-articular swelling on and about the knee. A defect may be palpated on the anterior patella. A straight-leg raise will be impossible to perform. Radiographs are needed for verification. Initial treatment will involve ice, elevation, and immobilization in a knee immobilizer. Nondisplaced patellar fractures are treated nonoperatively with a plaster cast

or knee immobilizer for four to six weeks. Partial weight-bearing is then allowed with a full rehabilitation program initiated. In a displaced fracture with major disruption to the extensor mechanism, surgery is indicated.

The basketball player may have a stress fracture of the medial tibial plateau. This may be due to repetitive overuse on a hard surface, or lack of adequate support in the shoes to absorb and disperse force. This individual should be referred to a physician for assessment.

ASSESSING THE KNEE COMPLEX

A high school football player is complaining of anterior knee pain during running, and in ascending and descending stairs. Knowing that the knee is a complex joint, can you limit the assessment to only the knee region? Why not?

The lower extremity works as a unit to provide motion. Several biomechanical problems at the foot directly impact strain on the knee. In addition, the knee plays a major role in supporting the body during dynamic and static activities. Furthermore, referred pain from the hip and lumbar spine may also be involved. As such, assessment of the knee complex must encompass an overview of the entire lower extremity.

HISTORY

What information should be gathered from the football player complaining of anterior knee pain during running and going up and down stairs. What questions can help identify the main components of the primary complaint?

Many conditions at the knee are related to family history, age, congenital deformities, mechanical dysfunction, and recent changes in training programs, surfaces, or foot attire. In addition to general questions covered in Chapter 4, specific questions related to the knee can be seen in **Field Strategy 8-6**.

The player reported that pain came on gradually and hurt during running and blocking drills when he attempts to maintain position against an oncoming opponent. It is particularly bothersome when descending stairs or after sitting for a long time. He rested for two days, iced the area, and took over-the-counter anti-inflammatory medication, but pain returned when activity resumed. Noth-

Hemarthrosis
Collection of blood within a joint or cavity

Patellar fractures are commonly caused by compression forces from a direct blow or tensile forces during an eccentric contraction of the quadriceps

A straight-leg raise will be impossible to perform with a patella fracture

Field Strategy 8–6. Developing a History of the Injury.

ing in the family history or medical history seems to be a factor.

OBSERVATION AND INSPECTION

In which position(s) do you want to observe this individual? Should you do a posture and gait analysis? Why? What specific congenital anomalies might contribute to pain at the knee?

Both legs should be clearly visible to check symmetry, any congenital deformity, swelling, discoloration, hypertrophy, muscle atrophy, or previous surgical incisions. The individual should wear running shorts to allow full view of the entire lower extremity. Ask the individual to bring the shoes they normally wear when pain is present. Inspect the sole, heel box, and general condition of the shoe for unusual wear, which would indicate a biomechanical abnormality that may be affecting the knee.

Place the injured knee on a folded towel or pillow at 30° flexion to relieve any strain on the joint structures. Inspect the injury site for obvious deformities, discoloration, swelling, scars that might indicate previous surgery, and note the general condition of the skin. Swelling proximal to the patella may indicate suprapatellar bursitis or quadriceps involvement. Swelling distal to the patella may indicate patellar tendinitis, fat pad contusion, or internal derangement. Posterior swelling may indicate a Baker's cyst, gastrocnemius strain, or venous thrombosis. Medial swelling over the pes anserinus may indicate bursitis or tendinitis. Quadriceps atrophy is usually a sign of a chronic injury. Compare the affected limb with the unaffected limb.

Faulty posture or congenital abnormalities can also increase stress on any joint. In an ambulatory patient, complete observations with a thorough postural exam. Specific areas to focus on are summarized in **Field Strategy 8-7**. After a static postural exam, observe the individual walking from an anterior, posterior, and lateral view. Ask the individual to do a deep knee squat, ascend, and descend stairs. Note any abnormalities in gait, favoring one limb, tibial torsion, increased Q-angle, or an inability to perform a fluid motion.

● *The individual appears to walk with a slight antalgic gait. Ascending stairs seems painful but an obvious antalgic gait and pained facial expression is noted when descending the stairs. A deep knee squat causes additional anterior knee pain. Slight redness and swelling are noticeable at the inferior patella pole.*

PALPATIONS

● *With pain centered on the anterior knee region, where should you begin to pal-*

 Field Strategy 8–7. Postural Assessment of the Knee Region.

Anterior View

1. Both thighs should look the same. Ask the person to contract the quadriceps. Check for hypertrophy or atrophy. Check for genu valgum (knock-kneed), genu varum (bow-legged), or tibial torsion. Women tend to be more prone toward genu valgum.
2. Both patellas should be at the same height and face straight forward. The Q-angle should appear to be bilaterally equal. If there is swelling at the knee, is it intra-articular (diffuse with patella floating high) or extra-articular (localized with the outline of the patella obscured)? Are the fibular heads level?
3. The medial and lateral malleoli should be level as compared to the opposite foot. Both feet should be angled equally. Tibial torsion may result in the foot either pointing inward ("pigeon toes"), or slightly lateral. Check for supination or pronation of the feet.
4. Check the skin for normal contours, discolored lesions, bruising, ecchymosis, and scars indicating a previous injury or surgery. Note any signs of circulatory impairment or varicose veins.
5. Ask the individual to do a deep knee squat and observe how posture is affected.

Posterior View

1. Are the gluteal and knee folds level? Do the hamstrings and calf muscles have equal bulk? Check the popliteal fossa for abnormal swelling that may indicate a Baker's cyst.
2. Does the Achilles tendon go straight down to the calcaneus. If it appears to angle out, excessive pronation of the foot may affect forces at the knee.

Side View

1. The knees should be slightly flexed (0 to 5°) with the plumb line passing through the center of the knee. Women may be prone to genu recurvatum (hyperextended knees) leading to lordosis. If joint swelling is present, the involved knee may assume a position of 15° to 25° of flexion.
2. Check the level of the tibial tuberosity for possible Osgood-Schlatter disease. If patella alta is present, the infrapatellar fat pad may become more prominent.

Seated Position; Anterior and Side Views

1. The patellas should face forward and rest on the distal femur. With patella alta, the patella will rest on the anterior surface of the femur. Laterally displaced patellas give the appearance of "frog's eyes" or "grasshopper's eyes," and may lead to patellofemoral problems.
2. Ask the person to extend both knees and note tibial movement and patellal tracking.

pate the various structures? During palpation, what factors are you looking for?

Bilateral palpations can determine temperature, swelling, point tenderness, crepitus, deformity, muscle spasm, and cutaneous sensation. Vascular pulses can be taken at the popliteal artery in the posterior knee, the posterior tibial artery behind the medial malleolus, and the dorsalis pedis artery in the dorsum of the foot. Proceed proximal to distal leaving the most painful area to last. With the individual non-weight bearing, place a pillow under the knee to relax the limb. You may need to change knee position to palpate certain structures more effectively. For example, meniscal lesions are best palpated at 45°; the joint line is more prominent at 90°.

Pain during palpation of bony structures may indicate a possible fracture. Compression, distraction, and percussion may also be used to detect fracture. For example, compression at the distal tibia and fibula causes distraction at the proximal tibiofibular joint. Percussion or tapping on the malleoli or use of a tuning fork may also produce positive signs at the fracture site. If you suspect a fracture, put the joint in a knee immobilizer, or summon EMS if a traction splint is necessary. Assess circulatory and neural integrity distal to the fracture site, and take vital signs.

Anterior Palpations

1. Quadriceps muscles, adductor muscles, and sartorius
2. Patellar surface, edges, and retinaculum
3. Patellar tendon, fat pad, tibial tuberosity, medial and lateral tibial plateaus, and bursa
4. Patella plica (medial to the patella with the knee flexed at 45°)
5. Medial femoral condyle and epicondyle, and medial collateral ligament
6. Pes anserinus
7. Iliotibial band, lateral femoral condyle and epicondyle, lateral collateral ligament, and head of fibula. The lateral collateral ligament can be further palpated by having the individual place the foot of the affected limb on the knee of the unaffected leg while palpating the lateral joint line **(Figure 8-24)**
8. With the knee flexed at 90°, palpate the tibiofemoral joint line, medial and lateral tibial plateaus, medial and lateral femoral condyles, and adductor muscles

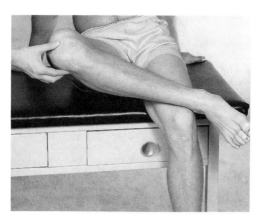

Fig. 8.24: To palpate the lateral collateral ligament, place the foot of the affected leg on the knee of the unaffected leg. Palpate the rope-like structure on the lateral joint line.

Pulses can be taken at the popliteal artery, posterior tibial artery, or dorsalis pedis artery

Posterior Palpations with Knee Slightly Flexed

1. Popliteal fossa for Baker's cyst and popliteal artery
2. Popliteus muscle in posterolateral corner
3. Hamstring muscles and gastrocnemius

Palpation for Swelling

At the knee, you must palpate for joint effusion. Two special tests may be used to determine if the swelling is intra-articular or extra-articular. Intra-articular swelling feels heavy and mushy because blood is often mixed with the synovial fluid. Extra-articular swelling is light and fluid, and can easily be moved between the fingers from one side to the another.

Brush or Stroke Test (Milking) for Joint Swelling

This test differentiates between synovial thickening and joint effusion. With effusion, the knee will assume a resting position of 15 to 25° of flexion which allows the synovial cavity the maximum capacity for holding fluid (6). Beginning below the medial joint line, stroke 2 or 3 times toward the individual's hip moving proximal to the suprapatellar pouch. With the opposite hand, stroke down the lateral side of the patella **(Figure 8-25)**. With effusion, you should observe a wave of fluid pass to the medial side of the joint and bulge just below the medial distal portion of the patella.

Patellar Tap ("Ballotable Patella") Test

This test indicates whether swelling is intra-articular or extra-articular. With the leg

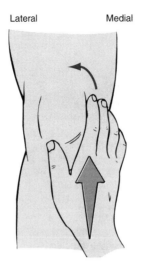
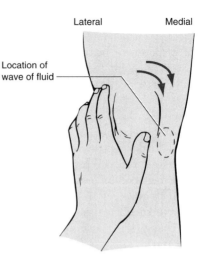

Lateral   Medial   Lateral   Medial

Location of
wave of fluid

Fig. 8.25: To assess joint swelling, stroke the medial side of the knee several times toward the hip. With the opposite hand, stroke down the lateral side of the patella and note any wave of fluid as it moves to the medial side of the joint.

relaxed, push the patella downward into the patellofemoral groove (**Figure 8-26**). If swelling is intra-articular, the fluid under the patella will cause it to rebound, exhibiting the outlines of the floating patella. If the swelling is extra-articular, a click, or definite stopping point will be felt when the patella strikes the patellofemoral groove. The outline of the patella will usually be obscured by extra-articular swelling, seen typically with a ruptured bursa.

🔦 *Pain increased on palpation of the inferior pole of the patella and proximal patellar tendon. Slight swelling and an increase in temperature was noted on either side of the proximal tendon.*

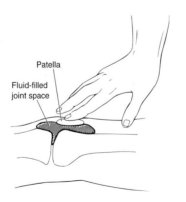

Patella

Fluid-filled
joint space

Fig. 8.26: To perform the patella tap ("ballotable patella") test, the leg should be relaxed. Gently push the patella downward into the groove. If joint effusion is present, the patella will rebound and float back up.

SPECIAL TESTS

❓ *Pain and swelling are limited to the inferior pole of the patella. What special tests can be performed to determine if the injury is muscular, capsular, or ligamentous?*

Perform special tests with the injured athlete in a comfortable position, preferably supine. Pain and muscle spasm can restrict motion and cause an inaccurate result. Do not force the limb through any sudden motions. It may be necessary to place a rolled towel under the knee to relieve strain on the joint structures.

Active Movements

Active movements can first be performed with the individual sitting on a table with the leg flexed over the end of the table, then repeated in a prone or supine position. Stabilize the thigh and as always, perform the most painful movements last to prevent painful symptoms from overflowing into the next movement. The following movements should be assessed at the knee:

1. Knee flexion (0 to 135°)
2. Knee extension (0 to 15°)
3. Medial rotation of the tibia on the femur (20 to 30°) with the knee flexed at 90°
4. Lateral rotation of the tibia on the femur (30 to 40°) with the knee flexed at 90°

Measuring range of motion at the knee with a goniometer is demonstrated in **Figure 8-27**.

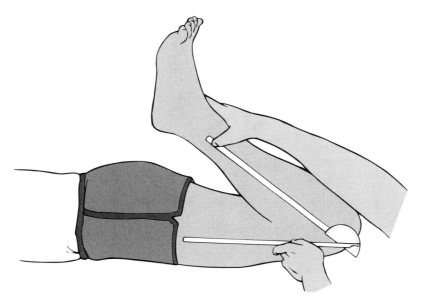

Fig. 8.27: Goniometry measurement for knee flexion and extension. Center the fulcrum over the lateral epicondyle of the femur. Align the proximal arm along the femur using the greater trochanter for reference. Align the distal arm in line with the lateral malleolus.

Passive Range of Motion

If the individual is able to perform full range of motion during active movements, apply gentle pressure at the extremes of motion to determine end feel. End feel for flexion is tissue approximation; extension, medial and lateral rotation is tissue stretch. Patella motion should be performed passively with medial and lateral movement and compared to the unaffected patella. The patella should move half its width in both directions with an end feel of tissue stretch (6). If the individual is unable to perform full active movements, passive movement is done through the range of motion.

Resisted Muscle Testing

Stabilize the hip and perform all resisted muscle testing in a seated position except hamstring testing, which is done in the prone position. To isolate the biceps femoris, place the tibia in external rotation and perform knee flexion against resistance. Internal tibial rotation and knee flexion tests the medial hamstrings. As the quadriceps extend the knee, observe any abnormal tibial movement or excessive pain from patellar compression. **Figure 8-28** demonstrates motions that should be tested (myotomes are listed in parentheses):

1. Knee extension (L_3)
2. Ankle plantar flexion (S_1)
3. Ankle dorsiflexion (L_4)
4. Knee flexion (S_1 and S_2)

Neurological Assessment

Assess neurologic integrity with isometric muscle testing of the myotomes, reflex testing, and sensation in the segmental dermatomes and peripheral nerve cutaneous patterns

Myotomes

Isometric muscle testing should be performed in the following motions to test specific segmental myotomes: hip flexion (L_1, L_2); knee extension (L_3); ankle dorsiflexion (L_4); toe extension (L_5); ankle plantar flexion, foot eversion, or hip extension (S_1); and knee flexion (S_2)

Reflexes

Reflexes in the lower extremity include the patella (L_3, L_4) and Achilles tendon reflex (S_1), and were covered in Chapter 7 (See **Figure 7-39**).

Cutaneous Patterns

In testing cutaneous sensation, run a sharp and dull object over the skin, i.e., blunt tip of taping scissors vs. flat edge of taping scissors. With their eyes closed or looking away, ask the individual if they can distinguish sharp and dull. The segmental nerve dermatome patterns for the knee are demonstrated in **Figure 8-29**. The peripheral nerve cuta-

End feel for flexion is tissue approximation; extension, medial and lateral rotation is tissue stretch

A

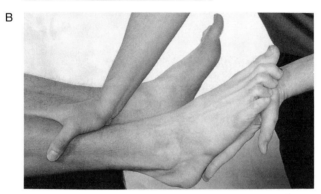
B

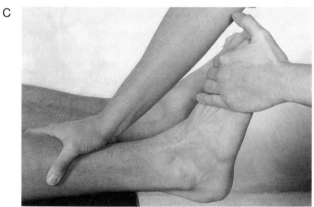
C

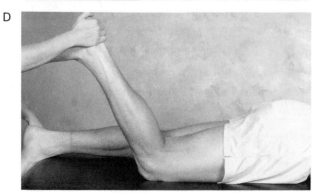
D

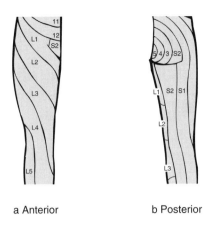

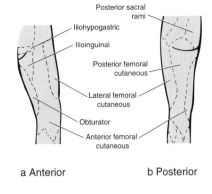

a Anterior   b Posterior

Fig. 8.29: Segmental nerve dermatome patterns.

Fig. 8.30: Peripheral nerve sensory distribution patterns.

neous distribution patterns are demonstrated in **Figure 8-30**.

Stress and Functional Tests

From information gathered during the history, observation, inspection, and palpation, determine which tests most effectively assess the condition. Perform only those tests you believe to be absolutely necessary.

Abduction (Valgus Stress) Test

With the individual supine and leg extended, place the heel of one hand on the lateral joint line. The other hand stabilizes the distal lower leg. Apply a lateral force (valgus stress) at the joint line with the lower leg stabilized in slight lateral rotation **(Figure 8-31A)**. If positive (i.e., the tibia abducts), primary damage to the tibial collateral ligament, posteromedial capsule, and posterior oblique ligament are indicated. To isolate the tibial

collateral ligament, flex the knee at 30° and repeat the valgus stress.

Adduction (Varus Stress) Test

The knee is placed in a similar position as the abduction test, however a medial force (varus stress) is applied at the knee joint **(Figure 8-31B)**. Laxity in full extension indicates major instability and damage to the fibular collateral ligament, popliteus, and posterolateral capsule. When testing at 20 to 30° of flexion, the true test for one plane lateral instability, a positive test indicates damage to the fibular collateral ligament.

Lachman's Test (Anteroposterior Drawer Test)

If you suspect anterior cruciate ligament damage, perform this test first because swelling, joint effusion, and muscle spasm may occlude the extent of instability if per-

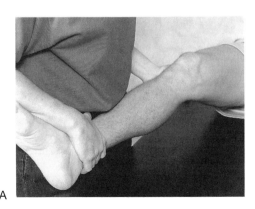

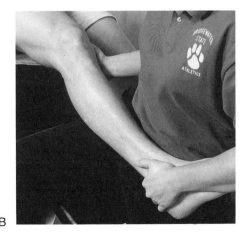

A   B

Fig. 8.31: (A) Valgus stress test. Flex the knee at 30° and apply a gentle valgus stress at the knee joint while moving the lower leg laterally. Repeat the test with the knee fully extended. (B) Varus stress test. Flex the knee at 30° and gently apply a varus stress at the knee joint while moving the lower leg medially. Repeat the test with the knee fully extended.

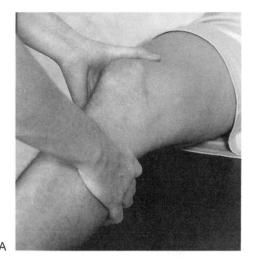

A

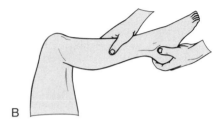

B

Fig. 8.32: Damage to the cruciate ligaments should be performed before swelling, joint effusion, and muscle spasm occlude the extent of instability. (A) Lachman test. Stabilize the thigh with one hand. With the other hand, apply firm pressure on the posterior proximal tibia in an attempt to move the tibia anteriorly. (B) The posterior "sag" test. Flex both hip and knees. Look from the side and compare the anterior contours of both legs. If one leg sags back and the prominence of the tibial tuberosity is lost, the posterior cruciate may be damaged.

formed later. Place the knee joint at 20 to 30° and stabilize the femur with one hand. Place the other hand over the proximal tibia and displace the tibia anteriorly **(Figure 8-32A)**. A positive sign results in a "mushy" or soft end feel when the tibia is moved anterior in relation to the femur. This indicates primary damage to the anterior cruciate ligament. With the tibia in slight internal rotation, anterior displacement indicates additional damage to the iliotibial tract, and anterior and middle lateral capsule. With the tibia in slight external rotation, anterior displacement indicates damage to the anterior cruciate ligament, tibial collateral ligament, and medial meniscus. The test can also be performed at 90° of knee flexion, called the drawer test. However, it is not as reliable as Lachman's test for two reasons. Lachman's test reduces tension in the hamstrings. The hamstrings along with secondary ligamentous structures provide more restraint at 90° preventing anterior displacement. Furthermore, increased pain is elicited in an acute injury at 90° flexion, thus masking the true extent of injury.

Gravity Drawer Test (Posterior "Sag" Sign)

Single-plane posterior instability is tested by flexing the hip and knee at 90°. In this position the tibia sags back on the femur if the posterior cruciate ligament is torn **(Figure 8-32B)**. It is important to note the sag, because it may produce a false-positive Lachman's test if the sag goes unnoticed.

McMurray's Test

With the individual supine, flex the knee completely against the chest, externally rotate the tibia, and slowly extend the knee and hip **(Figure 8-33)**. You are attempting to trap the

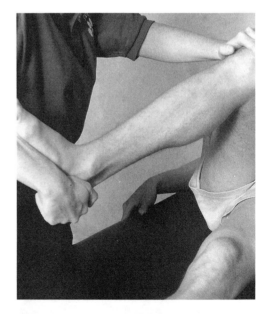

Fig. 8.33: To perform the McMurray test, flex the hip and knee. Stabilize the lower leg with one hand and laterally rotate the tibia. Place the other hand over the anterior knee with the fingers on the joint line. Slowly extend the leg. If there is a loose body in the medial meniscus this action will cause a snap or click. Internally rotating the leg and repeating the test with the thumb over the lateral joint line will test for lateral meniscus damage.

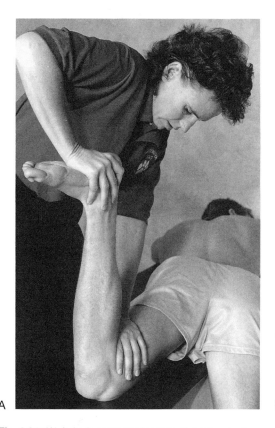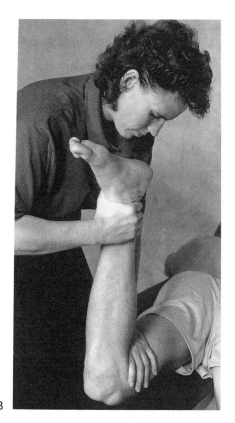

A   B

Fig. 8.34: (A) Apley's compression test. If rotation and compression cause pain, meniscal damage may be present. (B) Apley's distraction test. If rotation and distraction cause pain, ligamentous damage may be present.

displaced posterior horn of the medial meniscus in the joint, producing an audible and palpable click or thud. Return to the starting position. With internal rotation and extension of the knee and hip, the posterior horn of the lateral meniscus is trapped. Each test is repeated several times.

Apley's Compression Test

In a prone position with the knee flexed at 90°, stabilize the thigh and rotate the leg by applying downward compression in a medial and lateral direction **(Figure 8-34A)**. The test is positive if pain is produced. Pain should be relieved by repeating the test with the joint distracted **(Figure 8-34B)**. If rotation with distraction produces pain, the lesion is probably ligamentous. This compression test may or may not produce a positive sign, however, even though a meniscal tear is present.

Patella Compression or Grind Test

Place a rolled towel under the knee flexing it at about 20°. Compress the patella into the patellofemoral groove **(Figure 8-35A)**. The test is positive if pain is felt or a grinding

sound is heard, indicating pathology to the patellar articular cartilage.

Clarke's Sign

Using the web of your hand, place the hand just proximal to the superior pole of the patella **(Figure 8-35B)**. Ask the individual to contract the quadriceps while you gently push downward. If the individual can hold the contraction without pain, the test is negative. If the individual has pain, and is unable to hold the contraction, the test is positive for chondromalacia patellae. This test can elicit pain in any individual if the pressure is significant. Therefore, it is imperative to repeat the procedure several times with increasing pressure in full knee extension, and at 30°, 60°, and 90° of knee flexion.

Waldron Test

Palpate the patella while the individual does several slow deep knee bends. Note any crepitus, pain, "catching", or improper tracking of the patella. If any of these signs or symptoms occur simultaneously, the test is positive for chondromalacia patellae.

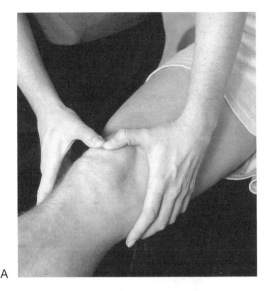 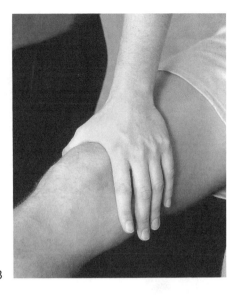

A   B

Fig. 8.35: (A) Pain on compression of the patella into the groove indicates pathology to the patella articular cartilage. (B) To elicit Clarke's sign, apply slight compression just proximal to the superior pole of the patella and ask the individual to contract the quadriceps. The test is positive for chondromalacia patella if the individual has pain or is unable to hold the contraction.

Patella Apprehension Test

With the knee in a relaxed position, push the patella laterally (**Figure 8-36**). If the individual voluntarily or involuntarily shows apprehension, it is a positive test for subluxating patella.

Ober's Test for Iliotibial Tract Contracture

The individual lies on their side with the lower leg slightly flexed at the hip and knee for stability. Stabilize the pelvis with one hand to prevent the pelvis from shifting posteriorly during the test. Passively abduct and slightly extend

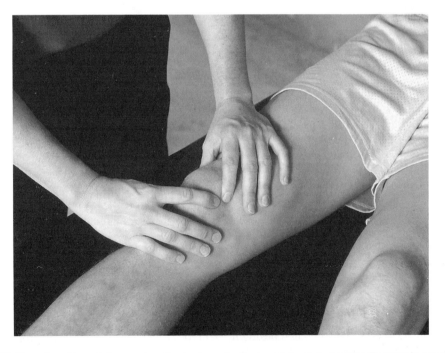

Fig. 8.36: To perform the patella apprehension test, gently displace the patella laterally. The test is a positive sign for subluxating patella if the individual shows apprehension.

the hip so the iliotibial tract passes over the greater trochanter (**Figure 8-37A**). Although the original Ober's test called for the knee to be flexed at 90°, the iliotibial tract has a greater stretch if the knee is extended. Slowly lower the upper leg. If the iliotibial band is tight, the leg will remain in the abducted position.

Noble Compression Test

This test is used with Ober's test to determine if iliotibial band friction syndrome is present near the knee (**Figure 8-37B**). The individual is supine on a table with the hip and knee flexed at 90°. The individual slowly lowers the leg and extends the knee. Apply pressure with the thumb directly over, or 1 to 2 cm proximal, to the lateral epicondyle of the femur. As the knee moves to 30° of knee flexion, the individual will report severe pain similar to that caused during activity.

Functional Tests

Functional tests should be performed before clearing the individual for return to participation. These tests should be performed pain-free without a limp or antalgic gait. Examples of functional tests include forward running, cross over stepping, running figure 8's or V-cuts, side step running, and karioca running. When appropriate, functional braces or protective supportive devices should be used to prevent reinjury.

During special tests you found increased pain and weakness during active and resisted knee extension. Passive knee flexion also led to pain in the anterior knee region. Neurologic assessment was normal, and other stress tests were negative. Did you determine

the individual may have patellar tendinitis? If so, you are correct. How will you manage this condition?

REHABILITATION OF KNEE INJURIES

What major components must be included in a knee rehabilitation program? How will you determine when the individual can return to sport participation?

A rehabilitation program attempts to minimize inflammation and the effects of immobilization by initiating early mobilization and controlled movement to allow healing tissues to be stressed gradually and progressively until normal joint function is restored. The rehabilitation program should restore motion and proprioception, maintain cardiovascular fitness, and improve muscular strength, endurance, and power predominantly through closed chain exercises. Sample exercise programs for specific injuries are listed in Field Strategies 8-2, 8-3, 8-4, and 8-5.

Restoration of Motion

After most knee injuries, some loss of motion will occur. Passive range of motion exercises can begin on the first day after injury. Continuous passive motion (CPM) machines are primarily used post-surgically at the knee, after knee manipulation, or after stable fixation of intrarticular and extrarticular fractures (See **Figure 5-26**). The unit moves the knee through a protected range of motion to stimulate the intrinsic healing process, maintain articular cartilage nutrition, reduce disuse

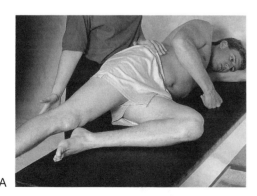

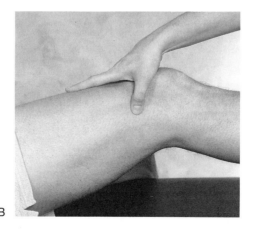

A   B

Fig. 8.37: (A) To perform Ober's test, passively abduct and slightly extend the hip. Slower lower the extended leg. If the iliotibial band is tight, the leg will remain in the abducted position. (B) To perform the Noble compression test, flex the hip and knee at 90°. Apply thumb pressure over the lateral epicondyle of the femur as the leg is extended. Pain at or near 30° flexion indicates iliotibial band syndrome.

effects, retard joint stiffness and muscle spasm, and benefit collagen remodeling, joint dynamics, and pain reduction (32,33). When a CPM machine is not needed, range of motion exercises, such as the wall slide, heel slide, assisted knee flexion and extension, half squats, or PNF stretching exercises can be performed **(Figure 8-38)**.

In addition to active and passive range of motion exercises at the tibiofemoral joint, stretching exercises to improve passive glide of the patellofemoral joint, particularly medial glide, can stretch tight lateral structures to correct patellar positioning and tracking **(Figure 8-39)**. Normal passive glide of the patellofemoral joint should be restored before full flexion exercises, resisted exercises, or bicycling is initiated.

Restoration of Proprioception and Balance

Proprioception and balance must be regained to return safely to sport participation. In the early stages following injury, exercises such as shifting one's weight while on crutches, straight leg raises, bilateral minisquats, or use of a BAPS board with support may be helpful. As balance improves, unassisted use of the BAPS board, running in place on a mini-tramp, or use of a slide board may be incor-

porated along with other closed chain exercises, such as those listed below.

Muscular Strength, Endurance, and Power

Early emphasis is placed on strengthening the quadriceps femoris musculature, particularly the vastus medialis and vastus medialis oblique (VMO). These muscles aid in the stabilization of the patella superiorly and medially. Isometric contractions, called quad sets, are performed at, or near, 0°, 45°, 60°, and 90° flexion. Isometric hip adduction exercises are also used to recruit the VMO, and can be performed by squeezing a rolled towel between the knees in a seated position (21).

Open-chain exercises may include straight leg raises in all directions, supplemented by ankle weights or tubing to increase resistance. Knee extension and knee flexion exercises may be done with free weights or on several commercially available isotonic or isokinetic machines.

Closed-chain exercises performed during weight bearing may include terminal knee extension **(Figure 8-40)**, step ups, step downs, lateral step ups, mini squats from 0° to 40°, leg presses on a machine from 0° to 60°, or use of a stepping machine or stationary bicycle. Several of these exercises were illus-

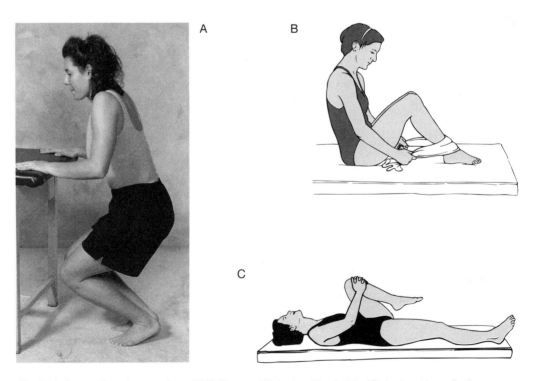

Fig. 8.38: Range of motion exercises. (A) Half squat. (B) Assisted heel slide. (C) Assisted knee flexion.

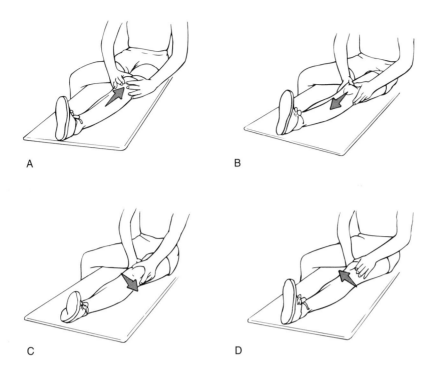

Fig. 8.39: Patella self-mobilization. (A) Proximal. B) Distal. (C) Medial. (D) Lateral.

trated in **Field Strategy 8-1**. Closed chain exercises can be made progressively more difficult by increasing the resistance, speed of movement, or changing the individual's visual feedback, i.e. looking at the ceiling, looking at the floor, or closing the eyes (34).

Plyometric jumping in the later stages of rehabilitation can use small boxes and directional changes to improve power and propri-

oceptive function. Because of the increased eccentric contraction and the associated muscle microtrauma that results from the power maneuvers, these exercises should only be performed two or three times weekly (34).

Cardiovascular Fitness

Cardiovascular fitness exercises can begin immediately after injury with use of an UBE

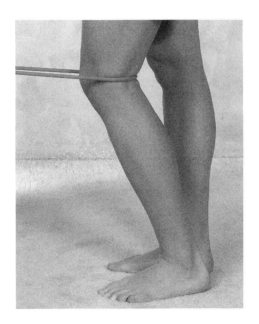
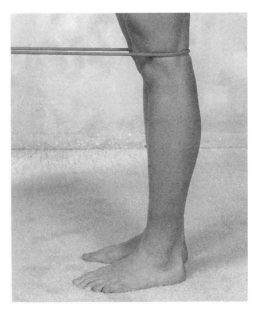

Fig. 8.40: Closed chain terminal extension. (A) Starting position. (B) Ending position.

or hydrotherapeutic exercise. Running in water and performing sport specific exercises in deep water can allow the individual to maintain sport specific functional skills in a non-weight bearing position. When range of motion is adequate, a stationary bicycle may be used. The seat should be adjusted so the knee is flexed 15° to 30°. The individual should be instructed to pedal with the ball of the foot using toe clips and pull through the bottom of the stroke. A low to moderate workload is recommended to reduce

---

 Field Strategy 8–8. Knee Evaluation.

History

Primary complaint including:
 Description and mechanism of current injury
 Onset of symptoms
 Changes in training, equipment, or shoes
Pain perception and discomfort
Disability and functional impairments from the injury
Previous injuries to the area
Family history

Observation and Inspection

Postural assessment
 Gait analysis
 Inspection of injured area for:
  Muscle symmetry   Hypertrophy or muscle atrophy
  Swelling   Visible congenital deformity
  Discoloration   Surgical incisions or scars

Palpation

Bony structures to determine a possible fracture
Soft tissue structures to determine:
  Temperature   Crepitus
  Swelling   Muscle spasm
  Point tenderness   Cutaneous sensation
  Deformity   Vascular pulses
Brush or stroke test, and patellar tap test for joint swelling

Special Tests

Active movements
 Passive range of motion
 Resisted muscle testing
Neurological testing
Stress and functional tests
 Abduction (valgus) and adduction (varus) stress tests
 Lachman test (anteroposterior drawer test)
 Gravity drawer test (posterior "sag" sign)
 McMurray's test
 Apley's compression/distraction test
 Patella compression test, Clarke's sign, Waldron's test
 Patella apprehension test
 Ober's test and Noble's compression test for iliotibial band tightness
 Functional tests

patellofemoral compressive forces. Other exercises, such as walking, light jogging, and functional activities can progress as tolerated. ● *The rehabilitation program should restore motion and proprioception, maintain cardiovascular fitness, and improve muscular strength, endurance, and power. The individual can return to sport participation after completing all functional tests pain-free and must be cleared by the supervising physician. These tests might include timed sprints, shuttle runs, agility runs, karioca runs, hop or vertical jump tests.*

SUMMARY

The knee is highly susceptible to stress during sport participation, particularly in running and jumping activities that involve deceleration and rotation. Congenital abnormalities, muscle imbalance, muscle dysfunction, and postural deviations can also predispose an individual to injury. During the assessment remember that referred pain may originate in the lumbar spine, hip, or ankle. **Field Strategy 8-8** lists the steps in assessing the knee region.

Refer the individual to a physician if any of the following conditions are suspected: obvious deformity suggesting a dislocation or fracture; significant loss of motion or locking of the knee; excessive joint swelling; gross joint instability; reported sounds, such as popping, snapping, clicking, or giving way of the knee; possible epiphyseal injuries; abnormal or absent reflexes; abnormal sensations in either segmental dermatomes or peripheral cutaneous patterns; absent or weak pulse; weakness in a myotome; or any unexplained or chronic pain. Any knee injury that disrupts an individual's play or performance should be diagnosed by a physician.

If the individual is referred to a physician, remove the person from activity and immobilize the limb. Immobilization may consist of a knee immobilizer or other splint to pad and protect the injured area. If necessary, fit the individual for crutches if they are unable to walk without a limp or pain. Apply ice therapy to control inflammation and swelling, and transport the individual in an appropriate manner. Individualize the rehabilitation program to address deficiencies discovered in the assessment. The individual should not return to competition until they can perform all functional tests without pain, and receive a medical clearance to participate.

REFERENCES

1. Soderberg, GL. *Kinesiology: Application to pathological motion*. Baltimore: Williams & Wilkins, 1986.
2. Beaupré, A, Choukroun, R, Guidouin, R, Garneau, R, Gerardin, H, and Cardou, A. 1986. Knee menisci: Correlation between microstructure and biomechanics. Clin Orthop & Rel Res, 208:72–75.
3. Norkin, CC, and Levangie, PK. *Joint structure and function: A comprehensive analysis*. Philadelphia: FA Davis, 1992.
4. Mueller, W. *The knee: Form, function and ligament reconstruction*. New York: Springer-Verlag, 1983.
5. Terry, GC, Hughston, JC, and Norwood, LA. 1986. The anatomy of the iliopatellar band and iliotibial tract. Am J Sports Med, 14(1):39–45.
6. McGee, DJ. *Orthopedic physical assessment*. Philadelphia: WB Saunders, 1987.
7. Jenkins, DB. *Hollinshead's functional anatomy of the limbs and back*. Philadelphia: WB Saunders, 1991.
8. Shiavi, R, Limbird, TL, Frazer, M, Stivers, K, Strauss, A, and Abramovitz, J. 1987. Helical motion analysis of the knee—II: Kinematics of uninjured and injured knees during walking and pivoting. J Biomech, 20(7):653–665.
9. Morrison, JB. 1970. The mechanics of the knee joint in relation to normal walking. J Biomech, 3(1):51–61.
10. Olmstead, TG, Wevers, HW, Bryant, JT, and Gouw, GJ. 1986. Effect of muscular activity on valgus/varus laxity and stiffness of the knee. J Biomech, 19(8):565–577.
11. Shrive, NG, Phil, D, O'Connor, JJ, and Goodfellow, JW. 1978. Load-bearing in the knee joint. Clin Orthop, 131:279–287.
12. Nordin, M, and Frankel, VH. "Biomechanics of the knee." In *Basic biomechanics of the musculoskeletal system*, edited by M Nordin and VH Frankel. Philadelphia: Lea & Febiger, 1989.
13. Reilly, DT, and Martens, M. 1972. Experimental analysis of the quadriceps muscle force and patellofemoral joint reaction force for various activities. Acta Orthop Scand, 43:126–137.
14. American Academy of Orthopaedic Surgeons. *Athletic training and sports medicine*. Park Ridge, IL: American Academy of Orthopaedic Surgeons, 1991.
15. Reid, DC. *Sports injury assessment and rehabilitation*. New York: Churchill Livingstone, 1992.
16. Cooper, DE, Arnoczky, SP, and Warren, RF. "Athroscopic meniscal repair." In *Clinics in sports medicine*, edited by KM Singer. vol. 9, no. 3. Philadelphia: WB Saunders, 1990.
17. Terry, GC. "The anatomy of the extensor mechanism." In *Clinics in sports medicine*, edited by JH Henry, vol. 8, no. 2. Philadelphia: WB Saunders, 1989.
18. Moss, RI, DeVita, P, and Dawson, ML. 1992. A biomechanical analysis of patellofemoral stress syndrome. J Ath Train, 27(1):64–69.
19. Lebsack, D, Gieck, J, and Saliba, E. 1990. Iliotibial band friction syndrome. J of Ath Train, 25(4):356–361.
20. Eisele, SA. 1991. A precise approach to anterior knee pain: More accurate diagnoses and specific treatment programs. Phys Sportsmed, 19(6):127–139.

21. Westfall, DC, and Worrell, TW. 1992. Anterior knee pain syndrome: Role of the vastus medialis oblique. J Spt Rehab, 1(4):317–325.
22. Spiker, JC, and Massie, DL. 1992. Comprehensive management of patellofemoral pain. J Spt Rehab, 1(3):258–263.
23. Hughston, JC "Patellar subluxation: A recent history." In Clinics in sports medicine, edited by JH Henry, vol. 8, no. 2. Philadelphia: WB Saunders, 1989.
24. Pezzullo, DJ, Irrgang, JJ, and Whitney, SL. 1992. Patellar tendonitis: Jumper's knee. J Sport Rehab, 1(1):56–68.
25. Roels, J, Martens, M, Mulier, JC, et al. 1978. Patellar tendinitis (jumper's knee). Am J Sports Med, 6(5):362,368.
26. Lucas, CA. 1992. Iliotibial band friction syndrome as exhibited in athletes. J Ath Train, 27(3):250–252.
27. Crawford, AH. 1976. Fractures about the knee in children. Orthop Clin North Am, 3:639–656.
28. Levi, JH, and Colemen CR. 1976. Fractures of the tibial tubercle. Am J Sports Med, 4(4):254–256.
29. Balmat, P, Vichard, P, and Pem, R. 1990. The treatment of avulsion fractures of the tibial tuberosity in adolescent athletes. Sports Med, 9(5):311–316.
30. Brown, DE. "Ankle and leg injuries." In The team physician's handbook, edited by MB Mellion, WM Walsh, and GL Shelton. Philadelphia: Hanley & Belfus, 1990.
31. Cameron, JC. "Osteochondritis dissecans, osteochondral fractures, and osteoarthritis of the knee." In Current therapy in sports medicine, edited by RP Welsh and RJ Shephard. Toronto: BC Decker, 1985.
32. Starkey, C. Therapeutic modalities for athletic trainers. Philadelphia: FA Davis, 1993.
33. O'Donoghue, PC, McCarthy, MR, Gieck, JH, and Yates, CK. 1991. Clinical use of continuous passive motion in athletic training. Ath Tr (JNATA), 26(3):200–208.
34. Harrelson, GL. "Knee rehabilitation." In Physical rehabilitation of the injured athlete, edited by JR Andrews and GL Harrelson. Philadelphia: WB Saunders, 1991.

Thigh, Hip, and Pelvis Injuries

After you have completed this chapter, you should be able to:

- Locate the important bony and soft tissue structures of the thigh, hip, and pelvis
- Describe the motions of the hip and identify the muscles that produce them
- Explain what forces produce loading patterns responsible for common injuries of the thigh, hip, and pelvis
- Identify measures that can prevent injury to the region
- Recognize specific injuries at the thigh, hip and pelvis
- Demonstrate a thorough assessment of the hip region
- Demonstrate general rehabilitation exercises for the region

Although the thigh, hip, and pelvis have a sturdy anatomical composition, this region can be subjected to large, potentially injurious forces when individuals engage in sports or exercise. For example, the soft tissues of the anterior thigh often sustain compressive forces, particularly during contact sports. Although the resulting contusions are not usually serious, mismanagement of these injuries can lead to more serious problems. Because activities of daily living rarely involve stretching of the hamstrings, this muscle group is particularly susceptible to strain. Inflexibility and a strength imbalance between the hamstrings and the more frequently exercised quadriceps contribute to a higher likelihood of hamstring strain. Because of their strong bony stability, the hip and pelvis are seldom injured. However, since the hip sustains repetitive forces of four to seven times body weight during walking and running, the joint is subjected to stress-related injuries (1).

This chapter begins with a review of the anatomy, kinematics, and kinetics of the thigh, hip, and pelvis. Next, preventative measures will be discussed, followed by information on basic injuries to the region. A step by step injury assessment process is then followed by examples of rehabilitation exercises for the region.

ANATOMY OF THE THIGH, HIP, AND PELVIS

❓ *Although the hip has a larger range of motion than the knee and ankle joints, injuries to the hip are less common than injuries to the other lower extremity joints. Why is this true?*

The thigh, hip, and pelvis have an extremely stable bony structure that is further reinforced by a number of large, strong ligaments and muscles. This region is anatomically well-suited for withstanding the large forces to which it is subjected during daily activities.

Bony Structure of the Thigh

The thigh consists of the femur, and the muscles and other soft tissue structures that surround it. The femur is a major weight-bearing bone and is the longest, largest, and strongest bone in the body (**Figure 9-1**). Its weakest component is the femoral neck, which is smaller in diameter than the rest of the bone, and weak internally because it is primarily composed of cancellous bone. The femur angles medially downward from the hip during the support phase of walking and running, enabling single leg support beneath the body's center of gravity. Because women have a wider pelvis, this angulation tends to be more pronounced in women.

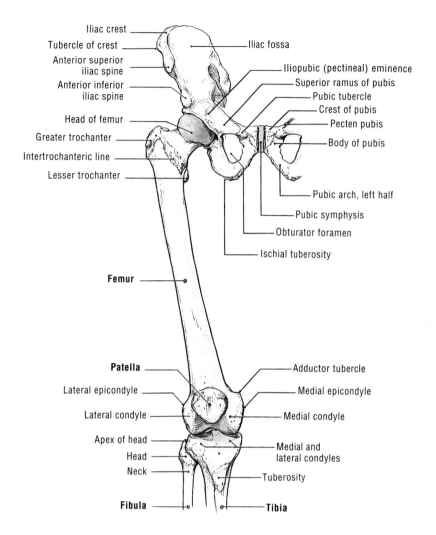

Iliac crest
Tubercle of crest
Anterior superior iliac spine
Anterior inferior iliac spine
Head of femur
Greater trochanter
Intertrochanteric line
Lesser trochanter

Iliac fossa
Iliopubic (pectineal) eminence
Superior ramus of pubis
Pubic tubercle
Crest of pubis
Pecten pubis
Body of pubis

Pubic arch, left half
Pubic symphysis
Obturator foramen
Ischial tuberosity

Femur

Patella
Lateral epicondyle
Lateral condyle
Apex of head
Head
Neck

Fibula

Adductor tubercle
Medial epicondyle
Medial condyle
Medial and lateral condyles
Tuberosity

Tibia

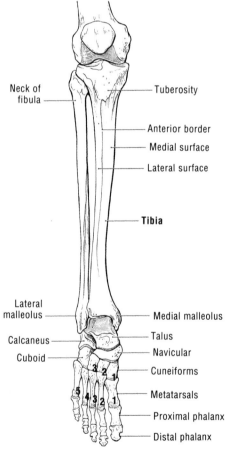

Neck of fibula
Tuberosity
Anterior border
Medial surface
Lateral surface

Tibia

Lateral malleolus
Medial malleolus
Calcaneus
Talus
Cuboid
Navicular
Cuneiforms
Metatarsals
Proximal phalanx
Distal phalanx

A

Fig. 9.1: The femur and pelvis. (A) Anterior view. (B) Posterior view.

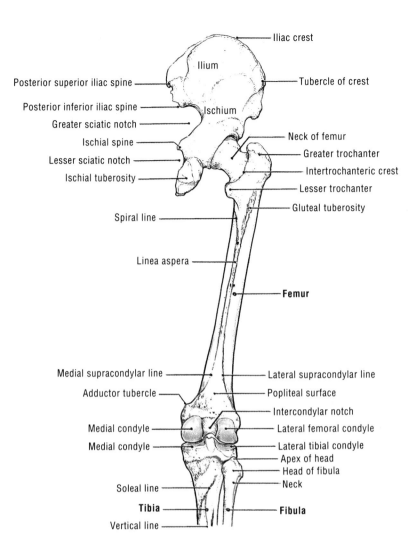

Iliac crest
Ilium
Posterior superior iliac spine
Tubercle of crest
Posterior inferior iliac spine
Ischium
Greater sciatic notch
Ischial spine
Neck of femur
Lesser sciatic notch
Greater trochanter
Ischial tuberosity
Intertrochanteric crest
Lesser trochanter
Spiral line
Gluteal tuberosity
Linea aspera
Femur
Medial supracondylar line
Lateral supracondylar line
Adductor tubercle
Popliteal surface
Intercondylar notch
Medial condyle
Lateral femoral condyle
Medial condyle
Lateral tibial condyle
Apex of head
Head of fibula
Soleal line
Neck
Tibia
Fibula
Vertical line

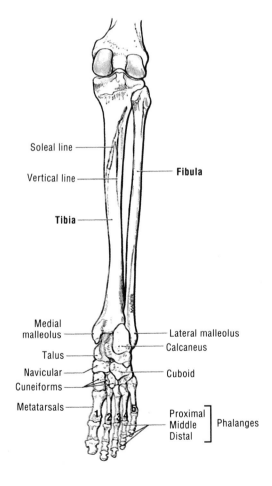

Soleal line
Vertical line
Fibula
Tibia
Medial malleolus
Lateral malleolus
Talus
Calcaneus
Navicular
Cuboid
Cuneiforms
Metatarsals
1 2 3 4 5
Proximal
Middle   Phalanges
Distal

B

The Hip Joint

The hip is the articulation between the concave acetabulum of the pelvis and the head of the femur. The acetabulum functions as a classic ball and socket joint (**Figure 9-1**). The acetabulum angles obliquely in an inferior, anterior, and lateral direction. Because the socket is deep, it provides considerable bony stability to the joint. Both articulating surfaces are covered with friction-reducing joint cartilage. The cartilage on the acetabulum is thickened around the periphery where it merges with the U-shaped fibrocartilaginous acetabular labrum, which further contributes to stability of the joint.

The Pelvis

The pelvis, or pelvic girdle, consists of a protective bony ring formed by four fused bones—the two innominate bones, the sacrum, and coccyx (**Figure 9-1**). The innominate bones articulate with each other anteriorly at the symphysis pubis, and with the sacrum posteriorly at the sacroiliac joints. Each innominate bone consists of three fused bones—the ilium, ischium, and pubis. Among these, the ilium forms the major portion of the innominate bone, including the prominent iliac crests. The anterior superior iliac spine (ASIS) is a readily palpable landmark. The posterior superior iliac spine (PSIS) is typically marked by an indentation in the soft tissues just lateral to the sacrum. The pelvis' functions include protecting the enclosed inner organs, transmitting loads between the trunk and lower extremity, and providing a site for a number of major muscle attachments.

Joint Capsule and Bursae

The joint capsule of the hip is large and loose. It completely surrounds the joint, attaching to the labrum of the acetabular socket. It also passes over a fat pad internally to join to the neck of the femur. Because the capsular fibers attaching to the femoral neck are arranged in a circular fashion, they are known as the zona orbicularis. The zona orbicularis is an important contributor to hip stability.

The joint capsule interior is covered by a synovial membrane, and several bursae are present. The most prominent bursae are the iliopsoas bursa and the deep trochanteric bursa. The iliopsoas bursa is positioned between the iliopsoas and articular capsule, serving to reduce the friction between these structures. The deep trochanteric bursa provides a cushion between the greater trochanter of the femur and the gluteus maximus at its attachment to the iliotibial tract.

Ligaments of the Hip

Several large, strong ligaments support the hip (**Figure 9-2**). The Y-shaped iliofemoral ligament, sometimes referred to as the Y ligament of Bigelow, strengthens the joint capsule of the hip anteriorly. The position of this ligament, extending from the AIIS to the intertrochanteric line on the femur, enables it to severely limit hip hyperextension. The pubofemoral ligament, also located anteriorly, connects the pubic ramus to the intertrochanteric line. The ischiofemoral ligament reinforces the hip posteriorly, extending from the ischium in a superior, lateral direction to the greater trochanter of the femur. Tension

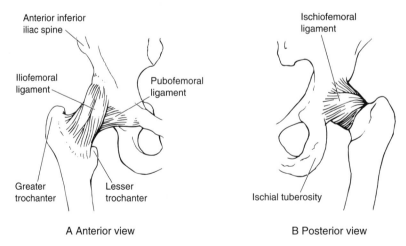

Fig. 9.2: The ligaments of the hip. (A) Anterior view. (B) Posterior view.

in these major ligaments act to twist the head of the femur into the acetabulum upon hip extension, as when a person rises from sitting to an upright, standing position. Other ligaments at the hip are of little functional importance.

Muscles of the Hip

A number of large, strong muscles cross the hip, enhancing its stability. The muscles of the hip are summarized in **Table 9-1** and the actions of the major muscles are discussed later in the chapter.

Nerves of the Thigh, Hip, and Pelvis

The major nerve supply to the thigh, hip, and pelvis arises from the lumbar and sacral plexi. The **lumbar plexus** is formed from the first four lumbar spinal nerves (**Figure 9-3**). It innervates portions of the abdominal wall and psoas major, with branches into the thigh region. The largest branch is the femoral nerve (L_2-L_4) that supplies muscles and skin of the anterior thigh. Another branch, the obturator nerve (L_2-L_4), provides innervation to the hip adductor muscles.

The **sacral plexus** is positioned just anterior to the lumbar plexus, and has some intermingling of fibers from the sacral and lumbar plexi. The lower spinal nerves, including L_4 through S_4, spawn the sacral plexus (**Figure 9-3**). Twelve nerve branches arise from the sacral plexus. The most major is the sciatic nerve (L_4, L_5, S_1-S_3), which is the largest and longest single nerve in the body. The sciatic nerve passes through the greater sciatic notch of the pelvis, courses through the gluteus maximus muscle, and then innervates the hamstrings and adductor magnus. The tibial and common peroneal nerves that branch from the sciatic nerve in the posterior thigh region, are discussed in Chapters 7 and 8.

Blood Vessels of the Thigh, Hip, and Pelvis

The external iliac arteries become the femoral arteries at the level of the thighs, providing the major blood supply to the lower extremity (**Figure 9-4**). The femoral artery gives off several branches in the thigh region, including the deep femoral artery, which serves the posterior and lateral thigh muscles, and the lateral and medial femoral circumflex

arteries, which supply the region of the femoral head.

💡 *The hip is the most stable joint in the body. Not only does it have a substantial amount of bony stability, but it is reinforced by several large, strong ligaments and muscles.*

KINEMATICS AND MAJOR MUSCLE ACTIONS OF THE HIP

❓ *Which muscles that move the hip also contribute to motion of the knee? What is the functional significance of these two-joint muscles?*

Since the hip is a ball and socket joint, the femur can move in all planes of motion. However, the massive muscles crossing the hip tend to limit range of motion, particularly in the posterior direction.

Pelvic Positioning

During many activities of daily living, the positioning of the pelvic girdle facilitates motion of the femur at the hip (**Figure 9-5**). For example, abduction of the leg during the preparatory phase of a kick in one of the martial arts, is made easier by a lateral tilt of the pelvis toward the side opposite the kicking leg. Likewise, flexion at the hip is assisted by **posterior pelvic tilt**, and extension at the hip is enhanced by **anterior pelvic tilt**.

Flexion

The major hip flexors are the iliacus and psoas major, referred to jointly as the iliopsoas because of their common attachment at the femur (**Figure 9-6**). Four other muscles cross the anterior aspect of the hip to contribute to hip flexion. These include the pectineus, rectus femoris, sartorius, and tensor fascia latae. Because the rectus femoris is a two-joint muscle active during both hip flexion and knee extension, it functions more effectively as a hip flexor when the knee is in flexion, such as when a person kicks a ball. The sartorius is also a two-joint muscle. Crossing from the ASIS to the medial surface of the proximal tibia just below the tuberosity, the sartorius is the longest muscle in the body.

Extension

The hip extensors are the gluteus maximus and the three hamstrings—the biceps femoris, semitendinosus, and semimembranosus (**Figure 9-6**). The gluteus maximus is

Lumbar plexus
Interconnected roots of the first four lumbar spinal nerves

The femoral nerve innervates the muscles and skin of the anterior thigh

The obturator nerve innervates the hip adductor muscles

Sacral plexus
Interconnected roots of the L_4-S_4 spinal nerves

The sciatic nerve is the largest, longest nerve in the body

The lateral and medial circumflex arteries encircle the femoral head, providing blood supply to the hip joint

Lateral movements of the femur are facilitated by lateral tilt of the pelvis toward the opposite side

Posterior pelvic tilt
Posterior sagittal plane tilt of the ASIS with respect to the pubic symphysis

Anterior pelvic tilt
Anterior sagittal plane tilt of the ASIS with respect to the pubic symphysis

The hamstrings contribute to both hip extension and knee flexion

Table 9–1. Muscles of the Hip.

Muscle	Proximal Attachment	Distal Attachment	Primary Action(s)	Nerve Innervation
Rectus femoris	Anterior inferior iliac spine (AIIS)	Patella	Hip flexion and knee extension	Femoral (L_2-L_4)
Iliopsoas			Hip flexion	L_1 and femoral (L_2-L_4)
(Iliacus)	Iliac fossa and adjacent sacrum	Lesser trochanter		
(Psoas major)	12th thoracic and lumbar vertebrae, and lumbar discs	Lesser trochanter		(L_1-L_3)
Sartorius	Anterior superior iliac spine (ASIS)	Upper medial tibia	Assists with flexion, abduction, and lateral rotation	Femoral (L_2,L_3)
Pectineus	Pectineal crest of pubic ramus	Medial proximal femur	Flexion and adduction	Femoral (L_2,L_3)
Tensor fascia latae	Anterior crest of the ilium and ASIS	Iliotibial band	Assists with flexion, abduction and medial rotation	Superior gluteal (L_4-S_1)
Gluteus maximus	Posterior ilium, iliac crest, sacrum, and coccyx	Gluteal tuberosity of the femur and iliotibial band	Hip extension and lateral rotation	Inferior gluteal (L_5-S_2)
Gluteus medius	Between posterior and anterior gluteal lines on the posterior ilium	Superior, lateral greater trochanter	Abduction	Superior gluteal (L_4-S_1)
Gluteus minimus	Between anterior and inferior gluteal lines on posterior ilium	Anterior surface of the greater trochanter	Medial rotation	Superior gluteal (L_4-S_1)
Gracilis	Anterior, inferior symphysis pubis	Medial, proximal tibia	Adduction	Obturator (L_3,L_4)
Adductor magnus	Inferior ramus of pubis and ischium	Entire linea aspera	Adduction	Obturator (L_3,L_4)
Adductor longus	Anterior pubis	Middle linea aspera	Adduction	Obturator (L_2,L_3)
Adductor brevis	Inferior ramus of the pubis	Upper linea aspera	Adduction	Obturator (L_3,L_4)
Semitendinosus	Medial ischial tuberosity	Proximal, medial tibia	Hip extension and knee flexion	Tibial (L_5,S_1)
Semimembranosus	Lateral ischial tuberosity	Proximal, medial tibia	Hip extension and knee flexion	Tibial (L_5,S_1)
Biceps femoris	Posterior lateral ischial tuberosity	Head of fibula and condyle of tibia		
(long head)	Lateral ischial tuberosity		Hip extension and knee flexion	Tibial (L_5–S_2)
(short head)	Lateral linea aspera		Knee flexion	Common peroneal (L_5,S_1)
Lateral rotators	Sacrum, ilium, and ischium	Posterior greater trochanter	Lateral rotation	L_5–S_2

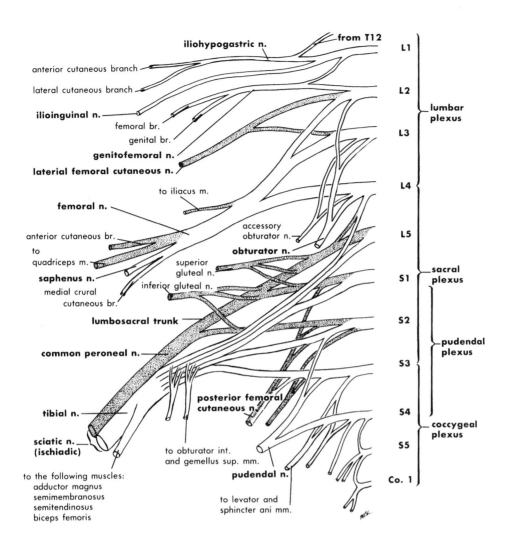

Fig. 9.3: The lumbar and sacral plexus.

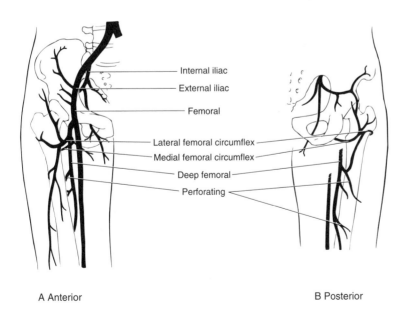

A Anterior

B Posterior

Fig. 9.4: The arterial supply to the hip and thigh region.

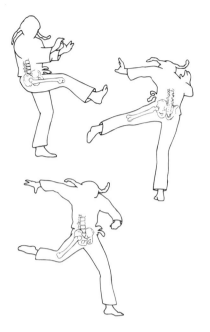

Fig. 9.5: Positioning of the pelvis facilitates motion of the femur.

usually active only when the hip is in flexion, such as during stair climbing or cycling, or when extension at the hip is resisted. The nickname "hamstrings" derives from the prominent tendons of the three muscles, which are readily palpable on the posterior aspect of the knee. The hamstrings cross both the hip and knee, contributing to hip extension and knee flexion.

Abduction

The gluteus medius is the major abductor at the hip with assistance from the gluteus minimus. The hip abductors are active in stabilizing the pelvis during single leg support of the body, and during the support phase of walking and running. For example, when body weight is supported by the right foot during walking, the right hip abductors contract isometrically and eccentrically to prevent the

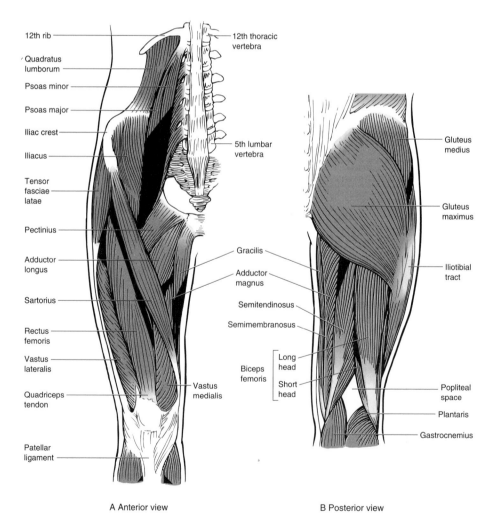

A Anterior view

B Posterior view

Fig. 9.6: The superficial muscles of the hip and thigh. (A) Anterior view. (B) Posterior view.

left side of the pelvis from being pulled downward by the weight of the swinging left leg. This allows the left leg to move freely through the swing phase without scuffing the toes. If the hip abductors are too weak to perform this function, then lateral pelvic tilt occurs with every step during gait.

Adduction

The hip adductors include the adductor longus, adductor brevis, and adductor magnus (**Figure 9-6**). These muscles are active during the swing phase of gait to bring the foot beneath the body's center of gravity for placement during the support phase. The relatively weak gracilis also assists with hip adduction. The hip adductors also contribute to flexion and internal rotation at the hip, especially when the femur is externally rotated.

Medial and Lateral Rotation of the Femur

Although several muscles contribute to lateral rotation of the femur, there are six muscles that function solely as lateral rotators. These are the piriformis, gemellus superior, gemellus inferior, obturator internus, obturator externus, and quadratus femoris (**Figure 9-7**). Lateral rotation of the femur of the swinging leg occurs during gait to accommodate the lateral rotation of the pelvis.

The major medial rotator of the femur is the gluteus minimus, with assistance from the tensor fascia latae, semitendinosus, semimembranosus, gluteus medius, and the four adductor muscles. The medial rotators are weak in comparison to the lateral rotators, with the estimated strength of the medial rotators approximately one third of the lateral

> The hip adductors also contribute to flexion and internal rotation at the hip

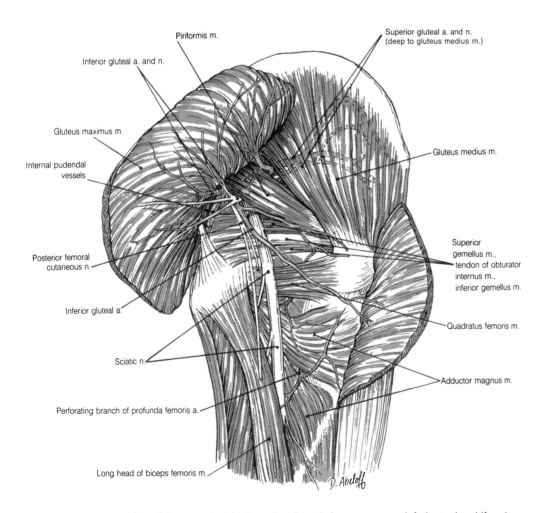

Piriformis m.

Inferior gluteal a. and n.

Gluteus maximus m.

Internal pudendal vessels

Posterior femoral cutaneous n.

Inferior gluteal a.

Sciatic n.

Perforating branch of profunda femoris a.

Long head of biceps femoris m.

Superior gluteal a. and n. (deep to gluteus medius m.)

Gluteus medius m.

Superior gemellus m., tendon of obturator internus m., inferior gemellus m.

Quadratus femoris m.

Adductor magnus m.

D. Abeloff

Fig. 9.7: The deep muscles of the posterior hip. Note that the sciatic nerve passes inferior to the piriformis muscle to enter the posterior thigh.

rotators (1). **Table 9-2** summarizes the muscles responsible for the various motions at the hip joint.

⬤ *When a muscle crosses two joints, the positions of both joints affect the amount of stretch or tension present in the muscle. Both joint positions therefore affect the extent to which a muscle can be stretched during a warm-up exercise, and the amount of force the muscle can produce upon contraction. This principle will have significance for injury assessment.*

KINETICS OF THE HIP

⬤ *What factors contribute to forces on the hip when a person is in a standing position? Do these forces increase or decrease during walking and running?*

Forces at the Hip during Standing

The hip is a major weight-bearing joint that is subject to extremely high loads during sport participation. During upright standing, with weight evenly distributed on both legs, the weight supported at each hip is one-half the weight of the body segments above the hip. However, the total load on each hip in this situation is greater than the weight supported because tension in the large, strong hip muscles further adds to compression at the joint.

Forces at the Hip during Gait

Compression on the hip is approximately the same as body weight during the swing phase of normal walking gait, but increases to at least six times body weight during the stance phase (2). Body weight, impact forces translated upward through the skeleton from the foot, and muscle tension all contribute to this compressive load. Forces on the hip increase along with walking or running speed. Use of a crutch or cane on the side opposite an injured lower limb is beneficial in that it serves to more evenly distribute the load between the legs throughout the gait cycle.

⬤ *Both body weight and tension in the hip muscles contribute to compression at the hip. During walking and running, impact forces are also translated upward through the skeleton from the foot, further increasing compression at the hip. As walking or running speed increases, the forces on the hip increase.*

PREVENTION OF INJURIES TO THE THIGH, HIP, AND PELVIS

⬤ *Muscles of the thigh, hip, and pelvis are used extensively in nearly every physical activity. What exercises will strengthen the muscles in this region to prevent injury?*

As with the knee and lower leg, several factors can prevent injury to the hip region. Wearing protective equipment, wearing shoes with adequate cushion and support, and participating in an extensive physical conditioning program can reduce the incidence of acute and chronic injuries to the region.

Table 9–2. Movement at the Hip and Associated Muscle Action.

Flexion	Extension	Abduction	Adduction	Medial Rotation	Lateral Rotation
Iliopsoas	Gluteus	Gluteus	Pectineus	Gluteus medius	Piriformis
Rectus	maximus	medius	Adductor	Gluteus minimus	Obturator
femoris	Biceps	Gluteus	brevis	Tensor fascia	internus
Pectinius	femoris	minimus	Adductor	latae	Obturator
Sartorius	Semitendinosus	Tensor fascia	longus		externus
Tensor	Semimembranosus	latae	Adductor		Superior
fascia	Adductor	Sartorius	magnus		gemelli
latae	magnus	Piriformis	Gracilis		Inferior gemelli
					Quadratus
					femoris
					Gluteus
					maximus

Protective Equipment

The hip joint is well protected within the pelvic girdle and is seldom injured. In collision and contact sports, however, the hip and buttock region requires special pads to protect vulnerable areas, such as the iliac crests, sacrum and coccyx, and genital region. Protective cups placed in the athletic supporter can protect the male genital region from projectiles. Special commercial pads may also be used to protect soft tissue structures in the thigh and upper leg. Photos of these items can be seen in Figure 6-18.

Physical Conditioning

Exercises to prevent injury to the thigh, hip, and pelvic region are primarily concerned with flexibility and strengthening muscles in the region. Exercises for the quadriceps, hamstrings, and tensor fascia latae were provided in Chapter 8. **Field Strategy 9-1** demonstrates additional exercises for the hip flexors, extensors, adductors, abductors, and medial and lateral rotators.

Shoe Selection

Shoes should adequately cushion impact forces, support, and guide the foot during the

---

 Field Strategy 9–1. Exercises to Prevent Injury at the Thigh, Hip, and Pelvis.

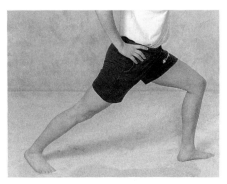

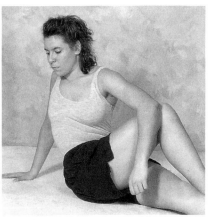

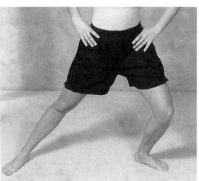

Field Strategy 8-1 demonstrated stretching exercises for the hamstrings, quadriceps, and iliotibial band and strengthening exercises for the muscles that cross the knee joint. In addition to these exercises, the following exercises can be performed.

1. Hip flexor stretch (Lunge). Place the leg to be stretched in front of you. Bend the contralateral knee as you move the hips forward. Keep the back straight. Alternative method: Place the foot on a chair or table and lean forward until a stretch is felt.

2. Lateral rotator stretch, seated position. Cross one leg over the thigh and place the elbow on the outside of the knee. Gently stretch the buttock muscles by pushing the bent knee across the body while keeping the pelvis on the floor.

3. Adductor stretch, standing position. Place the leg to be stretched on a chair or table. Slowly bend the contralateral knee. Keep the hips in a neutral or extended position.

(continued)

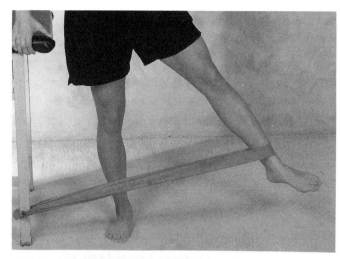

4. Theraband or tubing exercises. Secure Theraband or surgical tubing to a table. Perform hip flexion, extension, abduction, adduction, medial and lateral rotation in a single plane or in multidirectional patterns

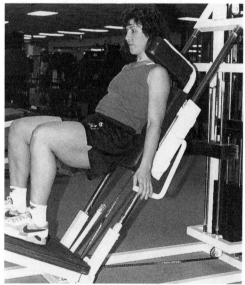

5. Full squats. A weight belt should be worn during this exercise. Place the feet at shoulder width or wider. Keep the back straight by keeping the chest out and the head up at all times. Flex the knees and hips to no greater than 90°. Begin the upward motion by extending the hips first

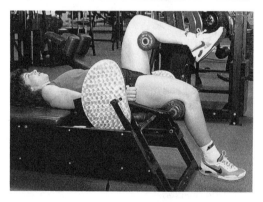

6. Hip extension. With the trunk stabilized and the back flat, extend the hip while keeping the knee flexed. Alternate legs

stance and final pushoff phase of running. Inadequate cushioning in the heel region can transmit forces up the leg, leading to inflammation of the hip joint or stress fractures to the femoral neck or pubis.

Muscles that move the hip must be flexible enough to prevent muscular strains. In addition, range of motion and strengthening exercises for the hip should be incorporated into a year-round physical conditioning program.

CONTUSIONS

❓ *A soccer player took a direct blow to the anterolateral thigh from an opponent's knee during a game. Immediate pain, loss of function, and mild swelling is evident. You want to control acute swelling with ice, compression, and elevation. In what position should the leg be placed to best achieve this objective?*

Contusions may occur anywhere in the hip region, but are typically seen on the crest of the ilium, called a hip pointer, and in the quadriceps muscle group, sometimes referred to as a charley horse. Direct impact to soft tissue, such as a kick to the thigh or a fall onto a hard surface, causes a compressive force to crush soft tissue. The condition may be mild and resolve itself in a matter of days, or the bleeding and swelling may be more extensive resulting in a large, deep hematoma that takes months to resolve. Football and hockey provide special athletic girdles that allow hip and thigh pads to be slipped conveniently into slots, thus protecting the area. These girdles can also be worn in other sports to prevent injury to this vulnerable area.

Quadriceps Contusion

A contusion to the quadriceps results in localized tenderness, swelling, and occasionally bruising or ecchymosis. The injury almost always merges into a muscle strain, with the two usually coexisting as a single injury. If the contusion is located adjacent to the intermuscular septum, pain and hemorrhage tend to resolve more rapidly. Contusions within the muscle itself are often associated with greater tearing, hemorrhage, pain, and a greater tendency toward morbidity. Severity of the injury is almost always underestimated and undertreated. The most common site for a quadriceps contusion is the anterolateral thigh.

Immediately after impact, pain and swelling may be extensive, and if severe, the individual will be unable to bear weight or fully flex the knee. In a mild contusion, the individual will have mild pain and swelling, and will be able to walk without a limp. Passive flexion beyond 90° may be painful, but resisted knee extension may cause less discomfort. In a moderate contusion, the individual can flex the knee only between 45 and 90°, and will walk with a noticeable limp. In a severe contusion, a sympathetic effusion frequently develops over a 24-hour period. Initially, there is little evidence of bruising, but within 24 hours, progressive bleeding and swelling occur, preventing knee flexion beyond 45°. There may be a palpable firm hematoma resulting in an inability to contract the quadriceps or do a straight leg raise (3).

Treatment involves ice application and a compressive wrap for the first 24 hours applied with the knee in maximal flexion (**Figure 9-8**). This position preserves the needed flexion and limits intramuscular bleeding and spasm (4). After 24 hours, gentle passive and active pain-free stretching with daily ice treatments are initiated. Isometric quadriceps strengthening can progress to active stretching and a progressive resistance strengthening program. High voltage galvanic stimulation may be helpful in the early stages. Ultrasound, hydrotherapy, and massage should be avoided in the early stages as they may irritate the inflammatory process, but may be used in later stages to aid recovery. **Field Strategy 9-2** explains the care of a quadriceps contusion.

Myos
itis Ossificans

Myositis ossificans is an abnormal ossification involving bone deposition within muscle tissue, and is seen in varying degrees in as many as 15% of individuals with severe quadriceps contusion (3). It may stem from a single traumatic blow, or several repeated blows to the quadriceps. The anterior and lateral thigh are common sites, however, it may

Contusions to the iliac crest are called hip pointers; those in the quadriceps muscle group are referred to as charley horses

Ultrasound, hydrotherapy, and massage should be avoided in the initial days of treatment as they may irritate the inflammatory process

Myositis ossificans
Ectopic ossification resulting in bone deposition within muscle tissue

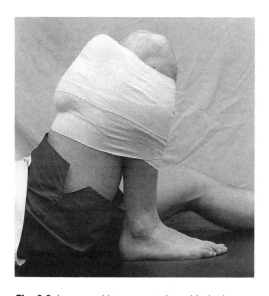

Fig. 9.8: Ice a quadriceps contusion with the knee in maximal flexion to place the muscles on stretch.

Field Strategy 9–2. Management of a Quadriceps Contusion.

Acute phase (first 24 to 48 hours)

- Apply ice packs and compression with knee flexed at 120°
- Crutches with non- or partial-weight bearing
- Pain-free passive stretching
- Pain-free gentle, active range of motion exercises
- Anti-inflammatory medication after 24 hours

Subacute Phase (2 to 5 days)

- Cryotherapy and passive stretching exercises
- Active range of motion exercises
- Pain-free resisted PNF strengthening exercises
- High voltage galvanic stimulation, hot packs, or hydromassage
- Swimming with gentle kicking exercises
- NSAIDs
- Partial weight bearing continued until 90° flexion is attained

Full Weight Bearing

- Discontinue crutches
- Continue active range of motion exercises
- Continue progressive resistance exercises
- Cycling or light jogging as tolerated
- High voltage galvanic stimulation
- Radiograph at 3 weeks to rule out myositis ossificans

Final Phase

- Range of motion within 10° of unaffected leg
- Bilaterally equal strength and endurance
- Work on jumping, starts, stops, changing directions, sprinting
- If progress is slow, consider bone scan
- Return to participation after passing functional tests
- Consider protective padding to prevent reinjury

also occur on the hip, groin, leg, and lateral aspect of the midhumerus. Although the precise mechanism that triggers the bone formation has yet to be established, it is thought that during resolution of the hematoma the inflammatory process falters as the existing fibroblasts involved in the repair process begin to differentiate into osteoblasts within a week after injury (5). The evidence of calcification on a radiograph becomes visible after three to four weeks. As the calcification continues to progress, a palpable firm mass can be felt in the deep tissues. After six to seven weeks, the mass generally stops growing and resorption occurs. However, total resorption may not fully occur, leaving a visible cortical-type bony lesion (**Figure 9-9**) (5).

Examination reveals a warm, firm, swollen thigh nearly 2 to 4 cm larger than the unaf-fected thigh. A palpable mass may limit passive knee flexion to 20 to 30°. Active quadriceps contractions and straight leg raises may be impossible. Refer this individual to a physician. Treatment will include ice, compression, elevation, crutches, protected rest, and non-steroidal anti-inflammatory drugs (NSAIDs) to reduce swelling. Periodic radiographs will generally be taken until the abnormal ossification matures. This typically occurs within 6 to 12 months (3). In cases where the mass fails to reabsorb completely, many individuals return safely to participation with adequate protection from subsequent blows. Surgery is only indicated in cases where activity is limited by pain, weakness, and decreased range of motion (5). Excision before the mass matures may result in reformation, sometimes larger than the original mass.

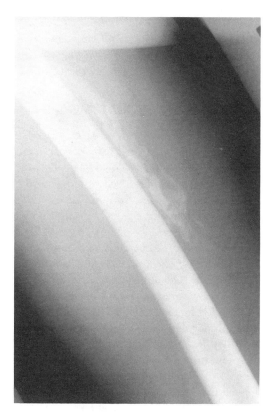

Fig. 9.9: With myositis ossificans, full resorption of the calcification may not occur leaving a visible cortical-type bony lesion.

Hip Pointers

Hip pointers are contusions to an unprotected iliac crest. Because of inadequate soft tissue padding, compression leads to severe crushing of soft tissues and may, in fact, fracture the iliac crest. Injury can occur anywhere along the iliac crest. Because so many trunk and abdominal muscles attach to the iliac crest, any movement of the trunk will be painful including coughing, laughing, and even breathing. Immediate pain, discoloration, spasm, and loss of function will prevent the individual from rotating the trunk or laterally flexing the trunk toward the injured side. In severe injury, the individual may be unable to walk or bear weight, even with crutches, because of the intense pain caused by muscular tension pulling on the injury site. Ice, compression, NSAIDs, and total inactivity should be initiated during the first two to three days following injury. Because the mechanism may also lead to a fracture of the iliac crest, refer the individual to a physician for follow-up radiographs. Heat therapy, ultrasound, transcutaneous electrical nerve

stimulation (TENS), and range of motion exercises may begin after inflammation is controlled. Gradual return to activity with a dense foam donut pad fitted into a custom-formed plastic shell can be used to protect the area from further injury.

The thigh should be maximally flexed during any ice treatment to reduce intramuscular bleeding and spasm. Re-evaluate range of motion following the ice treatment, and the next day to determine the degree of injury. What signs indicate if myositis ossificans may be present?

BURSITIS

A forty-seven-year-old woman is complaining of pain while running. Pain is localized on the posterolateral aspect of the hip near the greater trochanter and occasionally is accompanied by a snapping sensation. What structures are located in this area that might be irritated during repetitive running motions?

Bursitis is common in runners and joggers, and typically affects the trochanteric bursa, iliopsoas bursa, and ischial bursa. The trochanteric bursa can be repeatedly compressed between the greater trochanter and iliotibial tract during the running motion, leading to an aching pain that intensifies after exercise (**Figure 9-10**). Because streets are crowned to allow for run-off, the condition usually affects the down leg, referring to the leg closest to the gutter. Seen commonly in female runners because of the wider pelvis and larger Q angle, it is also seen in runners who cross their feet over the midline as they run, thereby functionally increasing the Q angle. A burning or deep, aching feeling is

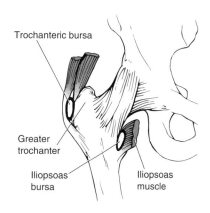

Fig. 9.10: Bursitis at the hip may involve the trochanteric bursa, iliopsoas bursa, or ischial bursa.

Hip pointers
Contusions caused by direct compression to an unprotected iliac crest that crushes soft tissue, and sometimes the bone itself

Any movement of the trunk will be painful, including coughing, laughing, and even breathing

Runners who cross the feet over their midline as they run, functionally increase the Q angle and can develop trochanteric bursitis

felt just posterior to the tip of the greater trochanter, and can be aggravated by contraction of the hip abductors against resistance, or during hip flexion and extension on weight bearing. Referred pain may move distally into the lateral aspect of the thigh.

The iliopsoas bursa can be irritated when the iliopsoas muscle repeatedly compresses the bursa against either the joint capsule of the hip or the lesser trochanter of the femur. Pain is felt more medial and anterior to the joint and cannot be easily palpated. Occasionally, pain can be elicited with passive rotary motions at the hip, or with resisted hip flexion, abduction, and external rotation (3,6).

Direct bruising from a fall can lead to compression of the ischial bursa. Although it is relatively uncommon, it must be differentiated from a hamstring tear at the tendinous attachment or an epiphyseal fracture.

Treatment for bursitis includes ice packs or ice massage, deep friction massage, protected rest, and NSAIDs. A postural examination and biomechanical analysis of the running motion can be done by trained professionals to determine if certain factors contributed to the individual's condition. Different shoes, orthotics, or altering the running technique may correct the problem and avoid recurrence. A flexibility program to stretch the involved muscle should be incorporated within the rehabilitation program. If the condition does not rapidly improve, a bone scan should be conducted to rule out possible femoral neck stress fractures, as these often mimic bursitis symptoms.

Chronic bursitis can lead to **snapping hip syndrome**, and is particularly prominent in dancers. The condition is characterized by a snapping sensation either heard or felt during motion. This may occur in dancers or gymnasts who laterally rotate and flex the hip joint while balancing on one leg during routines, or during foot strike while running as the iliotibial tract snaps over the greater trochanter. If the iliopsoas bursa is affected, the individual may complain of snapping in the medial groin. The condition is usually handled with anti-inflammatories and a stretching program. However, if the snapping is associated with pain or a sense of hip joint instability, the individual should be referred to a physician for follow-up care.

The runner probably has trochanteric bursitis due to the iliotibial tract snapping over the greater trochanter during the running motion. This individual should stretch the iliotibial tract and alter the direction in which she runs to prevent the same leg from being the down leg when running in the street.

SPRAINS AND DISLOCATIONS

A football player was tackled by an opponent when his hip and knee were flexed at 90°. The impact drove the femur posteriorly. The individual is now lying on the ground in great pain with the hip slightly flexed and internally rotated in a fixed position. From the player's position, you have determined that EMS should be immediately summoned. What can you do for the individual while the ambulance is on the way?

Hip joint sprains are rare because of the multitude of movements allowed at the ball and socket joint, and the level of protection provided by layers of muscles that add to its stability. Injury can occur in violent twisting actions or in catastrophic trauma when the knee is driven into a stationary object, such as in an automobile accident when the knee is driven into the dashboard. Traumatic hip dislocations in children are rare, but are more common than femoral neck fractures (7). This may be largely due to the pliable cartilage composition of the acetabula during the early to mid teen years.

Symptoms of a mild or moderate hip sprain mimic those of synovitis, or stress fractures about the hip. Pain is present on hip rotation. Radiographs or bone scans are usually taken to rule out degenerative joint disease, slipped femoral capital epiphysis, and femoral stress fractures. Treatment is symptomatic and may include cryotherapy, NSAIDs, rest, and protected weight bearing on crutches until walking is pain free.

Severe hip sprains and dislocations result in immediate intense pain, and an inability to walk or even move the hip. The hip remains in a characteristic flexed and internally rotated position indicating a posterior, superior dislocation (**Figure 9-11**). In suspecting this injury, initiate the emergency plan and summon EMS. Because the sciatic nerve may be damaged, assess nerve function. Run your fingers down both lower legs and ask the individual where you are touching the leg, and what it feels like. Do they have full or partial sensation? Monitor vital signs and treat for shock. It is imperative not to move the individual until the ambulance arrives. A possible

Snapping hip syndrome
A snapping sensation either heard, or felt during motion at the hip

Hip sprains and dislocations occur in violent twisting actions or in catastrophic trauma, such as when the flexed knee is driven into a stationary object

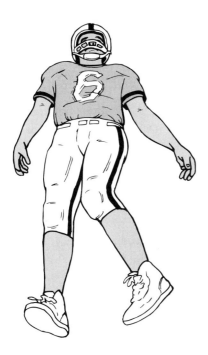

Fig. 9.11: Most hip dislocations drive the head of the femur posterior and superior leaving the leg in a characteristically flexed and internally rotated position.

fracture to the posterior rim of the acetabulum or head of the femur may be present. Movement may damage the blood supply to the head of the femur leading to avascular necrosis. Movement may also cause further damage to surrounding soft tissue structures, complicating joint reduction, thus lengthening the individual's recovery time. The ambulance attendants will splint the hip region and transport the individual to the nearest trauma center.

💡 *While the ambulance is en route, talk to the individual in a calm, reassuring voice, assess the ABC's, monitor the vital signs, check for nerve and circulatory impairment at the lower leg and ankle, and treat for shock. Do not move the individual.*

STRAINS

❓ *A middle distance runner is complaining of a tightness and pulling sensation just distal to the ischial tuberosity. It is uncomfortable when running on level ground, and very painful and tight when running up steep hills. What muscle group may be injured? What is your course of action?*

Muscular strains to the hip and thigh muscles are frequently seen not only in sport, but in many occupations involving repetitive motions. Strains may occur to the quadriceps, hamstrings, adductors (groin), or gluteal muscles. Inadequate stretching, warm-up, or conditioning, coupled with excessive tension forces in the musculotendinous unit can lead to a partial or total tearing of muscle fibers. Furthermore, spasm in the piriformis muscle can compress the sciatic nerve leading to sciatica-like pain and symptoms. Strains may range from mild to severe with the severity of symptoms paralleling the amount of disruption to the fibers. **Table 9-3** summarizes the signs and symptoms of muscular strains in the hip and thigh region.

Quadriceps Strain

A strain of the quadriceps is less common than strains to the hamstrings, although they do occur with regular frequency in sports such as basketball, football, hockey, rugby, and soccer. The rectus femoris is a two-joint muscle and is typically injured during explosive knee extension and hip flexion movements. The explosive muscular contraction can cause an avulsion fracture at the proximal attachment on the AIIS, or tear fibers near the proximal or distal musculotendinous junctions. Compressive forces from a helmet or knee can lead to a massive contusion as discussed earlier, and may lead to a complete rupture of the rectus femoris muscle belly, usually in the mid-thigh region (8). Because it is the most superficial muscle of the quadriceps, any disruption in its continuity is easily visible.

The individual may report a snapping or tearing sensation during an explosive jumping, kicking, or running motion. This is followed by immediate pain, loss of function, and if severe, an inability to bear weight. Assessment will reveal tenderness, swelling, a palpable defect if continuity is disrupted, discoloration, and pain on passive knee flexion, particularly past 90°. Pain and muscle weakness is elicited during resisted hip flexion with the knee flexed at 45° (**Figure 9-12**).

Hamstrings Strains

Hamstrings strains may be caused by a rapid contraction of the muscle during a ballistic action, or a violent stretch. This muscle group is the most frequently strained in the body (9,10). Common sites for muscle tears include the proximal musculotendinous

> The rectus femoris muscle is typically injured during explosive knee extension and hip flexion movements

> A snapping or tearing sensation during an explosive jumping, kicking, or running movement followed by immediate pain and muscle weakness signifies a quadriceps strain

Table 9–3. Muscular Strains and Associated Signs.

HISTORY

Quadriceps. Individual may report a snapping or tearing sensation at AIIS, or at mid-thigh during an explosive kicking, jumping, or running movement

Hamstrings. Individual has a history of poor posture, inflexibility, and muscle imbalance. Injury may occur when muscle function suddenly changes from a stabilizing knee flexor to an active hip extensor, such as in sprinting, and may occur mid-stride with sharp pain in the posterior thigh

Adductors. Individual may report that running straight ahead and backwards does not cause discomfort, but sliding sideways does

Gluteals. Individual will describe muscle overload or repetitive muscular contractions, such as in weight lifting or rowing in crew

Piriformis. History may include prolonged sitting, overuse, or a recent increase in activity. A dull ache in the midbuttock region that worsens at night may be accompanied by weakness and numbness extending down the back of the leg

OBSERVATION

Mild strain. No noticeable limp, but mild swelling is present

Moderate to severe strains. A noticeable limp and moderate swelling is present. Discoloration after a hamstring strain may be present in the popliteal fossa several days after injury

PALPATION

Mild strain. Mild point tenderness over the injury site

Moderate strain. Moderate pain over the injury site. A possible defect may be palpated if continuity of the muscle is disrupted. A warm tender mass indicates swelling

Severe strain. Severe pain and a defect in the muscle continuity will be palpable. A warm painful mass indicates swelling

SIGNS AND SYMPTOMS

Pain will be present with passive stretching and active muscle contraction of the involved muscle.

Severity of injury is gauged by the amount of limited motion. For example:

Quadriceps. 1st°—Passive knee flexion beyond 90° may be painful, but resisted knee extension will cause more discomfort; 2nd°—Passive knee flexion is limited to 45 to 90°. Knee extension is painful and weak. 3rd°—Pain and swelling limit passive knee flexion to <45°. Active hip flexion and knee extension is extremely painful and weak

This increment of disability is applied to other hip muscles in the following motions:

Hamstrings. Pain on passive hip flexion with knee extended. Pain on active knee flexion, and hip extension with the knee extended

Adductors. Pain on passive hip abduction and external rotation. Pain on active hip adduction

Gluteals. Pain on passive hip flexion. Pain on active hip abduction (gluteus medius & gluteus minimus) or hip extension (gluteus maximus)

Piriformis. Pain on passive hip flexion, adduction, and internal rotation. Pain on resisted external rotation

aponeurosis, an avulsion from the ischium, or a tear in the distal muscle belly, although this is rare. The more proximal the injury, the longer the healing time (3).

A hamstrings strain has a reputation of being both chronic and recurring. This is not necessarily due to neglect of hamstring stretching after injury, quite the contrary. Most sport participants are fully aware of limited motion after a strain and concentrate on regaining flexibility through an aggressive stretching program. However, these individu-

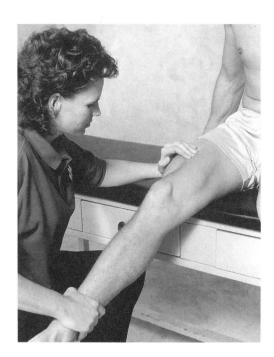

Fig. 9.12: To isolate a painful and weak rectus femoris muscle, do resisted hip flexion with the knee flexed at 45°.

als fail to adequately restrengthen the hamstrings, setting up a muscle imbalance with the quadriceps. During the initial swing phase of gait, the hamstrings act to flex the knee. In late swing, the hamstrings contract eccentrically to control knee extension and re-extend the hip in preparation for the stance phase. The hamstrings are also important dynamic stabilizers at the knee. Atrophy in the medial hamstrings (semitendinosus and semimembranosus) can contribute to anteromedial instability at the knee. Conversely, muscle atrophy of the biceps femoris can contribute to anterolateral instability at the knee. Collectively, hamstrings function antagonistically to resist the quadriceps, and thus may protect an injured or surgically-repaired anterior cruciate ligament (11).

Most strains can be prevented by early detection of inflexibility, poor posture, and muscle imbalance. Other factors, such as muscle fatigue, lack of neuromuscular control, overuse, and improper technique also contribute to a higher risk for injury (6). Discovery of predisposing factors should lead to a preseason flexibility and strengthening program to prevent injuries from occurring.

In mild strains, the individual will complain of tightness and tension in the muscle. Moderate strains will produce an accompanying tearing sensation leading to immediate pain and weakness in knee flexion. In more severe cases, a sharp pain will be present in the posterior thigh and may occur during mid-stride. The individual will limp and be unable to fully extend the knee. Pain and muscle weakness is elicited during active knee flexion. Frequently, profuse swelling and ecchymosis will become visible in the popliteal fossa one to two days after injury.

Adductor (Groin) Strain

Adductor strains are common in activities that require quick changes of direction, and in those requiring explosive propulsion and acceleration, such as hockey, football, soccer, the high jump, or in the breaststroke (3,12). The more severe strains are typically at the muscles' proximal attachment on the hip, particularly the adductor longus. Milder strains may occur more distally at the musculotendinous junction.

The individual will complain of sharp pain in the groin region followed by increased pain, stiffness, and weakness in hip adduction and flexion. Running straight ahead or backwards may be tolerable, but any side-to-side movement will lead to more discomfort and pain. Localized tenderness can be palpated on the ischiopubic ramus, lesser trochanter, or musculotendinous junction. Increased pain will be present during passive stretching with the hip extended, abducted, and externally rotated (13). Pain with hip flexion against resistance may be indicative of a strain to the rectus femoris or sartorius. Pain with hip adduction against resistance indicates adductor strain. Occasionally, a palpable defect may be found, indicating a more serious injury.

Groin pain may also be referred from problems in the bowel, bladder, testicle, kidney, abdomen, rectum, hip joint, sacroiliac joint, symphysis pubis, lymph nodes, or rectus abdominis muscle. In addition, stress fractures, avulsion injuries, osteitis pubis, tumors, avascular necrosis of the femoral head, hernias, and various forms of arthritis may also lead to pain in the groin region (13). In adolescents, epiphyseal injuries (slipped

Many individuals fail to restrengthen the hamstrings after injury, thereby setting up a muscle imbalance with the quadriceps

In a hamstring strain, the individual will limp and be unable to fully extend the knee

Adductor strains are common in activities that require quick changes of direction, and in those requiring explosive propulsion and acceleration

The person may be able to tolerate running straight ahead, but any side-to-side movement causes pain

Groin pain may be referred from the bowel, bladder, testicle, kidney, abdomen, rectum, hip joint, sacroiliac joint, symphysis pubis, tumors, avascular necrosis of the femoral head, hernias, and arthritis

capital femoral epiphysis), and apophyseal fractures may be overlooked and simply misevaluated as a groin strain. If assessed as an adductor strain, but the condition does not improve within two to five days, refer the individual to a physician for follow-up care.

Gluteal Muscles

The gluteal muscles are rarely injured because of their size and strength. These muscles may be injured, however, in activities that require muscle overload, such as in power weight lifting or rowing in crew. Symptoms will be the same as in other muscular strains. Passive stretching and resisted hip extension or abduction will cause discomfort.

Piriformis Syndrome

The individual may have a dull ache in the midbuttock region, pain that worsens at night, difficulty climbing stairs, and numbness down the posterior leg

The sciatic nerve passes through the sciatic notch beneath the piriformis muscle to travel into the posterior thigh (**Figure 9-7**). In about 10 to 15 percent of the population, the nerve passes through or above the muscle, subjecting the nerve to compression from trauma, hemorrhage, or spasm of the piriformis muscle (3). The incidence of piriformis syndrome has been reported to be six times more prevalent in women than men (14). Resulting symptoms may mimic a herniated lumbar disk problem with nerve root impingement. The individual may complain of a dull ache in the midbuttock region, pain that worsens at night, difficulty walking up stairs or on an incline, and weakness or numbness down the back of the leg. Low back pain is not usual. A history of prolonged sitting, overuse, a recent increase in activity, or buttock trauma may be reported (15).

Assessment will reveal point tenderness in the midbuttock region and weakness on hip abduction and external rotation. The individual may stand with the leg in slight external rotation. Pain can be elicited with the individual supine and the hip flexed, adducted and internally rotated, as this stretches the piriformis muscle. Straight leg raising may be limited and there may be a positive Faber's test (**see Figure 9-27**)

Treatment and Rehabilitation

In severe strains, a compression wrap should be applied from the toe to groin, as one applied only around the thigh region may lead to venous thrombosis and/or distal edema

Treatment for muscle strains involves immediate ice, compression, elevation, protected rest, and NSAIDs. Whenever possible, muscles should be iced in a stretched position and crutches used if the individual walks with a limp.

In severe strains, a compression wrap may be indicated from the toe to groin. Isolated compression around the thigh region may lead to venous thrombosis and/or distal edema (6).

After the acute inflammatory phase has progressed to resolution of the hematoma, pain-free gentle stretching and isometric contractions can begin with cryotherapy and electrical modalities (3,16). Active stretching, progressive resistance exercises, soft tissue mobilization, and swimming, cycling, mild jogging, and stair climbing can begin when the region is pain-free and range of motion is within 10° of the uninvolved limb. Many of the stretching and strengthening exercises were discussed in **Field Strategy 8-1** and **9-1**. When jogging is comfortable, skipping and rope jumping may begin. Rapid stops, starts, and changing directions are not allowed until the individual can achieve full pain-free motion. The individual should not be returned to sport participation until normal muscle strength and power are achieved. With a severe quadriceps strain, carefully monitor the progress to ensure that myositis ossificans is not occurring. Protective padding of the area may reduce the risk of reinjury from direct trauma.

Did you determine the runner strained the hamstrings? If so, you are correct. This individual should incorporate a stretching program after the acute phase is concluded, and should strengthen the hamstrings to prevent reoccurrence.

VASCULAR DISORDERS

A baseball player was struck on the medial side of the distal thigh with a line drive. Ice, compression, and elevation significantly reduced the initial swelling and discoloration but now, several days later, the individual is complaining of an aching, burning pain and superficial tenderness over the area. How can you account for this delayed burning pain? What vascular structures pass through this area that may have been damaged in the blow? What further treatment is necessary?

Vascular disorders should be suspected in injuries caused by compression, or in an injury where no physical findings support the continued discomfort

Vascular disorders should be suspected in any lower extremity injury caused by compression from high velocity-low mass projectiles, and in an injury where no physical findings support the continued discomfort. Fractures to the hip or femur can cause significant damage to deep lying arteries, leading to a loss of blood and hypovolemic shock.

Muscle strains or contusions can also disrupt the vascular system. If an acute problem exists in circulation, the lower leg and foot may appear pale, cyanotic, be cool to the touch, or have diminished or total loss of sensitivity. Immobilization of the limb and transportation to the nearest trauma center is a priority to restore proper circulation to the involved extremity.

Legg-Calvé-Perthes Disease

Legg-Calvé-Perthes disease, or avascular necrosis of the proximal femoral epiphysis, is a self-limiting congenital disorder seen in young children, especially males ages three to eight (3,6). It is considered to be an **osteochondroses** condition of the femoral head, caused by diminished blood supply to the capital region of the femur (**Figure 9-13**). The individual will limp, and pain may be referred to the groin or knee region.

Examination will reveal a decreased range of motion in hip abduction, extension, and external rotation due to muscle spasm in the hip flexors and adductors. This condition should be suspected in this age group when pain in the groin, anterior thigh, or knee region cannot be explained. If pain persists for more than one week after initial acute care, or if the individual continues to limp after activity, immediate referral to a physician is needed. Early recognition can pre-

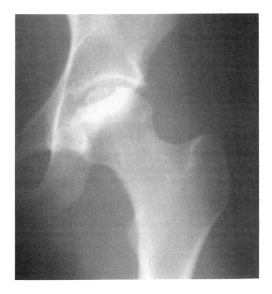

Fig. 9.13: Osteochondrosis of the left femoral head (Legg-Calvé-Perthes disease). Note the destruction of the articular cartilage. In mild cases, no restriction of activity is indicated.

vent the adolescent from having severe hip problems, osteoarthritis, or permanent disability later in life. Confirmation of the condition is made through radiographs, bone scans, or magnetic resonance imagings (MRI's). Treatment can be quite extensive, sometimes taking one to two years, and may involve immobilization, non-weight bearing, and possible surgery to prevent any further deformity of the femoral head due to the avascular necrosis.

Venous disorders

A direct blow from a high-velocity loss mass projectile, such as a baseball, softball, puck, or helmet, may damage a vein causing thrombophlebitis or phlebothrombosis. **Thrombophlebitis** is an acute inflammation of a vein; **phlebothrombosis** is a thrombosis, or clotting, in a vein without overt inflammatory signs and symptoms. Superficial thrombophlebitis is the preferred term for inflammation of superficial veins. The term deep venous thrombosis is preferred for problems with deep veins.

Superficial thrombophlebitis may present itself as acute, aching or burning pain, and superficial tenderness. It is usually more painful than deep venous thrombosis and may be associated with varicose veins (17). Treatment involves external support with compression stockings or elastic bandages, ambulation and lower extremity exercises, periodic elevation of the extremity, and avoidance of long-term sitting or standing in one position. Deep venous thrombosis is typically asymptomatic and may not become apparent until a pulmonary embolism occurs. A **pulmonary embolism** results when a blood clot travels through the circulatory system to lodge in a blood vessel in the lungs. The calf veins are more frequently involved, but the popliteal, superficial femoral, and ileofemoral vein segments are also commonly involved (17). The most reliable signs are chronic swelling and edema in the involved extremity, and a positive Homan's sign (See **Figure 9-31**). Treatment will involve anticoagulant therapy and bed rest with the foot of the bed elevated to maximize venous drainage until signs and symptoms, particularly edema, subside. Surgical intervention may be necessary to prevent a pulmonary embolism.

💡 *An aching, burning pain and superficial tenderness is present several days after*

Legg-Calvé-Perthes disease
Avascular necrosis of the proximal femoral epiphysis seen especially in young males ages 3 to 8

Osteochondroses
Any condition characterized by degeneration or aseptic necrosis of the articular cartilage due to limited blood supply

Treatment may take one to two years and involve immobilization, non-weight bearing, and occasionally surgery to prevent further damage to the femoral head

Thrombophlebitis
Acute inflammation of a vein

Phlebothrombosis
Thrombosis, or clotting, in a vein without overt inflammatory signs and symptoms

Pulmonary embolism
Occurs when a blood clot travels through the circulatory system to lodge in a blood vessel in the lungs

injury, despite adequate acute care. This individual should be referred to a physician for assessment, since delayed treatment could cause serious complications. Anytime an aching, burning sensation is unexplained, always refer the individual to a physician.

HIP FRACTURES

❓ *During the take-off on a high jump an individual experienced a painful snap on the anterior iliac crest. Pain increased on palpation of the ASIS during active hip flexion, and while placing the ankle of the involved leg on the contralateral knee. What might have occurred to this person? How will you manage this injury?*

Major fractures to the pelvic girdle and hip often result from severe direct trauma. This may occur when an individual is thrown from a horse onto hard ground, when a hockey player collides with the side boards, or in rugby or football when another player falls on top of a downed player. In sports where this might occur, such as football and hockey, the pelvic region is usually adequately protected by padding to prevent such injuries. As such, traumatic pelvic fractures are seldom seen in sport participation. Fractures that may be seen in this region include avulsion and apophyseal fractures, epiphyseal fractures, and stress fractures.

Avulsion Fractures

Avulsion fractures follow violent or explosive muscular contractions against a fixed resistance, sudden deceleration or stretching of the involved muscle, or as a result of direct trauma. Sprinters, hurdlers, kickers, gymnasts, dancers, and other individuals who perform rapid, sudden acceleration and deceleration moves are at risk for these injuries. Common sites for avulsion fractures include the ASIS with the sartorius being displaced, AIIS with the rectus femoris being displaced, ischial tuberosity with the hamstrings being displaced, and the lesser trochanter with the iliopsoas being displaced (**Figure 9-14**). Many of these apophyseal sites do not unite with the bone until ages 18 to 25. As such, these sites continue to be prone to fracture during an individual's competitive interscholastic and intercollegiate years.

The individual will complain of sudden acute localized pain that may radiate down the muscle. Examination will reveal severe

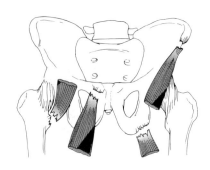

Fig. 9.14: Several major muscles attach to the pelvis, but can be avulsed from their bony attachment during muscular action. Can you name the muscles illustrated here?

pain, swelling, bruising, and tenderness directly over the tendinous attachment on the bony landmark. Pain is increased with passive stretching of the involved muscle, and during active and resisted motion. Depending on the fracture site, immobilization from an elastic compression spica wrap may limit motion and decrease pain. After fitting the individual with crutches, refer the adolescent or young adult to a physician for radiograph examination. Ice, rest, modified activity, and protected weight bearing with crutches for four to six weeks will provide adequate healing for an undisplaced fracture. Range of motion exercises should be discouraged until the fracture has healed, but isometric exercises can be performed if pain-free. Once healed, restoration of range of motion and strength should be initiated with gradual return to activity. If returned to vigorous activity too soon, a bony prominence may form at the site of the avulsion. In a complete displaced avulsion fracture, a gap may be palpated between the tendon's attachment and bone. Fractures of this type require surgical repair.

Epiphyseal Fractures

An epiphyseal fracture seen in adolescent boys age 8 to 15 occurs across the capital femoral epiphysis—the growth plate at the femoral head (**Figure 9-15**). The condition is seen in obese, or rapidly growing, slender boys. Although it may occur in conjunction with a hip dislocation or subluxation, it typically originates as a congenital disorder that develops over time. As the proximal femoral growth plate deteriorates, the individual begins to develop a painful limp with groin pain. Pain may also be referred to the anterior

---

Avulsion fractures occur during explosive muscular contractions against fixed resistance, or during rapid acceleration

---

In a complete displaced avulsion fracture, an obvious defect may be palpated between the bone and tendon's attachment

---

An epiphyseal fracture should be suspected when knee or thigh pain cannot be supported by physical findings

---

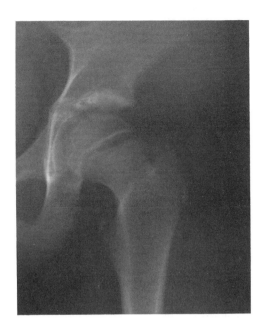

Fig. 9.15: An epiphyseal fracture seen in adolescents age 12 to 15 occurs through the growth plate at the femoral head. With this fracture, the patient will be unable to internally rotate the femur.

thigh or knee region. This condition should always be suspected when knee or thigh pain cannot be supported by any physical findings.

The condition leads to synovitis of the hip and an accompanying psoas major spasm. The individual will feel more comfortable holding the leg in slight flexion. During passive hip flexion, the leg tends to move into external rotation and slight abduction rather than staying in the midline. The individual will be unable to internally rotate the femur or stand on one leg. If the obturator nerve is damaged during the fracture, an aching pain may be referred to the groin, medial thigh, or knee. Radiographs of the hip will confirm the condition, and rule out other possible conditions, such as tumors, bone cysts, and underlying osteochondromas that may also lead to hip pain (6). In nearly all cases, surgery is indicated.

Stress Fractures

Stress fractures to the pubis, femoral neck, and proximal third of the femur are seen in individuals who do extensive jogging or aerobic dance activities. These fractures frequently occur after an excessive increase in one's activity level in which exertion to the point of muscle fatigue occurs (18). An aching pain is localized in the anterior groin

or thigh region, increasing after weight-bearing activity, but is relieved with rest. Night pain is a frequent complaint. Deep palpation in the inguinal area will produce discomfort. Increased pain on the extremes of hip rotation and an inability to stand on the involved leg may indicate a femoral neck stress fracture (3).

Bone scans are frequently used for early diagnosis to prevent delayed treatment. Subsequent radiographs will show periosteal bone formation and a faint fracture line. If diagnosed early enough, rest is indicated for at least two to three months with no weight-bearing activity until the fracture is completely healed (19). Swimming can be performed to maintain cardiovascular fitness, however, the whip kick and scissors kick should be avoided. Displaced stress fractures to the femoral neck require pin fixation to prevent a complete fracture and avascular necrosis of the femoral head from occurring (20,21).

Osteitis pubis is a stress fracture caused by continued stress on the symphysis pubis from repeated overload of the adductor muscles, or from repetitive stress activities, such as long-distance running. Pain is localized over the symphysis pubis and increases with activity. Treatment is symptomatic with ice, protected rest, and anti-inflammatory medication until the condition is resolved.

Displaced and Nondisplaced Pelvic Fractures

Major fractures to the pelvis seldom occur in sport participation, except in activities such as equestrian sports, hockey, rugby, skiing, or football. This crushing injury produces severe pain, total loss of function, and in many cases, severe loss of blood leading to **hypovolemic shock**. Fractures may involve more than one break in the ring, leading to pelvic instability and serious complications. The extent of blood loss is often obscured because hemorrhage occurs within the pelvic cavity, and as such, is not visible. In addition, possible internal injuries to the genitourinary system, such as rupture of the bladder or laceration of the urethra may also occur. In dramatic, severe fractures, this internal damage and subsequent shock may lead to death.

A possible pelvic fracture can be determined with slight compression to the sides of the ilium and the ASIS. Fractures to the acetabulum can be detected by gently placing upward pressure on the femur against the

Stress fractures often occur after an increase in one's activity level in which exertion to the point of muscle fatigue occurs

Swimming can be done to maintain cardiorespiratory fitness, however, avoid the whip and scissors kick

Osteitis pubis
Stress fracture to the pubic symphysis caused by repeated overload of the adductor muscles, or repetitive stress activities

Major pelvic fractures produce severe pain, total loss of function, and severe loss of blood that can lead to hypovolemic shock and subsequent death

Hypovolemic shock
Shock caused by excessive loss of whole blood or plasma

acetabulum (**Figure 9-16**). If a fracture is suspected, summon EMS. Monitor vital signs frequently and watch for signs of internal hemorrhage and shock. Cover the individual with a blanket to maintain body temperature. When EMS arrives, place the individual on a long spine board in the position in which they were found. The foot of the board is elevated 8 to 12 inches to reduce pooling of blood and fluids in the pelvic region and lower extremities during transportation to the nearest trauma center.

Femoral Fractures

Fractures to the femoral shaft can be very serious because of potential damage to the neurovascular structures from bony fragments. Femoral shaft fractures are caused by tremendous impact forces, such as shearing or torsion forces when an alpine skier falls, or from direct compressive forces in football, hockey, or rugby. Fractures may be open or closed with significant bleeding at the fracture site. Signs and symptoms of a displaced fracture include a shortened limb deformity, severe angulation with the thigh externally rotated, swelling into the soft tissues, severe pain, and total loss of function. Non-displaced fractures will reveal extreme pain on palpation, crepitation, weakness, spasm, and swelling. Bilateral comparison with the unaffected leg can differentiate a possible fracture from a quadriceps contusion.

It is not unusual that significant bleeding in the thigh will also lead to hypovolemic shock, similar to that seen in pelvic fractures. Be alert to this factor and treat for shock. Vascular damage may lead to impaired circulation distal to the injury, causing a pale, cold, pulseless foot. Treatment involves initiating the emergency procedures plan. This fracture is best immobilized in a traction splint (See **Figure 3-4**), and should be applied by trained personnel. Any bleeding should be covered with a dry, sterile dressing to protect the area from further contamination. Distal neurovascular function should be assessed immediately and monitored frequently. Palpate a pulse at the posterior tibial artery and dorsalis pedis artery. Look for pale skin at the foot and feel for cool skin temperature. Stroke the dorsum and plantar aspect of both feet, and ask the individual if the feeling is the same on the involved leg as on the uninvolved leg. The leg should be totally immobilized and the individual transported immediately to the nearest trauma center. **Table 9-4** summarizes signs and symptoms of the various fractures seen in the pelvis and thigh region.

Pain was palpated directly on the ASIS and increased with active hip flexion. This is probably a result of an avulsion fracture to the ASIS from an explosive contraction of the sartorius muscle. Immobilize the region with an elastic compression hip spica wrap, fit the individual with crutches, and refer the individual immediately to a physician.

Signs and symptoms of displaced femoral fracture:
  deformity and severe angulation with the thigh externally rotated
  swelling into the soft tissues
  shortened limb
  total loss of function
  severe pain

Vascular damage may lead to a pale, cold, pulseless foot

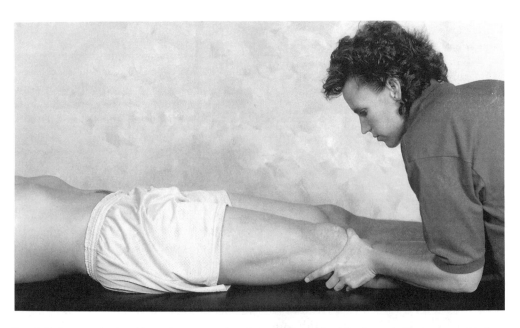

Fig. 9.16: Increased pain with gentle compression along the long axis of the femur indicates a possible fracture of the femur or acetabulum.

Table 9–4. Fractures and Associated Signs.

Fracture	Common Sites	History	Observation	Palpation	Signs and Symptoms
Avulsion and apophyseal	ASIS, AIIS, ischial tuberosity, lesser trochanter	Violent or explosive muscular contraction against fixed resistance or by direct trauma	Possible swelling at site	Severe pain and tenderness directly over bony landmark	Increased pain with active motion in involved muscle
Epiphyseal	Capital femoral epiphysis	May occur in conjunction with dislocation or subluxation. May describe hip subluxation. pain in groin, medial thigh or knee	Joint may appear normal	May not provide significant findings	Unable to internally rotate the thigh
Stress	Pubis, femoral neck, proximal third of femur	Repeated muscle overload or excessive increased activity level, especially in females. Pain is worse before and after activity, but relieved with rest	Joint may appear normal	May have point tenderness over the fracture site	Possible limp as fracture progresses
Pelvic girdle	Wing of ilium or acetabulum	Severe crushing or compression injury	May show signs of shock	Severe pain directly over fracture site. + pelvic gapping test. + compression test along long axis of femur	Total loss of function. May show signs of shock
Femoral	Shaft of femur or femoral neck	Severe shearing, torsion, or direct compressive force	Deformity and severe angulation with thigh externally rotated; shortened limb; swelling into soft tissues	Severe pain and crepitation at fracture site; + compression test along long axis of femur	Total loss of function. May show signs of shock. May have vascular damage leading to pale, cold, pulseless foot

ASSESSMENT

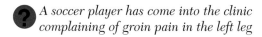

A soccer player has come into the clinic complaining of groin pain in the left leg during running and kicking motions. Can you assume the injury is only related to muscle disruption? Why not?

The lower extremity works as a unit to transmit load from the upper body to the ground through a closed kinetic chain. In the closed chain, the foot, ankle, leg, and hip also absorb force from the ground and dissipate the stress throughout the various structures. When excessive loads and stress exceed the tissues' yield point, injury occurs. Furthermore, the hip is a common site for referred pain from visceral, low back, and knee conditions. As such, evaluations must be inclusive, particularly with adolescents complaining of groin pain. In the absence of direct trauma to the hip, or in situations where improvement is not seen in two to five days, always refer the individual to a physician to rule out serious underlying conditions.

HISTORY

What information should be gathered from the individual complaining of vague groin pain during running and kicking activities? What questions can identify the four main components of the primary complaint?

Many conditions at the hip may be related to family history, age, congenital deformity, improper biomechanical execution of skills, and recent changes in training programs, surfaces, or foot attire. You should gather information on the mechanism of injury, associated symptoms, the progression of the symptoms, any disabilities that may have resulted from the injury, and related medical history. In addition to general questions discussed in Chapter 4, specific questions related to the thigh, hip, and pelvis region can be seen in **Field Strategy 9-3**.

The seventeen-year old soccer player has been plagued with chronic pain in the groin region since mid-season. Pain increases throughout practice and is very painful when the left leg is used to kick, or to push off from when changing directions quickly. Going up and down stairs is also uncomfortable. A few days rest with ice treatments did help, but pain returned when participation was started again. Nothing in the family history or past related medical history seems to be a factor.

OBSERVATION AND INSPECTION

Would a posture and gait analysis be indicated with this individual? Why? What specific postural factors might contribute to pain in the hip and pelvic region?

In the examination room, the individual should wear running shorts to allow full view of the lower extremity. However, this may not be possible in an acute injury that occurs on the field, such as in football or hockey where protective equipment or the uniform may obstruct the view. In these cases, determination of the condition may rest more heavily on palpation and special tests. With individuals who are non-ambulatory, complete all observations, inspection, and palpations for possible fractures and dislocations prior to moving the individual.

Observe for symmetry in the region. Note any visible congenital deformity (excessive femoral torsion, abnormal positioning of the patella, toeing in, toeing out), swelling, discoloration, hypertrophy, muscle atrophy, or previous surgical incisions. If time permits, a full postural assessment and gait analysis should be completed. The individual should be viewed from an anterior, lateral, and posterior position. Specific areas on which to focus in this region are summarized in **Field Strategy 9-4**. After completing a static exam, observe the individual walking from an anterior, posterior, and lateral view. Note any abnormalities in gait. Ask the person if any actions cause pain or discomfort. In adolescent boys who limp, ask when the limp started. Does the pain or limp come and go? What activities make it worse, better? You are investigating the possibility of a congenital defect in the femoral head with these questions and observations. Inspect the specific injury site for obvious deformities, discoloration, edema, scars that might indicate previous surgery, and note the general condition of the skin. Always do bilateral comparison.

You observed no postural abnormalities in the standing position. Pain increased when standing only on the affected leg. Slight discoloration and swelling are present in the groin region on the anterior proximal thigh.

PALPATIONS

With pain centered on the anterior groin region, think for a minute where you will begin to palpate the various structures. Should you start in the groin or begin away from the painful area?

Bilateral palpations can determine temperature, swelling, point tenderness, crepitus, deformity, muscle spasm, and cutaneous sensation. Vascular pulses can be taken at the femoral artery in the groin, popliteal artery in

Field Strategy 9–3. Developing a History of the Injury.

Current Injury Status

1. Where is the pain (or weakness) located? Can you point to the area that is the most uncomfortable? On a scale of 1 to 10 with 10 being very severe, how would you rate your pain (weakness)? What type of pain is it? Does the pain radiate? (Hip pain may be referred pain so ask additional questions if you suspect a visceral, low back, lumbar, or knee problem).
2. Did the pain come on gradually (overuse) or suddenly (acute)? How long has it been a problem? Was the pain greatest when the injury first occurred or did it get worse the second or third day? What have you done for the condition? Does it hurt when you walk, run, twist, or change directions?
3. If you have an acute problem identify the mechanism of injury. Ask: What were you doing at the time of the injury? What position was the leg in when the injury occurred? Was there direct trauma? If the injury came on gradually ask: Have you had recent changes in your training methods, such as an increase in frequency, duration, or intensity of training, or changes in shoes, equipment, or running surface?
4. Did you hear any sounds during the incident? Any snapping, tearing, or cracks? (Snapping may indicate bursitis; tearing may indicate a muscle strain). Can you bear weight on the leg? Was there any swelling or discoloration at the time of injury? Have you had any muscle spasms or numbness since the injury? How soon did it occur? What did you do for it?
5. What actions or motions bring on the pain? Is it worse in the morning, during activity, after activity, or at night? Does it wake you up at night? When the pain sets in, how long does it last? Has there been any improvement in your condition?
6. Are there certain activities you are unable to perform because of the pain? Which ones? How old are you? (Remember some problems are age-related). Which leg is dominant?

Past Injury Status

1. Have you ever injured your hip or low back before? When? How did that occur? Who evaluated and cared for the injury? What have you done since then to strengthen the area and prevent recurrence? Did you have any difficulty returning to your full functional status?
2. Have you had any medical problems recently? (Look for problems that may refer pain to the area from the abdominal viscera or lumbar spine). Are you on any medication? Do you have any musculoskeletal problems elsewhere in the body? What shoes do you wear? (These may lead to changes in gait or technique that transfer abnormal forces to structures in the involved limb).

the posterior knee, and posterior tibial artery and dorsalis pedis artery in the foot (See **Figures 7-17** and **8-4**). Proceed proximal to distal, but leave the most painful area to last. Have the individual non-weight bearing, preferably on a table. When the individual is face down or prone on the table, always place a pillow under the hip and abdominal area to reduce strain on the low back region.

Pain during palpation of bony structures may indicate a displaced avulsion fracture or femoral shaft fracture. Compression, distraction, percussion or use of a tuning fork on specific bony landmarks may also be used to determine a possible fracture. For example, to determine a possible fracture to the acetabulum, femoral neck or head, slowly apply a compressive force to the hip through the longitudinal axis of the femur by pushing through the femoral condyles (See **Figure 9-16**). A possible pelvic fracture can be determined with the pelvic gapping test (See **Figure 9-18**). If you suspect a fracture, immediately assess circulatory and neural integrity distal to the fracture site, summon EMS, take vital signs, and treat for shock.

Anterior Palpations

1. Iliac crest, ASIS, tensor fascia latae, and sartorius
2. Inguinal ligament, lymph nodes, symphysis pubis, greater trochanter, trochanteric bursa, and abductors (gluteus medius and gluteus minimis)

> Vascular pulses may be taken at the femoral artery in the groin, popliteal artery in the posterior knee, and posterior tibial artery and dorsalis pedis artery in the foot

> Use the pelvic gapping test to help determine a possible hip fracture

Field Strategy 9–4. Postural Assessment of the Hip Region.

Anterior View

1. The iliac crests should be level. Leg length discrepancies may alter the height on one side leading to lateral pelvic tilt. Ask the person to stand on one leg and view the level of the iliac crests
2. The anterior superior iliac spines should be level and an equal distance from the center of the body
3. The greater trochanters should be level
4. Both thighs should look the same. Ask the athlete to contract the quadriceps. Check for hypertrophy or atrophy. Check the patella's relative position and alignment, and note any internal or external rotation of the thigh
5. Check the skin for normal contours, discolored lesions, bruising, ecchymosis, and scars indicating a previous injury or surgery. Note any signs of circulatory impairment or varicose veins

Posterior View

1. The iliac crests should be level
2. The posterior superior iliac spines should be level and an equal distance from the center of the body. Uneven skin depressions may indicate lateral pelvic tilt
3. The gluteal and knee folds should be level
4. The ischial tuberosities should be level. The hamstrings and calf muscles should have equal bulk
5. Check the popliteal fossa for abnormal bruising that may indicate a recent hamstring strain

Lateral View

1. Check to see if there is excessive lumbar lordosis or flat back caused by anterior or posterior pelvic tilt, respectively. Anterior pelvic tilt may also be indicative of hip flexion contractures. Is genu recurvatum (hyperextension of the knees) present?
2. Check for any skin abnormalities, bruising, discoloration, or scars indicating previous injuries or surgery

3. Femoral triangle, femoral artery, psoas bursa, and flexor and adductor muscles (pectineus, adductor brevis, adductor longus, adductor magnus, and gracilis)
4. Quadriceps muscles (vastus lateralis, rectus femoris, vastus medialis, vastus intermedius)

Posterior Palpations

1. Iliac crest and PSIS
2. Ischial tuberosity, ischial bursa, hamstring muscles (lateral-biceps femoris; medial-semitendinosus and semimembranosus), and greater trochanter
3. Sacroiliac, lumbosacral, and sacrococcygeal joints

Painful palpation in the anterior groin area extended from the inguinal ligament and femoral triangle distal for about three inches. The area was warm to the touch *and slightly swollen. No other painful or warm sites were palpable.*

SPECIAL TESTS

Pain and discoloration are isolated in the anteromedial groin region. What special tests can be performed to determine if the injury is muscular, capsular, or neurovascular?

Always perform any special tests in a comfortable position for the patient and begin with gentle stress. Pain and muscle spasm may prevent an accurate assessment of the extent of weakness or instability, but do not force the limb through any sudden motions, nor cause any undue pain. Proceed cautiously through the examination.

Active Movements

Active movements can be performed in a seated or prone position with the most painful movements done last. The following movements should be assessed with a hip injury:

1. Knee extension (0 to 15°)
2. Lateral rotation (40 to 60°)
3. Medial rotation (30 to 40°)
4. Hip flexion (110 to 120°) with knee flexed
5. Abduction (30 to 50°)
6. Adduction (30°)
7. Knee flexion (0 to 135°)
8. Hip extension (10 to 15°)

Measuring range of motion at the hip with a goniometer is demonstrated in **Figure 9-17**.

Passive Range of Motion

If the individual is able to perform full range of motion during active movements, apply gentle pressure at the extremes of motion to determine end feel. The end feel for hip flexion and adduction is tissue approximation; hip extension, abduction, and medial and lateral rotation is tissue stretch. Passive movements at the pelvic joint also stress the ligamentous structures at these joints and will be discussed in this section.

Gapping Test

With the individual supine, apply a cross-arm pressure down and outward to the anterior superior iliac spines with your thumbs (**Figure 9-18**). Unilateral gluteal or posterior leg pain may indicate a sprain to the anterior sacroiliac ligaments. Sharp pain elsewhere along the pelvic ring with outward pressure, or with bilateral compression of the iliac crests may indicate a pelvic fracture.

> The end feel for hip flexion and adduction is tissue approximation; hip extension, abduction, and medial and lateral rotation is tissue stretch

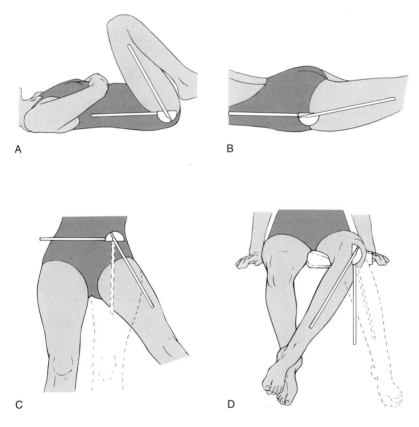

Fig. 9.17: Goniometry measurements for the hip. (A) Hip flexion. Center the fulcrum over the greater trochanter of the femur. Align the proximal arm with the lateral margin of the pelvis. Align the distal arm along the lateral midline of the femur using the lateral epicondyle as reference. (B) Hip extension. Alignment is the same as for measuring hip flexion except the individual is prone. (C) Hip abduction and adduction. Center the fulcrum over the anterior superior iliac spine (ASIS) of the extremity being measured. Align the proximal arm along an imaginary horizontal line extending to the other ASIS. Align the distal arm along the middle of the femur using the midline of the patella for reference. (D) Hip medial and lateral rotation. Center the fulcrum over the anterior aspect of the patella. Align the proximal arm perpendicular to the floor. Align the distal arm using the crest of the tibia and a point midway between the two malleoli for reference.

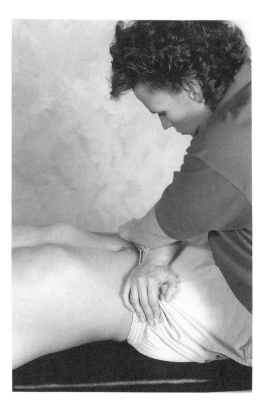

Fig. 9.18: To perform the gapping test, apply a cross-arm pressure down and outward to the ASIS with your thumbs. Although the test is used to detect a sprain of the sacroiliac joints, can you think of what other significant injury may lead to increased pain with this type of pressure on the bony landmarks?

"Squish" Test

With the individual supine, push both ASISs downward and inward at a 45° angle. This action stresses the posterior sacroiliac ligaments, and is positive if pain is present.

Sacroiliac Rocking ("Knee-to-Shoulder") Test

In a supine position, fully flex the individual's knee and hip toward the opposite shoulder, then adduct the hip **(Figure 9-19)**. The sacroiliac joint is rocked by flexion and adduction of the hip. A positive test causes pain at the sacroiliac joint.

Approximation test

In a side-lying position, apply a downward force over the iliac crest **(Figure 9-20)**. The movement causes forward pressure on the sacrum. A positive test will produce pain or a feeling of pressure on the sacroiliac joints, indicating a possible sprain to the sacroiliac joint. Sharp pain along the pelvic ring may indicate a fracture.

Resisted Muscle Testing

Stabilize the hip during manual muscle testing to prevent any muscle substitution. Begin

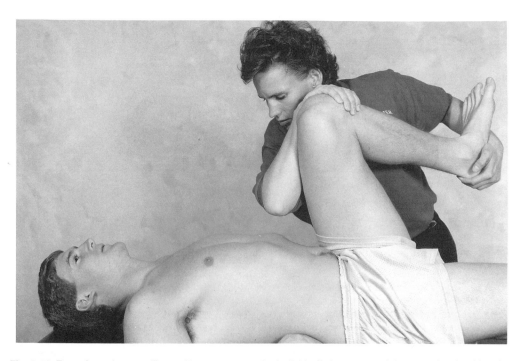

Fig. 9.19: To perform the sacroiliac rocking test, move the individual's knee toward the opposite shoulder. A positive sign is pain in the sacroiliac joint.

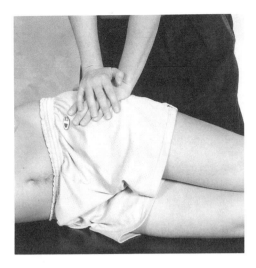

Fig. 9.20: To perform the approximation test, apply a downward force over the iliac crest. Increased pain or a feeling of pressure on the sacroiliac joints indicates a possible joint sprain. Sharp pain may indicate a possible pelvic fracture.

A

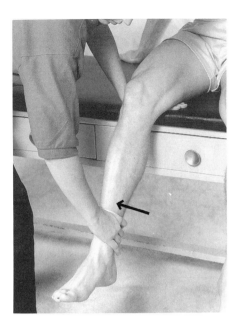

with the muscle on stretch and apply resistance throughout the full range of motion. Note any muscle weakness when compared to the uninvolved limb. As always, painful motions should be delayed until last. **Figure 9-21** demonstrates motions that should be tested (myotomes are listed in parentheses):

1. Knee extension (L_3)
2. Lateral rotation of the hip
3. Medial rotation of the hip
4. Hip flexion (L_2)
5. Hip abduction
6. Hip adduction
7. Knee flexion (S_1 and S_2)
8. Hip extension (S_1)

Neurological Assessment

Neurological integrity can be assessed with the use of myotomes, reflexes, and segmental dermatomes and peripheral nerve cutaneous patterns.

Myotomes

Isometric muscle testing in the loose packed position should be performed in the following motions to test specific segmental myotomes: hip flexion (L_1, L_2); knee extension (L_3); ankle dorsiflexion (L_4); toe extension (L_5); ankle plantar flexion, foot eversion, or hip extension (S_1); and knee flexion (S_2).

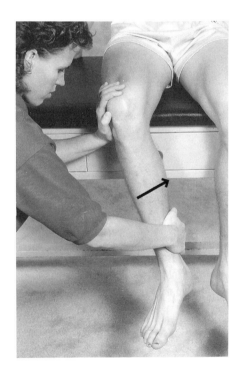

B

Fig. 9.21: Resisted manual muscle testing. (A) Knee extension. (B) Lateral rotation.

Testing of these motions are demonstrated in **Figure 7-37** and **Figure 9-21**.

Reflexes

There are no specific reflexes to test the pelvic or hip area. Other reflexes in the lower extremity, demonstrated in **Figure 7-38** include the patella (L_3, L_4), and Achilles tendon reflex (S_1).

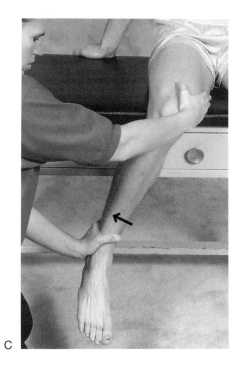

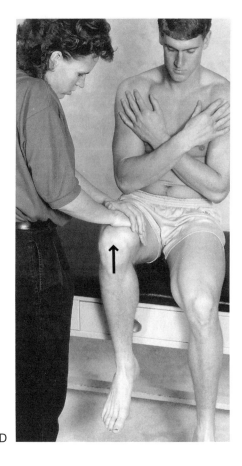

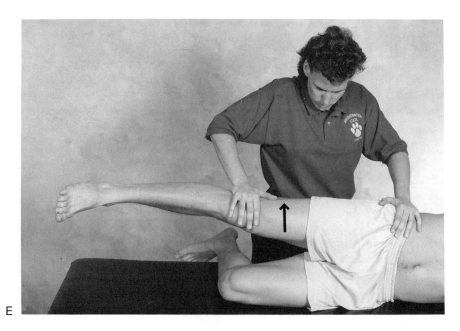

Fig. 9.21: (C) Medial rotation. (D) Hip flexion. (E) Abduction.

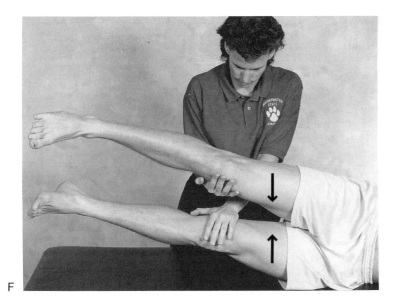

F

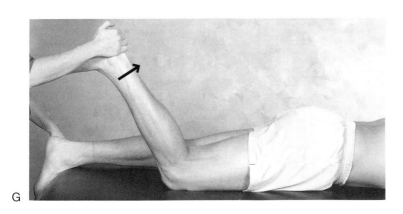

G

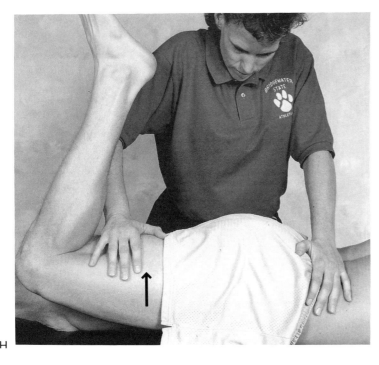

H

Fig. 9.21: (F) Adduction. (G) Knee flexion. (H) Hip extension.

Cutaneous patterns

In testing cutaneous sensation, run a sharp and dull object over the skin, i.e., blunt tip of taping scissors vs. flat edge of taping scissors. With their eyes closed or looking away, ask the individual if they can distinguish sharp and dull, and pinpoint the area being tested. The segmental nerve dermatome patterns for the thigh, hip, and pelvic region are demonstrated in **Figure 9-22**. The peripheral nerve cutaneous distribution patterns are demonstrated in **Figure 9-23**.

Stress and Functional Tests

Always be alert to possible congenital defects and epiphyseal injuries when dealing with adolescents. As you progress through the assessment process, perform only those tests you believe to be absolutely necessary.

Leg Length Measurement

Anatomical discrepancy in true leg length as a result of a shortened lower limb is taken in a supine position with the pelvis square, level, and balanced. The legs should be parallel to each other with the heels approximately six to eight inches apart. Measure between the distal edge of the ASIS to the distal aspect of the lat-

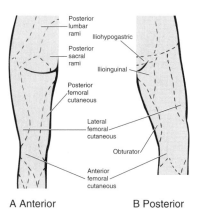

A Anterior   B Posterior

Fig. 9.23: Peripheral nerve cutaneous patterns for the thigh, hip, and pelvic region.

eral malleolus of each ankle (**Figure 9-24**). Measurement to the lateral malleolus is more commonly used than the medial malleolus, since it is less likely to be affected by muscle bulk and contractures in the hip abductors and adductors. A difference of 1.0 to 1.5 cm is considered normal. Functional discrepancies as a result of lateral pelvic tilt, flexion or adduction deformities are measured from the umbilicus to the medial malleolus of each ankle.

Thomas Test for Flexion Contractures

In a supine fully extended position, observe any noticeable lumbar lordosis. If contractures are present, you may be able to slip your hand under the low back. Ask the individual to flex the uninvolved leg to the chest and hold it in that position. This should flatten the lumbar region. If the test is negative, the straight leg will remain in contact with the table. If the test is positive, however, the straight leg (involved leg) will rise off the table (**Figure 9-25**). Both legs are tested and compared.

Kendall Test for Rectus Femoris Contracture

The individual lies supine on the table with both knees flexed at 90° over the edge of the table. The individual flexes the unaffected knee to the chest and holds it in that position. The other knee should remain flexed at 90°. If the knee slightly extends, a contracture in the rectus femoris may be present on that leg (**Figure 9-26**). If the results are positive, palpate the muscle for tightness to confirm the contracture. If there is no palpable tightness, the condition may be due to tight joint struc-

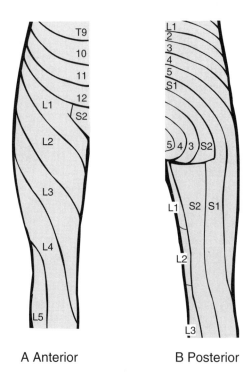

A Anterior   B Posterior

Fig. 9.22: Segmental nerve dermatome patterns for the thigh, hip, and pelvic region.

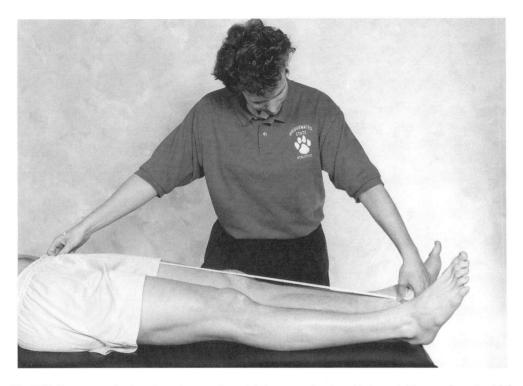

Fig. 9.24: To measure leg length, make sure the pelvis is square, level, and balanced. Measure from the ASIS to the distal point of the medial or lateral malleolus of each ankle.

tures (capsular or ligamentous). If the hip abducts during the test, it may be due to iliotibial band tightness. Ober's test and the Noble compression test should then be performed bilaterally (See **Figure 8-41**).

Faber (Patrick) Test

In a supine position, rest the foot and ankle of the involved leg on the contralateral knee.

The flexed leg is then slowly lowered into abduction (**Figure 9-27**). The final position of *f*lexion, *ab*duction, and *external r*otation (Faber) at the hip should place the involved leg on the table or at least near a horizontal position with the opposite leg. If the leg is unable to relax to this position and remains above the opposite leg, it may indicate a iliopsoas spasm, tight piriformis muscle, or hip joint contracture. Overpressure on the knee

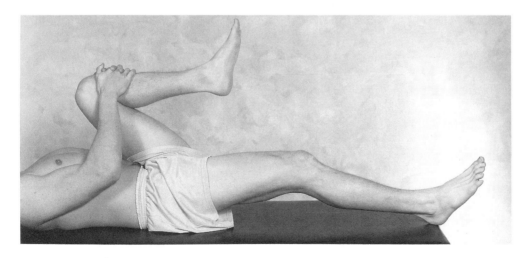

Fig. 9.25: To perform a Thomas test for flexion contractures, ask the individual to flex the uninvolved leg to the chest and hold it. A positive test occurs when the extended leg moves up off the table indicating hip flexion contractures.

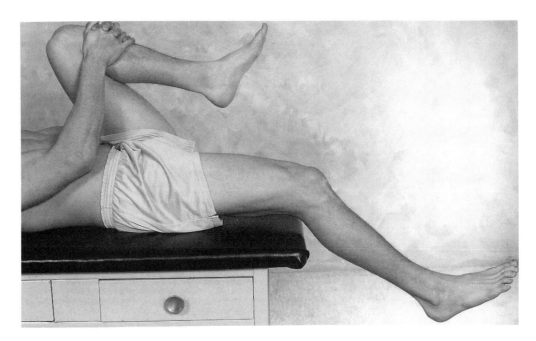

Fig. 9.26: The Kendall test is similar to the Thomas test, except the individual lies supine with both knees flexed over the edge of the table. The uninvolved leg is flexed to the chest and held. A positive test occurs when the leg flexed over the end of the table, extends.

of the involved leg and the contralateral iliac crest may produce pain in the sacroiliac joint on the side of the involved leg, denoting possible pathology.

Hamstrings Contracture Test

In a seated position on a table, flex the hip bringing one leg against the chest to stabilize the pelvic region. Ask the individual to touch

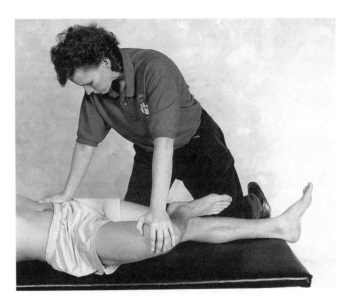

Fig. 9.27: To perform the Faber (Patrick) test, have the individual rest the foot and ankle of the involved leg on the contralateral knee. Apply overpressure on the knee and contralateral iliac crest. Pain in the sacroiliac joint on the side of the involved leg indicates possible pathology.

the toes of the extended leg (**Figure 9-28**). If unable to do so, this indicates tight hamstrings on the extended leg. Test both legs and compare.

Straight Leg Raising (Lasègue's) Test

Although this test is typically used to stretch the dura mater of the spinal cord to assess possible intervertebral disc lesions, it is also used to rule out tight hamstrings. In a supine position, passively flex the individual's hip while keeping the knee extended until the individual complains of tightness or pain (**Figure 9-29**). Slowly lower the leg until the pain or tightness disappears. Then, dorsiflex the foot, have the individual flex the neck, or perform both actions simultaneously. Pain that increases with dorsiflexion and neck flexion, or both, indicates stretching of the dura mater of the spinal cord. Pain that does not increase with dorsiflexion or neck flexion usually indicates tight hamstrings. If both legs are passively raised simultaneously, and pain occurs prior to 70° of flexion, it indicates sacroiliac joint problems.

Sign of the Buttock Test

This test determines the presence of pathology in the buttock region, such as a bursitis, tumor, or abscess that may restrict hip flexion. The passive unilateral straight leg raising test is performed as above. If a restriction is reached in hip flexion, flex the individual's knee to see if hip flexion will increase (**Figure 9-30**). If a problem exists in the lumbar spine, hip flexion will increase, denoting a negative buttock test. A positive buttock test is determined when hip flexion does not increase after the knee if flexed.

Homan's Sign

To test for deep venous thrombosis, place the individual supine on a table. Passively dorsiflex the foot of the involved leg with the knee extended (**Figure 9-31**). Pain in the calf indicates a positive Homan's Sign. Tenderness may also be elicited with palpation of the calf. In addition, pallor or swelling in the leg may be accompanied by an absence of the dorsalis pedis pulse (22).

Functional tests

Functional tests should be performed before clearing any individual for re-entry into sports participation. The individual should be able to perform activities pain-free with no limp or antalgic gait. Examples of functional activities include walking, going up and down stairs, jogging, squatting, jumping, running straight ahead, running sideways, and changing directions while running. Whenever possible, protective equipment or padding should be used to prevent reinjury.

You have completed assessing the soccer player. You found pain and weakness on active and resistive hip adduction, flexion, and medial rotation. Bilateral normal results were found in end feels, passive range of motion (PROM), cutaneous sensation, and

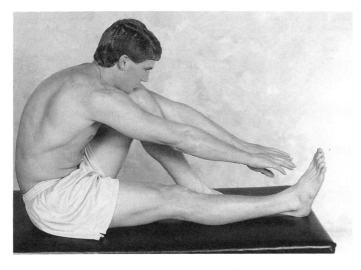

Fig. 9.28: To test for possible hamstring contractures, have the individual flex one hip against the chest to stabilize the pelvic region. The test is positive if the individual cannot touch the toes of the extended leg.

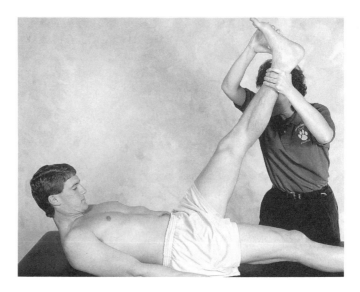

Fig. 9.29: Passively flex the individual's hip while keeping the knee extended until pain or tension is felt in the hamstrings. Slowly lower the leg until the pain or tension disappears. Then, dorsiflex the foot, have the individual flex the neck, or do both simultaneously. If pain does not increase with dorsiflexion of the ankle or flexion of the neck, it indicates tight hamstrings.

stress tests. Did you determine the individual had an adductor strain? If so, you are correct.

REHABILITATION OF THE HIP

? *The soccer player is doing ice therapy to control inflammation and pain. What range of motion exercises and strengthening exercises should be included in the rehabilitation program?*

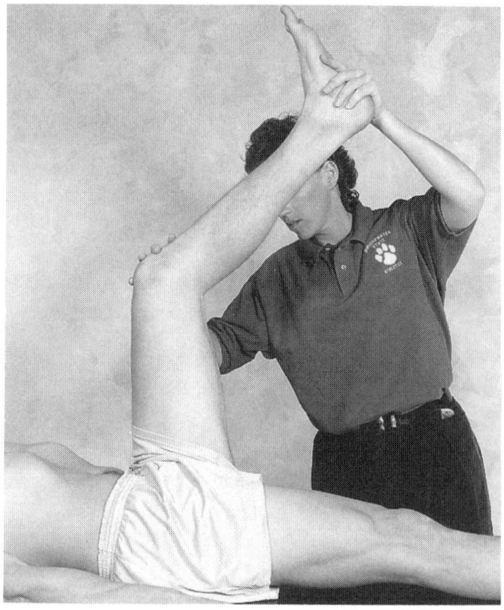

Rehabilitation for the hip area should restore motion and proprioception, improve muscular strength, endurance and power, and maintain cardiovascular fitness. In addition to focusing on muscles that move the hip, exercises should also involve the quadriceps and hamstrings muscle groups.

Restoration of Motion

Range of motion exercises for the hip region should focus on the hip flexors, extensors, abductors, adductors, medial and lateral rotators, and the quadriceps and hamstrings.

Fig. 9.30: To perform the sign of the buttock test, do a unilateral straight leg raising test. If a restriction is felt, flex the knee. If hip flexion increases, a problem may exist in the lumbar spine. A positive buttock test occurs when hip flexion does not increase.

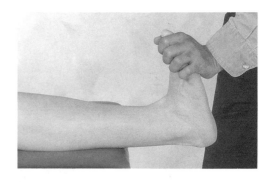

Fig. 9.31: To perform the Homan's sign, passively dorsiflex the foot with the knee extended. Pain in the calf indicates a possible deep venous thrombosis.

Many of the stretching exercises were demonstrated in **Field Strategy 8-1**, **Figure 8-41**, and in **Field Strategy 9-1** . These exercises can be active or passive, and should include proprioceptive neuromuscular facilitation (PNF) stretching techniqes.

Restoration of Proprioception and Balance

Proprioception and balance is regained in the early stages of exercise with activities such as shifting one's weight while on crutches, doing straight leg raises while weight bearing on one leg, performing bilateral minisquats, and using the BAPS board, slide board, or minitramp. Straight leg raises can be further supplemented with ankle weights and surgical tubing or Theraband. Attaching the tubing to the opposite limb on which you are working can develop balance in one limb while strengthening the other. Movement patterns can work in a single plane or in multidirectional patterns.

Muscular Strength, Endurance, and Power

Isometric exercises may be used early to strengthen the muscle groups. Open chain exercises, such as straight leg raises can be completed in a single plane or in multidirectional patterns, and can be supplemented with ankle weights or tubing. Closed chain exercises may include minisquats and modified lunges, and should progress to full squats and lunges. Resistance may be added with hand-held weights, a weighted bar, or use of a leg press machine. A variety of commercial isotonic and isokinetic machines are available to strengthen the individual muscle groups, utilizing open and closed chain technique.

Cardiovascular Fitness

Cardiovascular fitness exercises can include early use of an upper body ergometer (UBE) or hydrotherapeutic exercise. Running in water and performing sport specific exercises in deeper water can allow the individual to maintain sport specific functional skills in a non-weight bearing position. When range of motion is adequate, a stationary bike should be used, beginning with a light to moderate load, increasing the load as tolerated. A slide board may also be used. Light jogging can begin with one quarter speed, and progress to half speed, three quarter speed, and full

sprints. Plyometric exercises including jumping, skipping, and bounding can be combined with running, side-to-side running, or cutting and changing directions. Timed sprints, shuttle runs, karioca runs, hops or vertical jump tests may be used to measure return to full activity. At that time, the individual should have bilaterally equal range of motion, balance, muscular strength, endurance, and power, and an appropriate level of cardiovascular fitness for their specific sport.

The soccer player should focus on range of motion exercises for the hip adductors and hip flexors in addition to general range of motion exercises for the entire hip region. Furthermore, exercises for the hip muscles should include closed chain exercises to improve muscular strength, endurance, and power. Proprioception, balance, and cardiovascular fitness should be at or better than the preinjury level.

SUMMARY

The thigh and pelvic region is highly susceptible to compression forces from direct trauma and tensile forces from explosive muscular contractions. These forces lead to a high incidence of contusions and muscular strains. Although a tremendous amount of stress is placed on the hip and pelvic joints during running and jumping activities, joint injuries are rare. Muscle imbalance and dysfunction, congenital abnormalities, or postural deviations can, however, predispose an individual to injury. **Field Strategy 9-5** lists the steps in assessing the thigh, hip and pelvic region.

During the assessment, remember that the individual may be experiencing referred pain from the abdominal, lumbar, or knee region. Furthermore, in an adolescent, congenital defects, epiphyseal and apophyseal injuries are common. Refer the individual to a physician if any of the following conditions are suspected: obvious deformity suggesting a dislocation or fracture; significant loss of motion or a palpable defect in a muscle; severe joint disability that may be evident by a noticeable limp; excessive soft tissue swelling; possible epiphyseal and apophyseal injuries; any groin pain that does not improve within five to seven days; any abnormal or absent reflexes; abnormal sensations in either the segmental dermatomes or peripheral cutaneous patterns; absent or weak pulse; or weakness in a myotome. Radiographs, bone scans, or MRI's

Field Strategy 9–5. Hip Evaluation.

History

Primary complaint including:
 Description and mechanism of current injury
 Onset of symptoms
Pain perception and discomfort
Disability and functional impairments from the injury
Previous injuries to the area
Family history

Observation and Inspection

Postural assessment
 Gait analysis
 Inspection of injured area for:

Muscle symmetry	Hypertrophy or muscle atrophy
Swelling	Visible congenital deformity
Discoloration	Surgical incisions or scars

Palpation

Bony structures to determine a possible fracture
Soft tissue structures to determine:

Temperature	Deformity
Swelling	Muscle spasm
Point tenderness	Cutaneous sensation
Crepitus	Vascular pulses

Special Tests

Active movement
 Passive range of motion

Gapping test	"Squish" test
Sacroiliac rocking test	Approximation test

Resisted manual muscle testing
Neurologic testing
Stress and functional tests
 Leg length measurement
 Contracture tests

Thomas test	Kendall rectus femoris test
Faber test	Hamstrings test

 Straight leg raising
 Sign of the buttock test
 Homan's sign
 Functional tests

can be used to rule out underlying bone cysts, tumors, osteochondromas, or congenital defects that could lead to permanent disability.

If the individual is referred to a physician for care, remove the player from any activity and immobilize the limb in a comfortable position, or fit the individual with crutches if they are unable to walk without pain or a limp. Apply ice therapy to control inflammation and swelling, and transport the individual in an appropriate manner. Prior to return to activity, the individual should have medical clearance from the supervising physician, and have passed all functional tests pain-free without a limp or antalgic gait.

REFERENCES

1. Johnston, RC. 1973. Mechanical considerations of the hip joint. Arch of Surg, 107:411–417.

2. Nordin, M, and Frankel, VH. *Basic biomechanics of the musculoskeletal system*. Philadelphia: Lea and Febiger, 1989.

3. Reid, DC. *Sports injury assessment and rehabilitation*. New York: Churchill Livingstone, 1992.

4. Aronen, JG, and Chronister, RD. 1992. Quadriceps contusions: Hastening the return to play. Phys Sportsmed, 20(7):130–136.

5. Estwanik, JJ, and McAlister, JA. 1990. Contusions and the formation of myositis ossificans. Phys Sportsmed, 18(4):53–64.

6. Esposito, PW. "Pelvis, hip and thigh injuries." In *The team physician's handbook*, edited by MB Mellion, WM Walsh, and GL Shelton. Philadelphia: Hanley and Belfus, 1990.

7. Downing, JF, Nicholas, JA. 1991. Four complex joint injuries. Phys Sportsmed, 19(10):81–97.

8. Garrick, JG, and Webb, DR. *Sports injuries: Diagnosis and management*. Philadelphia: WB Saunders, 1990.

9. Garrett, WE, Califf, JC, Bassett, FH. 1984. Histochemical correlates of hamstring injuries. Am J Sports Med, 12(2):98–103.

10. Brubaker, CE, James, SL. 1974. Injuries to runners. Am J Sports Med, 2(3):189–194.

11. Engle, RP. 1988. Hamstring facilitation in anterior instability of the knee. J of Ath Tr, 23(3):226–228, 285.

12. Loosli, AR, and Quick, J. 1992. Thigh strains in competitive breaststroke swimmers. J of Sport Rehab, 1(1):49–55.

13. Estwanik, JJ, Sloane, B, and Rosenberg, MA. 1990. Groin strain and other possible causes of groin pain. Phy Sportsmed, 18(2):55–65.

14. Pace, JB, and Nalge, D. 1976. Piriformis syndrome. West J Med, 124(6):435–439.

15. Rich, BS, and McKeag, D. 1992. When sciatica is not disk disease: Detecting piriformis syndrome in active patients. Phys Sportsmed, 20(10):105–115.

16. Keskula, DR, and Tamburello, M. 1992. Conservative management of piriformis syndrome. J of Ath Tr, 27(2):102–110.

17. Price, SA, and Wilson, LM. *Pathophysiology: Clinical concepts of disease processes*. St. Louis: Mosby Year Book, 1992.

18. Fullerton, LR, and Snowdy, HA. 1988. Femoral neck stress fractures. Am J Sports Med, 16(4):365–377.

19. Hershman, EB, Lombardo, J, and Bergeld, JA. "Femoral shaft stress fractures in athletes." In *Clinics in sports medicine*, edited by JT Watson and JA, Bergfeld, vol. 9, no. 1. Philadelphia: WB Saunders, 1990.

20. Johansson, C, Kenman, I, Tornkvist, H, and Eriksson, E. 1990. Stress fractures of the femoral neck in athletes: The consequence of a delay in diagnosis. Am J Sports Med, 18(5):524–528.

21. Visuri T, Vara, A, and Meurman, KOM. 1988. Displaced stress fractures of the femoral neck in young male adults: A report of twelve operative cases. J Trauma 28(11):1562–1569.

22. Magee, D. *Orthopedic physical assessment*. Philadelphia: WB Saunders, 1992.

Injuries to the Upper Extremity

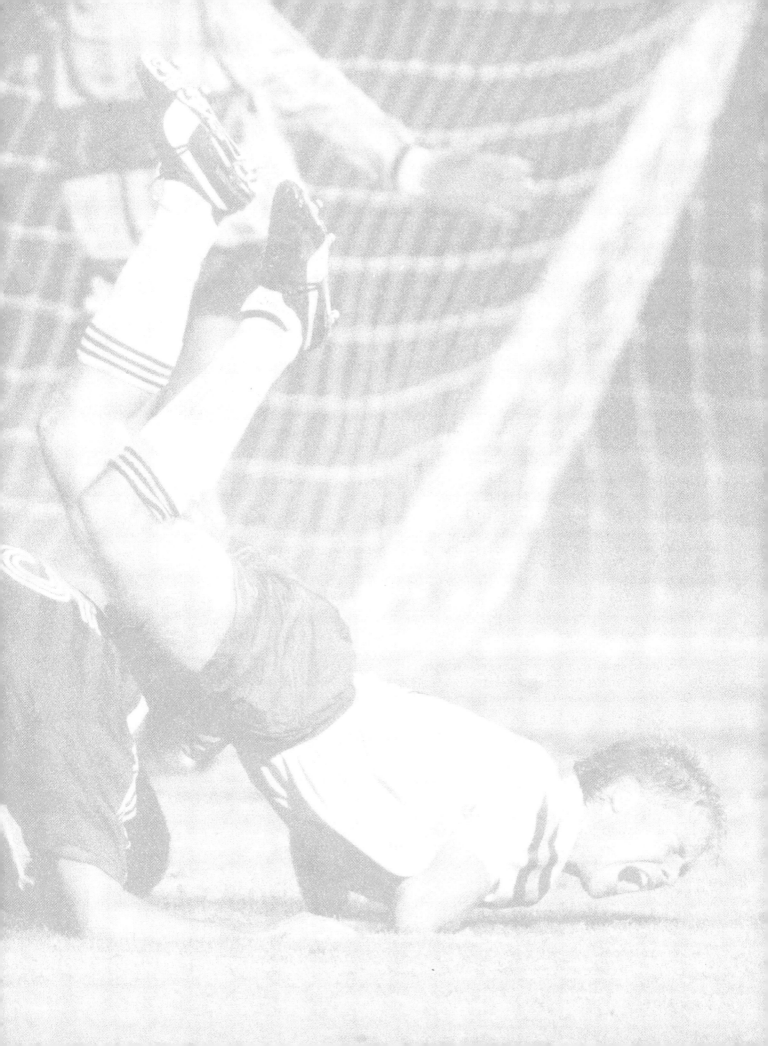

Yoshitaka Ando, B.S., L.A.T.,C.

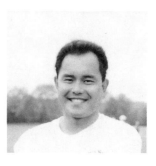

I came to the United States from Japan to play American football and learn to speak fluent English. During a high school game, I got injured, and was taken care of by a student trainer who was finishing his degree at Northeastern University. In talking with him and my guidance counselor, I decided to pursue a career in athletic training at Bridgewater State College.

As a high school athletic trainer, I order, fit, clean, and inspect all protective equipment, develop pre-season conditioning programs for the sports, and provide on-site medical coverage for the high school athletes. A team physician and physical therapist work directly with me to provide a very comprehensive health care program for the athletes. In addition to the daily management of the training room, I also provide a fair amount of counseling to athletes on weight control, nutrition, substance abuse, and other health issues.

Our school has around 1000 students, 600 of which participate on athletic teams. Many of these individuals are three-season athletes. We have 15 competitive sports with nearly all sports fielding three separate teams. In our league, six of the eight high schools have NATA-certified athletic trainers, so we know our athletes are getting good health care coverage. Communication among the trainers is excellent. After an away event, I always get a call from the on-site trainer to let me know if anything happened to my athletes, and I return the courtesy to my other colleagues.

Working at this school is really a delight. The parents, superintendent, athletic director, and coaches really appreciate the service I provide them. My budget is adequate, and if I really need something that the school can't provide, the Booster's Club is right there to help. The athletes also see this tremendous support and appreciate what I do for them. Many go on to play at the college level, and continually return during home games just to say hi.

One thing about working with so many teams is that you need to be in multiple places at the same time. We know that's impossible, but our on-site communication is excellent. Although my athletic director doesn't expect to see me before noon, I come in early in the morning to update my files on the computer, clean the coolers and water bottles, and make my phone calls to the physicians and other league trainers. I work six days a week, and during the winter the days can be very long, but I wouldn't trade it for anything.

If you would like to work at the high school level, I would suggest doing a clinical rotation there to find out what it's all about. Your taping skills have to be excellent due to the incredible volume of people you have to tape and get out on the field ready for practice. You also have to remember that you are working with minors, children under 18, so you can't take anything for granted. All injury assessments must be thorough and complete, and you have to develop a good follow-up system to recheck injuries and develop easy rehabilitation programs that the students can do on their own. Developing a good working relationship with the parents is also a must. They can be your best ally or your worst nightmare. You have to make yourself visible and demonstrate your professional style by always placing the health of the athletes in the forefront. Each day is a new challenge, especially when you realize you are there to safeguard these young athletes. You know it's worth that extra effort, and I wouldn't trade it for the world.

Yoshitaka Ando is a full-time athletic trainer at Lincoln-Sudbury Regional High School in Sudbury, Massachusetts. As a regional high school trainer, he provides health care coverage to over 600 high school athletes throughout the year.

Shoulder Injuries

After you have completed this chapter, you should be able to:

- Locate the important bony and soft tissue structures of the shoulder
- Describe the major motions at the shoulder and identify the muscles that produce them
- Explain what forces produce the loading patterns responsible for common injuries at the shoulder
- Explain general principles and exercises used to prevent injuries to the shoulder
- Recognize and manage specific injuries in the shoulder region
- Demonstrate a thorough assessment of the shoulder region
- Demonstrate general rehabilitation exercises for the shoulder complex

The loose structure of the shoulder complex enables extreme mobility but provides little stability. As a result, the shoulder is much more prone to injury than the hip. The shoulder is involved in 8 to 13% of all sport-related injuries, with reports indicating complaints of shoulder pain among up to 50% of competitive swimmers (1,2). Shoulder injuries are a major concern in activities involving an overhead motion, such as in baseball, swimming, tennis, volleyball, and weight lifting. These activities place significant demands on the shoulder and other joints of the upper extremity leading to many acute and chronic conditions. Common injuries include sprains, rotator cuff strains, bursitis, bicipital tendinitis, and impingement syndromes. Dislocations of the shoulder articulations are not uncommon, particularly in contact sports such as wrestling or football.

This chapter begins with a review of the anatomy of the shoulder region, followed by a synopsis of the kinematics and kinetics of the shoulder joints. Discussion on prevention of injuries is followed by an overview of common injuries to the shoulder complex. Injury management for specific injuries and the assessment process are then followed by examples of rehabilitation exercises.

ANATOMY REVIEW OF THE SHOULDER

A volleyball player is complaining of throbbing pain on the anterior aspect of the shoulder of the hitting arm. The pain intensifies following practice sessions. What anatomical structure(s) might be the source of this pain?

The shoulder region encompasses five separate articulations—the sternoclavicular (SC) joint, acromioclavicular (AC) joint, coracoclavicular joint, glenohumeral joint, and the scapulothoracic joint. The articulation referred to specifically as the shoulder joint is the glenohumeral joint, whereas the other articulations are joints of the shoulder girdle. The sternoclavicular and acromioclavicular joints enhance motion of the clavicle and scapula that position the glenohumeral joint to provide a greater range of motion for the humerus.

Sternoclavicular Joint

As the name suggests, the sternoclavicular (SC) joint is the articulation of the superior sternum, or manubrium, with the proximal clavicle (**Figure 10-1**). The SC joint is a synovial joint surrounded by a joint capsule that is thickened anteriorly and posteriorly. Four ligaments reinforce the capsule, including the interclavicular, costoclavicular, and anterior and posterior sternoclavicular ligaments.

The SC joint is a ball and socket joint that enables rotation of the clavicle with respect to the sternum. The joint allows motion of the distal clavicle in superior, inferior, anterior, and posterior directions, along with some forward and backward rotation of the

> The glenohumeral joint is the major joint of the shoulder

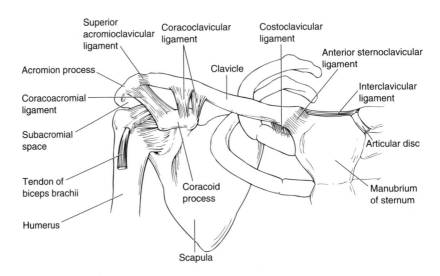

Fig. 10.1: The bony and ligamentous structure of the shoulder girdle.

The sternoclavicular joint enables rotation of the clavicle with respect to the sternum during motions, such as shrugging the shoulders or reaching above the head

The head of the humerus not only rotates, but can move linearly across the surface of the glenoid fossa during arm movements

Glenoid labrum
Soft tissue lip around the periphery of the glenoid fossa that adds stability to the glenohumeral joint

clavicle. Thus, rotation occurs at the SC joint during motions such as shrugging the shoulders, reaching above the head, and performing most swimming strokes. Because the first rib is joined by its cartilage to the manubrium just inferior to the joint, motion of the clavicle in the inferior direction is restricted. The close packed position for the SC joint occurs with maximal shoulder elevation.

Acromioclavicular Joint

The acromioclavicular (AC) joint consists of the articulation of the acromion process of the scapula with the distal end of the clavicle (**Figure 10-1**). This is an irregular diarthrodial joint with limited motion permitted in all three planes. The joint is enclosed by a capsule, though the capsule is thinner than that of the SC joint. The strong superior and inferior acromioclavicular ligaments cross the joint, providing stability. The coracoacromial ligament, sometimes referred to as the "arch" ligament, also attaches to the inferior lip of the AC joint to serve as a buffer between the rotator cuff muscles and the bony acromion process. The coracoclavicular ligament, with its conoid and trapezoid branches, resists independent upward movement of the clavicle, downward movement of the scapula, and anteroposterior movement of the clavicle or scapula. The close packed position of the AC joint occurs when the humerus is abducted at 90°.

Coracoclavicular Joint

The coracoclavicular joint is a syndesmosis formed by the binding together of the cora-

coid process of the scapula and the inferior surface of the clavicle by the coracoclavicular ligament (**Figure 10-1**). Very little movement is permitted at this joint.

Glenohumeral Joint

The glenohumeral joint is the articulation between the glenoid fossa of the scapula and the head of the humerus. Although the joint enables a greater total range of motion than any other joint in the human body, it is lacking in bony stability (**Figure 10-2**). This is partially because the hemisphere-shaped head of the humerus has three to four times the amount of surface area of the shallow glenoid fossa. Because the glenoid fossa is also less curved than the humeral head, the humerus not only rotates, but moves linearly across the surface of the glenoid fossa when humeral motion occurs (3).

The glenoid fossa is somewhat deepened around its perimeter by the **glenoid labrum**, a narrow rim of fibrocartilage around the edge of the fossa (**Figure 10-2**) (4). The glenohumeral joint capsule is joined by the superior, middle, and inferior glenohumeral ligaments on the anterior side, and the coracohumeral ligament on the superior side. Although joint displacements can occur in anterior, posterior, and inferior directions, the strong coracohumeral ligament protects against superior dislocations.

The tendons of four muscles, including the supraspinatus, infraspinatus, teres minor, and subscapularis also join the joint capsule (**Figures 10-3, 10-4**). These muscles are referred

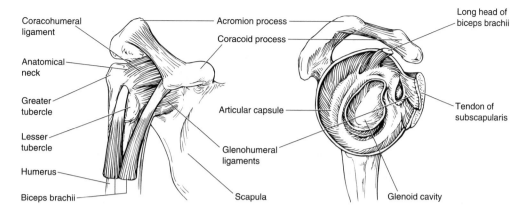

Fig. 10.2: The glenohumeral joint.

to as the SITS muscles, after the first letter of the muscles' names. They are also known as the **rotator cuff** muscles, because they all act to rotate the humerus and their tendons merge to form a collagenous cuff around the joint. Tension in the rotator cuff muscles helps to hold the head of the humerus against the glenoid fossa, further contributing to

Rotator cuff
The SITS muscles (supraspinatus, infraspinatus, teres minor, and subscapularis) hold the head of the humerus in the glenoid fossa and produce humeral rotation

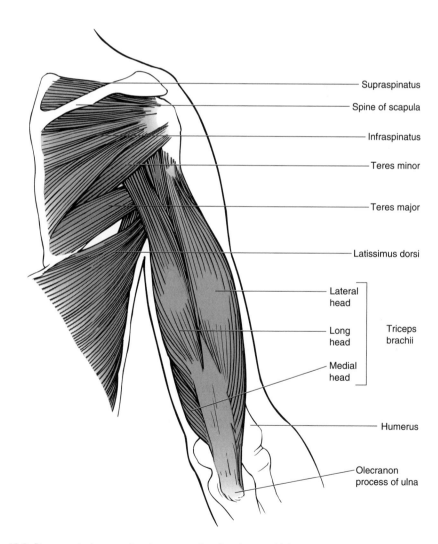

Fig. 10.3: Deep posterior muscles that move the glenohumeral joint.

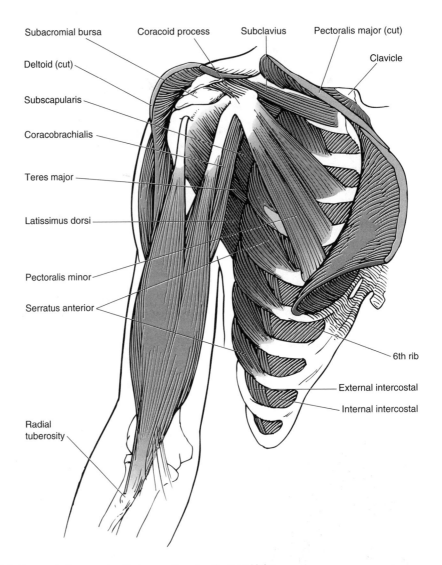

Subacromial bursa — Coracoid process — Subclavius — Pectoralis major (cut)

Clavicle

Deltoid (cut)

Subscapularis

Coracobrachialis

Teres major

Latissimus dorsi

Pectoralis minor

Serratus anterior

6th rib

External intercostal

Internal intercostal

Radial tuberosity

Fig. 10.4: Deep anterior muscles that move the glenohumeral joint.

joint stability. The joint is most stable in its close packed position when the humerus is abducted and laterally rotated.

Scapulothoracic Joint

Because muscles attaching to the scapula permit its motion with respect to the trunk or thorax, this region is sometimes described as the scapulothoracic joint. Muscles attaching to the scapula include the levator scapula, rhomboids, serratus anterior, pectoralis minor, subclavius, deltoid, subscapularis, supraspinatus, infraspinatus, teres major, teres minor, coracobrachialis, the short head of the biceps brachii, long head of the triceps brachii, and the trapezius (**Figures 10-3,4,5,6**).

The scapular muscles perform two functions. The first is stabilization of the shoulder region. For example, when a barbell is lifted

from the floor, the levator scapula, trapezius, and rhomboids develop tension to support the scapula, and in turn, the entire shoulder, through the acromioclavicular joint. The second function is to facilitate movements of the upper extremity through appropriate positioning of the glenohumeral joint. During an overhand throw, for example, the rhomboids contract to move the entire shoulder posteriorly as the arm and hand move backward during the preparatory phase. As the arm and hand then move forward to execute the throw, tension in the rhomboids is released to permit forward movement of the shoulder, enabling medial rotation of the humerus.

Muscles of the Shoulder

A large number of muscles cross the glenohumeral joint, as shown in **Table 10-1**. Iden-

The scapular muscles stabilize and/or position the scapula to facilitate movement at the glenohumeral joint

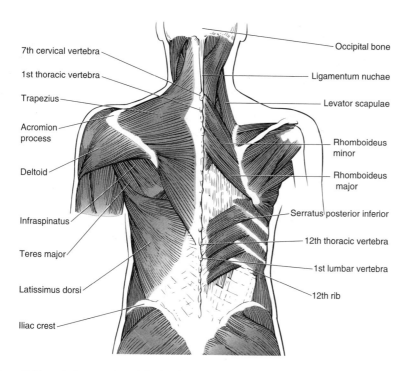

7th cervical vertebra

1st thoracic vertebra

Trapezius

Acromion process

Deltoid

Infraspinatus

Teres major

Latissimus dorsi

Iliac crest

Occipital bone

Ligamentum nuchae

Levator scapulae

Rhomboideus minor

Rhomboideus major

Serratus posterior inferior

12th thoracic vertebra

1st lumbar vertebra

12th rib

Fig. 10.5: Superficial posterior muscles of the back.

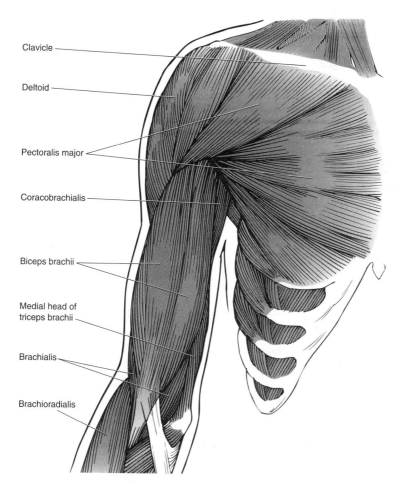

Clavicle

Deltoid

Pectoralis major

Coracobrachialis

Biceps brachii

Medial head of triceps brachii

Brachialis

Brachioradialis

Fig. 10.6: Superficial anterior muscles of the shoulder.

Table 10–1. Muscles of the Shoulder.

Muscle	Proximal Attachment	Distal Attachment	Primary Action(s)	Nerve Innervation
Deltoid	Outer third of the clavicle, top of the acromion, and scapula spine	Deltoid tuberosity of the humerus		Axillary (C_5, C_6)
(Anterior)			Flexion, horizontal adduction	
(Middle)			Abduction, horizontal abduction	
(Posterior)			Extension, horizontal abduction	
Pectoralis major		Lateral aspect of the humerus just below the head		
(Clavicular)	Medial two-thirds of the clavicle		Flexion, horizontal adduction	Lateral pectoral (C_5-T_1)
(Sternal)	Anterior sternum and cartilage of 1st six ribs		Extension, adduction, horizontal adduction	Medial pectoral (C_5-T_1)
Supraspinatus	Supraspinous fossa	Greater tuberosity of the humerus	Abduction	Suprascapular (C_5, C_6)
Coracobrachialis	Coracoid process of the scapula	Medial anterior humerus	Horizontal adduction	Musculocutaneous (C_5-C_7)
Latissimus dorsi	Lower six thoracic, all lumbar vertebrae, posterior sacrum, iliac crest, lower three ribs	Anterior humerus	Extension, adduction	Thoracodorsal (C_6-C_8)
Teres major	Lower, lateral, dorsal scapula	Anterior humerus	Extension, adduction, inward rotation	Subscapular (C_5, C_6)
Infraspinatus	Infraspinous fossa	Greater tubercle of the humerus	Outward rotation, horizontal abduction	Subscapular (C_5, C_6)
Teres minor	Posterior, lateral border of scapula	Greater tubercle and adjacent shaft of humerus	Lateral rotation, horizontal abduction	Axillary (C_5, C_6)
Subscapularis	Entire anterior surface of scapula	Lesser tubercle of the humerus	Inward rotation	Subscapular (C_5, C_6)
Biceps brachii		Tuberosity of the radius		Musculocutaneous (C_5-C_7)
(Long head)	Upper rim of the glenoid fossa		Assists with abduction	
(Short head)	Coracoid process of the scapula		Assists with flexion, adduction, inward rotation, and horizontal adduction	
Triceps brachii (Long head)	Just inferior to the glenoid fossa	Olecranon process of the ulna	Assist with extension and adduction	Radial (C_5-T_1)

tifying actions of these muscles is complicated by the fact that due to the large range of motion at the shoulder, the action produced by contraction of a given muscle may change with the orientation of the humerus.

Bursae

The shoulder is surrounded by several bursae, including the subcoracoid, subscapularis, and the most important, the subacromial. The subacromial bursa lies in the subacromial space where it is surrounded by the acromion process of the scapula and the coracoacromial ligament above and the glenohumeral joint below **(Figure 10-4)**. The bursa cushions the rotator cuff muscles, particularly the supraspinatus, from the overlying bony acromion. This bursa may become irritated when repeatedly compressed during overhead arm action.

Nerves of the Shoulder

Innervation of the upper extremity arises from the **brachial plexus**, a complex web of neural pathways branching primarily from the lower four cervical (C_5-C_8) and the first thoracic (T_1) spinal nerves **(Figure 10-7)**. The ventral rami, or roots, of these nerves divide into upper, middle, and lower trunks, which separate into anterior and posterior divisions, then divide into lateral, medial, and posterior cords. This network of nerve branches extends from the neck anteriorly and laterally, passing between the clavicle and first rib at approximately one third of the length of the clavicle proximal to the glenohumeral joint. Injuries to the clavicle in this region can damage the brachial plexus.

Major nerves arising from the brachial plexus that supply the shoulder region are the axillary (C_5, C_6), musculocutaneous (C_5-C_7),

Brachial plexus
A complex web of spinal nerves (C_5-T_1) that innervate the upper extremity

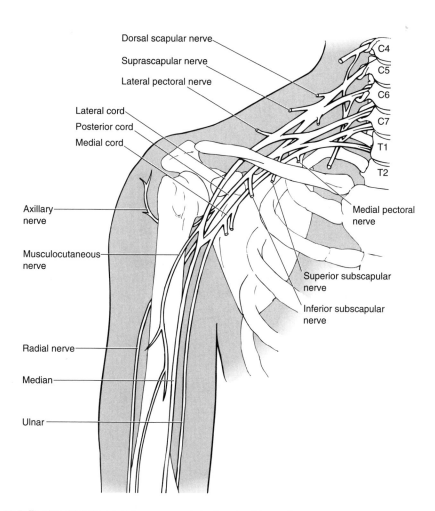

Dorsal scapular nerve
Suprascapular nerve
Lateral pectoral nerve
Lateral cord
Posterior cord
Medial cord
Axillary nerve
Musculocutaneous nerve
Radial nerve
Median
Ulnar
C4
C5
C6
C7
T1
T2
Medial pectoral nerve
Superior subscapular nerve
Inferior subscapular nerve

Fig. 10.7: The brachial plexus and nerve supply to the shoulder region.

dorsal scapular (C$_5$), subscapular (C$_5$, C$_6$), suprascapular (C$_5$, C$_6$), and pectoral nerves (C$_5$-T$_1$) **(Figure 10-7)**. The nerve-muscle associations are presented in **Table 10-1**.

Blood Vessels of the Shoulder

The subclavian artery passes beneath the clavicle to become the axillary artery, providing the major blood supply to the shoulder **(Figure 10-8)**. Branches of the axillary artery include the thoracoacromial trunk, lateral thoracic artery, subscapular artery, and thoracodorsal artery, as well as the anterior and posterior humeral circumflex arteries that supply the head of the humerus.

💡 *Forceful overhead arm movement such as spiking a volleyball, can, when performed repetitively, irritate the subacromial bursa, coracoacromial ligament, or supraspinatus tendon leading to pain and inflammation.*

KINEMATICS AND MAJOR MUSCLE ACTIONS OF THE SHOULDER COMPLEX

❓ *Why would an injury to the sternoclavicular joint impair an individual's ability to throw a ball?*

The shoulder is the most freely moveable joint in the body, with motion capability in all three planes **(Figure 10-9)**. Sagittal plane movements of the humerus at the shoulder include flexion, or elevation of the arm in an anterior direction, extension, or return of the arm from a position of flexion to the side of the body, and hyperextension, or elevation of the arm in a posterior direction. Frontal plane movements consist of abduction, or elevation of the arm in a lateral direction, and adduction, or return of the arm from a position of abduction to the side of the body. Transverse plane movements of the horizontally extended arm are termed horizontal adduction when the arm is moved medially, and horizontal abduction when the arm is moved laterally. The humerus can also rotate medially and laterally.

Throwing

Throwing and related motions produce a variety of both acute and chronic injuries to the shoulder. As with gait, throwing kinematics vary from individual to individual, even across overarm, sidearm, and underarm styles of the throw. To further complicate matters, some sport skills, casually referred to as throwing, actually involve more of a pushing motion than a throwing motion. An example is putting the shot.

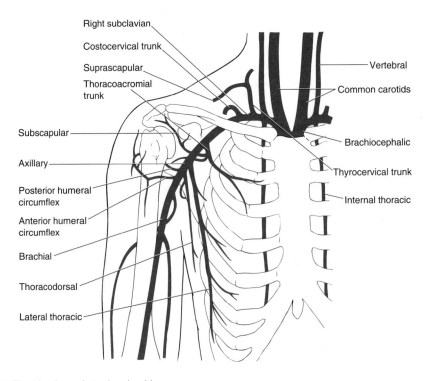

Right subclavian
Costocervical trunk
Suprascapular
Thoracoacromial trunk
Vertebral
Common carotids
Subscapular
Brachiocephalic
Axillary
Thyrocervical trunk
Posterior humeral circumflex
Internal thoracic
Anterior humeral circumflex
Brachial
Thoracodorsal
Lateral thoracic

Fig. 10.8: The blood supply to the shoulder.

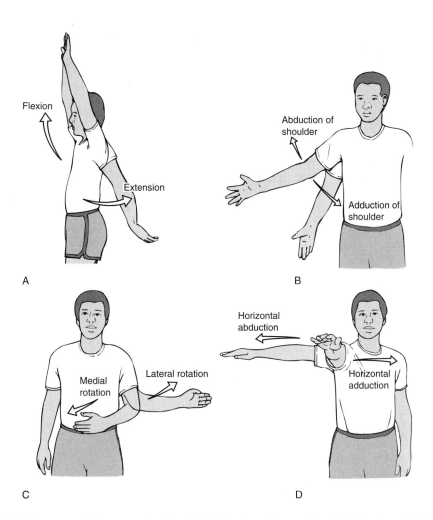

Fig. 10.9: Movements of the arm at the shoulder. (A) Flexion and extension. (B) Abduction and adduction. (C) Medial and lateral rotation. (D) Horizontal abduction and adduction. Combined movements are called circumduction.

Nevertheless, overarm throwing can be described in three phases. Although skillful throwing involves the coordinated action of the entire body, this description focuses on the shoulder girdle and glenohumeral joint. In the preparatory or cocking phase, the arm and hand are drawn behind the body, through horizontal abduction, hyperextension, and lateral rotation of the humerus **(Figure 10-10A)**. To facilitate this motion, the rhomboids contract to pull the scapula and the glenohumeral joint posteriorly. During the acceleration or delivery phase, the ball is brought forward and released **(Figure 10-10B)**. This involves horizontal adduction, flexion, and medial rotation of the humerus. The rhomboids relax to enable anterior movement of the glenohumeral joint. During this phase, the thrower may also intentionally pronate or supinate the forearm to place a spin on the ball. Because

throwing can involve a whip-like action of the arm, large stresses can be placed on the tendons, ligaments, and epiphyses of the throwing arm during delivery. The follow-through phase occurs after ball release and consists primarily of a snap-like flexion of the wrist, with the shoulder girdle and glenohumeral joint relatively stabilized **(Figure 10-10C)**.

Coordination of Shoulder Movements

The extensive range of motion afforded by the shoulder is partially due to the loose structure of the glenohumeral joint, and partially due to the proximity of the other shoulder articulations and the movement capabilities they provide. Movement at the shoulder typically involves some rotation at all three shoulder joints. For example, as the arm is elevated past 30° of abduction or 60° of flex-

Movement at the shoulder typically involves some rotation at all three shoulder joints

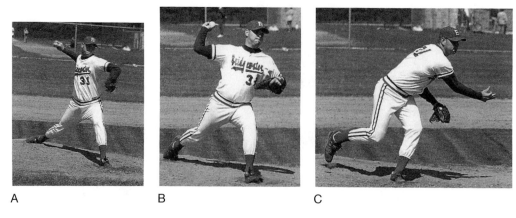

Fig. 10.10: The overarm throwing motion. (A) Preparatory or cocking phase. (B) Acceleration or delivery phase. (C) Follow-through phase.

Scapulohumeral rhythm
Coordinated rotational movement of the scapula that accompanies abduction and adduction of the humerus

ion, the scapula also rotates, contributing approximately one third of the total rotational movement of the humerus (5). This important coordination of scapular and humeral movements, known as **scapulohumeral rhythm**, enables a much greater range of motion at the shoulder than if the scapula were fixed **(Figure 10-11)**. Also contributing to the first 90° of humeral elevation is the elevation of the clavicle through approximately 35 to 45° of motion at the sternoclavicular joint (6). The acromioclavicular joint contributes to overall movement capability as well, with rotation occurring during the first 30° of humeral elevation, and then again as the arm is moved past 135° (7).

Glenohumeral Flexion

The muscles that cross the glenohumeral joint anteriorly are positioned to contribute to flexion **(Figure 10-4, 10-6)**. The anterior deltoid and the clavicular pectoralis major are the primary shoulder flexors, with assistance provided by the coracobrachialis and short head of the biceps brachii. Since the biceps also crosses the elbow joint, it is capable of exerting more force at the shoulder when the elbow is in full extension.

Glenohumeral Extension

When extension is unresisted, the action is caused by gravity. Eccentric contraction of

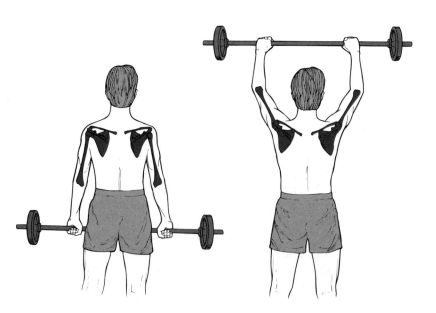

Fig. 10.11: The coordinated movement of the scapula needed to facilitate motion of the humerus is known as scapulohumeral rhythm.

the flexor muscles serves as a controlling or braking mechanism. When resistance to extension is offered, the posterior glenohumeral muscles act, including the sternocostal pectoralis, latissimus dorsi, and teres major, with assistance provided by the posterior deltoid and long head of the triceps brachii (**Figure 10-3, 10-5**).

Glenohumeral Abduction

The muscles superior to the glenohumeral joint produce abduction and include the middle deltoid and supraspinatus (**Figure 10-3**). During the contribution of the middle deltoid, from approximately 90° through 180° of abduction, the infraspinatus, subscapularis, and teres minor produce inferiorly directed force to neutralize the superiorly directed dislocating force produced by the middle deltoid. This action serves an important function in preventing impingement of the supraspinatus and subacromial bursa.

Glenohumeral Adduction

As with extension, adduction in the absence of resistance results from gravitational force with the abductors controlling the speed of motion. When resistance is present, adduction is accomplished through the action of the muscles positioned on the inferior side of the glenohumeral joint, including the latissimus dorsi, teres major, and sternocostal pectoralis (**Figure 10-5**). The short head of the biceps and long head of the triceps contribute minor assistance. When the arm is elevated above 90°, the coracobrachialis and subscapularis also assist.

Lateral and Medial Rotation of the Humerus

Lateral rotators of the humerus lie on the posterior aspect of the humerus, including the infraspinatus and teres minor, with assistance provided by the posterior deltoid. Muscles on the anterior side of the humerus contribute to medial rotation. These include the subscapularis and teres major, with assistance from the pectoralis major, anterior deltoid, latissimus dorsi, and the short head of the biceps (**Figure 10-3**). **Table 10-2** provides a summary of muscles that act on the arm.

Although the glenohumeral joint provides most of the range of motion needed to throw a ball, a forceful movement of the upper extremity requires the coordinated contribution of motion from all joints in the shoulder complex. Consequently, an injury to one joint can affect the ability of the other joints to work effectively.

KINETICS OF THE SHOULDER

For what reason is the shoulder considered to be a major load-bearing joint?

Although the articulations of the shoulder girdle are interconnected, the glenohumeral joint sustains much greater loads than the other shoulder joints. This is primarily because the glenohumeral joint provides mechanical support for the entire arm. Although the weight of the arm is only approximately 9% of body weight, the length of the horizontally extended arm creates large torques that must be countered by the shoulder muscles. When these muscles contract to support the extended arm, large compressive forces are generated inside the joint. The compressive force acting on the articulating surfaces of the glenohumeral joint when the arm is abducted to 90° has been estimated to reach 90% of body weight. Although this load is reduced by about half when the elbow is maximally flexed due to the shortened moment arm, the shoulder is considered to be a major load-bearing joint (4).

Muscles that attach to the humerus at small angles with respect to the glenoid fossa contribute more to shear than to compression at the joint. These muscles serve the important role of stabilizing the humerus in the fossa when the contractions of the powerful muscles that move the humerus might otherwise dislocate the joint. Maximum shear force has been found to be present at the glenohumeral joint when the arm is elevated approximately 60° (4).

The length and weight of the horizontally extended arm combine to generate a large torque that must be counteracted by the muscles of the glenohumeral joint. Contraction of these muscles creates compression on the joint.

PREVENTION OF SHOULDER INJURIES

The shoulder complex enables extreme mobility but provides little stability. As a result, injuries are common to the region. What measures can you take to protect and

During abduction, the infraspinatus, teres minor, and subscapularis produce inferiorly directed force to neutralize the superiorly directed dislocating force from the middle deltoid

When the arm is abducted to 90°, it has been estimated that the load exerted on the glenohumeral joint can reach 90% of body weight

Table 10–2. Muscles Producing Movement at the Glenohumeral Joint.

Flexion	Extension	Abduction	Adduction	Medial Rotation	Lateral Rotation
Deltoid (anterior)	Deltoid (posterior)	Deltoid (middle)	Pectoralis major (sternal)	Pectoralis major	Infraspinatus
Pectoralis major (clavicular)	Latissimus dorsi	Supraspinatus	Latissimus dorsi	Latissimus dorsi	Teres minor
Coracobrachialis (posterior)	Pectoralis major (sternal)	Biceps brachii (long head)	Teres major	Teres major	Deltoid
Biceps brachii (short head)	Teres major		Coracobrachialis	Subscapularis	Supraspinatus
	Triceps brachii (long head)		Infraspinatus	Deltoid (anterior)	
			Biceps brachii (short head)		
			Triceps brachii (long head)		

Muscles Producing Movement of the Scapula.

Elevation	Depression	Abduction	Adduction	Superior Rotation	Inferior Rotation
Trapezius (upper)	Trapezius (lower)	Pectoralis minor	Trapezius (middle and lower)	Serratus anterior	Rhomboids
Levator scapulae	Pectoralis minor	Serratus anterior	Rhomboids	Trapezius (upper and lower)	Levator scapulae
Serratus anterior (superior fibers)	Latissimus dorsi				Pectoralis minor
					Latissimus dorsi

strengthen the musculature to reduce the risk for injury?

Acute and chronic injuries to the shoulder complex are common in sport participation. Many contact and collision sports do require some protective equipment, but in most cases, flexibility and physical conditioning, along with proper technique are the primary factors that can reduce the risk of injury to this vulnerable area.

Protective Equipment

Contact and collision sports, such as football, lacrosse, and ice hockey require use of shoulder pads. These pads protect exposed bony protuberances from high velocity-low mass forces, and low velocity-high mass forces. **Field Strategy 6-3** outlined guidelines in fitting football shoulder pads. Although shoulder pads do prevent some soft tissue injuries

to the region, they do not protect the glenohumeral joint from excessive motion. As a result, special commercial restraints are often added to the pads to prevent excessive abduction at the glenohumeral joint (**Figure 6-10**). These restraints can prevent or reduce the severity of glenohumeral sprains. Protective padding can also be applied to vulnerable areas, and is typically secured with an elastic tape or wrap.

Physical Conditioning

Flexibility and strengthening are of major importance in reducing risk of injury to the shoulder complex. Limited range of motion and lack of flexibility can predispose an individual to joint sprains and muscular strains. Warm-up exercises should focus on general joint flexibility, and may be performed alone or with a partner utilizing proprioceptive neuromuscular facilitation (PNF) stretching techniques. Individuals using the throwing motion in their sport should increase range of motion in external rotation, as it has been shown to increase the velocity of the throwing arm and decrease shearing forces on the glenohumeral joint (7). Several flexibility exercises for the shoulder complex are demonstrated in **Field Strategy 10-1**.

Strengthening programs should focus on muscles acting on both the glenohumeral and scapulothoracic region. In throwers, a weakened supraspinatus is often present. Concentric and eccentric contractions with light resistance in the first 30° of abduction can be used to strengthen this muscle. The infraspinatus is also frequently weak and atrophied in a chronic shoulder problem. Strength in the infraspinatus, teres minor, and posterior shoulder musculature is necessary to: (a) begin the cocking phase of throwing, (b) fix the shoulder girdle during the acceleration phase, and (c) provide adequate muscle tension through eccentric contractions for smooth deceleration through the follow-through phase (7). To strengthen the infraspinatus, teres minor, posterior deltoid, trapezius and rhomboids, move the arm through a resisted diagonal pattern of external rotation and horizontal abduction. Push-ups are also helpful in strengthening the scapulothoracic musculature. Other exercises to strengthen the shoulder complex are demonstrated in **Field Strategy 10-2**.

Proper Skill Technique

As mentioned above, coordinated muscle contractions are necessary for smooth execution of the throwing motion. Any disruption in the sequencing of integrated movements can lead to additional stress on the glenohumeral joint and surrounding soft tissue structures. High speed photography is often used to assess proper throwing mechanics in baseball pitchers. These movies record a series of throwing mechanics that could lead to early detection of improper technique. High speed photography can also be used in other sports, such as volleyball, tennis, softball, and swimming to detect improper technique.

In addition to proper throwing technique, participants in contact and collision sports should be taught the shoulder roll method of falling, rather than falling on an outstretched arm. This technique reduces direct compres-

sion of the articular joints and disperses the force over a wider area.

Flexibility at the glenohumeral joint is necessary to provide adequate range of motion to perform throwing-like activities. In addition, adequate strength in the glenohumeral and scapulothoracic muscles allow for a synchronized throwing action that can reduce stress on the glenohumeral joint and reduce the incidence of many shoulder injuries.

SPRAINS TO THE SHOULDER COMPLEX

A baseball player is complaining that his shoulder feels "dead" in the cocking phase of the throwing motion. Pain increases during acceleration. Muscular endurance and strength is not at the level it was earlier in the season. What structures may be involved in this injury? How will you manage this condition?

Ligamentous injuries to the SC joint, AC joint, and glenohumeral joint typically occur as a result of compression, tension, and shearing forces. These forces may stem from a direct blow, falling on the point of the shoulder, falling on an outstretched arm, receiving a force on the top of the shoulder producing tensile forces between two structures, or by repetitive direct or indirect trauma, such as that caused by the throwing motion (**Figure 10-12**). Acute sprains to the sternoclavicular, acromioclavicular, and glenohumeral ligaments are commonly seen in hockey, rugby, football, soccer, equestrian sports, and the martial arts.

Sternoclavicular Joint Sprain

The SC joint is the main axis of rotation for movements of the clavicle and scapula. Nearly all injuries are due to compression from a direct blow. However, indirect forces, such as falling on an outstretched arm, or an opposition force directed on the shoulder while lying on the side, can also damage joint structures. This indirect force drives the shoulder forward and inward disrupting the costoclavicular and sternoclavicular ligaments. The disruption typically drives the proximal clavicle superior, medial, and anterior causing anterior displacement.

First degree injuries are characterized by point tenderness and mild pain over the SC joint with no visible deformity and little disability. Second degree injuries involving

Indirect forces can drive the proximal clavicle superior, medial, and forward causing an anterior displacement

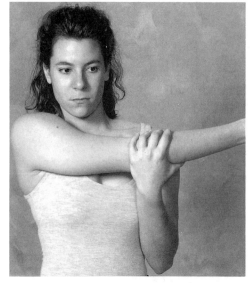

A

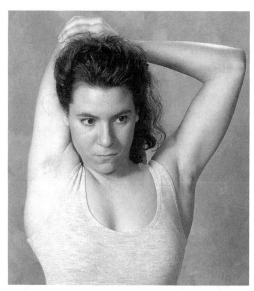

B

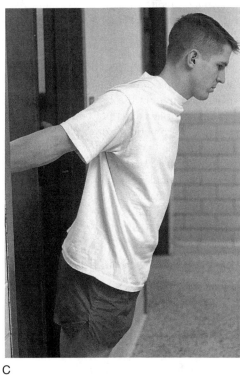

C

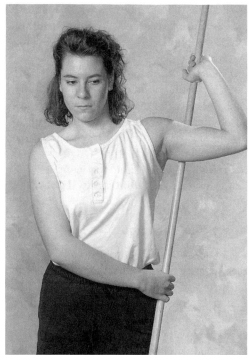

D

A. Posterior capsular stretch. Horizontally adduct the arm across the chest while the opposite hand assists the stretch

B. Inferior capsular stretch. Hold the involved arm over the head with the elbow flexed. Use the opposite hand to assist in the stretching. Add a side stretch

C. Anterior and posterior capsular stretch. Hold onto both sides of a doorway with your hands behind you. Let the arms straighten as you lean forward. Repeat with your hands in front of you as you lean backward

D. Medial and lateral rotators. Using a towel, bat, or racquet, pull the arm to be stretched into medial rotation. Repeat in lateral rotation

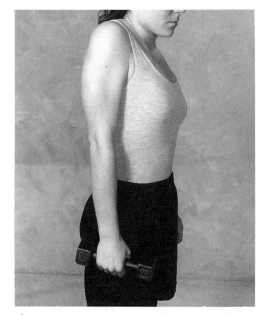

A

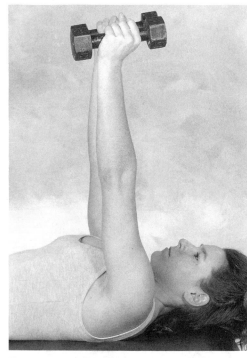

B

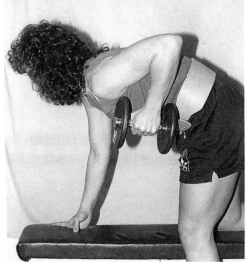

C

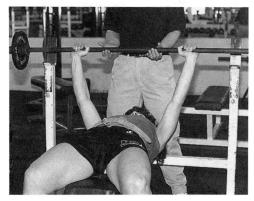

D

A. Shoulder shrugs. Elevate the shoulders toward the ears and hold. Pull the shoulders back, pinch the shoulder blades together, and hold. Relax and repeat

B. Scapular abduction (protraction). Thrust the weight directly upward lifting the posterior shoulder from the table. Relax and repeat

C. Scapular adduction (retraction). Do bent-over rowing while flexing the elbows. At the end of the motion, pinch the shoulder blades together and hold

D. Bench press or incline press. Use a weight belt and spotter. Place the hands shoulder width apart and push the barbell directly above the shoulder joint

(continued)

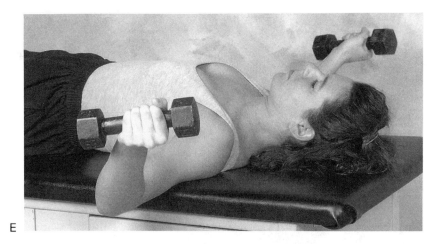

E

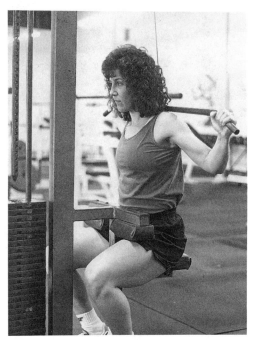

F

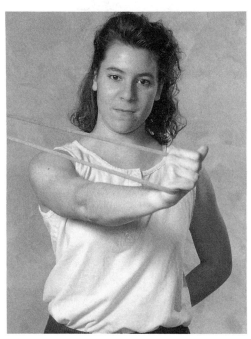

G

E. Bent arm lateral flies, supine position. With the elbows slightly flexed, bring the dumbbells directly over the shoulders. Lower the dumbbells until they are parallel to the floor, then repeat. An alternative method is to move the dumbbells in a diagonal pattern. In the prone position, the exercise strengthens the trapezius (trap flies)

F. Lat pull downs. In a seated position, grasp the handle and pull the bar behind the head. An alternative method is to pull the bar in front of the body

G. Surgical tubing. With the tubing secured, work in diagonal functional patterns

---

> Posterior displacement of the clavicle can lead to hoarseness, difficulty swallowing, diminished pulse, or respiratory distress

stretching or rupturing of ligamentous tissue cause bruising, swelling, and significant pain over the joint line. The individual will be unable to horizontally adduct the arm without considerable pain. Third degree sprains indicate total disruption of the joint, and may

involve a fracture resulting in a prominent displacement of the sternal end of the clavicle.

Posterior displacement, although rare, is more serious than anterior displacement because of the potential injury to the esophagus, trachea, and subclavian artery (**Figure 10-13**).

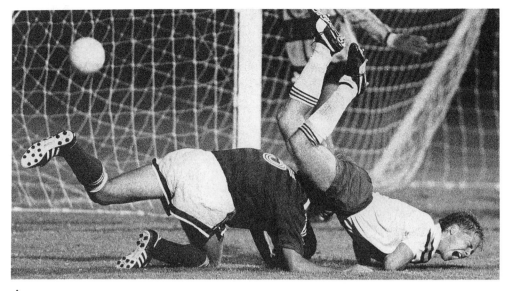

A

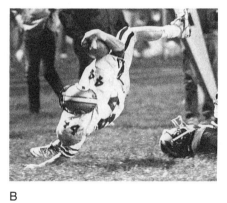

B

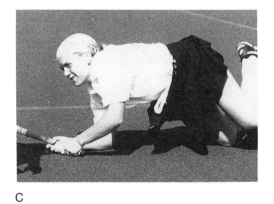

C

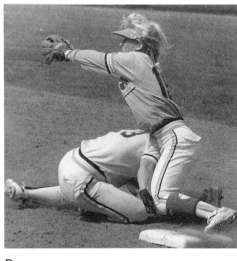

D

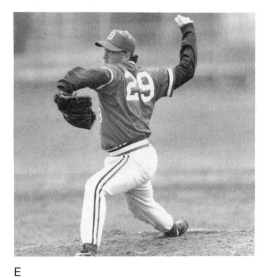

E

Fig. 10.12: Common mechanisms of injury. (A) Direct impact with the ground. (B) Falling on the point of the shoulder. (C) Falling on an outstretched arm. (D) Impact on the top of the shoulder. (E) Repetitive direct or indirect trauma.

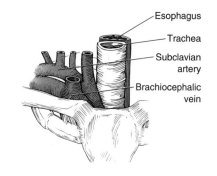

Fig. 10.13: The esophagus, trachea, subclavian artery, and brachiocephalic vein can be damaged in a posterior sternoclavicular sprain.

A depression can be palpated between the sternal end of the clavicle and manubrium. The individual will complain of pain with shoulder protraction, and may have hoarseness, difficulty swallowing, shortness of breath, or be gasping for air. A diminished radial pulse at the wrist may be present. Posterior displacement can become life-threatening. As such, the primary and secondary survey should include continued assessment of the ABC's.

First and second degree sprains of the SC joint are immobilized with a sling and swathe, a figure-of-eight elastic wrap, or clavicular strap with a sling. Third degree sprains require immediate reduction of the dislocation by trained medical personnel. **Field Strategy 10-3** summarizes the management of sternoclavicular sprains.

Acromioclavicular Joint Sprain

The AC joint is weak and easily injured by a direct blow, a fall with impact taken on the point of the shoulder (called a shoulder pointer), and occasionally from a force transmitted up the long axis of the humerus during a fall on an outstretched arm. In a first degree injury, minimal swelling and tearing of the acromioclavicular ligament is present. No deformity in displacement of the clavicle is seen and palpation reveals only mild discomfort over the joint line (**Figure 10-14**). Pain will be present on abduction past 90°. In a second degree injury, the superior and inferior acromioclavicular ligaments are torn, leading to some subluxation of the joint surfaces, but the coracoclavicular ligament is still intact, although it can also be partially torn. The clavicle rides above the level of the acromion and swelling is present over the joint line (**Figure 10-15**). Pain increases when a steady downward pressure is exerted on the distal clavicle and in an anteroposterior direction. A palpable gap or minor step is present over the joint line. Point tenderness along the distal border of the clavicle may indicate some tearing of the trapezius and deltoid attachments. Tenderness may also be elicited over the coracoclavicular ligament if it has been torn. Horizontal adduction causes increased pain and may elicit a snapping sound at the AC joint.

A third degree injury indicates complete ligamentous disruption of the acromioclavicular and coracoclavicular ligaments. There is obvious swelling, bruising, and a step deformity present at the distal clavicle. Extensive mobility and pain in the area may signify tearing of the deltoid and trapezius muscle attachments at the distal clavicle. Immediate

> Horizontal adduction causes increased pain and may elicit a snapping sound at the AC joint

Field Strategy 10–3. Management of a Sternoclavicular Sprain.

Signs and Symptoms	Mild-1°	Moderate-2°	Severe-3°
Deformity	None	Slight prominence of medial end of the clavicle	Gross prominence of medial end of the clavicle
Swelling	Slight	Moderate	Severe
Palpable pain	Mild	Moderate	Severe
Movement	Usually unlimited, but may have discomfort with movement	Unable to abduct the arm or horizontally adduct the arm across the chest without noticeable pain	Limited as in 2°, but pain will be more severe
Treatment	Ice, rest, immobilize with sling and swathe	Ice, rest, immobilize with figure-of-eight or clavicular strap with sling for 3 to 4 weeks. Initiate strength program after 3 to 4 weeks	Figure-of-eight immobilizer with scapulas retracted. Refer to physician

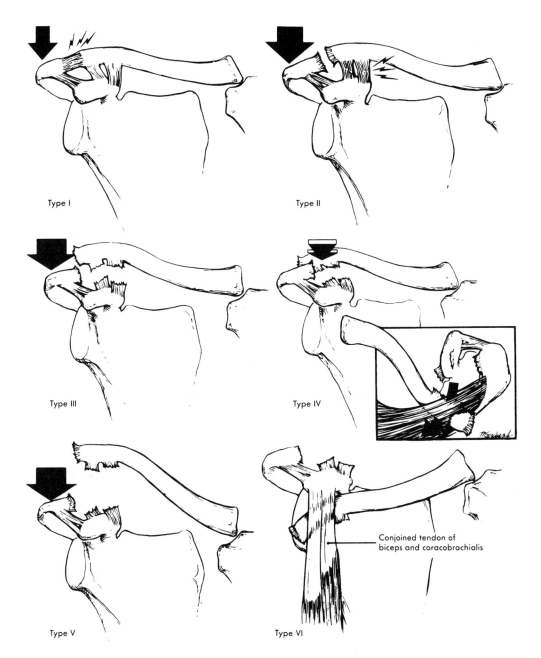

Type I

Type II

Type III

Type IV

Type V

Type VI

Conjoined tendon of
biceps and coracobrachialis

Fig. 10.14: Acromioclavicular sprains.

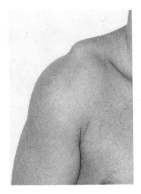

Fig. 10.15: With an acromioclavicular separation, the distal clavicle is elevated.

referral to a physician is warranted, as radiographs provide a more accurate measurement of the separation between the distal clavicle and acromion, and can rule out a fracture.

First and second degree injuries are treated conservatively with ice and range of motion exercises as tolerated. Immobilization is necessary only if pain is present. The individual may return to certain activities earlier than others, but the area should be padded to protect it from further insult. Most third degree injuries are treated nonoperatively with ice treatments during the first 72 hours to control pain and inflammation followed by

Immobilization is necessary only if pain is present

moist heat therapy. Recent studies have shown that nonsurgical treatment is superior in restoring normal shoulder function the first year following injury (8,9). Gentle range of motion exercises can begin at two weeks followed by a period of resisted exercises to strengthen the atrophied muscles and increase joint mobility. **Field Strategy 10-4** summarizes management of acromioclavicular sprains.

In severe cases where total disruption of the supporting ligaments has occurred, the intra-articular disk is damaged, or an intra-articular fracture is involved, open or arthroscopic intervention may be necessary. Immobilization may extend to four to six weeks followed by a gradual rehabilitation program. Complete sport participation is usually not permitted before 12 weeks postsurgery.

Glenohumeral Joint Sprain

Damage to the glenohumeral joint can occur when the arm is forcefully abducted (i.e., when making an arm tackle in football), or abducted and externally rotated. In nearly all cases (95%), the anterior capsule is stretched or torn from its attachment to the anterior glenoid. This results in the humeral head slipping out of the glenoid fossa in an anterior-inferior direction **(Figure 10-16)**. A direct blow or forceful movement that pushes the humerus posteriorly can also result in damage to the joint capsule. Instability leads to a glenohumeral joint sprain or dislocation, and can be acute or recurrent.

In a first degree injury, the anterior shoulder is particularly painful to palpation. Although passive range of motion should not be restricted, pain occurs during glenohumeral movement, especially when the mechanism of injury is reproduced. Active range of motion may be slightly limited, but pain will not occur on adduction or internal rotation, such as will occur with a muscular strain. A second degree sprain will produce some joint laxity. Pain is usually severe; active and passive range of motion—particularly abduction—is limited, and there may be swelling or bruising (8).

Treatment depends on the severity of pain and limited motion. Cryotherapy, rest, non-

Field Strategy 10–4. Management of an Acromioclavicular Sprain.

Signs and Symptoms	Mild-1°	Moderate-2°	Severe-3°
Deformity	None, ligaments are still intact	Slight elevation of lateral clavicle; AC ligaments are disrupted, but coracoclavicular is still intact	Prominent elevation of clavicle; AC ligaments and coracoclavicular ligaments are disrupted
Swelling	Slight	Moderate	Severe
Palpable pain	Mild over joint line	Moderate with downward pressure on distal clavicle; palpable gap or minor step present; snapping may be felt on horizontal adduction	Severe on palpation and downward displacement of acromion process; definite palpable step deformity present
Movement	Usually unlimited, but may have some discomfort on abduction over 90°	Unable to abduct the arm or horizontally adduct the arm across the chest without noticeable pain	Limited as in 2°, but pain will be more severe
Stability	No instability	Some instability	Demonstrable instability
Treatment	Ice, NSAIDs, and return to activity as tolerated with protection	Ice, NSAIDs, immobilize with sling 1 to 4 weeks if pain is present. Return to activity with protection	Ice, immobilize, and refer to physician

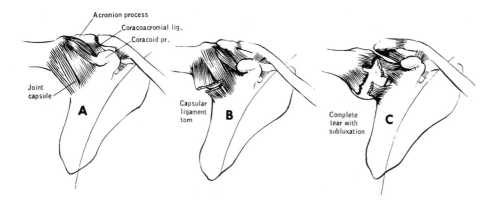

Fig. 10.16: Glenohumeral sprains. (A) Normal abduction with some stretching of the fibers. (B) Forced external rotation and abduction with minimal tears to the joint capsule leading to a moderate or second degree sprain. (C) Continuation of the forced movement causes a third degree sprain or shoulder dislocation.

steroidal anti-inflammatory drugs (NSAIDs), and immobilization with a sling during the initial 12 to 24 hours can reduce pain and inflammation. Once hemorrhage has subsided, early emphasis on pain-free range of motion exercises, elastic band strengthening and PNF exercises should be stressed. Exercises to regain full external rotation and abduction should be delayed at least three weeks to allow adequate time for capsular healing (8). A more extensive resistance program can be started as soon as the individual can tolerate it. In certain sports, particularly football, a functional brace such as the one seen in **Figure 6-10** can limit abduction and external rotation to prevent recurrence.

Glenohumeral Dislocations

Anterior dislocations to the glenohumeral joint may result from a blow to the posterolateral aspect of the shoulder. More commonly, however, indirect excessive forces push the arm into abduction, external rotation, and extension. The capsule and capsular ligaments are significantly damaged as the head of the humerus is forced out of the glenoid fossa in an anterior-inferior direction to locate adjacent to the coracoid process **(Figure 10-17)**. The labrum may be damaged or avulsed from the anterior lip of the glenoid as the humerus slides forward **(Bankart lesion)**.

There is intense pain with the initial dislocation, although recurrent dislocations may be less painful. Tingling and numbness may extend down the arm into the hand. The individual may become very frightened and apprehensive. With a first time dislocation,

the injured arm is often held in slight abduction (20 to 30°) and external rotation, and is stabilized against the body by the opposite hand. Visually, a sharp contour on the affected shoulder with a prominent acromion process can be seen when compared to the smooth deltoid outline on the unaffected shoulder **(Figure 10-18)**. The humeral head may be palpated in the axilla anterior to the acromion resting adjacent to the coracoid process. The individual will not allow passive horizontal adduction or internal rotation of the arm (i.e., the arm cannot be brought across the chest). Assessment of both the axillary nerve and artery is imperative since both structures are vulnerable to injury in a dislocation. A pulse may be taken on the medial proximal humerus over the brachial artery, or at the radial artery in the wrist. The axillary nerve innervates the teres minor and deltoid muscle and provides sensory innervation to the skin on the upper lateral arm. This nerve is assessed by stroking the skin on the upper lateral arm in the region of the deltoid muscle. Ask the individual if it feels the same on both arms. Because the deltoid is not only a key shoulder abductor, but also contributes to shoulder flexion and extension, damage to this nerve can be devastating (10).

Management of a first time dislocation requires immediate reduction by a physician, since many are often associated with a fracture. Treat the injury as a fracture and immobilize the arm in a comfortable position. To prevent unnecessary movement of the humerus, place a rolled towel or thin pillow between the thoracic wall and humerus prior to applying a sling. Ice is applied to control hemorrhage and muscle spasm as the indi-

Bankart lesion
Avulsion or damage to the anterior lip of the glenoid as the humerus slides forward in an anterior dislocation

In a first time dislocation, the injured arm is held in slight abduction and external rotation, and may be stabilized against the body with the opposite hand

The axillary nerve and artery can be damaged in a shoulder dislocation

Treat a first time dislocation as a fracture and immobilize the arm in a comfortable position

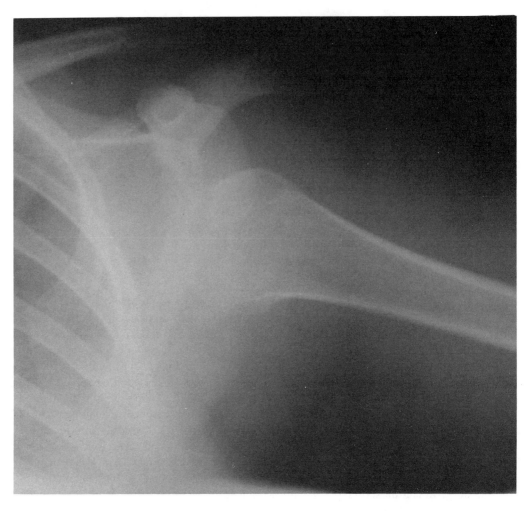

Fig. 10.17: In a typical anterior dislocation, the head of the humerus is forced out of the glenoid fossa and comes to rest adjacent to the coracoid process.

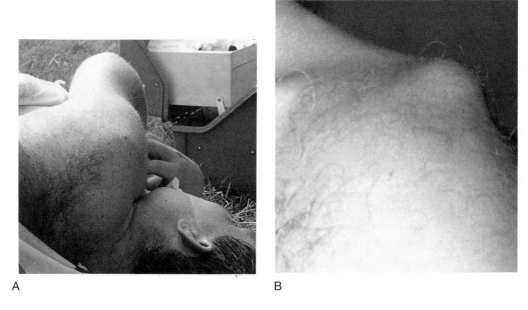

A   B

Fig. 10.18: Suspect an anterior dislocation if you observe a prominent acromion process, a flat contour of the deltoid musculature, or if the athlete carries the arm away from the side. (A) Lying down position. (B) Standing position.

vidual is transported to the nearest medical facility.

After reduction, the shoulder is immobilized in adduction and internal rotation. The immobilizer may be removed for prescribed exercises or bathing, but should not be removed for sleeping. Adjustable binders on the shoulder brace enable the therapist to redefine the limits of movement and eliminate the risk of premature movement into a range of motion restricted by the injury (11). Cryotherapy is used to reduce swelling and pain. Resisted isometric and stretching exercises should be started immediately after the acute phase has ended. Theraband exercises below 90° of abduction can be incorporated early in the program to maintain and improve strength (12). Interferential current stimulation is used to reduce inflammation, stimulate muscle re-education, promote deep tissue circulation, and minimize fibrotic infiltration (11). Strength development of the lateral rotators can reduce strain on the anterior structures of the joint by pulling the humeral head posteriorly during lateral rotation of the shoulder, thus reducing anterior instability (13,14). Strong scapula stabilizers (e.g., trapezius, rhomboids, serratus anterior), are also believed to improve anterior stability by placing the glenoid in the optimal position to perform the skill techniques required. Isokinetic internal rotation and adduction can begin within three to four weeks and advance as tolerated. Complete shoulder rehabilitation exercises are not started until five to six weeks after removal of the shoulder brace. **Field Strategy 10-5** lists several exercises to include in a chronic glenohumeral dislocation rehabilitation program.

Occasionally a posterior dislocation occurs from a fall on, or blow to, the anterior surface of the shoulder, or a fall on the outstretched arm that is flexed, adducted, and internally rotated (15,16). The humeral head slides posteriorly past the glenoid fossa to lodge in the posterior rotator cuff musculature. Because of the tension in these muscles, the dislocation may reduce spontaneously without the person even realizing the shoulder has been dislocated, making evaluation difficult. If dislocated, the individual will complain of pain radiating to the tip of the shoulder along the axillary nerve cutaneous pattern. The entire arm will be carried tightly against the chest and across the front of the trunk in rigid adduction and internal rotation. When

viewed from the side, the anterior shoulder will appear flat, the coracoid process will become prominent, and a corresponding bulge may be seen posteriorly if not masked by a heavy deltoid musculature (8,16). Any attempt to abduct or externally rotate the arm produces severe pain. Because the biceps brachii is unable to function in this position, the individual will be unable to supinate the forearm with the shoulder flexed (15). Treatment is the same as with an acute anterior dislocation with immobilization in a sling, and immediate transportation to a physician.

Recurrent Subluxations and Dislocations

Acute dislocations or repetitive trauma can significantly damage supporting structures of the glenohumeral joint leading to recurrent subluxations and dislocations. In recurrent injuries, anterior dislocations are more common than anterior subluxations. In contrast, posterior subluxations are more common than dislocations (17).

In recurrent anterior subluxations or dislocations the mechanism of injury is the same as previously noted in acute dislocations, i.e., forced abduction, external rotation, and extension. However, as the number of occurrences increases, the forces needed to produce the injury decrease. The characteristic deformity of acute dislocations will be present, but associated muscle spasm, pain, and swelling typically seen in acute cases will lessen with each occurrence. The individual is aware of the shoulder displacing because the arm will give the sensation of "going dead," commonly referred to as the **dead arm syndrome**. Often it is reduced by the individual or with the help of a teammate.

Recurrent posterior subluxations are common in activities such as the follow-through phase of throwing, or a racquet swing, ascent phase of push-ups or bench pressing, linebacker recoil, certain swimming strokes, or during crew sweep strokes (15). Many individuals voluntarily induce subluxation by positioning the arm in flexion, adduction, and internal rotation. Pain is usually the major complaint with crepitation and/or clicking when the arm shifts into the appropriate position.

Under the direction of a physician, initial treatment involves reducing the dislocation or subluxation quickly and safely. Conserva-

In a posterior dislocation, the individual may not realize the shoulder has dislocated, but may complain of pain radiating to the tip of the shoulder along the axillary nerve cutaneous pattern

Any attempt to abduct or externally rotate the arm will produce severe pain

In recurrent injuries, anterior dislocations are more common than anterior subluxations. In contrast, posterior subluxations are more common than dislocations

Dead arm syndrome
Common sensation felt with a recurrent anterior shoulder dislocation

Recurrent posterior subluxations are common in activities, such as the follow-through phase of throwing, ascent phase of push-ups or bench pressing, linebacker recoil, or during crew sweep strokes

Field Strategy 10-5. Exercises for a Chronic Glenohumeral Dislocation.

Exercises should begin as soon as pain subsides. A chronic condition will likely have little or no loss of mobility. Therefore, the program should focus on strength development.
Isometric exercises. Pain-free exercises should be performed hourly with 20 to 30 repetitions.

A. With the glenohumeral joint in a neutral position, do medial and lateral rotation, flexion, extension, and abduction isometric exercises against a wall. Perform adduction by pressing against a pillow in the axilla

B. With the arm abducted at 90°, perform horizontal abduction and adduction against a doorway

Progressive resistance exercises. Exercises should be controlled while focusing on the line of movement. Begin with gravity as resistance, progress to light dumbbells or sandbags, surgical tubing, then overhead exercises with moderate resistance.

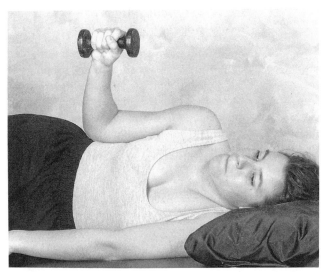

C. Sidelying medial and lateral rotation. With the elbow flexed, perform lateral and medial rotation

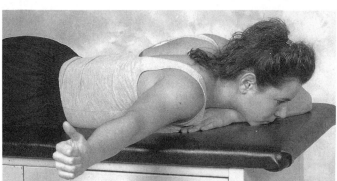

D. Prone horizontal abduction (90°). The arm hangs over the table with the hand rotated outward. Raise the arm and laterally rotate the humerus until it is parallel to the floor

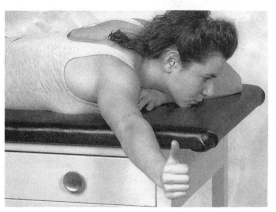

E. Prone horizontal abduction (100°). With the arm abducted at 100°, raise the arm and laterally rotate the humerus

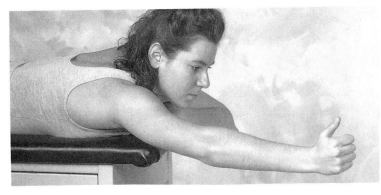

F. Prone flexion and extension. With the hand rotated outward as far as possible, raise the arm forward into flexion. Repeat, moving the arm into extension

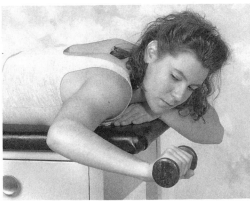

G. Prone medial and lateral rotation. With the shoulder abducted 90° and the elbow flexed, perform lateral and medial rotation. Repeat in the supine position

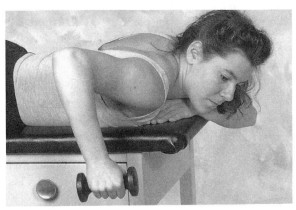

H. Prone rows (scapular adduction). With the shoulder abducted 90° and the elbow flexed, raise the arm off the table as if pinching the shoulder blades together. Do not raise the chest off the table

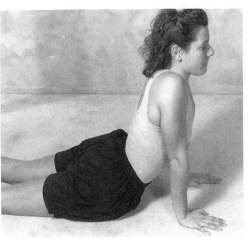

I. Wall push-ups and press-ups
J. PNF diagonal patterns with surgical tubing
K. Lat pull downs
L. Bent arm lateral flies (Pec flies)
M. Biceps and triceps curls
N. Shoulder shrugs
O. Ball exercises. Bounce a ball at 90° of shoulder flexion against a wall to promote scapular stability and proprioception for the glenohumeral joint
P. Push ups. Place two to three boxes of varying height on the floor. Move between the boxes by placing one hand at a time on top of the box constantly moving to the right. Repeat by moving back to the left

tive treatment with rest and immobilization involves avoiding any voluntary episodes of movement or positions likely to cause a subluxation or dislocation, restoring shoulder motion, and strengthening the rotator cuff muscles. If persistent instability occurs, surgery may be indicated.

Multidirectional shoulder instability (MDI) occurs when damage is done in more than one plane. Acutely, most if not all anterior and posterior dislocations are associated with some pre-existing inferior laxity, or laxity in the opposite direction (15). Pain and/or clicking can occur during simple tasks, such as picking up a box or suitcase. Treatment is initially conservative with 50 to 70% responding favorably to rehabilitation and activity modification. Surgical repair is indicated for individuals who do not respond to conservative measures.

The baseball player complained that the shoulder felt "dead" in the cocking position of the throwing motion. Did you determine that he may have a recurrent anterior subluxation, commonly referred to as the dead arm syndrome? If so you are correct.

OVERUSE INJURIES

A volleyball player has severe pain during spiking drills that is getting worse. The player is unable to actively abduct the arm between 70 to 120° without excruciating pain. What structures may be involved in this injury? How can you determine if the subacromial bursa is involved?

Although an acute injury can occur to soft tissue structures, injuries at the shoulder more commonly occur as a result of repetitive overhead motions that impinge the muscles, bursae, and nerves between non-yielding bony and soft tissue structures. The proximal attachments of the rotator cuff muscles on the scapula are slightly caudal to the distal attachments on the humerus, relative to the glenoid fossa. Normally, this depressive function prevents the humeral head from migrating upward and impinging the supraspinatus tendon and subacromial bursa between the acromion, the coracoacromial ligament, and the greater tubercle of the humerus. Repeated over-stretching of the rotator cuff musculature and long head of the biceps brachii results in excessive joint laxity. The tendons are incapable of depressing the humeral head in the glenoid fossa during overhead motion. As a result, the rotator cuff/biceps must work harder to maintain the

joint in its normal anatomical position. Fatigue sets in faster, leading to further reliance upon the joint capsule for stability. The middle deltoid muscle consequently pulls the humeral head superiorly during abduction, resulting in impingement and subsequent wear and tear on the supraspinatus tendon and subacromial bursa (18). This compressive impingement can lead to a rotator cuff strain, impingement syndrome, bursitis, and bicipital tendinitis.

Rotator Cuff Injuries

A single indirect force can lead to an acute tear of the muscles (supraspinatus, infraspinatus, teres minor, and subscapularis). Acute tears may result when the arm is violently pushed into abduction, such as when an ice hockey player is pushed face forward into the boards and uses the arms to cushion the impact. The individual may hear the cuff tear and complain of acute sharp pain in the anterosuperior shoulder. Strength in abduction is significantly impaired, and surgical repair is usually indicated. More commonly however, the supraspinatus tendon is impinged just proximal to the greater tubercle of the humerus, leading to chronic, degenerative, partial- or full-thickness tears in the tendon (**Figure 10-19**). Partial tears are usually seen in young individuals with total tears typically seen in adults over 30 years of age (19).

Chronic tears in young individuals often result from repetitive microtraumatic episodes. In older age groups, chronic tears can lead to cuff thinning, degeneration, and finally, total rupture of the supraspinatus tendon. Pain is difficult to locate, but in early stages, pain is usually described as deep in the shoulder and present at night. Initially, there is pain with activity, usually only in the impingement position, but as repetitive trauma continues, pain becomes progressively worse. Pain increases when the arm is in 30° horizontal adduction and then moves through active and resisted movement between 70 and 120° of abduction (20). As the condition progresses, it eventually leads to extreme discomfort and inability to perform simple shoulder movements. For example, with a complete tear of the supraspinatus tendon the individual will be unable to actively abduct the arm against minimal resistance. A defect or crepitus in the supraspinatus tendon may be palpated just anterior to the acromion process when the arm is extended at the glenohumeral joint.

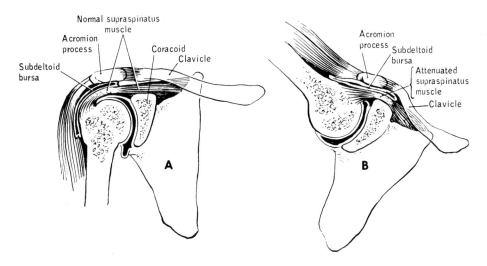

Fig. 10.19: Supraspinatus tendon during abduction. (A) Normal position. (B) Abducted position. Repetitive overhead motions can impinge the muscle or tendon between non-yielding bony and soft tissue structures resulting in a chronic rotator cuff injury.

An arthrogram or radiograph may be indicated, but if the tear is incomplete, treatment will remain conservative with cryotherapy, NSAIDs, rest and activity modification. When the condition is severe, all activities that lead to pain should be avoided until the individual is pain-free. Maintain mobility with stretching exercises. Isometric and isokinetic strengthening exercises should work the scapula rotators, rotator cuff, and trunk musculature below the level of discomfort.

Special attention should be given to the infraspinatus muscle, as it is the only muscle in a position to generate a significant inferior pull on the humeral head (8). To strengthen the infraspinatus and supraspinatus, place the individual prone on a table with the arm in maximum external rotation and abducted 90° and 100°, respectively (20). Exercises such as pull-ups or push-ups should be avoided in the early stages of rehabilitation, as they can impinge the rotator cuff, thus complicating the condition (21).

Once stiffness and discomfort have been overcome, rapid resumption of a strength program for the scapula rotators and rotator cuff muscles can begin throughout the full range of motion. However, the condition may flare up, prolonging rehabilitation. Surgery is not indicated unless little improvement is seen after 9 to 12 months of rehabilitation, or if daily activities are severely hampered (18). Even with surgical repair of the tendon, at least one year of intensive rehabilitation is still needed for full return of integrity, espe-

cially in those sports where maximum stress is applied to the repaired area. **Field Strategy 10-6** outlines several exercises to include in a rehabilitation program for a rotator cuff injury.

Impingement Syndrome

Impingement syndrome not only involves the rotator cuff muscles but can include damage to the glenoid labrum, long head of the biceps brachii, and subacromial bursa. Like rotator cuff tears, damage is typically due to repetitive overhead activity, such as in throwing, overhead serving, spiking a volleyball, javelin throw, or certain swimming strokes, namely freestyle, backstroke, and butterfly. The condition is sometimes called "painful arc" syndrome, or among competitive swimmers, *"swimmer's shoulder"*.

Pain occurs during rapid overhead movements from external rotation into internal rotation, particularly when glenohumeral abduction is between 70 and 120° (hence the name painful arc). Swimming strokes use adduction and internal rotation with excessive propulsion forces (22,23). With hypermobile shoulder joints, this motion may allow subclinical anterior subluxations to occur, thus damaging the glenoid labrum. This anterior lesion may be frayed but not detached, resulting in a roughened leading edge that may mechanically catch during overhead motions. As such, swimmers may feel a snapping sensation or clicking when

Impingement syndrome
Chronic condition caused by repetitive overhead activity that damages the glenoid labrum, long head of the biceps brachii, and subacromial bursa

Field Strategy 10–6. Exercises for a Rotator Cuff Injury.

Wand and T-bar exercises. Hold the stretch for 5 to 10 seconds and repeat 10 to 20 repetitions per session. Initially, range of motion exercises can be performed two to three times daily.

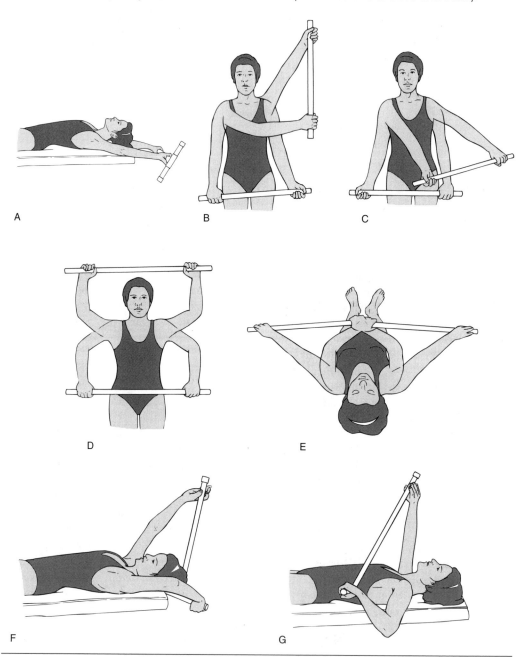

A   B   C

D   E

F   G

moving through the pull phase of the stroke, or sense that the shoulder is "going out".

Examination may reveal diffuse pain depending on which structure is inflamed. It can occur anteriorly over the coracoacromial ligaments, laterally at the insertion of the supraspinatus, posteriorly at the insertion of the infraspinatus and teres minor, or over the long head of the biceps tendon (24). Atrophy of the shoulder muscles with subsequent weakness in the supraspinatus and biceps brachii may also be present. Because forced scapular protraction leads to further impingement and pain in the structures, the individual may be unable to sleep at night on the involved side. Depending on the severity,

Field Strategy 10–6. Exercises for a Rotator Cuff Injury. *(continued)*

Wand and T-bar exercises. Hold the stretch for 5 to 10 seconds and repeat 10 to 20 repetitions per session. Initially, range of motion exercises can be performed two to three times daily.

A. Supine shoulder flexion. Grasp the wand with both hands palm down at waist height. Raise the wand directly overhead leading with the uninvolved arm until a stretch is felt in the involved shoulder. If an impingement syndrome is present, this exercise can be performed palm up
B. Shoulder abduction. Hold the wand with the involved arm palm up, uninvolved arm palm down. Push the wand sideward and upward toward the involved side with the uninvolved arm until a stretch is felt in the involved shoulder
C. Shoulder adduction/horizontal adduction. Reverse hand positions from exercise 2. Pull the wand toward the uninvolved side until a stretch is felt in the involved shoulder
D. Shoulder internal/external rotation. Keeping both palms down, abduct the shoulders and flex the elbows. Move the wand upward toward the head, then return to waist level
E. Shoulder horizontal abduction/adduction. Keeping both palms down, push the wand across the body with the uninvolved arm, then pull back across the body. Do not allow the trunk to twist
F. Supine external rotation. Abduct the shoulder and flex the elbow to 90°. Grip the T-bar in the hand on the involved arm. Use the opposite arm to push the involved arm into external rotation. Perform external rotation with the arm abducted at 135° and 180°
G. Supine internal rotation. With the arms in the same position as in exercise 6, use the uninvolved arm to push the involved arm into internal rotation

Progressive resistance exercises. Refer to Field Strategy 10–5 for progression of these exercises.

H Prone external rotation
I. Prone horizontal abduction at 90° and 100° (palm down)
J. Prone shoulder extension (palm down)
K. Prone shoulder flexion (thumb up). Raise the arm parallel to the floor at a 45° angle to the body
L. Prone rows. This can be performed in varying angles
M. Scapular adduction
N. Sidelying external rotation
O. Standing shoulder shrugs
P. Standing empty can exercise (supraspinatus). With the elbow extended and internally rotated, raise the arm parallel to the floor at a 30° angle to the body
Q. Standing Theraband exercises in external rotation
R. Military press

positive results may be elicited in the supraspinatus test, "empty can test," and impingement tests (see Assessment).

Treatment involves restricting motion below 90° of abduction and using cryotherapy, NSAIDs, and rest until inflammation is controlled. Ultrasound, EMS, interferential therapy, ice, and heat can supplement treatment. Stretching exercises in external rotation are important at 90°, 135°, and 180° of abduction. Progressive resistance exercises should concentrate on the deep scapula rotators and posterior rotator cuff muscles. Swimmers present a special problem. Because rest translates into detraining, other steps may need to be taken to allow contin-ued activity. The intensity and quantity of training need to be reduced, and paddle work eliminated. Stroke mechanics should be assessed to determine if changes are needed to reduce shoulder stress (22,23). Stages of impingement syndrome and its management are summarized in **Field Strategy 10-7.**

Bursitis

Bursitis is commonly seen in swimmers, baseball, softball, and tennis players (24). It is not generally an isolated condition, but rather is associated with other injuries, such as a rotator cuff tear, impingement syndrome, or in older individuals with pre-existing degenerative changes in the rotator cuff.

> Because of forced scapular protraction, the individual may be unable to sleep at night on the involved side

> With swimmers, intensity and quantity of training need to be reduced, and paddle work eliminated

Stage 1	Condition is typically seen in individuals under 25 years old and is reversible.
	Localized hemorrhage and edema is present in the supraspinatus tendon.
	Minimal pain (like a toothache) with activity, but no restriction/weakness of motion.
	Be aware that atrophy of the rotator cuff muscles may be present.
Stage 2	Condition is typically seen in individuals between 25 and 40 years old.
	Marked reactive tendinitis with significant pain between 70° and 120° abduction.
	Inflammation may affect the biceps brachii tendon and subacromial bursa leading to thickening and fibrotic changes in the structures.
	Limited range of motion in external rotation and abduction.
	Possible clicking sounds on resisted adduction and internal rotation.
Stage 3	History of chronic long-term shoulder pain with significant weakness.
	Rotator cuff tear is usually less than 1 centimeter.
	May have prominent capsular laxity with multidirectional instability.
	Noticeable atrophy of the supraspinatus and infraspinatus muscles.
	Arthroscopy may show a damaged labrum.
Stage 4	Rotator cuff tear is greater than 1 centimeter.
Treatment	Use selective rest. Concentrate on motions that do not cause pain for four to six weeks.
	Cryotherapy initially; later contrast with moist heat therapy twice/day.
	NSAIDs may be prescribed by the physician.
	EMS, ultrasound, interferential current, and TENS may be helpful.
	Study skill technique and correct movements that produce shoulder stress.
	Eliminate partner stretching.
	Wand and T-bar exercises can improve sport specific mobility, but should not encourage hypermobility.
	Isometric and Theraband exercises can be performed within a comfort zone to maintain muscle tone at least two to three times daily.
	Use low weights and high repetitions.
	Special attention should be directed toward strengthening the infraspinatus to control superior displacement of the humeral head.
	After four to six weeks incorporate isokinetics at high speeds and Theraband exercises in diagonal patterns.
	Eliminate overhead weight training.
	For swimmers, eliminate use of hand paddles.
	Begin a gradual return to activity as long as the symptoms do not recur.

> The subacromial bursa is the largest and most commonly traumatized bursa in the shoulder region

The subacromial bursa is the largest and most commonly traumatized bursa in the shoulder region. Located between the coracoacromial ligament and the underlying supraspinatus muscle, this bursa provides the shoulder with some inherent gliding ability **(Figure 10-4)**. During the throwing motion this bursa can become inflamed when impinged between the unyielding structures in the subacromial space.

Frequently, a sudden onset of pain at the shoulder is reported during the initiation and acceleration of the throwing motion. Inability to sleep, especially on the affected side occurs because of forced scapular protraction leading to further impingement of the bursa. Pain

> A sudden onset of pain is felt during the initiation and acceleration of the throwing motion

is often referred to the distal deltoid attachment. Point tenderness can be elicited on the anterior and lateral edges of the acromion process. A painful arc will exist between 70 and 120° of passive abduction.

Treatment is symptomatic and includes cryotherapy or heat, NSAIDs, and activity modification. Unfortunately, by the time many individuals seek care for this condition, it has already existed for two to three months. In advanced stages, adhesions form within the bursa leading to chronic inflammation and extended periods of disability. Added problems of reduced extensibility of the bursa cause limited range of motion in external rotation and abduction of the glenohumeral joint. A physician may inject a corticosteriod solution into the subacromial space to relieve the symptoms (24). Before injections are considered however, other underlying conditions, such as a rotator cuff tear, impingement syndrome, or bicipital tendinitis must be ruled out. Exercises to strengthen the area should avoid movements above 90°, particularly in a position of internal rotation. The rotator cuff should be strengthened to prevent elevation of the humeral head during any overhead movement.

Bicipital Tendinitis

Injury to the biceps brachii tendon often occurs from repetitive overuse during rapid overhead movements involving excessive elbow flexion and supination activities such as in racquet sports, shot-putters, baseball/softball pitchers, football quarterbacks, swimmers, and javelin throwers. Irritation of the tendon occurs as it passes back and forth in the intertubercular (bicipital) groove of the humerus. Partial subluxation of the tendon may be due to laxity of the traverse humeral ligament, a poorly developed lesser tubercle, or both. A direct blow to the tendon or tendon sheath can lead to bicipital tenosynovitis. Anterior impingement syndrome associated with overhead rotational activity may also damage the tendon.

Pain and tenderness over the bicipital groove moves when the shoulder is internally and externally rotated. In internal rotation the pain stays medial; in external rotation the pain is located in the midline or just lateral to the groove. Pain may also be elicited when the tendon is passively stretched in extreme shoulder extension with the elbow extended and forearm pronated. Resisted supination of a flexed elbow while externally rotating the shoulder will increase pain, as will forward shoulder flexion of the extended, supinated elbow.

Treatment involves restriction of rotational activities that exacerbate symptoms. Because of potential vascular impingement of the biceps tendon when the shoulder is at the side, the arm should be propped or wedged into slight abduction if immobilized in a sling. In early stages, cryotherapy, NSAIDs, ultrasound, EMS, or interferential therapy can control inflammation. Icing before and after activity is combined with a gradual program of stretching and strengthening as soon as pain subsides.

Biceps Tendon Rupture

A total rupture of the biceps tendon can occur from forceful flexion of the arm against excessive resistance, as in weight lifters or gymnasts, or through forceful movement of the arm while the biceps muscle is contracted. More commonly however, prolonged tendinitis can make the tendon vulnerable to forceful rupture during repetitive overhead motions, such as is commonly seen in swimmers. The rupture occurs as a result of the avascular portion of the proximal tendon constantly passing over the head of the humerus during the execution of the stroke. This condition is often seen in degenerative tendons in older individuals, and in those who have had previous corticosteroid injections into the tendon.

The individual will often hear and feel a snapping sensation, and experience intense pain at the time of the rupture. Ecchymosis and a visible, palpable defect can be seen in the muscle belly when the individual flexes the biceps with the arm in abduction and external rotation (**Figure 10-20**). If the muscle mass moves distally as a result of a proximal long head rupture, a "Popeye" appearance is clearly visible. Partial ruptures may produce only slight muscular deformity but will still be associated with pain and weakness in elbow flexion and supination.

Surgical repair is not usually suggested for the non-competitive athlete or older participant. Many individuals can return to normal sport activity after completing an appropriate rehabilitation program. Surgical repair and fixation is indicated for competitive athletes in order to restore elbow flexion and forearm supination strength needed for competitive sports participation.

Thoracic Outlet Compression Syndrome

Thoracic outlet compression syndrome is a condition when nerves and/or vessels become compressed in the root of the neck or the axilla (**Figure 10-21**). Several disorders are included under the broad title of this condition, including cervical rib syndrome, scalenus-anticus syndrome, Wright's hyperabduction syndrome, and costoclavicular syndrome (25,26). It is often aggravated in activities that require overhead rotational stresses while muscles are loaded, such as in weight lifting and swimming.

With bicipital tendinitis, pain over the bicipital groove moves when the shoulder is internally and externally rotated

A total rupture of the biceps tendon can occur from forceful flexion of the arm against excessive resistance, or through forceful movement of the arm while the biceps muscle is contracted

Thoracic outlet syndrome
Condition whereby nerves and/or vessels become compressed in the root of the neck or axilla leading to numbness in the arm

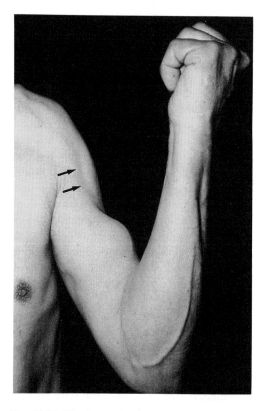

Fig. 10.20: Biceps tendon rupture.

If a nerve is compressed, an aching pain or numbness in the side or back of the neck extends across the shoulder down the medial arm to the ulnar aspect of the hand. Weakness in grasp and atrophy of the hand muscles may also be present. If arterial or venous vessels are compressed, signs and symptoms vary. Venous involvement produces edema, limb stiffness, venous engorgement of the arm with cyanosis, and occasionally thrombophlebitis. Arterial involvement results in a rapid onset of coolness, numbness in the entire arm, and fatigue after exertional overhead activity. The radial pulse may be obliterated when taken with the arm extended and externally rotated while the individual elevates the chin, turns the head toward the arm, and holds the breath (See Adson's maneuver Figure 10-40). Referral to a physician is necessary for more extensive assessment to rule out serious vascular involvement.

Conservative treatment involves assessing muscle strength and posture. Noted deficits should lead to an appropriate retraining program to develop strength and muscle balance in the shoulder girdle and facilitate the maintenance of a corrected posture. If the condi-

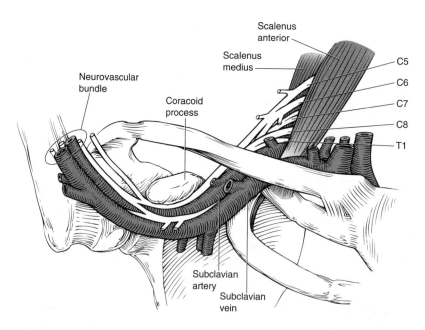

Fig. 10.21: Thoracic outlet syndrome may be caused when the neck musculature is over-developed. The scalenus anticus and subclavian muscles can compress the neurovascular bundle as it passes through the root of the neck, or the neurovascular bundle can be stretched when the arm is hyperabducted and externally rotated. Congenital anomalies, such as a cervical rib or elongated transverse process of C7 may also lead to the condition.

tion was precipitated by a sudden increase in activity, treatment involves anti-inflammatory medication, activity modification, and a reassessment of the training program. Return to full activity may occur after range of motion and strength in the shoulder musculature has been regained.

💡 *The volleyball player had pain during active movement between 70 and 120° abduction. A possible impingement syndrome may have occurred because of the repetitive overhead spiking drills. To distinguish this condition from an isolated bursitis, move the limb through a passive range of motion. If pain still persists in the painful arc, the bursa is also inflamed.*

FRACTURES TO THE SHOULDER REGION

❓ *A young gymnast lost her balance on a dismount and fell onto the point of the right shoulder. The shoulder is sagging down and forward. There is a noticeable bump in the mid-clavicular region. Shoulder movement is limited because of severe pain. What possible condition might you suspect?*

Most fractures to the shoulder region result from a fall on the point of the shoulder, rolling over onto the top of the shoulder, or indirectly by falling on an outstretched arm. In sport, clavicular fractures are more common than fractures to the scapula and proximal humerus.

Clavicular Fractures

The clavicle connects the axial skeleton and appendicular skeleton of the upper extremity. The medial two thirds of the clavicle is convex anteriorly; its lateral third is concave anteriorly, producing the characteristic S-shaped configuration (**Figure 10-1**). It is highly susceptible to compressive forces with midclavicular breaks accounting for nearly 80% of all fractures (**Figure 10-22**). Most fractures are caused by a blow or fall on the point of the shoulder, a direct blow to the bone by an opponent or object, or falling on an outstretched arm.

The sternocleidomastoid muscle pulls the proximal bone fragment upward, allowing the distal shoulder to collapse downward and medial (**Figure 10-23**). Swelling and ecchymosis will be present. A deformity may be visible and palpable at the fracture site. Greenstick fractures typically seen in adolescents will also produce a noticeable deformity. Pain occurs with any shoulder motion, and may radiate into the trapezius area. In older adults, fractures of the distal clavicle may involve tears of the coracoclavicular ligament resulting in an increased deformity. Complications, although rare, may arise if bony fragments penetrate local arteries or nerves.

Immediate treatment involves immobilization in a sling and swathe. After assessment by the physician, a figure-eight brace or

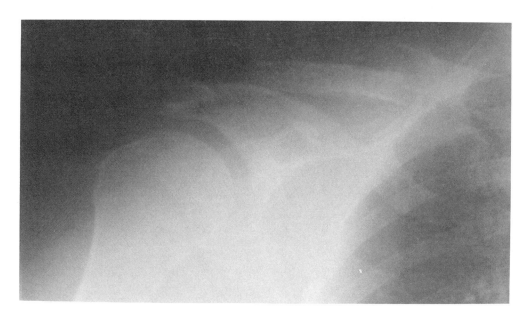

Fig. 10.22: Midclavicular fracture.

Scapular fractures may involve the body, spine and acromion process, coracoid process, or glenohumeral joint

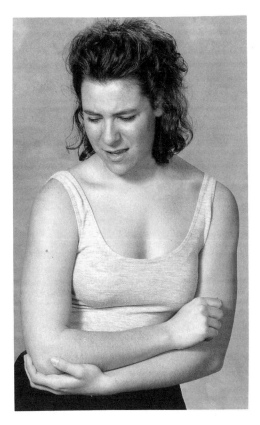

Fig. 10.23: Because the sternocleidomastoid muscle displaces the proximal bone fragment upward, the shoulder will appear to sag downward and medially.

Scapular Fractures

This flat bone is surrounded by muscles that not only protect it, but allow it to glide and recoil along the posterior ribs. Upon impact, force is dissipated through the surrounding soft tissues, thus reducing the incidence of fracture. Nearly 80% of all scapular fractures are associated with other traumatic injuries not typically seen in sport participation. Fractures from extrinsic forces have been reported in football players who were struck by an opponent's helmet directly on the scapula, and in pole vaulters and high jumpers who missed the padded landing pit. Other fractures may be due to axial loading from a fall on an outstretched arm with simultaneous forceful contraction of the serratus anterior.

Scapular fractures may involve the body, spine and acromion process, coracoid process, or glenohumeral joint. Fractures to the body and spine result in minimal displacement and exhibit localized hemorrhage, pain, and tenderness. The individual is reluctant to move the injured arm and prefers to maintain it in adduction. Avulsion fractures to the coracoid process result from direct trauma, or forceful contraction of the pectoralis minor or short head of the biceps brachii. Fractures to the glenoid area are associated with shoulder subluxations and dislocations. In this case, treatment is dictated by the shoulder dislocation rather than the fracture, and often requires open reduction and internal fixation or shoulder reconstruction.

The majority of fractures do not require reduction but should be immediately immobilized with a sling and swathe and referred to a physician. Cryotherapy is used during the first 48 hours to minimize hematoma formation. Complications may arise from scarring

strapping is used to pull the shoulder backward and upward for six to eight weeks (**Figure 10-24**). A sling may supplement the brace to reduce sagging of the arm due to gravity. Although this immobilization prevents movement in nearly all planes, it will not prevent scapular elevation. As a result, healing may be delayed and an excessive callus formation may form at the fracture site.

Scarring and adhesions in muscles overlying the scapula can lead to other muscles compensating for the limited motion leading to overuse injuries

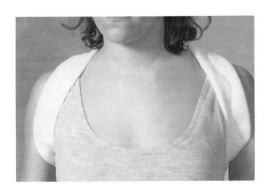
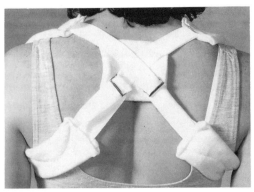

Fig. 10.24: Figure-eight clavicular straps. (A) Anterior view. (B) Posterior view.

and adhesions in the muscles overlying the scapula. Other muscles in the region must then compensate for this limited scapular motion leading to overuse injuries. The amount of adhesions in the area can be reduced with an early program of passive and active stretching exercises.

Epiphyseal and Avulsion Fractures

Strength of the epiphyseal plate is only one fifth that of the joint capsule and supporting ligaments (27). Epiphyseal centers around the shoulder region remain unfused for a longer span of time than is typically seen at other epiphyseal sites. For example, the medial clavicular growth plate does not close until age 25, and is often misdiagnosed as a sternoclavicular subluxation/dislocation. The proximal humeral epiphysis does not close until age 18 to 21 years of age (28). As a result, rotation and compressive forces can lead to epiphyseal fractures in high school and college age individuals. Many of these injuries involve the proximal humeral epiphysis.

Little league shoulder is associated with a fracture of the proximal humeral growth plate **(Figure 10-25)**. This fracture can occur during one throw, but more commonly occurs from a change in the bone resulting from repetitive rotational stresses placed on the shoulder during pitching (29). Catchers may also get this fracture since they throw the ball as hard and often as pitchers, but with less of a windup. Pain may be elicited with deep palpation in the axilla. X-rays are necessary to see the widened epiphyseal line and demineralization. Treatment is conservative with symptoms disappearing after three to four weeks of rest. If activity is resumed too quickly, the condition may recur.

Avulsion fractures to the coracoid process can be seen in a young individual when forceful, repetitive throwing places too much stress on the growth plate. Careful initial assessment and subsequent referral to a physician can help identify these fractures.

Fractures of the lesser tubercle are often associated with posterior glenohumeral dislocations. Fractures of the greater tubercle may be seen in anterior glenohumeral dislocations when the rotator cuff muscles hold fast, avulsing the tubercle. These fractures often require open reduction/internal fixation, particularly when the tubercle cannot be maintained in a stable position.

> Epiphyseal centers around the shoulder region remain unfused for a longer span of time than is typically seen

> **Little league shoulder**
> Fracture of the proximal humeral growth plate in adolescents caused by repetitive rotational stresses during the act of pitching

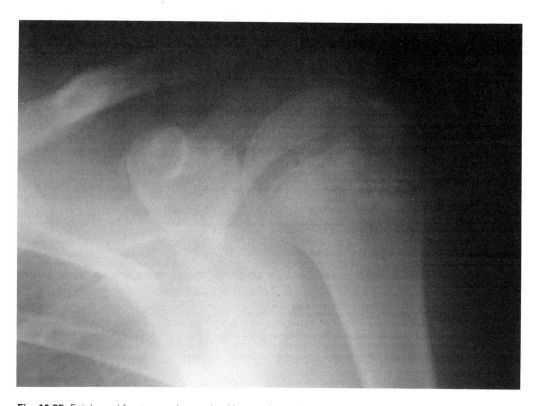

Fig. 10.25: Epiphyseal fracture to the proximal humeral growth center.

Humeral Fractures

Humeral fractures result from violent compressive forces from a direct blow, a fall on the upper arm, or a fall on an outstretched hand with the elbow extended. Fractures to the proximal humerus occur in a region between the surgical neck and midshaft, with the surgical neck being the most common site. A fracture at the surgical neck may display an appearance similar to a dislocation (**Figure 10-26**). Pain, swelling, hemorrhage, discoloration, an inability to move the arm, an inability to supinate the forearm, and possible paralysis may be present. The arm is often held splinted against the body (29). Fortunately, these fractures are often impacted, which facilitates closed reduction and allows early mobilization after three to four weeks of immobilization (8).

During the throwing motion, the pectoralis major or latissimus dorsi can cause excessive rotational torque through the muscular attachments, fracturing the mid-portion of the humerus. These spiral fractures are commonly seen in softball players (29). Fractures to this area can be very serious because of the close proximity of major nerves and vessels running along the bone that may be damaged from jagged bone fragments. As such, immobilization of the limb should be in a rigid or vacuum splint. Assess the neural integrity by stroking the skin on the palm and dorsum of the hand. Ask the individual if it

> Fractures in the mid-portion of the humerus can damage major nerves and vessels running along the bone

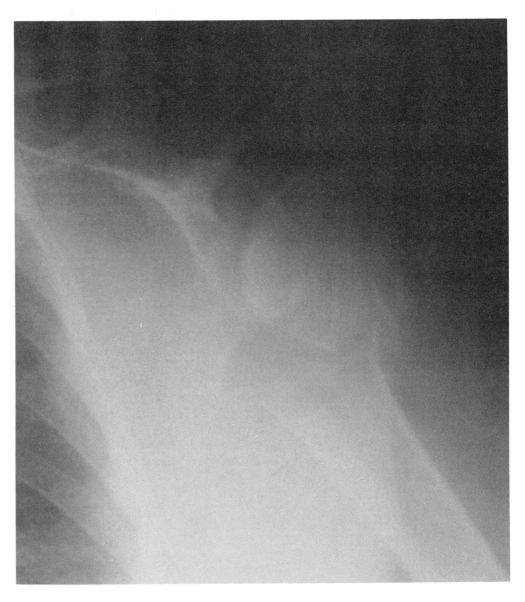

Fig. 10.26: Fracture to the surgical neck of the humerus.

feels bilaterally the same on both sides of the hands. Take a radial pulse, check skin temperature at the hand, and blanch the fingernails and note capillary refill. Immediate referral to a physician is indicated.

After a fall on the point of the shoulder, the arm of the gymnast appeared to sag downward and forward, and had a visible bump in the mid-clavicular region. Any shoulder movement caused severe pain. If you determined a possible clavicular fracture, you are correct. How should the arm be immobilized?

ASSESSMENT

A baseball player is complaining of pain in the right arm every time the arm is abducted above 90°. Pain is localized on the anterior shoulder and aggravated with horizontal adduction. What biomechanical factors are involved in this injury? How will you assess this individual?

The shoulder complex is a complicated region to assess because of the number of important structures located in such a small area. Furthermore, the biomechanical demands on each structure during overhead motion is not fully understood, so identification of all injured structures is difficult. As a result, each joint must be methodically assessed to determine limitation of function in an injured individual. Although there are several recognized methods of evaluation, differences in the order of questioning or performing special tests will depend on personal preference. The emphasis, however, remains the same: performing a thorough, complete objective assessment of the area.

Improper biomechanical skill technique is a leading cause of many acute and overuse injuries at the shoulder. Assessment of the individual's sport specific techniques may determine if improper technique contributed to the injury. By correcting minor mechanical flaws in technique and identifying flexibility and strength deficits, many shoulder injuries can be prevented. Also keep in mind that pain may be referred from the cervical region, heart, spleen, lungs, and other internal organs to the shoulder region (See **Figure 4-7**).

HISTORY

What information should be gathered from the baseball player complaining of anterior shoulder pain during shoulder abduction and horizontal adduction?

Questions about a shoulder injury should focus on the current primary complaint, past injuries to the region, and other factors that may have contributed to the current problem (referred pain, alterations in posture, change in technique, or overuse). Many conditions may be related to family history, age, improper biomechanical execution of skills, and recent changes in training programs. Keep questions open-ended to allow the individual to fully describe the injury. In addition to the general questions discussed in Chapter 4, specific questions related to the shoulder region can be seen in **Field Strategy 10-8**.

The baseball player has averaged six games per week for the past two and a half months. During the day he directs the swimming program at a local health club and swims three to five miles/day. The pain started gradually two months ago. It hurts to raise the arm and wakes him up at night when he sleeps on the affected side. Although he has had a sore shoulder numerous times before, he has never seen a physician. However, it is particularly painful now.

OBSERVATION AND INSPECTION

After taking a thorough history, what specific factors should be observed in the postural exam and during inspection of the injury site?

On-the-field assessment may be somewhat limited due to uniforms and protective equipment that may obstruct the region from observation and assessment. Initially, you may have to slide your hands under the pads to palpate the region to determine the presence of a possible fracture or major ligament damage. If necessary, the pads should be cut and gently removed to more fully expose the area. After the initial exam, the individual may need to be removed from the field to complete a more comprehensive assessment in the examination room.

In an ideal clinic situation, women should wear a bathing suit or halter top so the entire shoulder and arm can be fully exposed. Complete a postural exam looking for faulty posture or congenital abnormalities that could place additional strain on the anatomical structures. The individual should be viewed from the anterior, lateral, and posterior views. During movement, look for symmetry and fluid scapular motion. Inspect the specific

Field Strategy 10–8. Developing a History of the Injury.

Current Injury Status

1. Where is the pain (or weakness) located? Can you point to the area that is the most uncomfortable? On a scale of 1 to 10 with 10 being very severe, how would you rate your pain (weakness)? What type of pain is it (dull ache, throbbing, sharp,intermittent, "red-hot" or burning)?
2. Did the pain come on gradually (overuse problem) or suddenly (acute problem)? How long has it been a problem? Was the pain greatest when the injury first occurred or did it get worse the second or third day? What have you done for the condition?
3. If you have an acute problem, identify the mechanism of injury. Ask: What were you doing at the time of the injury? Was there a direct blow? Did you fall? How (outstretched arm, rolling over the shoulder, side of the shoulder, etc.)? If the injury came on gradually ask: What different activities have you been doing in the last week? (Look for changes in frequency, duration, intensity, type, or method.) Have you had any recent changes in your equipment?
4. Did you hear any sounds during the incident? Any snaps, pops, or cracks? Did you notice any swelling, discoloration, muscle spasms, or numbness with the injury?
5. What actions or motions bring on the pain? Is it worse in the morning, during activity, after activity, or at night? Does it wake you up at night? How does the arm feel during activity? In what part of the arm motion does it hurt the worse? Does it tire easily? When the pain sets in, how long does it last?
6. Are there certain activities you are unable to perform because of the pain? Which ones?
7. How old are you? (Remember that many shoulder problems are age-related.) Which hand is dominant?

Past Injury Status

1. Have you ever injured your shoulder before? When? How did that occur? Who evaluated and cared for the injury? What was done for the injury? Did you have any difficulty returning to your full functional status?
2. Have you had any medical problems recently? (You are looking for problems that may refer pain to the area from visceral organs, heart, and lungs.) Are you on any medication? Do you have any musculoskeletal problems elsewhere in the body? (These may result in changes in gait or technique that transfer abnormal forces to structures in the shoulder)

> Intra-articular swelling would prevent the athlete from fully adducting the arm against the body

injury site for obvious deformity, swelling, discoloration, symmetry, hypertrophy, muscle atrophy, or previous surgical incisions. Compare the affected limb with the unaffected limb. Specific areas to focus on in this region are summarized in **Field Strategy 10-9**.

No anomalies are observed during the postural exam. Slight swelling is present on the anterior lip of the acromion process and over the bicipital groove.

PALPATIONS

Pain and swelling appear to be confined to the anterior shoulder. Where should palpations begin, and what specific factors are you looking for?

Bilateral palpations can determine temperature, swelling, point tenderness, crepitus, deformity, muscle spasm, and cutaneous sensation. Increased skin temperature could indicate inflammation or infection. Decreased skin temperature could indicate a reduction in circulation. Swelling should be differentiated between localized extra-articular swelling and joint effusion. In the shoulder, intra-articular swelling would prevent full adduction of the arm against the body. Crepitus may indicate an inflamed subacromial bursa, bicipital tenosynovitis, or an irregular articular surface. Vascular pulses can be taken at the radial and ulnar arteries in the wrist, brachial artery on the medial arm, or axillary artery in the armpit.

Fractures can be assessed through palpation of pain at the fracture site, compression of the humeral head against the glenoid fossa, compression along the long axis of the humerus, percussion on a specific bony landmark, or by using a tuning fork. If a fracture or dislocation is suspected, immediately assess circulatory and neural integrity distal to the site. Take a pulse at the sites indicated

Field Strategy 10–9. Postural Assessment of the Shoulder Region.

Anterior View

1. Check that the neck and head are in the midline of the body
2. Follow the clavicles distally and note any deformity that may indicate a possible fracture
3. Look to make sure both shoulders have a well-rounded deltoid cap with no prominent acromion process present
4. Check the level of the shoulders. The dominant side will usually be lower than the non-dominant side.
5. Note any scars or muscular atrophy, particularly in the supraspinatus or infraspinatus
6. Note the color of the hand. This may indicate a vascular problem

Posterior View

1. Note any abnormal prominence of bony structures or muscle atrophy. Are the scapula at the same height and resting at the same angle?
2. Are the spines of the two scapula and inferior angles bilaterally even?
3. Note any "winging" of the scapula.
4. Note the presence of any scoliosis, or lateral curvature of the spine.
5. Is there any swelling or discoloration present?

Lateral View

1. Note the attitude of the head and neck in relation to the shoulders. Is the head jutting forward or backward?
2. Note any kyphosis (rounded shoulders)

above, and stroke the palm and dorsum of both hands and ask the individual if it feels the same bilaterally. Immobilize the extremity in an appropriate sling or splint, monitor vital signs, and refer the individual to the nearest medical facility.

Stand behind the individual to begin bilateral palpations moving proximal to distal. Leave the most painful area last.

Anterior Palpations

1. Sternocleidomastoid muscle
2. Sternoclavicular joint, interclavicular ligament, sternoclavicular ligament, and sternal end of the clavicle
3. Clavicle and costoclavicular ligament
4. AC joint, acromion process and acromioclavicular ligament
5. Corocoid process, pectoralis minor, short head of the biceps brachii, and coracoacromial ligament
6. Pectoralis major and anterior deltoid muscle
7. Greater tuberosity, and distal attachments of the supraspinatus, infraspinatus, and teres minor
8. Biceps brachii muscle and tendon. Palpate the bicipital groove with the arm in exter-

nal rotation. The lesser tubercle is medial to the groove where the subscapularis is attached
9. Subacromial bursa and supraspinatus tendon with the arm extended

Lateral Palpations

1. Middle deltoid muscle and greater tubercle
2. Glenohumeral capsule

Posterior Palpations

1. Posterior deltoid and trapezius muscles
2. Spine of the scapula, medial and lateral borders, and inferior angle
3. Rhomboid muscles, latissimus dorsi, serratus anterior, levator scapulae, and scaleni

Crepitus and point tenderness were elicited just anterior to the acromion process when the arm was passively flexed and extended. The bicipital groove was also point tender. The anterior shoulder was warm to the touch and swelling was noted anterior to the acromion process and over the bicipital groove.

SPECIAL TESTS

There are several painful areas. How will you determine what structures have been injured, and how severe this injury is?

Perform special tests in a comfortable position for the patient and begin with gentle stress. It is common at the shoulder to have painful arcs. Note what range of motion is the most painful. Do not force the limb through any sudden motions, nor cause undue pain. Proceed cautiously through the assessment.

Active Movements

Perform active range of motion at the neck first, since pain is frequently referred from the cervical region into the shoulder

Active movements may be performed in a seated or prone position with the most painful movements done last. Perform active range of motion at the neck first, since pain is frequently referred from the cervical region into the shoulder. Neck flexion, extension, rotation, and lateral flexion should be assessed for fluid motion and presence of pain. If pain is elicited on active motion at the neck, immediately complete a full neck evaluation. If findings are significant, immobilize the neck in a cervical collar and refer the individual to a physician.

If no problems are noted during neck movement, continue with the shoulder evaluation. Ask the individual to perform gross movement patterns at the shoulder. Watch the arms from an anterior and posterior view. When standing behind the individual make sure the scapula and humerus move together in a freely coordinated motion. Move the unaffected arm first to determine what is normal motion. The following gross movement patterns are collectively referred to as Apley's Scratch Test:

Ask the individual to perform gross movement patterns while you watch the arms from an anterior and posterior view

1. **Medial rotation and adduction**. Reach in front of the head and touch the opposite shoulder (**Figure 10-27A**)
2. **Medial rotation, extension, and adduction**. Reach behind the back and touch the inferior angle of the opposite scapula (**Figure 10-27B**)
3. **Abduction, flexion, and lateral rotation**. Reach behind the head and touch the superior angle of the opposite scapula (**Figure 10-27C**)

In addition, the following tests may also be performed to assess glenohumeral and scapulothoracic movement:

1. **Abduction and upward/downward rotation of the scapula**. Abduct the arms to 90°, supinate the forearm, and continue abduction until the palms meet above the head (**Figure 10-28A**)
2. **Abduction and lateral rotation**. Clasp the fingers together, move the palms behind the head, and push the elbows posterior (**Figure 10-28B**)

The advantage of these simple tests is to quickly assess bilateral symmetry in gross motor movements. Any deficit can be easily seen and investigated in further detail. The following individual motions can also be assessed at the shoulder:

1. Shoulder abduction (170 to 180°)
2. Shoulder flexion (160 to 180°)
3. Shoulder extension (50 to 60°)
4. Lateral or external rotation (80 to 90°)
5. Medial or internal rotation (60 to 100°)
6. Adduction (50 to 70°)
7. Horizontal abduction/adduction (130°)
8. Upward/downward rotation of the scapula

Goniometry measurements for the glenohumeral joint are illustrated in **Figure 10-29**.

Passive Range of Motion

If the individual is able to perform full range of motion during active movements, apply gentle pressure at the extremes of motion to determine end feel. Tissue stretch is the normal end feel for shoulder flexion, extension, lateral rotation, medial rotation, abduction, and horizontal abduction. Adduction is tissue approximation. Horizontal adduction can be tissue stretch or tissue approximation. Abduction of the shoulder can be bone to bone or tissue stretch.

Resisted Muscle Testing

Stabilize the hip and trunk during muscle testing to prevent any muscle substitution. Begin with the muscle on stretch and apply resistance throughout the full range of motion. Note any lag, muscle weakness, or painful arc. Delay working those muscles that cause extreme pain until the final phase of muscle testing. **Figure 10-30** demonstrates resisted motions that should be tested (myotomes are listed in parentheses).

1. Elevation of the scapula (C_4)
2. Depression of the scapula

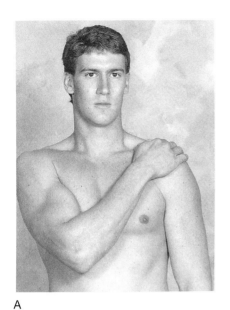

A

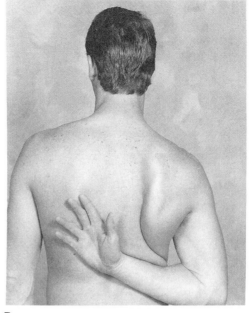

B

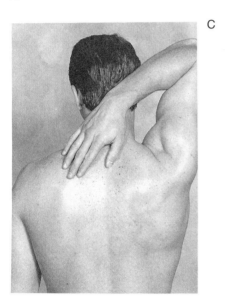

C

Fig. 10.27: Apley's scratch test to determine range of motion. (A) Internal rotation and adduction. (B) Internal rotation, extension, and adduction. (C) Abduction, flexion, and external rotation.

3. Protraction of the scapula
4. Retraction of the scapula
5. Forward flexion of the humerus at the shoulder
6. Extension of the humerus at the shoulder
7. Abduction of the humerus at the shoulder (C_5)
8. Adduction of the humerus at the shoulder
9. Lateral rotation of the humerus at the shoulder
10. Medial rotation of the humerus at the shoulder
11. Flexion of the forearm at the elbow (C_6)
12. Extension of the forearm at the elbow (C_7)

Neurological Assessment

Neurological integrity can be assessed with the use of myotomes, reflexes, and segmental dermatomes and peripheral nerve cutaneous patterns.

Myotomes

Isometric muscle testing should be performed in the following motions to test specific myotomes in the upper extremity: scapular elevation (C_4), shoulder abduction (C_5), elbow flexion and/or wrist extension (C_6), elbow extension and/or wrist flexion (C_7), thumb extension and/or ulnar deviation

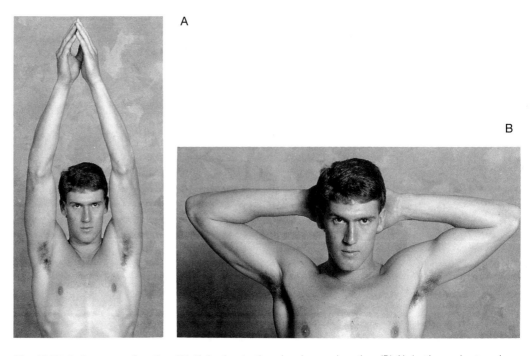

Fig. 10.28: Active range of motion. (A) Abduction testing glenohumeral motion. (B) Abduction and external rotation of the humerus and scapular retraction.

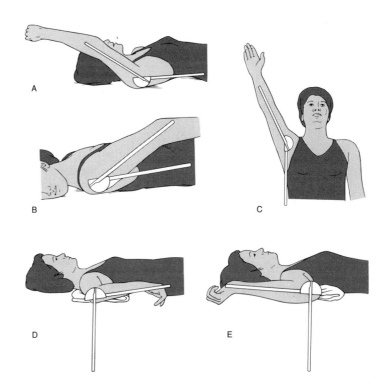

Fig. 10.29: Goniometry measurements. (A) Shoulder flexion. Align the proximal arm with the mid-axillary line of the thorax with the fulcrum close to the acromion process. Align the distal arm along the humerus in line with the lateral epicondyle of the humerus. (B) Shoulder extension. Use the same landmarks used for shoulder flexion. (C) Shoulder abduction. The proximal arm is parallel to the midline of the sternum with the fulcrum close to the acromion process. Align the distal arm with the humerus using the medial epicondyle for reference. (D and E) Lateral and medial rotation. Flex the elbow at 90° with the fulcrum centered over the olecranon process. The proximal arm is placed perpendicular to the floor with the distal arm aligned with the olecranon process and ulnar styloid process.

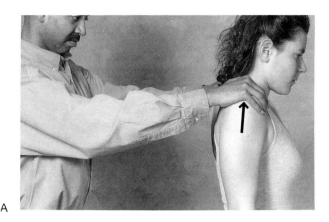

A

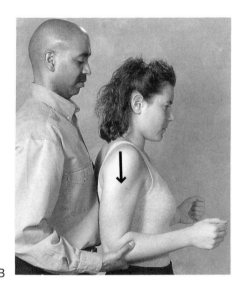

B

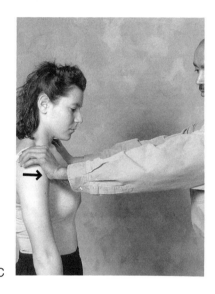

C

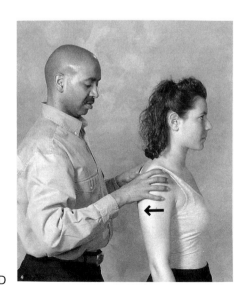

D

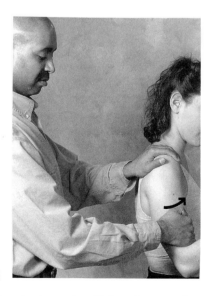

E

Fig. 10.30: Manual muscle testing. (A) Scapular elevation. (B) Scapular depression. (C) Scapular protraction. (D) Scapular retraction. (E) Shoulder flexion. *(continued)*

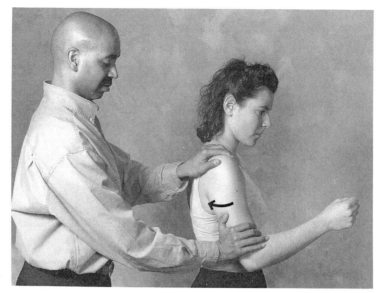

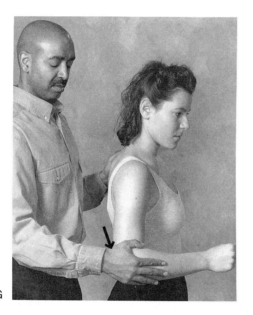

Fig. 10.30 (*continued*): (F) Shoulder extension. (G) Shoulder abduction. (H) Shoulder adduction.

($\mathbf{C_8}$), and abduction and/or adduction of the hand intrinsics ($\mathbf{T^1}$). These tests are demonstrated in **Figures 10-30** and **12-37**.

Reflexes

Reflexes in the upper extremity include the biceps ($\mathbf{C_5}$-$\mathbf{C_6}$) and triceps ($\mathbf{C_7}$). The biceps reflex is tested with the individual's arm flexed and supported by the examiner's forearm. Place your thumb over the biceps tendon and strike the thumb with the reflex hammer using a quick downward thrust (**Figure 10-**

31A). A normal response is slight elbow flexion. The triceps reflex is tested with the individual's arm abducted and extended with the elbow flexed. Place the triceps tendon on slight stretch and tap the triceps tendon with the reflex hammer (**Figure 10-31B**). A normal response is slight elbow extension.

Cutaneous Patterns

The segmental nerve dermatome patterns for the shoulder region are demonstrated in **Fig-**

In the upper extremity the biceps and triceps reflexes can be tested

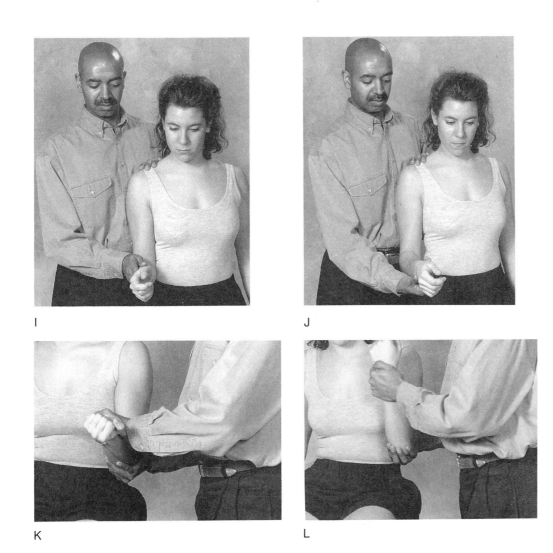

I   J

K   L

Fig. 10.30 (*continued*): (I) Shoulder external rotation. (J) Shoulder internal rotation. (K) Elbow flexion. (L) Elbow extension.

ure 10-32. The peripheral nerve cutaneous patterns are demonstrated in **Figure 10-33**. Test bilaterally for altered sensation with sharp and dull touch by running the open hand and fingernails over the neck, shoulder, anterior and posterior chest walls, and down both sides of the arms.

Stress and Functional Tests

At this point in the assessment, the history, observations, palpations, range of motion, and neurological assessment should have established a strong suspicion of what structures may be damaged. In using stress and functional tests, perform only those tests that are absolutely necessary.

Serratus Anterior Weakness

Weakness of the serratus anterior, often called winging of the scapula, is determined by having the individual perform a push-up against the wall (**Figure 10-34**). If the muscle is weak, or the long thoracic nerve is involved, the medial border of the scapula will pull away from the chest wall.

Acromioclavicular (AC) Distraction/Compression

If the AC joint is unstable, downward traction on the upper extremity will lead to downward movement of the acromion process away from the clavicle. Grasp the arm in one hand while palpating the joint with the other hand. Apply steady downward traction (**Figure 10-35A**). A positive test will produce pain and/or joint movement. Horizontal adduction of the humerus across the chest compresses the AC joint and will also lead to increased pain if the joint is injured (**Figure 10-35B**).

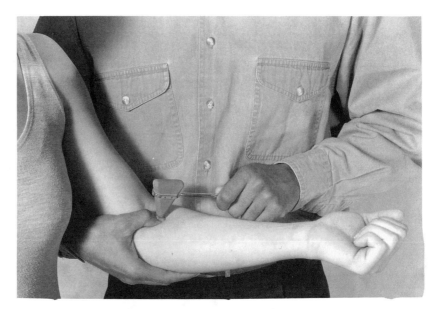

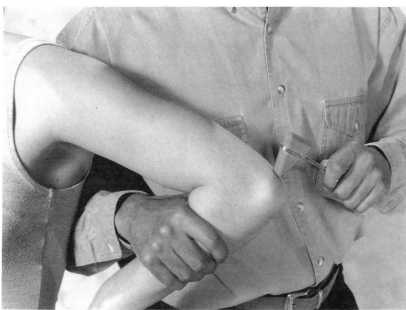

Fig. 10.31: Reflex testing. (A) Biceps reflex (C_5, C_6). (B) Triceps reflex (C_7).

Apprehension Test for Anterior Shoulder Dislocation

In a supine position, slowly abduct and externally rotate the individual's humerus **(Figure 10-36A)**. If the individual will not allow passive movement to the extremes of motion, or apprehension or alarm is shown in the facial expression, it is a positive sign. This motion should always be done slowly to prevent recurrence of a dislocation.

Posterior Apprehension Test

In a supine position, move the arm into forward flexion and internal rotation. Apply a steady downward force on the elbow **(Figure 10-36B)**. A positive sign indicating a possible posterior dislocation is verified by a look or feeling of apprehension, or alarm on the individual's face.

Drop-arm Test

To test the integrity of the supraspinatus muscle and tendon, abduct the shoulder to 90° with no humeral rotation. Ask the individual to slowly lower the arm to the side. If positive, the arm will not lower smoothly, or increased pain will occur during the motion. An alternative test is to abduct the arm again at 90° with no rotation, and ask the individual to hold that

C3
4
5
T1
2
3
4
5
T1
C5
C6
C7
C8
C3
4
5
6
7
8
T1
2
3
4
5
6
7
8
9
10
11
12

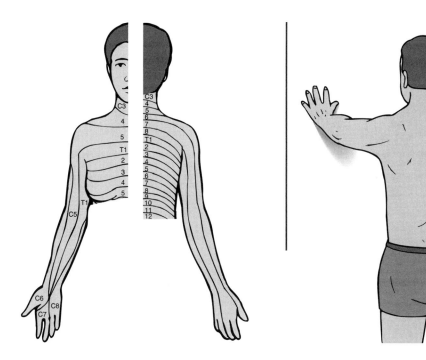

Fig. 10.32: Dermatome patterns for the shoulder region.

Fig. 10.34: Winging of the scapula can result from weakness in the serratus anterior or injury to the long thoracic nerve.

Branches from cervical plexus
Axillary
Branches from medial cord of brachial plexus
Radial
Median antebrachial cutaneous
Radial
Ulnar
Median

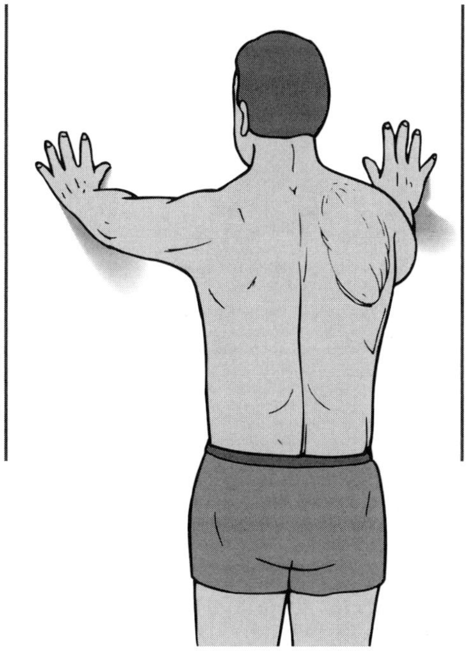

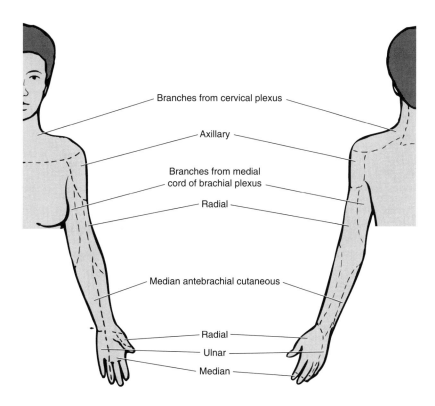

Fig. 10.33: Cutaneous patterns for the peripheral nerves.

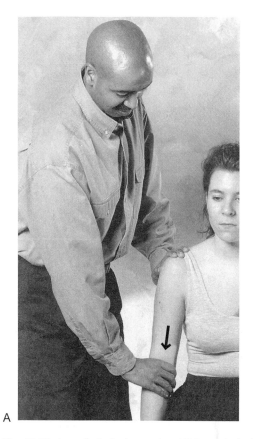
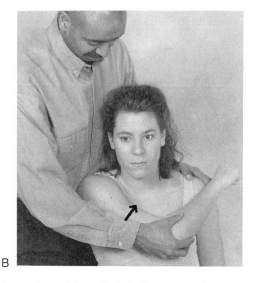

Fig. 10.35: Acromioclavicular treating. (A) Acromioclavicular traction. (B) Acromioclavicular compression.

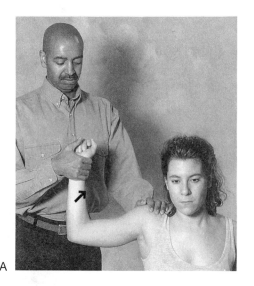
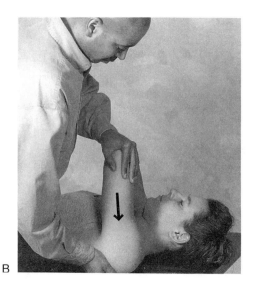

Fig. 10.36: Glenohumeral dislocation. (A) Anterior apprehension test. (B) Posterior apprehension test.

position. Apply downward resistance to the distal end of the humerus (**Figure 10-37A**). A positive test is indicated if the individual is unable to maintain the arm in the abducted position.

Centinela Supraspinatus Muscle Test

Position both arms in abduction at 90°, horizontally adduct the arm approximately 30 to 60°, and internally rotate the humerus with the thumbs pointing downward ("empty can position") (**Figure 10-37B**). Apply downward pressure proximal to the elbows and look for pain and/or weakness. The arms should rebound to the 90° abducted position. A positive test indicates a tear to the supraspinatus muscle or tendon.

Anterior Impingement Test

Internally rotate and abduct the humerus through shoulder flexion while depressing the scapula, thus jamming the greater tubercle underneath the anteroinferior border of the acromion process. Return the arm to 90° of abduction (with the elbow flexed at 90°), and then horizontally adducted across the chest while maintaining internal rotation of the humerus (**Figure 10-38**). Pain or apprehension on the individual's face may indicate an overuse injury to the supraspinatus or biceps brachii tendon.

Transverse Humeral Ligament Test

To test for a torn transverse humeral ligament place the shoulder in 90° of abduction and

A
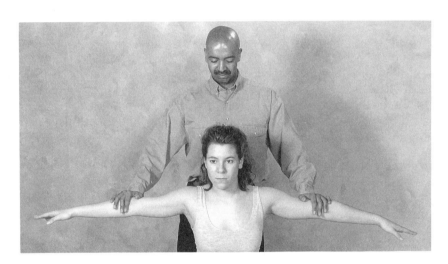

B
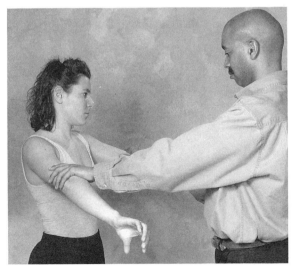

Fig. 10.37: Supraspinatus testing. (A) To perform the drop-arm test, abduct the humerus to 90°. Apply mild downward pressure on the distal humerus. (B) To perform the Centinela supraspinatus muscle test, horizontally adduct the arm approximately 30°–60° with the humerus internally rotated. Apply mild downward pressure on the distal humerus.

external rotation with the elbow flexed at 90°. Place your fingers over the bicipital groove. An audible and/or palpable snap, which may be accompanied with pain, will occur as the arm is moved into internal rotation (**Figure 10-39A**).

Yergason's Test for Bicipital Tendinitis

Flex the elbow at 90° and stabilize the arm against the body with the forearm pronated. Ask the individual to supinate the forearm, flex the elbow, and externally rotate the humerus. Simultaneously resist the motion with one hand while applying downward traction on the elbow with the other hand (**Figure 10-39B**). The test is positive if pain is elicited over the bicipital groove or the tendon snaps out of the groove.

Speed's Test for Bicipital Tendinitis

In this test the tendon moves over the bone during motion, rather than only placing tension on it, thus providing a more effective, accurate result. Supinate the arm with the elbow fully extended. Place one hand over the bicipital groove and resist forward flexion of the arm with the other hand. A positive test

will result in tenderness over the groove (**Figure 10-39C**).

Thoracic Outlet Compression Syndrome Tests

After locating a radial pulse, ask the individual to turn the head toward the affected shoulder and extend the head while you slowly extend and laterally rotate the humerus (**Figure 10-40**). The individual is instructed to take a deep breath and hold it. A diminished or absent pulse indicates a positive test. An alternative position is to have the individual rotate the head to the opposite side and hyperextend the neck.

Functional Tests

Occasionally, functional movements are the only activities that reproduce the signs and symptoms. Throwing a ball, performing a swimming stroke, or doing an overhead serve or spike may replicate the painful pattern. Based on your knowledge of the mechanics of the motion, you may be able to narrow down the few definitive results of the assessment to determine the actual injury. These movements are also commonly used to determine

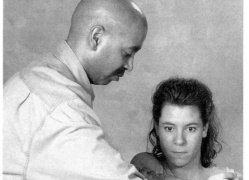

A   B

Fig. 10.38: Anterior impingement test. (A) Internally rotate and abduct the humerus through shoulder flexion while depressing the scapula. (B) Flex the elbow and internally rotate the humerus. Move the arm into horizontal adduction. Pain or apprehension on the individual's face indicates a possible overuse injury to the supraspinatus or biceps brachii tendon.

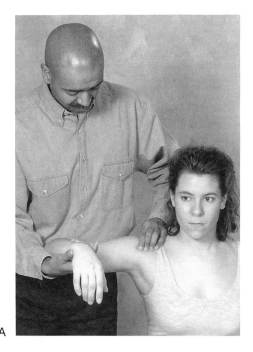

A

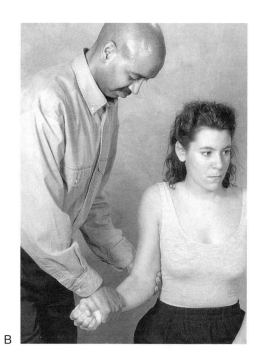

B

Fig. 10.39: (A) To perform the transverse humeral ligament test, place the extended arm in 90° of abduction and external rotation. Place your fingers over the bicipital groove and move the arm into internal rotation. An audible or palpable snap, which may be accompanied by pain, will occur during internal rotation if positive. (B) The Yergason's test is performed by stabilizing the flexed arm against the body with the forearm pronated. Ask the individual to supinate the forearm, flex the elbow, and externally rotate the humerus while you apply resistance. Simultaneously apply downward traction on the elbow with the other hand. The test is positive if pain is elicited over the bicipital groove or the tendon snaps out of the groove.

when the individual can return to sport participation. All functional patterns should be fluid, and pain-free.

You found a painful arc of motion between 60 and 120° of abduction and flexion of the glenohumeral joint during active, passive, and resisted motion. Pain increased when the arm was horizontally adducted as the greater tubercle of the humerus slid under the acromion process. Positive results were found with the drop-arm test, Centinela supraspinatus test, impingement test, Yergason's, and Speed's test. Neurological tests were normal. If you determined this individual has an impingement syndrome involving the supraspinatus tendon, subacromial bursa, and long head of the biceps brachii, you are correct.

REHABILITATION

The baseball player has a painful shoulder as a result of an impingement syndrome. What will be your priority of care to rehabilitate this injury and return the player to full functional status?

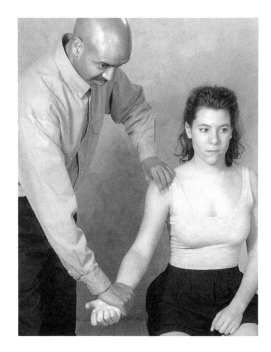

Fig. 10.39: (C) Speed's test is more accurate. Supinate the hand with the elbow fully extended. With one hand over the bicipital groove, resist forward flexion of the arm. A positive test will result in tenderness over the bicipital groove.

A   B

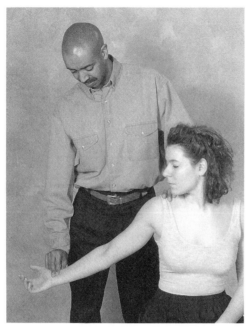 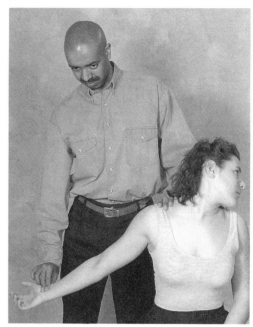

Fig. 10.40: Thoracic outlet compression syndrome. (A) Adson's maneuver. Extend and externally rotate the humerus while the individual extends the head. (B) Halstead's maneuver. Apply slight traction to the arm while the individual hyperextends the neck and rotates the head to the opposite side.

Rehabilitation of the shoulder region must involve range of motion and strengthening exercises for the entire shoulder complex in a functional progression. Progress within any program is dictated by the type and severity of injury, amount of immobilization, and the supervising physician's treatment plan. In a general sense, restoration of active range of motion should precede strengthening exercises that focus on specific strength deficits. Strengthening exercises for the scapular stabilizers should not be overlooked, since they play a key role in each phase of the throwing motion. In addition to restoring range of motion and strength, proprioception and cardiovascular fitness levels must be maintained.

Restoration of Motion

Gentle range of motion exercises, such as Codmans' circumduction and pendulum swings, are often used immediately after injury (**Figure 10-41**). The exercise is performed by making small circles and a pendulum motion in flexion and extension, and horizontal abduction and adduction. The range of motion increases as pain-free motion is regained. Exercises can progress to active assistive T-bar exercises in the supine position

(**Field Strategy 10-6**). In throwing activities, the range of motion needed to adequately complete the cocking phase exceeds 90° of external rotation when the arm is abducted 90° (20). Special attention should be focused on regaining this additional range of motion, but not to the point of hypermobility. A rope and pulley system can augment active assistive glenohumeral flexion and abduction. Shoulder shrugs performed in three directions (superior, anterior, and posterior) can increase scapular range of motion.

Restoration of Proprioception and Balance

Closed chain exercises may be performed immediately after injury. Shifting body weight from one hand to the other may be performed on a wall, table top, or unstable surface, such as a foam mat or BAPS board. Push-ups and exercises in a frontal and sagittal plane can be performed on a ProFitter or slide board, if available. Step-ups can be completed on a box, stool, or Stair Master. This activity can progress to stepping up and down on boxes of differing heights arranged so the exercise is performed in diagonal patterns, circles, figure 8's, or any other pattern.

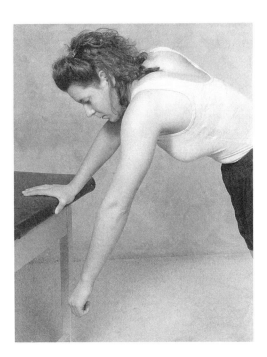

Fig. 10.41: Codman's exercises. Begin with small circular motions increasing the diameter as pain free range of motion occurs. Pendulum motion is also performed in flexion and extension, and horizontal abduction and adduction.

Use of free weights can develop balance, coordination and skill in moving through diagonal patterns. It is imperative, however, to include a transference of proprioceptive training to the actual throwing motion. This is accomplished with a slow, deliberate rehearsal of the throwing motion incorporating visual feedback through the use of mirrors or videotape. As the motion is performed, biomechanical errors are corrected. When motion is perfected, speed of movement and distance of throw is gradually increased. A sample throwing program is listed in **Field Strategy 10-10**.

Muscular Strength, Endurance, and Power

Gentle resisted isometric exercises can begin immediately after injury or after surgery while the arm is still immobilized (**See Field Strategy 10-5**). With the glenohumeral joint in a resting position, apply a slow mild overload. A disadvantage of isometric exercise is that strength gains are relatively specific to the joint angle at which the exercise is performed. Therefore, to strengthen the joint, isometric contractions must be performed at

multiple positions. As the individual improves, a more moderate isometric overload is applied. Finally, a higher, rapid unexpected resistance is provided at various positions including the end of the range of motion required for throwing.

Once range of motion approximates normal for the individual, open chain kinetic exercises can be performed in a prone, sidelying, supine, or standing position to add gravity as resistance. Many of these exercises were listed and explained in **Field Strategy 10-5** and **10-6**. A sandbag or dumbbell can be used for added resistance. The individual should complete 50 to 100 repetitions with a one pound weight, and should not progress in resistance until 100 repetitions are achieved. Resistance should be limited to five pounds, as this decreases the chance of rotator cuff inflammation during the strengthening program (30). Careful attention should be directed to a potential painful arc of motion during concentric and eccentric contractions, as pain can add additional insult to the injury. Therefore, work within a pain-free arc of motion with light resistance to the point of fatigue.

Muscular strength and endurance can be developed through PNF-resisted exercises in diagonal patterns to mimic functional skills, or surgical tubing can be used through a functional pattern. As strength improves, free weights or machine weight exercises for the upper body is incorporated. Many of these exercises were demonstrated in **Field Strategy 10-2**.

Plyometric exercises may involve catching a weighted ball utilizing a quick eccentric stretch of the muscle to facilitate a concentric contraction in throwing the ball. The exercise can progress through various one- and two-arm chest passes and overhead passes. A mini-tramp may also be used to do plyometric bounding push-ups.

Cardiovascular Fitness

General body conditioning should be maintained throughout the rehabilitation program. Several examples of programs were provided in **Field Strategy 5-9**, and included use of a jump rope, Stair Master, treadmill, and upper body ergometer (UBE). 💡 *The baseball player should increase range of motion in external rotation, restore strength in the rotator cuff and scapu-*

Although free weights can develop balance, coordination, and skill, it is imperative to transfer the proprioceptive training to the actual throwing or functional motion needed for the specific sport

Muscular strength and endurance can be developed through PNF-resisted diagonal patterns that mimic functional skills, or with surgical tubing

Field Strategy 10–10. Functional Throwing Program for the Shoulder.

Stretching Program. In addition to exercises in Field Strategy 10-1, A-B and 10-6, A-G, the following should be performed:

1. PNF stretching exercises for all motions at the shoulder
2. Pectoralis major and minor. Stand in corner with forearms on the wall. Lean the chest to the wall until a stretch is felt
3. All fours back stretch. While on all fours, arc the back until a stretch is felt
4. Trunk rotation, supine position. Lift one leg over the other to touch the opposite hand
5. Wrist flexion and extension stretching

Progressive resistance exercises.

1. Trunk exercises
   a. Stomach crunches with slight rotation
   b. With a medicine ball, do trunk twists with a partner
   c. On all fours, raise one arm and the opposite leg
2. Triceps and biceps curls
3. Posterior musculature. Field Strategy 10-5, D-G
4. Medial and lateral rotation with tubing, standing position
5. Supraspinatus. If weak, concentrate on "setting the shoulder" and initiating the supraspinatus through the first 30° of abduction
6. Scapular stabilization. Field Strategy 10-5, H-J and O-P
7. Standing empty can exercise
8. Lat pull downs
9. Wrist curls in supination and pronation
10. Throwing motion with tubing with full synchronous motion
11. Isokinetics to train at higher velocities

Throwing program. Begin only when flexibility, strength, and synchronous of motion of the shoulder complex is normal. All exercises should be asymptomatic.

1. Mirror throwing. With 1 pound weight, exaggerate the throwing motion with slow controlled concentric and eccentric movement.
2. Short distance throwing. Throw 20 to 30 feet beginning with five minutes progressing to 15 to 20 minutes. Form is more important than velocity. Videotape the movement for analysis
3. Long distance arc throwing. When able to throw comfortably for 15 to 20 minutes, gradually increase throwing distance to 150 feet. Form is still more important than velocity
4. Form pitching. Prior to beginning this phase, the individual must have completed short- and long-distance throwing program. Begin throwing off the mound. Proper mechanics are important. Gradually increase velocity. Begin with fast balls only. As near maximum velocity is reached on fast ball, begin working on breaking ball and other pitches.

lothoracic musculature, regain proprioception and balance, and restore proper throwing mechanics through a functionally progressive throwing program.

SUMMARY

The extreme mobility needed to perform common athletic skills and techniques, coupled with lack of stability in the glenohumeral joint sets the stage for many acute and chronic shoulder injuries. The shoulder complex does not function in an isolated fashion; rather a series of joints work together in a coordinated manner to allow complicated patterns of motion. Because of this, injury to one structure can affect other structures. This makes assessment of a shoulder injury very complicated. **Field Strategy 10-13** demonstrates the progression of a shoulder assessment.

Always keep in mind that pain may be referred from other areas of the body, particularly the heart, lungs, visceral organs, and cervical neck region. Any significant finding should be referred to a physician. Examples of these significant injuries may include: obvi-

Field Strategy 10–11. Shoulder evaluation.

History

Primary complaint including:
  Description and mechanism of current injury
  Onset of symptoms
Pain perception and discomfort
Disability and functional impairments from the injury
Previous injuries to the area
Family history

Observation and Inspection

Postural assessment
Inspection of injured area for:
  Muscle symmetry   Hypertrophy or muscle atrophy
  Swelling   Visible congenital deformity
  Discoloration   Surgical incisions or scars

Palpation

Bony structures to rule out fracture
Soft tissue structures to determine:
  Temperature   Deformity
  Swelling   Muscle spasm
  Point tenderness   Cutaneous sensation
  Crepitus   Vascular pulses

Special Tests

Active range of motion with gross motor movement
  Scapular motions and scapulohumeral rhythm
  Glenohumeral motions; watch for painful arc
Passive range of motion
Resisted manual muscle testing
Neurologic testing
Stress and functional tests
  Serratus anterior weakness
  Acromioclavicular (AC) distraction/compression
  Glenohumeral joint instability
  Apprehension test for anterior/posterior dislocation
  Rotator Cuff
    Drop-arm test
    Centinela supraspinatus muscle test
    Anterior impingement test
  Biceps brachii injury
    Transverse humeral ligament test
    Yergason's test for tendinitis
    Speed's test for tendinitis
  Thoracic outlet compression syndrome tests
  Functional tests

ous deformity suggesting a suspected fracture, separation, or dislocation, significant loss of motion or weakness in the myotomes, joint instability, abnormal sensations in either the segmental dermatomes or peripheral cutaneous patterns, absent or weak pulse distal to the injury, or any significant unexplained pain.

If a decision is made to refer the individual to a physician, remove the individual from activity and immobilize the limb in a sling and swathe, or another commercial product that adequately pads and supports the limb. Apply cryotherapy to reduce inflammation and swelling, and transport the individual in an appropriate manner.

Functional tests should be performed before clearing the individual for re-entry into sports participation. Upper extremity sport specific skills should be performed pain-free in all movements. Along with successful completion of functional and proprioception testing, each individual should have bilaterally equal strength, flexibility, muscular endurance, and a high cardiovascular level before returning to sport participation. Whenever possible, protective equipment or padding should be used to prevent reinjury.

REFERENCES

1. Johnson, RE, and Rust, RJ. 1985. Sports related injury: An anatomic approach, part 2. Minn Med, 68:829–831.
2. Norkin, CC, and Levangie, PK. *Joint structure and function: A comprehensive analysis*. Philadelphia: FA Davis, 1992.
3. Poppen, KN, and Walker, PS. 1976. Normal and abnormal motion of the shoulder. J Bone Joint Surg [Am], 58:195–201.
4. Kent, BE. 1971. Functional anatomy of the shoulder complex: A review. J Am Phys Ther Assoc, 51:867–888.
5. Zuckerman, JD, and Matsen, FA. "Biomechanics of the shoulder." In *Basic Biomechanics of the Skeletal System*, edited by M Nordin and VH Frankel. Philadelphia: Lea & Febiger, 1989.
6. Tibone, JE. "Shoulder problems of adolescents: How they differ from those of adults." In *Clinics in sports medicine*, edited by FV Jobe, vol. 2, no. 2, Philadelphia: WB Saunders, 1983.
7. Irrgang, JJ, Witney, SL, and Harner, CD. 1992. Nonoperative treatment of rotator cuff injuries in throwing athletes. J Spt Rehab, 1(3):197–222.
8. Reid, DC. *Sports injury assessment and rehabilitation*. New York: Churchill Livingstone, 1992.
9. Bach, BR, VanFleet, TA, and Novak, PJ. 1992. Acromioclavicular injuries: Controversies in treatment. Phys Sportsmed, 20(12):87–101.
10. Bryan, WJ, Schauder, K, and Tullos, JS. 1986. The axillary nerve and its relationship to common sports medicine shoulder procedures. Am J of Spts Med, 14(2):113–116.
11. Sawa, TM. 1992. An alternate conservative management of shoulder dislocation and subluxation. J Ath Train, 27(4):366–369.
12. Grana, WA, Holder, S, and Schelberg-Karnes, E. 1987. How I manage acute anterior shoulder dislocations. Phys Sportsmed, 15(4):88–93.
13. Blackburn, TA, McLeod, WD, White, BW, and Wofford, L. 1990. EMG analysis of posterior rotator cuff exercises. Ath Train, 25(1):40–45.
14. Cain, PR, Mutschler, TA, Fu, FA, and Kwon Lee, S. 1987. Anterior stability of the glenohumeral joint: A dynamic model. Am J Sports Med, 15(2):144–148.
15. Richardson, AB. "Overview of soft tissue injuries of the shoulder." In *The upper extremity in sports medicine*, edited by JA Nicholas, EB Hershman, and MA Posner. St. Louis: CV Mosby, 1990.
16. Norwood, LA, and Terry, GC. 1984. Shoulder posterior subluxation. Am J of Spts Med, 12(1):25–30.
17. Skyhar, JF, Warren, RF, and Altchek, DW. "Instability of the shoulder." In *The upper extremity in sports medicine*, edited by JA Nicholas, EB Hershman, and MA Posner. St. Louis: CV Mosby, 1990.
18. Nash, HL. 1988. Rotator cuff damage: Reexamining the causes and treatments. Phys Sptsmed, 16(8):129–135.
19. Warren, RF. "Surgical considerations for rotator cuff tears in athletes." In *Shoulder surgery in the athlete*, edited by DW Jackson. Rockville, MD: Aspen Systems. 1985.
20. Irrgang, JJ, Whitney, SL, and Harner, CD. 1992. Nonoperative treatment of rotator cuff injuries in throwing athletes. J Sport Rehab, 1(3):197–222.
21. Mulligan, E. 1988. Conservative management of shoulder impingement syndrome. Ath Train, 23(4):348–353, 413.
22. McMaster, WC. 1986. Painful shoulder in swimmers: A diagnostic challenge. Phys Sportsmed, 14(12):108–122.
23. McMaster, WC. 1986. Anterior glenoid labrum damage: A painful lesion in swimmers. Am J of Spts Med, 14(5):383–387.
24. McCarthy, P. 1989. Managing bursitis in the athlete: An overview. Phys Sportsmed, 17(11):115–125.
25. Karas, SE. "Thoracic outlet syndrome." In *Clinics in Sports Medicine*, edited by EB Hershman, vol. 9, no. 2. Philadelphia: WB Saunders, 1990.
26. Pianka, G, and Hershman, EB. "Neurovascular injuries." In *The upper extremity in sports medicine*, edited by JA Nicholas, EB Hershman, and MA Posner. St. Louis: CV Mosby, 1990.
27. Andrish, JT. "Upper extremity injuries in the skeletally immature athlete." In *The upper extremity in sports medicine*, edited by JA Nicholas, EB Hershman, and MA Posner. St. Louis: CV Mosby, 1990.
28. Ireland, ML, and Andrews, JR. "Shoulder and elbow injuries in the young athlete." In *Clinics in sports medicine*, edited by LJ Micheli, vol 7, no. 3. Philadelphia: WB Saunders, 1988.
29. Julin, MJ, and Mathews, M. "Shoulder injuries." In *The team physician's handbook*, edited by MB Mellion, WM Walsh, and GL Shelton. Philadelphia: Hanley & Belfus, 1990.
30. Stone, JA, Lueken, JS, Partin, NB, Timm, KE, and Ryan, EJ. 1993. Closed kinetic chain rehabilitation for the glenohumeral joint. J Ath Train, 28(1):34–37.

Chapter 11

Upper Arm, Elbow, and Forearm Injuries

After you have completed this chapter, you should be able to:

- Locate the important bony and soft tissue structures in the upper arm, elbow and forearm
- Describe the motions at the elbow and identify muscles that produce them
- Explain what forces produce the loading patterns responsible for common injuries in the upper arm, elbow, and forearm
- Describe measures used to prevent injuries to the upper arm, elbow, and forearm
- Recognize and manage common injuries in the upper arm, elbow, and forearm
- Demonstrate a thorough assessment of the elbow region
- Demonstrate common rehabilitation exercises for the elbow

The arms perform lifting and carrying tasks, cushion the body during collisions, and lessen body momentum during falls. Performance in many sports is also contingent on the ability of the arms to effectively swing a racquet or club, or to position the hands for throwing and catching a ball. Although dislocations of the elbow are not as common as dislocations of the glenohumeral joint, those that do occur among individuals under age 30 are more likely to arise during participation in sports (1). And, with the exception of the knee, the elbow is believed to be the joint most commonly subjected to overuse injuries (2). Common extensor tendinitis, also known as lateral epicondylitis or "tennis elbow," and medial epicondylitis, or "little league elbow" are examples of overuse injuries.

This chapter begins with a review of anatomy, and an overview of the kinematics and kinetics of the upper arm, elbow, and forearm. Discussion on measures to prevent injury to the region is followed by information on common injuries and their management. Finally, the injury assessment process is presented, and followed by examples of rehabilitation exercises.

ANATOMY REVIEW OF THE ELBOW

❓ *A tennis player is complaining of pain on the lateral side of the elbow that is* *exacerbated during the execution of ground strokes. What anatomical structures are likely to be inflamed?*

Although the elbow may be generally thought of as a simple hinge joint, the elbow actually encompasses three articulations—the humeroulnar, humeroradial, and proximal radioulnar joints (**Figure 11-1**). Several strong ligaments bind these articulations together, and a single joint capsule surrounds all three joints.

Humeroulnar Joint

The hinge joint at the elbow is the humeroulnar joint, where the trochlea of the humerus articulates with the reciprocally-shaped trochlear fossa of the ulna. Motion capabilities are primarily flexion and extension, although in some individuals, particularly women, a small amount of overextension is allowed. The joint is most stable in the close packed position of extension.

Humeroradial Joint

The humeroradial joint lies lateral to the humeroulnar joint. This articulation is formed between the spherical capitellum of the humerus and proximal radius. The humeroradial joint is a gliding joint, with motion restricted to the sagittal plane by the adjacent humeroulnar joint. The close

> The humeroulnar hinge joint is considered to be *the* elbow joint

Epicondylitis
Inflammation and microrupturing of the soft tissues on the epicondyles of the distal humerus

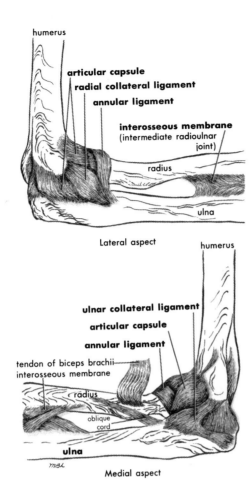

Fig. 11.1: The bones and major ligaments of the elbow.

Lateral aspect

humerus
articular capsule
radial collateral ligament
annular ligament
interosseous membrane
(intermediate radioulnar joint)
radius
ulna

Medial aspect

humerus
ulnar collateral ligament
articular capsule
annular ligament
tendon of biceps brachii
interosseous membrane
radius
oblique cord
ulna

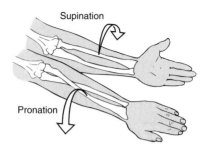

Fig. 11.2: Pronation involves the rotation of the radius around the ulna.

Supination
Pronation

fully supinated position, however, the functional significance of the carrying angle is questionable. Nevertheless, the size of the carrying angle at the elbow is one of the skeletal differences between females and males, and is attributed to differences in the shape of the trochlea. With the elbow fully extended and the forearm fully supinated, the carrying angle ranges from approximately 10 to 15° in adults, and is generally greater in females than in males (3).

Ligaments of the Elbow

The elbow is reinforced by the ulnar (medial) and radial (lateral) collateral ligaments, and by the annular ligament (**Figure 11-1**). The two collateral ligaments are strong and fan-shaped and consist of anterior, intermediate,

packed position is with the elbow flexed at 90° and the forearm supinated about 5°.

Proximal Radioulnar Joint

The annular ligament binds the head of the radius to the radial notch of the ulna, forming the proximal radioulnar joint. This is a pivot joint, with forearm pronation and supination occurring as the radius rolls medially and laterally over the ulna (**Figure 11-2**). The closed packed position is at 5° of forearm supination.

Carrying Angle

The angle between the longitudinal axes of the humerus and the ulna when the arm is in anatomical position is known as the **carrying angle (Figure 11-3)**. The angle is so-named because it causes the forearm to angle away from the body when a load is carried in the hand. Given that loads are typically carried with the forearm in a neutral, rather than a

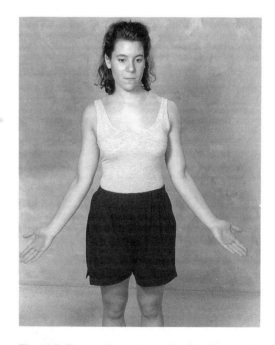

Fig. 11.3: The carrying angle at the elbow is generally larger among women than among men.

and posterior fiber bundles. The annular ligament provides support for the adjacent proximal radioulnar joint.

Muscles of the Elbow

A number of muscles cross the elbow, including several that also cross the shoulder, or extend down into the hand and fingers. The tendinous attachments of muscles near the medial and lateral aspects of the elbow are often irritated and inflamed by repetitive stresses associated with poor technique or overtraining in sports such as tennis, golf, and baseball pitching. The muscles considered to be primary movers of the elbow are summarized in **Table 11-1**.

Nerves of the Elbow

The major nerves of the elbow and forearm region descend from the brachial plexus and include the musculocutaneous (C_5-C_7), median (C_5-T_1), ulnar (C_8-T_1), and radial

Table 11–1. Muscles of the Elbow.

Muscle	Proximal Attachment	Distal Attachment	Primary Action(s)	Nerve Innervation
Biceps brachii		Tuberosity of the radius	Flexion; assists with supination	Musculocutaneous (C_5,C_6)
(Long head)	Superior rim of the glenoid fossa			
(Short head)	Coracoid process of the scapula			
Brachioradialis	Upper two-thirds lateral supra-condylar ridge of humerus	Styloid process of the radius	Flexion	Radial (C_5,C_6)
Brachialis	Anterior lower half of the humerus	Anterior coronoid process of ulna	Flexion	Musculocutaneous (C_5,C_6)
Pronator Teres		Lateral midpoint of the radius	Assists with flexion and pronation	Median (C_6,C_7)
(Humeral head)	Medial epicondyle of the humerus			
(Ulnar head)	Coronoid process of the ulna			
Pronator quadratus	Lower fourth of the anterior ulna	Lower fourth of the anterior radius	Pronation	Anterior interosseous (C_8,T_1)
Triceps brachii		Olecranon process of the ulna	Extension	Radial (C_6-C_8)
(Long head)	Just inferior to the glenoid fossa			
(Lateral head)	Upper half of the posterior humerus			
(Medial head)	Lower two-thirds of posterior humerus			
Anconeus	Posterior, lateral epicondyle of the humerus	Lateral olecranon and posterior ulna	Assists with extension	Radial (C_7,C_8)
Supinator	Lateral epicondyle of humerus and adjacent ulna	Lateral upper third of radius	Supination	Posterior interosseous (C_5,C_6)

nerves (**C₅-T₁**) (**Figure 11-4**). The musculocutaneous nerve provides motor supply to the flexor muscles of the anterior arm, and sensory innervation to the skin of the lateral forearm. The median nerve supplies most of the flexor muscles of the anterior forearm, and the skin on the palmar aspect of the hand including the thumb, index finger, middle finger, and the lateral half of the ring finger. The ulnar nerve provides innervation to the flexor carpi ulnaris and the medial half of the flexor digitorum profundus, and skin on the medial border of the hand including the little finger and medial half of the ring finger. The radial nerve, the largest branch of the brachial plexus, passes anteriorly to the lateral epicondyle at the elbow, then divides into the superficial and deep branches to continue along the posterolateral aspect of the forearm. The radial nerve supplies all the arm and forearm extensor muscles, and the skin on the posterior aspect of the arm and forearm. Specific nerve-muscle associations are shown in **Table 11-1**.

> The brachial artery supplies blood to the elbow

Blood Vessels of the Elbow

The major arteries of the elbow and forearm region are the brachial, ulnar, and radial arteries (**Figure 11-5**). The brachial artery courses down the medial side of the arm, providing blood supply to the flexor muscles of the arm. The deep brachial artery branches off to supply the triceps brachii. At the elbow the brachial artery forms an anastomosis to supply the elbow joint. The main branch of the brachial artery crosses the anterior aspect of the elbow where the brachial pulse can be readily palpated. Distal to the elbow, the brachial artery splits into the ulnar and radial arteries. The ulnar artery supplies the medial forearm and via one of its branches, the common interosseous artery, supplies the deep flexors and extensors of the forearm. The radial artery, which courses along the anterior aspect of the radius, supplies the lateral forearm muscles. Pulses can be taken for both arteries on the anterior aspect of the wrist (**See Figure 4-13**).

💡 *The tendinous attachments of the extensor muscles crossing the lateral aspect of the elbow can become irritated and inflamed through improper technique or repetitive overuse in tennis, golf, or throwing. The extensor carpi radialis brevis tendon is often implicated.*

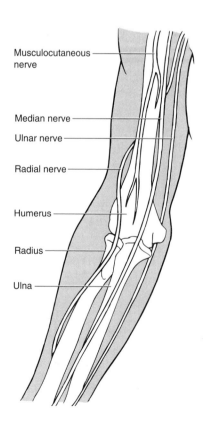

Fig. 11.4: The nerves of the elbow region.

Labels: Musculocutaneous nerve; Median nerve; Ulnar nerve; Radial nerve; Humerus; Radius; Ulna

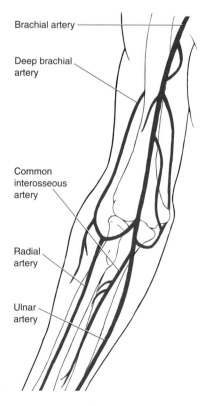

Fig. 11.5: The arteries of the elbow region.

Labels: Brachial artery; Deep brachial artery; Common interosseous artery; Radial artery; Ulnar artery

KINEMATICS AND MAJOR MUSCLE ACTIONS OF THE ELBOW

? *Why is the effectiveness of some elbow flexor muscles affected by the position of the radioulnar joint?*

The three associated joints at the elbow allow motion in two planes. Flexion and extension are sagittal plane movements that occur at the humeroulnar and humeroradial joints, and pronation and supination are longitudinal rotational movements that take place at the proximal radioulnar joint.

Flexion and Extension

The elbow flexors include those muscles crossing the anterior side of the joint (**Figure 11-6**). The primary elbow flexor is the brachialis. Because the distal attachment of the brachialis is the coronoid process of the ulna, the muscle is equally as effective when the forearm is in supination or pronation. Another elbow flexor, the biceps brachii, has both long and short heads attached to the radial tuberosity via a single common tendon. The muscle contributes effectively to flexion when the forearm is supinated, because it is slightly stretched. When the forearm is pronated, the muscle is less taut and consequently less effective. The brachioradialis, a third elbow flexor, is most effective when the

forearm is in a neutral position (midway between full pronation and full supination).

The triceps is the major elbow extensor (**Figure 11-7**). Although the three heads have separate proximal attachments, they attach to the olecranon process of the ulna through a common distal tendon. The small anconeus also assists with extension at the elbow.

Pronation and Supination

Pronation and supination of the forearm occur when the radius rotates around the ulna. There are three radioulnar articulations—the proximal, middle, and distal radioulnar joints. The proximal and distal joints are pivot joints. The middle radioulnar joint is a syndesmosis, with an elastic interconnecting membrane permitting supination and pronation, but preventing longitudinal displacement of one bone with respect to the other.

The primary pronator muscle is the pronator quadratus, which attaches to the distal ulna and radius (**Figure 11-8**). The pronator teres, which crosses the proximal radioulnar joint, assists with pronation.

As the name suggests, the supinator is the muscle primarily responsible for supination (**Figure 11-9**). During resistance and/or

> The primary elbow flexor is the brachialis

> Pronation and supination of the forearm involves the pivoting of the radius around the ulna

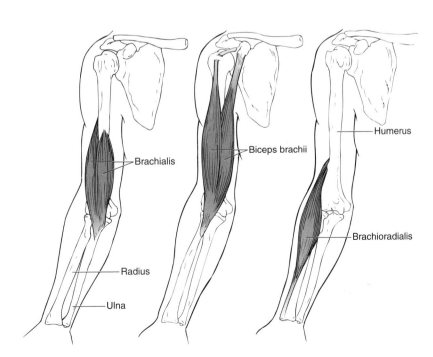

Fig. 11.6: The primary flexor muscles of the elbow. (A) Brachialis. (B) Biceps brachii. (C) Brachioradialis.

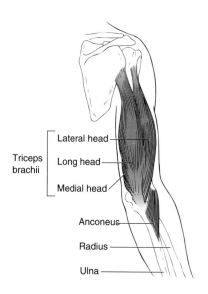

Fig. 11.7: The primary extensor muscles of the elbow are the triceps brachii and anconeus.

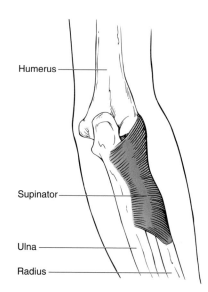

Fig. 11.9: The primary supinator of the elbow is the supinator muscle.

when the elbow is flexed, the biceps also participates in supination.

💡 *Muscles function most effectively when slightly stretched. Thus, the biceps brachii is most effective when the forearm is fully supinated, and the brachioradialis is most effective when the forearm is in a neutral position.*

KINETICS OF THE ELBOW

❓ *An individual has sustained a fracture to the proximal radial head. When the bone*

has healed sufficiently for the individual to begin rehabilitation exercises, are flexion and extension exercises equally safe?

Although the elbow is not considered to be a weight-bearing joint, it sustains significant loads during daily activities. For example, it has been estimated that the compressive load at the elbow reaches 300 N (67 lb) during activities such as dressing and eating, 1700 N (382 lb) when the body is supported by the arms when rising from a chair, and 1900 N (427 lb) when pulling a table across the floor (3). Although no estimates for the load on the elbow during participation in sport or exercise have been published, it is likely that even greater loads are present during the execution of selected sport skills. Large forces are generated by muscles crossing the elbow during forceful pitching and throwing motions, as well as during many resistance training exercises and weight lifting. During the execution of many skills in gymnastics and wrestling, the elbow functions as a weight-bearing joint.

Since the attachment of the elbow extensors to the ulna is closer to the joint center than the attachments of the elbow flexors on the radius and ulna, the extensor moment arm is shorter than the flexor moment arm. This means that the elbow extensors must generate more force than the elbow flexors to produce the same amount of joint torque. This translates to greater joint compression forces during extension than during flexion when movements with comparable speed and force requirements are executed.

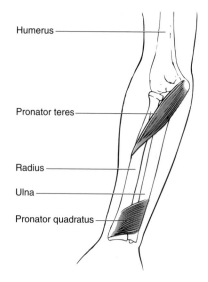

Fig. 11.8: The primary pronators of the elbow are the pronator quadratus and pronator teres.

> Higher joint compression forces occur during extension than during flexion

💡 *Because extension causes greater elbow joint compression than flexion, particular caution is in order when extension exercises are used to rehabilitate a fracture in the elbow region.*

PREVENTION OF ELBOW INJURIES

❓ *The arms perform lifting and carrying tasks, cushion the body during collisions, and lessen body movements during falls. What measures can be taken to protect and strengthen the region to prevent injuries?*

The elbow is often subjected to compressive forces when the arm is placed in such a position to cushion a fall or lessen body impact with another object. Microtraumatic forces caused by repetitive valgus and varus stresses can also lead to overuse injuries, many of which are related to poor skill technique. Few sports require protective equipment at the elbow. Therefore, physical conditioning and proper skill technique are major factors in preventing injury to this region.

Protective Equipment

Standard shoulder pads may not extend far enough to protect the upper arm. Many football lineman have an additional biceps pad attached to the shoulder pads, or use a padded knee pad to protect this vulnerable area. Hockey and lacrosse players also have special pads to protect the elbow during falls and collisions. A commercially available padded elbow sleeve or neoprene sleeve is worn in many sports to protect the olecranon from direct trauma and abrasions, particularly when playing on artificial turf. The sleeves extend into the forearm for added protection. Counterforce braces (**Figure 6-12**), commonly seen in racquet sports, reduce muscle tensile forces that can lead to medial or lateral epicondylitis. Braces, such as the one demonstrated in **Figure 6-13** add compression and support to the elbow to reduce excessive varus and valgus forces.

Physical Conditioning

Several muscles that move the shoulder also cross the elbow. Likewise, several muscles that move the wrist and fingers also cross the elbow. Therefore, flexibility and strengthening exercises must focus on muscles that move the shoulder, elbow, and wrist. General flexibility exercises for the shoulder can be used in conjunction with warm-up exercises that mimic specific sport skills. For example, a tennis player may begin the warm-up session with slow, controlled forehand and backhand strokes, gradually increasing intensity. A pitcher or outfielder may begin with short, controlled throws, increasing the distance and intensity as the arm is warmed up.

Strengthening exercises for the shoulder can be combined with those listed in **Field Strategy 11-1**. These exercises are designed to improve general strength in elbow flexion and extension, forearm pronation and supination, wrist flexion and extension, and radial and ulnar deviation. Begin with light resistance and progress to a heavier resistance.

Proper Skill Technique

Nearly all overuse injuries are directly related to repetitive throwing-type motions that produce microtraumatic tensile forces on the elbow and surrounding soft tissue structures. Analysis of the specific movement can detect improper technique in the acceleration and follow-through phase that place excessive stress on the elbow leading to joint sprains and muscular strains. High speed photography may aid in this analysis. As discussed in the shoulder chapter, participants in all sports should also be taught the shoulder roll method of falling. Falling on an extended hand or elbow may conduct excessive compressive forces to the region, leading to a fracture or dislocation.

💡 *Strengthening the musculature at the shoulder, elbow, and wrist, along with using proper throwing technique, and wearing protective pads can prevent many injuries.*

CONTUSIONS

❓ *A football player is complaining of pain on impact with his right arm during blocking. Palpation reveals a hardened mass of soft tissue over the distal anterior arm that is very tender and sore. There is good bilateral strength but the pain is getting worse. What potentially serious condition might develop? How will you manage this condition?*

Direct blows to the upper arm and lateral side of the forearm are frequently associated with contact and collision sports. For volleyball players, the very nature of the sport leads to trauma on the radial side of the forearm (**Figure 11-10**). Contusions can involve any aspect of the elbow region including injury to the ulnar nerve as it passes through the ulnar

Many individuals wear padded elbow sleeves or neoprene sleeves to protect the olecranon from direct trauma and abrasions, particularly when playing on artificial turf

Improper technique in the acceleration and follow-through phase of throwing can place excessive stress on the elbow leading to joint sprains and muscular strains

Field Strategy 11–1. Exercises to Prevent Injury to the Elbow Region.

Begin all exercises with light resistance using dumbbells or surgical tubing.

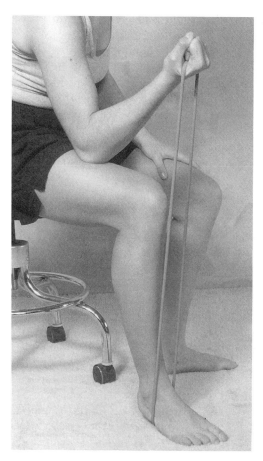

A. Biceps curl. Support the involved arm on the leg and bend the elbow into full flexion. This can be performed bilaterally in a standing position with a barbell

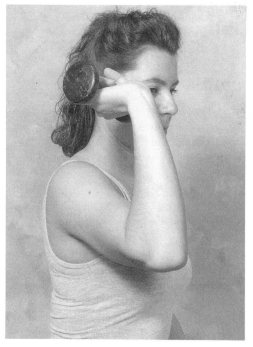

B. Triceps curl. Raise the involved arm over the head, supporting the elbow with the opposite hand. Extend the involved arm at the elbow. This can be performed bilaterally in a supine or standing position with a barbell

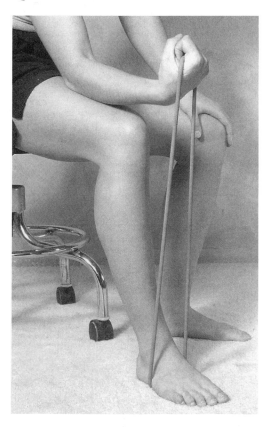

C. Wrist flexion. Support the involved forearm on a table with the hand off the edge. With the palm facing up, slowly do a full wrist curl and return to the starting position. Repeat

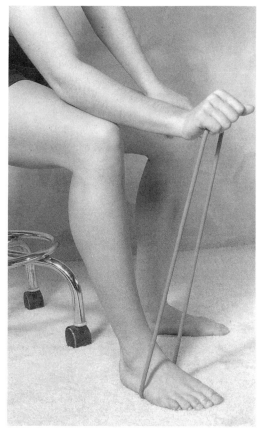

D. Wrist extension. Support the involved forearm on a table with the hand off the edge. With the palm facing down, slowly do a full reverse wrist curl and return to the starting position. Repeat

(continued)

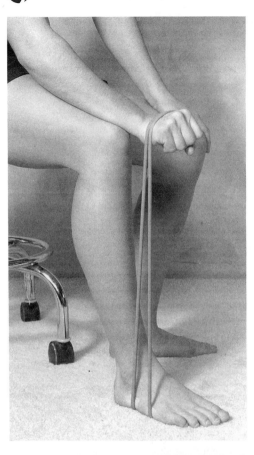

E. Forearm pronation/supination. Support the involved forearm on a table or your leg with the hand over the edge. With surgical tubing or a hand dumbbell, roll the forearm into pronation, then return to supination. Adjust the surgical tubing and repeat the exercise stressing the supinators. Be sure the elbow remains stationary

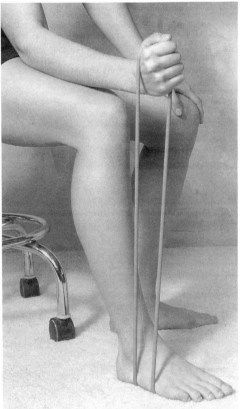

F. Ulnar/radial deviation. Support the involved forearm on a table or your leg with the hand over the edge. With surgical tubing or a hand dumbbell, contract the appropriate muscle group. An alternate method is to stand with the arm at the side holding a hammer or weighted bar. Raise the wrist in ulnar deviation. Repeat in radial deviation

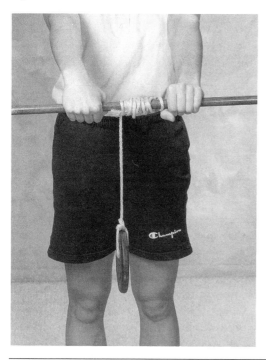

G. Wrist curl-ups. To exercise the wrist extensors, grip the bar with both palms facing down. Slowly wind the cord onto the bar until the weight reaches the top, then slowly unwind the cord. Reverse hand position to work the wrist flexors

groove. Bruising can lead to internal hemorrhage, rapid swelling, and hematoma formation that can limit range of motion. Chronic blows may also result in a fibrous mass or heavy callus on the bone. Individuals at risk for contusions should wear padded elbow and forearm pads.

In the anterior arm, resulting hemorrhage from direct blows, a fracture, or dislocation can lead to the development of **ectopic bone** in either the belly of the muscle (myositis ossificans) or as a bony outgrowth (exostosis) of the underlying bone. Because of the proximity of the brachialis muscle belly to the joint, it is a common site for the development of myositis ossificans after trauma. Another vulnerable site is just proximal to the deltoid's distal attachment on the lateral aspect of the humerus where the bone is least padded by muscle tissue. Standard shoulder pads do not extend far enough to protect the area, and the edge of the pad itself may contribute to the injury. The developing mass seldom interferes with arm function, although it can become painful and disabling if the radial nerve is contused, leading to transitory paralysis of the extensor forearm muscles.

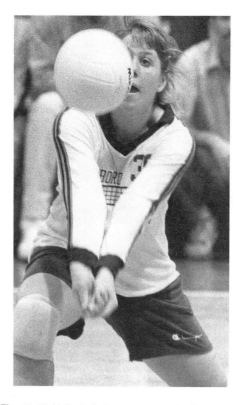

Fig. 11.10: Volleyball players contuse the forearms during the early part of the season from repetitive compression on soft tissue structures.

Ectopic bone
Proliferation of bone ossification in an abnormal place

The humerus is very vulnerable to direct trauma over the brachialis and at the distal attachment of the deltoid muscle

"Tackler's (blocker's spur) exostosis" commonly seen in football linemen is not a true myositis ossificans. This is because the ectopic formation is not infiltrated into the muscle, but rather is an irritative exostosis arising directly from the bone. A painful bony mass, usually in the form of a spur with a sharp edge, can be palpated on the anterolateral aspect of the humerus. Surgical excision of the calcification is seldom necessary because function is not usually impaired. The area should be protected with a special pad during participation. However, if function is adversely affected, surgery should be delayed until the calcification is mature, usually in 12 to 18 months, as it may redevelop.

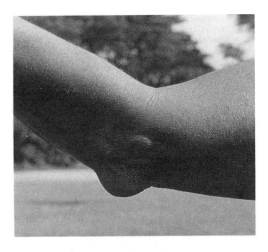

Fig. 11.11: When the olecranon bursa ruptures, a discrete, sharply demarcated goose egg is visible directly over the olecranon process.

Contusions are usually not disabling, but complications such as excessive hemorrhage, nerve damage, and fracture should be ruled out. Acute care should involve ice, compression, elevation, and rest, followed by nonsteroidal anti-inflammatory drugs (NSAIDs) and gentle, pain-free range of motion exercises. Aggressive stretching and strengthening exercises should be avoided (4). If conservative measures do not alleviate the condition, refer the individual to a physician for x-rays. Visible radiograph changes in the muscle can be noted after two to three weeks. As the condition progresses and becomes chronic, a painful **periostitis** and **fibrositis** may develop.

The football player may be developing myositis ossificans in the brachialis muscle. Standard acute care should be followed by referral to a physician for further assessment and possible radiographs.

OLECRANON BURSITIS

A wrestler has acute swelling about an inch in diameter on the proximal posterior ulna. What condition is present, and how will you manage it?

The olecranon bursa is the largest bursa in the elbow region. Injury may occur during a fall on a flexed elbow, by constantly leaning on one's elbow ("student's elbow"), by repetitive pressure and friction (as is common in wrestling), or by infections (5,6). The acutely inflamed bursa will present with rapid swelling, although it may be relatively painless **(Figure 11-11)**. The swelling may stem from bleeding or seepage of fluid into the bursal sac. Depending on the degree of acute inflammation, there may be heat and redness

associated with the swelling. Acute management involves ice, rest, and a compressive wrap applied for the first 24 hours.

Occasionally the bursa can become infected regardless of acute trauma to the area. In this case the area will be hot to the touch and inflamed. The individual will show traditional signs of infection, including **malaise**, fever, pain, restricted motion, tenderness, and swelling at the elbow. The physician may aspirate the bursa and take a culture of the fluid. The elbow is immobilized in a sling, and continuous hot packs and appropriate antibiotics are typically prescribed.

Chronic bursitis is managed with cryotherapy, NSAIDs, and protected from further insult with proper padding. In long-term cases of chronic bursitis, as with an infection, the bursa sac may be aspirated or totally excised, although there is a risk of poor wound healing over the olecranon process.

Did you determine that the wrestler had acute olecranon bursitis? Standard acute care should resolve the condition, however, additional padding can prevent recurrence.

SPRAINS

After practice, a javelin thrower is complaining of acute pain on the medial aspect of the elbow. Palpation reveals point tenderness over the medial joint line, but only mild discomfort during active and passive movement. How can you determine if the ulnar collateral ligament is injured?

At the elbow, acute tears to ligamentous and joint structures are rare, but may occur during a fall on an extended hand, producing a hyperextension injury, or through a valgus/varus tensile force. More commonly, however, repetitive trauma leads to chronic irritation and tearing of the ligaments, particularly the ulnar collateral ligament. Injury may vary from a partial tear (first degree sprain) to a total rupture of the supporting ligaments (third degree sprain). The ulnar collateral ligament is more vulnerable to injury, and is often associated with damage to the ulnar nerve. Examination will reveal point tenderness on the joint line, and increased pain and instability with the valgus stress test applied to the elbow at 15 to 20° flexion (See **Figure 11-23**). Ice, compression, NSAIDs, and rest is followed by early protected range of motion exercises. Surgery is indicated only for major tears.

Anterior Capsulitis

Anterior joint pain caused by hyperextension is more commonly attributed to acute anterior capsulitis, rather than as a result of chronic repetitive throwing. Microtears in the capsule are usually not sufficient to cause dislocation (7). The individual will have diffuse anterior elbow pain after a traumatic episode with deep tenderness on palpation, particularly on the anteromedial side. A strain to the pronator teres should be ruled out, as well as entrapment of the median nerve as it courses through the pronator teres. When this occurs, tingling or numbness of the thumb and index finger are usually noted.

Dislocations

Dislocations at the elbow are second only to glenohumeral dislocations, with most occurring in individuals younger than 20, with a peak incidence in late adolescence (8). In children younger than 10 years, it may be the most frequently dislocated joint. The mechanism of injury is usually hyperextension, or a sudden violent, unidirectional valgus or varus blow resulting in a shearing force to the elbow that drives the ulna posterior or posterolateral (5,9). The ulnar collateral ligament is usually ruptured, and there may be an associated fracture of the radial head, coranoid process, or olecranon process of the ulna. The anterior capsule, brachialis muscle, and the flexor and extensor muscle masses may also be disrupted (8). Damage to the

ulnar nerve may lead to numbness in the little finger. Damage to the brachial artery may lead to an acute forearm compartment syndrome.

Immediately on impact, a snapping or cracking sensation is followed by severe pain, rapid swelling, total loss of function, and an obvious deformity (**Figure 11-12**). The arm is frequently held in flexion with the forearm appearing shortened. The olecranon and radial head are palpable posteriorly, as is a slight indentation in the triceps just proximal to the olecranon. Immediate immobilization and transportation to the nearest medical facility is warranted, since early reduction minimizes the amount of muscle spasm. Management of an elbow dislocation is discussed in **Field Strategy 11-2**.

Closed reduction under general anesthesia is necessary. In cases where the forearm flexors, extensors, and annular ligament have maintained their integrity with no associated fracture, limited immobilization and early range of motion exercises have proven quite successful. There is however, a 9 to 14% chance of recurrent dislocation due mainly to the instability that results from disruption of the ulnar collateral ligament at the time of the initial dislocation (10). Elbow dislocations involving fractures of the radial head or capitellar fracture dislocations are more complex and require internal fixation.

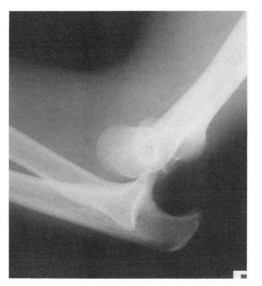

Fig. 11.12: Posterior dislocations produce a snapping or cracking sensation followed by immediate severe pain, rapid swelling, and total loss of function.

Signs and Symptoms

Snapping or cracking sensation.

Immediate severe pain with rapid swelling primarily on the medial aspect of the elbow along with total loss of function.

An obvious deformity is present as the olecranon is pushed posteriorly and the normal isosceles triangular relationship between the epicondyles and olecranon is not present.

The elbow will be slightly flexed and supported, if possible, by the uninjured arm.

Pain is predominantly localized over the medial aspect of the elbow.

If there is an associated fracture, crepitation may be palpated.

Management

This injury should be regarded as an emergency!

Apply ice immediately to the area to reduce swelling and inflammation.

Assess the radial pulse, skin color, and blanching of the nails to rule out circulatory impairment.

Assess motor and sensor function. If the patient is able, ask the person to flex, extend, and abduct and adduct the fingers. With the individual looking away, stroke the palm and dorsum of the hand in several different locations with a blunt and sharp object. Ask the individual to identify where you are touching, and if it is sharp or dull.

Because of the risk of an associated fracture, immobilize the area with a vacuum splint or other appropriate splint without causing additional pain for the individual.

Take vital signs, recheck the pulse and sensory functions, and treat for shock.

Transport immediately to the nearest medical facility.

In adolescents, subluxation or dislocation of the proximal radial head is often associated with an immature annular ligament. Distraction with rotation, such as when a young child is swung by the arms, can cause the radial head to slip out of the supporting annular ligament. Although this injury can occur in adults, it is not common but tends to recur. Immobilization for three to six weeks in flexion is usually necessary (5).

During the assessment, a positive valgus stress test at 15 to 20° of elbow flexion should indicate a tear to the ulnar collateral ligament. Standard acute care is followed by early range of motion exercises to minimize disability.

STRAINS

A rower is complaining of vague anterior arm pain aggravated during the pull portion of the stroke. Palpation elicits point tenderness on the distal anterior arm and resisted elbow flexion and supination increases pain. What muscles may be involved here? How will you handle this condition?

Muscular strains commonly result from inadequate warm-up, excessive training past the point of fatigue, and inadequate rehabilitation of previous muscular injuries. Less commonly, they may occur as a result of a single massive contraction or sudden over-stretching.

Elbow Flexor and Extensor Strains

Injury to the brachialis or biceps brachii will result in point tenderness on the anterior distal arm. Pain will increase with passive elbow extension and resisted elbow flexion. A total rupture of the biceps tendon is usually associated with forceful shoulder flexion against excessive resistance, as in weight lifters or gymnasts, and was discussed in Chapter 11.

Occasionally a direct blow to the posterior elbow, or an uncoordinated triceps contraction during a fall can result in an acute rupture of the tendon. In addition to the tendon rupture, 80% of all injuries involve an olecranon avulsion fracture (7). Although rare, spontaneous ruptures of the tendon can occur, but these are usually associated with systemic diseases or steroid use. With triceps strains, passive flexion and resisted elbow extension will produce discomfort. In more moderate strains, acute pain and swelling, and a palpable defect will be present. In a total rupture, weakness or loss of active motion occurs.

With triceps strains, passive flexion and resisted elbow extension produce increased pain

Forearm Flexor/Extensor Strains

Injury to the common flexor/extensor group of the forearm muscles is usually self-limiting, requiring only modified rest, ice, compression, and activity modification. Gentle stretching of the muscles is combined with strengthening exercises, such as those listed in **Field Strategy 11-1**. Major tears or ruptures seldom occur, and will have considerable ecchymosis, a palpable defect, and limited, weak motion. This individual should be referred to a physician, as surgery may be indicated.

Management of Strains

Treatment involves standard acute care with ice, compression, elevation, and protected rest. If a palpable defect is noted or an avulsion fracture is suspected, immobilization in a sling is followed by referral to a physician for possible surgical reattachment. Activity modification, NSAIDs, and a gradual active range of motion and strengthening exercise program should be initiated as tolerated. **Field Strategy 11-3** summarizes management of muscular strains.

The rower may have a strain to the biceps brachii or brachialis muscle that is aggravated during elbow flexion on the pull phase of the stroke. Ice, compression, and protected rest should be accompanied with stretching and strengthening exercises for the elbow flexors.

OVERUSE CONDITIONS

A little league baseball pitcher is complaining of pain on the medial elbow aggravated during the acceleration phase of throwing. Palpation reveals point tenderness on the medial epicondyle of the humerus, and pain during active elbow flexion and forearm pronation. What condition(s) might be present? How will you manage the injury?

The throwing mechanism discussed in Chapter 10 can also lead to overuse injuries at the elbow (See **Figure 10-10**). During the cocking phase of throwing, the elbow is

---

 Field Strategy 11–3. Management of Muscular Strains.

Acute management

Control inflammation, swelling, and pain with ice, compression, elevation, NSAIDs, and rest is necessary

Prevent progression of the injury by reducing stresses appropriately with activity modification, biomechanical analysis of skill performance, or equipment modification

Rehabilitation

Use daily applications of ice, ultrasound, EMS, interferential current, or thermotherapy to precede exercise

Restore range of motion. Do not forget to assess flexibility at the shoulder region since limitations there may increase stress at the elbow

Perform isometric exercises throughout a pain-free range of motion

Progress to isotonic exercises with light resistance, building from one to five lbs throughout a pain-free range

Add surgical tubing exercises as tolerated

Ice the injured muscle after each exercise session followed by stretching exercises

When pain-free, ensure adequate warm-up and gradual return to functional exercises. If the individual is in a throwing activity, begin functional throwing with a light toss over a distance of 20 to 30 feet for 5 minutes progressing to 15 to 20 minutes

When the individual can throw for 15 to 20 minutes, gradually increase the distance to 150 feet

When proper throwing mechanics are present, gradually increase velocity

Improve neuromuscular control with closed kinetic chain exercises, such as shifting a weighted ball in the hand, push-ups, press-ups, or walking on the hands in a push-up position between boxes of varying height

Continue a strengthening and stretching program as return to activity is initiated

flexed at approximately 45° with the wrist extended. As the body is brought rapidly forward during the acceleration phase, the elbow and hand are left behind prestressing structures at the elbow, particularly the ulnar collateral ligament. As acceleration of the upper body continues, the shoulder flexors and medial rotators contract. Simultaneously the elbow extensors and wrist flexors contract to add velocity to the throw. This results in a whipping action that produces significant stress on the medial elbow. Ball release begins the follow-through and deceleration phase where the elbow continues in extension and the forearm moves into pronation. The forearm must pronate regardless of the pitch delivered, only timing differs. In relation to the standard fastball, pronation occurs sooner in a screwball and later in the curveball (11). Some supination does occur during a curveball. During deceleration, eccentric contractions of the long head of the biceps brachii, supinator, and extensor muscles decelerate the forearm into pronation. Additional stress occurs on structures around the olecranon as pronation and extension jam the olecranon into its fossa (5).

Epicondylitis is a common chronic condition seen in activities involving pronation and supination, such as in tennis, javelin throwing, pitching, volleyball, or golf. Often the individual will reveal a pattern of poor technique, fatigue, and overuse.

Medial Epicondylitis

Medial epicondylitis is caused by repeated medial tension/lateral compression (valgus) forces. The tension forces lead to microtears in the wrist flexor/pronator muscle group at the common tendinous attachment on the medial epicondyle. In adolescents aged 9 to 14, this condition can lead to tension stress on the growth plate, known as "**little league elbow**" (2). Use of this term, however, to describe all medial pain negates the fact that other individuals, such as golfers, gymnasts, javelin throwers, tennis players, wrestlers, and weight lifters are susceptible to the condition. In addition to muscular injury, medial tension overload can lead to other extra-articular injuries, such as an ulnar collateral ligament sprain, ulnar traction spurring, ulnar neuritis, or a partial or complete avulsion of the medial epicondyle (7,19). Simultaneously, the lateral joint line experiences compressive

forces, while shear forces are generated posteriorly in the olecranon fossa. This action can result in lateral epicondylitis, radial head injury, or capitellar osteochondral injuries. Posterior stresses may lead to triceps strain, synovial impingement, olecranon fractures, or loose bodies and degenerative joint changes (2,5).

An acute injury seen in pitchers on cold days following inadequate warm-up involves a moderate to severe sprain of the ulnar collateral ligament. During acceleration a "pop" may be heard indicating the ligament has been torn. Although the individual may perceive this injury as a single episode, in reality it may have been the "final straw" that led to the acute injury. Many individuals will report a history of medial pain for months or years before the acute episode. Still others report previous corticosteroid injections into the medial aspect of the elbow which weakens the ulnar collateral ligament leading to rupture (10).

Valgus stress forces that lead to medial epicondylitis often produce a combined flexor muscle strain, ulnar collateral ligament sprain, and ulnar neuritis. Assessment will reveal swelling, ecchymosis, and point tenderness directly over the humeroulnar joint, or on the medial epicondyle. Pain is usually severe and aggravated by resisted wrist flexion and pronation, and a valgus stress applied at 15 to 20° of elbow flexion. If the ulnar nerve is involved, tingling and numbness may radiate into the forearm and hand, particularly the fourth and fifth fingers.

Most extra-articular conditions can be managed with ice, NSAIDs, and immobilization in a sling for two to three weeks. Transcutaneous electric nerve stimulation (TENS), high-voltage galvanic stimulation, ultrasound, and interferential current is used to decrease pain and inflammation. Early painless range of motion exercises and gentle resisted isometric exercises should progress to isotonic strengthening and use of surgical tubing. A functional brace may limit valgus stress and allow early resumption of strenuous activities (**Figure 6-13**). In moderate injuries, throwing or overhead motions should be avoided for up to 6 to 12 weeks (7). With intra-articular injuries, ulnar nerve problems, or moderate to severe cases of pain or instability, referral to a physician is indicated. **Field Strategy 11-4** describes management of medial elbow pain.

Field Strategy 11–4. Management of Medial Elbow Pain.

Initially pain or spasm of the flexor/pronator muscles will occur during activity. This may progress to an aching pain over the medial epicondyle after activity.

Later stages will produce sharp pain during activity, particularly during the throwing motion.

Point tenderness can be elicited over or just distal to the medial epicondyle of the humerus.

Pain will increase with resisted wrist flexion or forearm pronation, and passive stretching of the wrist flexors.

Swelling may be present and may limit elbow extension.

If the ulnar nerve is involved, numbness and tingling may radiate into the forearm and hand, particularly into the medial half of the fourth finger and all of the fifth finger.

Management

Ice, compression, elevation, NSAIDs, and rest can limit pain and inflammation.

If an avulsion fracture of the medial epicondyle or apophyseal fracture in the adolescent is suspected, refer the individual to a physician.

Avoid all activities that lead to pain. Immobilization in a sling may be necessary if simple daily activities cause pain. The individual can continue to perform activities that do not aggravate the condition.

Ice massage, contrast baths, ultrasound therapy, EMS, interferential current, and friction massage over the flexor tendons may also supplement the treatment plan.

Rehabilitation

The goal is to restore full strength, flexibility, and endurance in the wrist flexors and pronators.

Maintain range of motion and strength at the wrist and shoulder.

Stretching exercises should be done within pain-free motions and should include wrist flexion/extension, forearm pronation/supination, and radial and ulnar deviation.

Begin with fast contractions using light resistance. Perform tennis ball squeezes and other strengthening exercises within pain free ranges. Add surgical tubing as tolerated. Work up to three to five sets of ten repetitions per session before moving on to heavier resistance.

Incorporate early closed chain exercises such as press-ups, wall push-ups, or walking on the hands.

Continue to work on active range of motion and strengthening exercises for all shoulder, elbow, and wrist motions.

Do a biomechanical analysis of the throwing motion to determine proper technique, and make adjustments as necessary.

After return to protected activity, continue stretching exercises before and after practice. Ice after practice to control any inflammation. Return to full activity as tolerated.

Lateral Epicondylitis

Pain over the lateral epicondyle denotes extensor tendon overload, predominantly with the extensor carpi radialis brevis. Although commonly known as "tennis elbow" or lateral epicondylitis, it is more correctly called "common extensor tendinitis." The condition arises from four primary mechanisms: use of power grips, impact forces, excessive use of a curveball, but more routinely, eccentric loading of the extensor muscles. The strong gripping action in a power grip requires synergistic action of the wrist extensors and finger flexors. Impact forces are transmitted via the grip in a tennis racquet or bat leading to repetitive microtrauma. Overuse of the curveball can lead to a strain of the supinator muscle. Excessive forearm pronation and wrist flexion during the deceleration phase of the throwing motion or a tennis stroke can produce excessive eccentric loading of the extensor muscles (**Figure 11-13**) (6,10). Gripping a racquet too tightly, improper grip size, excessive string tension, excessive racquet weight or stiffness, faulty backhand technique, putting top spin on backhand strokes, or hitting the ball off-center all contribute to this condition (6).

> Common extensor tendinitis may be caused by excessive power grips, impact forces, excessive use of a curveball, or eccentric loading of the extensor muscles

Increased pain with resisted wrist extension, a coffee cup test, and the tennis elbow test indicates common extensor tendinitis

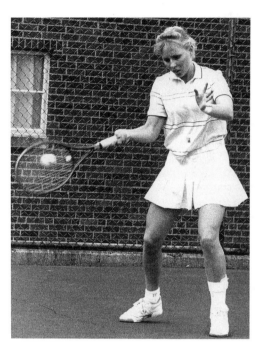

Fig. 11.13: Eccentric loading of the elbow extensor muscles occurs with excessive forearm pronation and wrist flexion during the deceleration phase of a tennis stroke or a throwing motion.

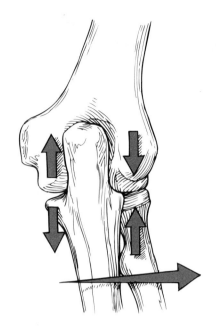

Fig. 11.14: An excessive valgus force can lead to both medial tensile stress and lateral compression stress, causing injury to both sides of the joint.

Entrapment of the ulnar nerve may lead to a sharp pain radiating down the medial aspect of the forearm as if you had "hit your crazy bone"

Pronator syndrome
Median nerve is entrapped by the pronator teres leading to pain on activities involving pronation

Pain will be over or just distal to the lateral epicondyle that may radiate into the forearm extensors during and after activity. Pain will increase with resisted wrist extension, the "Coffee cup" test (pain increases while picking up a full cup of coffee), and with the tennis elbow test (See **Figure 11-24**). Initially, ice, compression, NSAIDs, rest, and support will alleviate symptoms. A counterforce strap placed two to three inches distal to the elbow joint can limit excessive muscular tension placed on the epicondyle, and is usually sufficient to eliminate symptoms **(Figure 6-11)**. **Field Strategy 11-5** describes management of common extensor tendinitis.

Impingement and Neural Entrapment Injuries

Valgus stress, coupled with an extension overload in the deceleration and follow-through phase of the throwing motion, can impinge the olecranon against the medial edge of the olecranon fossa **(Figure 11-14)**. The resulting shearing force places stress on the ulnar nerve, the radius-capitellum joint, and olecranon fossa. Strong compressive and shearing forces on the lateral side of the joint can damage the radial head, capitellum, or both, leading to radiocapitellar chondromalacia or

osteochondritis dissecans capitellum. Symptoms that indicate a serious impingement problem include the inability to fully extend the elbow, sharp pain as the elbow snaps into extension, catching or locking of the elbow, aching pain following practice, joint effusion, crepitation during pronation and supination, and loose body sensation (7). In mild cases, the physician may recommend rest and

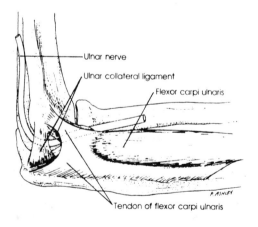

Fig. 11.15: As the ulnar nerve passes through the cubital tunnel between the ulnar collateral ligament and the olecranon fossa, it passes under the two heads of the flexor carpi ulnaris. This tendon is slack during extension, but becomes taut during flexion, contributing to ulnar nerve compression.

Field Strategy 11–5. Management of Common Extensor Tendinitis.

Signs and Symptoms

Initially, pain or spasm of the extensor muscles during activity will occur. This progresses to an aching pain over the lateral epicondyle after activity ceases.

Later stages will produce sharp pain during activity and during simple activities, such as lifting a coffee mug or carrying a heavy book.

Point tenderness can be palpated over or just distal to the lateral epicondyle.

Pain increases with active wrist extension, supination, and radial deviation of the wrist.

Pain increases with passive stretching of the wrist extensor tendons or resisted finger extension.

Management

Ice, compression, elevation, NSAIDs, and rest to limit pain and inflammation.

Immobilize in a splint with some wrist extension to allow for functional use of the hand while preventing aggravation of the wrist extensors. Allow the elbow to move freely.

Cryotherapy, ultrasound, thermotherapy, EMS, interferential current, and friction massage over the extensor tendons may be helpful.

Avoid strong gripping activities and activities that produce pain in the area, but allow the individual to perform those activities that do not irritate the region.

Rehabilitation

Restore full strength, flexibility, and endurance in the wrist extensors.

Stretching exercises should be done within pain-free motion and include wrist flexion/extension, forearm pronation/supination, and radial and ulnar deviation.

Begin with fast contractions using light resistance. Do isotonic strengthening exercises, and add surgical tubing exercises as tolerated.

The individual should experience a mild burning sensation as the muscles are exercised, but exercise should stop if pain sets in. Work up to three or five sets of ten repetitions per session before moving on to heavier resistance.

Caution the individual that overdoing the program may irritate the condition.

Continue to work on active range of motion and strengthening exercises for all shoulder, elbow, and wrist motions.

Incorporate early closed chain exercises, such as press-ups, wall push-ups, or walking on the hands.

Do a biomechanical analysis of the skills to determine if improper technique may have contributed to the problem and make appropriate changes.

After return to activity, continue stretching exercises before and after practice. Ice after practice to control any inflammation. Return to full activity as tolerated.

NSAIDs, but with severe cases joint debridement is indicated.

The ulnar nerve passes behind the medial epicondyle of the humerus through the cubital tunnel to rest against the posterior portion of the ulnar collateral ligament (**Figure 11-15**). Here the nerve is subjected to compression and tensile stress, which may be caused by trauma (acute or chronic), cubital valgus deformity, irregularities within the ulnar groove, or subluxation as a result of a lax ulnar collateral ligament (5,12). The individual will complain of sharp pain along the medial aspect of the elbow, radiating as if they were "hitting the crazy bone". Palpation in the ulnar groove will generally reproduce symptoms, differentiating this injury from a strain or sprain. Tingling and numbness is typically felt in the ring and little finger with weakness also seen in grip strength.

The median nerve travels across the cubital fossa, passes between the two heads of the pronator teres and the two heads of the flexor digitorum superficialis, and gives off its largest branch, the anterior interosseous nerve. Compression may be due to hypertro-

Wrist drop
Weakness and/or paralysis of the wrist and finger extensors due to damage to the radial nerve

Chronic nerve damage may require surgery to release any pressure or constriction on the nerve

Forearm splints
Chronic strain to the forearm muscles

Forearm splints will lead to an aching pain in the forearm that increases when weight bearing on the hands

Hemorrhage or edema cause pressure within the compartment leading to pressure on neurovascular structures and tissues within that space

phied muscles, particularly the pronator teres, or compression from fibrous arches near the flexor digitorum superficialis muscle, bicipital aponeurosis, or the supracondylar process (5,7). Often called "**pronator syndrome**," pain is felt in the anterior proximal aspect of the forearm, and is aggravated with pronation activities.

The radial nerve may be damaged during midshaft humeral fractures. Less frequently, direct trauma or entrapment occurs at the elbow as it passes anterior to the cubital fossa, pierces the supinator muscle, and runs posterior again into the forearm. The terminal branch, the posterior interosseous nerve, supplies all the deeper-lying extensor muscles of the forearm. When injured, symptoms often mimic lateral epicondylitis. An aching lateral elbow pain may radiate up and down the arm. Significant point tenderness can be elicited over the supinator muscle. Resisted supination is generally more painful than resisted wrist extension. Extensor weakness of the wrist, called **wrist drop**, may be seen in extreme cases.

Treatment for neural entrapment depends on frequency, duration, intensity, magnitude, and cause of the problem (5). If recognized early, complete rest and NSAIDs can help acute cases. If the injury is secondary to direct blows a pad can protect the area. Occasionally, chronic nerve damage may require surgery to release any pressure or constriction on the nerve.

Forearm Splints

In the forearm, particularly among gymnasts, chronic forearm strains can result in a condition called "**forearm splints**". The condition is also seen in skaters and skiers who fall repeatedly on the wrist, and in divers who enter the water with the wrists hyperextended to decrease the entry splash. Forearm splints are often seen in the early season, and may be due to lack of forearm strength, irritation of the radioulnar syndesmosis, periostitis, or myositis (13). An aching pain in the forearm is exacerbated when weight bearing on the hands. Palpation reveals point tenderness on the dorsum of the hand between the distal radius and ulna, and proximal row of the carpals. Extreme discomfort is felt when the wrist and fingers are maximally extended. A radiograph may be necessary to rule out carpal fracture, injury to the distal radial epiphysis, aseptic necrosis of the carpal bones,

lunate subluxation, or actual bony impingement that blocks the individual's wrist extension (6).

Treatment is conservative with ice, NSAIDs, and activity modification. A wrist splint may be worn to limit wrist extension and reduce tension on the wrist flexors. After symptoms have disappeared, a stretching and strengthening program should be initiated with a gradual return to full activity.

Compartment Syndrome

The deep fascia of the forearm encloses the flexor and extensor muscle groups in a common sheath. The two groups are separated into compartments by an interosseous membrane between the radius and ulna. The wrist and finger flexors are in the anterior compartment; the wrist and finger extensors are in the posterior compartment. The condition is often secondary to an elbow fracture or dislocation, crushing injury, forearm fracture, postischemic edema, or excessive muscular exertion, as in weight lifting. Hemorrhage or edema cause increased pressure within the compartment leading to excessive pressure on neurovascular structures and tissues within the space (14). Onset is usually rapid, and recognized by swelling, discoloration, absent or diminished distal pulse, and subsequent onset of sensory changes and paralysis. Severe pain at rest, aggravated by passive stretching of the muscles in the compartment signals a potential problem. Immediate referral to a physician is necessary since a fasciotomy may be needed to decompress the area.

💡 *The little league pitcher may have medial epicondylitis due to excessive valgus forces generated during the throw. Standard acute care is followed by early range of motion exercises to prevent joint stiffness and adhesions. If sensory changes occur on the ulnar aspect of the hand, indicating possible ulnar nerve involvement, this individual should see a physician.*

FRACTURES

❓ *A gymnast lost his grip on the horizontal bar and fell to the floor on a flexed elbow. Immediate pain and deformity is evident just proximal to the elbow. How will you assess possible damage to the neurovascular structures of the arm?*

Displaced and undisplaced fractures to the humerus, radius, and ulna usually result from violent compressive forces from direct trauma, such as impact with a helmet or implement, a fall on a flexed elbow or outstretched hand with or without a valgus/varus stress, or tensile forces associated with throwing. Because major nerves and vessels run along the bones, serious neurovascular injury can result from the jagged bone fragments. Fractures to the growth plates are common in adolescent baseball/softball pitchers and javelin throwers. Stress fractures have been reported in gymnasts and weight lifters.

Epiphyseal and Avulsion Fractures

A rapid strong contraction of the flexor-pronator muscle group can lead to an avulsion fracture of the medial epicondyle of the humerus, and is typically seen in children between the ages of 5 and 15 (5). Pain can be severe with point tenderness, swelling, and ecchymosis directly on the medial epicondyle. The fracture is managed conservatively with rest and immobilization for as little as two to three weeks. However, throwing is usually not allowed for 6 to 12 weeks.

Chronic valgus stress, such as that produced in the throwing motion, can also lead to separation of the apophysis of the medial epicondyle. Referred to as "little league elbow", the tension stress is related to throwing curve balls and other breaking pitches that require forceful pronation. Signs and symptoms include point tenderness, swelling, and an inability to move into full elbow extension.

Fracture to the secondary growth center of the lateral epicondyle is similar to the medial epicondyle fracture and is usually not a serious condition. Treatment involves immobilization with a sling.

Stress Fractures

Stress fractures to the diaphysis of the ulna can occur during intensive weight lifting. Bilateral distal radial and ulnar fractures have been found in young individuals who lift heavy weights or lose control of the barbells, resulting in added shear stress (15). For this reason, adolescents in a weight-lifting program should be properly instructed and supervised to prevent injury.

Displaced and Undisplaced Fractures

Supracondylar fractures, caused by falling on an outstretched hand, occur largely in children. A catastrophic complication from this fracture is ischemic necrosis of the forearm

muscles known as **Volkmann's contracture**. The brachial artery or median nerve can be damaged by the fractured bone ends leading to major circulatory or neural impairment to the forearm and hand. As a result, the hand is cold, white, and numb. Severe pain in the forearm is aggravated by passive extension of the fingers. These symptoms indicate a serious problem. Immediately immobilize the arm in a vacuum splint and transport the individual to a physician. Do not assume that the presence of a radial or ulnar pulse indicates adequate circulation to the forearm muscles.

Fracture of the olecranon process of the ulna results from direct trauma, such as being struck with a field hockey or lacrosse stick, or falling on a flexed elbow. The tension of the triceps pulls the bone fragment superiorly. Because this fracture is intra-articular, it does not respond to conservative treatment and requires surgical intervention.

The head of the radius may be fractured as a result of a valgus stress that tears the ulnar collateral ligament leading to traumatic compressive and shearing stress on the radial head (**Figure 11-14**). The individual may not have severe pain or a displacement of bony fragments. Tenderness can be elicited on palpation of the radial head, and swelling can be seen lateral to the olecranon. Flexion and extension may or may not be limited. However, pronation and supination will be painful and restricted. Early range of motion exercises can prevent joint stiffness. However, if more than one-third of the articular surface is involved, if there is more than 30 degrees angulation, or more than 3 mm or more of fracture gap, open reduction is recommended (5).

The "**nightstick fracture**" is seen in football and hockey players, and is caused by a direct blow to the forearm that fractures the ulna. After closed reduction, splinting or casting for 7 to 10 days is needed to allow initial swelling and discomfort to subside. However, if a radial head dislocation or distal radial ulnar joint subluxation is present, open reduction and internal fixation is necessary (16).

In gymnastics a unique forearm fracture occurs as a result of wearing leather grips with enclosed dowels (14,15). These dowels help grip the horizontal bar. Instead of allowing the individual to continue around the circle during a giant swing maneuver, the leather grip "catches" or grabs onto the bar and holds the hand in position causing the

A forearm fracture [...] to gymnasts [...] result of we[...] grips wit[...]

Fractures of the humerus can damage the brachial artery or median nerve leading to major circulatory or neural impairment in the forearm and hand

With a fracture of the radial head, pronation and supination will be very painful

Nightstick fracture
Fracture to the ulna due to a direct blow commonly seen in football players

Any fracture to the humerus should involve a full neurologic and circulatory assessment

forearm to "wrap around" and sustain multiple fractures. Severe pain and disability with this fracture require immediate immobilization in a vacuum splint and referral to a physician.

Fracture Management

Fractures should be suspected in all elbow and forearm injuries. Palpation, compression, traction, and percussion can assist in determining possible fractures, and are explained in **Field Strategy 11-6**. In addition, a neurological and circulatory assessment should be conducted. If the radial nerve is damaged, forearm supination and extension at the elbow, wrist, or fingers is weak, and sensory changes may occur on the dorsum of the hand. If the median nerve is damaged, active wrist and finger flexion is weak, and sensory changes may occur on the palm of the hand. If the ulnar nerve is damaged, ulnar deviation and finger abduction and adduction is weak, and sensory changes may occur on the ulnar border of the hand. Pulses can be taken at the wrist at the ulnar and radial arteries, or blanch the fingernails and note capillary refill.

The gymnast fell on a flexed elbow and now has deformity just proximal to the elbow. Immobilize the arm in a vacuum splint and take a pulse at the radial and ulnar artery, check capillary refill at the fingernails, and check bilateral sensation on the palm and dorsum of the hand.

ASSESSMENT OF THE ELBOW

Two weeks ago a wrestler injured his elbow during a takedown exercise when a strong posterolateral force was applied to the elbow. He iced periodically throughout the night, and wrestled the next day with only mild discomfort. He has iced daily and has had the elbow strapped for support, but noticed muscle weakness when pulling his opponent toward him, and an inability to fully extend the elbow without sharp pain. Numbness is present in the little finger and ulnar aspect of the right hand. How will you conduct the evaluation?

The elbow's primary role is to position the forearm and hand in the most appropriate position to perform efficient motion. Biomechanical errors in throwing technique at the shoulder can place additional stress at the elbow. Because use of equipment is often associated with overuse problems, find out if

the individual uses a bat, racquet, field hockey or lacrosse stick, or other implement. Check for proper grip size, excessive string tension, excessive racquet weight or stiffness, and assess skill technique to rule out possible contributing factors. During the evaluation, keep in mind that pain may be referred from the cervical region, shoulder, or wrist. As in any assessment, both elbows should be fully visible to allow for bilateral comparison.

HISTORY

What questions need to be asked to determine the wrestler's primary complaint? Could age, gender, or the sport-specific skills be a factor in this injury?

To gather information about the primary complaint, ask questions that focus on the individual's perception of pain, weakness, or sensory changes. When was the problem first noticed? Is it acute or has the problem progressively gotten worse? Ask specific questions related to equipment, technique, recent changes in training intensity, frequency, or duration. Is there any noticeable locking, catching, or general muscle weakness? Are there specific actions that aggravate the condition, such as throwing? In addition to the general questions discussed in Chapter 4, specific questions to ask in an elbow evaluation are listed in **Field Strategy 11-7**.

The 16-year old wrestler had several strong posterolateral forces applied to his locked elbow in an attempt to take him down onto the mat. He has a dull, tingling sensation on the ulnar aspect of the right hand, pain and weakness in wrist flexion, and an inability to fully extend the elbow without sharp pain in the olecranon fossa.

OBSERVATION AND INSPECTION

What specific factors should be observed during the assessment? Would it be advantageous to also assess the shoulder and wrist?

Both arms should be clearly visible for bilateral comparison. With an acute injury, it is critical early in the assessment to recognize possible fractures and dislocations. If the individual is in great pain, unable, or unwilling to move the elbow, complete the assessment in a position most comfortable for the individual. First observe the position of the arm. Is there a noticeable deformity? How is the individual holding the arm? If swelling is

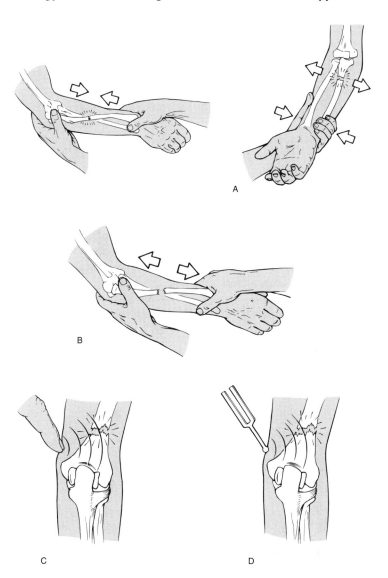

A. Compression. Palpate the region for any pain, deformity, crepitus, or loose bodies. Ask the individual if they heard any cracking sounds that might indicate a possible fracture Apply gentle compression along the long axis of the bone. Then encircle the distal ulna and radius with your hand and give mild compression. This will produce some distraction at the proximal end of the ulna and radius. Increased pain in either position indicates a possible fracture

B. Distraction. Slowly distract the bones. If pain is eased, this may indicate a possible fracture. If pain increases, it indicates soft tissue damage

C. Percussion. Gently tap the superficial bony landmarks. Vibrations will travel along the bone and cause increased pain at the fracture site. For example, tap the following sites:
    Humerus—medial and lateral epicondyles
    Ulna—olecronan process and distal styloid process
    Radius—distal styloid process

D. Tuning fork. Tap a tuning fork and place the base on the superficial bone sites mentioned above. Increased pain indicates a possible fracture

Any positive signs indicate the possibility of a fracture. Immobilize the limb in a vacuum splint or other appropriate splint or sling, and transport the individual to the nearest trauma center.

Current Injury Status

1. If it is an acute problem, identify the mechanism of injury. Ask: What were you doing at the time of the injury? How did the injury occur? What was the direction of the force? Did you hear any sounds during the incident? Any snaps, cracks, or pops? If the injury came on gradually ask: What different activities have you been doing in the last week? (Look for frequency, duration, intensity, type, method, or excessive throwing motion, use of a racquet, or other implement)

2. Where is the pain (or weakness) located? What type of pain is it? Is it constant or intermittent? Did the pain come on gradually or suddenly? What actions bring on the pain? Is it worse in the morning, during activity, after activity, or at night? What actions relieve the pain? Are there any activities that you are unable to perform because of the pain or weakness?

3. Was there any swelling or discoloration at the time of the injury? How soon did it occur? What was done for the injury? Have you had any muscle spasms, numbness, tingling, or burning sensations in the forearm or hand? Does the pain radiate up or down the arm?

4. How old are you? (Remember that common extensor tendinitis (tennis elbow) often occurs in older individuals or in individuals that do a great deal of flexion and extension in their jobs. Dislocation of the radial head is seen in young children who have had the arm jerked in a distractive manner).

Past Injury Status

1. Have you ever injured the elbow before? How did that occur? Who evaluated and treated the injury? What has been done to strengthen the area and prevent recurrence? Was there any difficulty in returning to full functional status?

2. Does the injury appear to be the same or similar to the previous injury? In what ways is it different?

3. Have you had any medial problems recently that might contribute to this pain or weakness? (Look for problems that refer pain to the region)

Resting position
Slightly flexed position of the elbow that allows for maximal volume to accommodate any intra-articular swelling

Cubital valgus
Angle of an extended elbow that deviates toward the radial side more than 20°

Cubital varus
Angle of an extended elbow that deviates less than 10° toward the radial side

present in the joint, the individual may be unable to fully extend the elbow, resulting in a slightly flexed position. This **resting position** allows the joint to have maximal volume to accommodate intra-articular swelling. Note the position of the olecranon relative to the epicondlyes of the humerus. In a normal flexed position, the olecranon process and two epicondyles of the humerus should form an isosceles triangle (**Figure 11-16**). In an extended position, the olecranon process and two epicondyles form a straight line. Any positive sign that indicates a possible fracture should be treated accordingly. Immobilize the arm in a vacuum splint or sling and transport the individual to a physician.

When no possible fracture or dislocation is present, the individual can be placed in anatomical position to determine the carrying angle (**Figure 11-3**). Normally the individual should have a slight valgus angle with the forearm fully supinated and elbow extended.

Angles greater than 20° are referred to as **cubital valgus**; angles less than 10° are referred to as **cubital varus**. The elbow is then placed in the position of function: 90° of flexion with the hand held halfway between supination and pronation (**Figure 11-17**). Inspect the region for symmetry, any abnormal deformity, muscle atrophy, hypertrophy, swelling, discoloration, or previous surgical incisions.

An abnormal carrying angle does not exist in either arm. Joint effusion and swelling is visible on the posteromedial aspect of the humerus over the cubital tunnel and medial epicondyle. No other visible signs are apparent.

PALPATIONS

Weakness is evident during wrist flexion, and swelling is visible on the medial and posteromedial aspect of the humerus. Fur-

A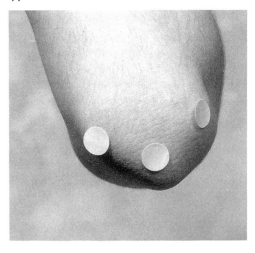
B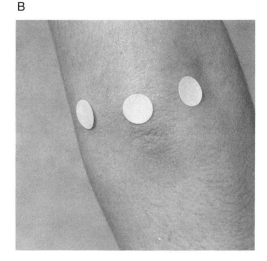

Fig. 11.16: In observing symmetry of the elbow, note the relationship of the olecranon process and epicondyles. (A) In flexion they form an isosceles triangle. (B) In extension they form a horizontal line.

thermore, the individual is unable to fully extend the elbow without sharp pain. Where will you begin palpations so the discomfort is not compounded?

Bilateral palpations should determine temperature, swelling, point tenderness, crepitus, deformity, muscle spasm, and cutaneous sensation. Vascular pulses can be taken at the radial and ulnar arteries at the wrist, and at the brachial artery in the cubital fossa. Begin palpations proximal to distal leaving the most painful areas to last. Support the injured arm during palpations and compare bilaterally. To determine a possible fracture, refer to **Field Strategy 11-6**.

Anterior Palpations

1. Cubital fossa bounded by the pronator teres medially and brachioradialis laterally with the biceps tendon, median nerve, and brachial artery within the fossa
2. Coracoid process and head of radius

Lateral Palpations

1. Lateral supracondylar ridge and brachioradialis muscle
2. Lateral epicondyle, common wrist extensors, and supinator muscle
3. Radial collateral ligament
4. Annular ligament and head of the radius. This is facilitated by supination and pronation of the forearm

Posterior Palpations

1. Triceps muscle
2. Olecranon process and olecranon fossa. This is facilitated with the elbow flexed at 45° to relax the triceps
3. Olecranon bursa. Grasp the skin overlying the olecranon process and note any thickening or presence of loose bodies
4. Ulnar nerve in the cubital tunnel
5. Ulnar border distal to the styloid process at the wrist

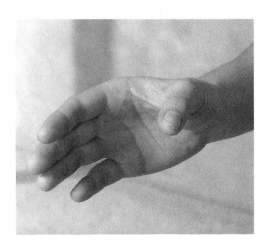

Fig. 11.17: The position of function at the elbow is 90° of flexion with the hand held halfway between supination and pronation with the 'thumb up.'

Medial Palpations

1. Medial supracondylar ridge
2. Medial epicondyle and common wrist flexor-pronator tendons and muscles
3. Ulnar collateral ligament

🔵 *Swelling and point tenderness were elicited on the medial epicondyle, medial joint line, medial olecranon process, and medial superior ridge of the olecranon fossa. Palpation in the cubital tunnel caused an extremely painful tingling sensation to travel down the ulnar aspect of the forearm into the little finger.*

SPECIAL TESTS

❓ *Swelling and pain appear to be centered on the medial aspect of the humerus and involve the medial border of the olecranon process and olecranon fossa. Furthermore, it appears the ulnar nerve may be involved. How will you proceed to confirm your suspicions about the extent of this injury?*

If a fracture or dislocation is suspected, do not attempt any special tests. Immobilize the arm in an appropriate splint and refer the individual to a physician. For other injuries, do only those tests necessary to assess the current injury.

Active Movements

As with previous assessments, bilateral comparison with the uninvolved arm should always be completed. In addition, painful active movements should be performed last to prevent painful symptoms from overflowing into the next movement. The following movements should be assessed:

1. Flexion at the elbow (140 to 150°)
2. Extension at the elbow (0 to 10°)
3. Supination of the forearm (90°)
4. Pronation of the forearm (90°)
5. Flexion of the wrist (80 to 90°)
6. Extension of the wrist (70 to 90°)

During elbow extension remember that some females can extend as much as 5 to 15° below the straight line. Bilateral comparison will verify if this extra motion is normal for this individual. In performing active pronation and supination, instruct the individual to flex the elbow to 90° and secure the elbow next to the body to avoid any glenohumeral motion. The individual can hold a pencil in the closed fist and perform both motions in a continuous pattern. Goniometry measurements are demonstrated in **Figure 11-18**.

Passive Range of Motion

If the individual is able to perform full range of motion during active movements, apply gentle overpressure at the extremes of motion to determine end feel in both arms for bilateral comparison. Flexion at the elbow provides an end feel of tissue approximation. In extension, end feel is bone to bone. Supination and pronation have an end feel of tissue stretch. If the individual is unable to perform full active movement, passive movement can determine the available range of motion and end feel.

Resisted Muscle Testing

Stabilize the individual's elbow against the body. Begin with the muscle on stretch and apply resistance proximal to the wrist throughout the full range of motion. Do bilateral comparison with the uninvolved side. To avoid any finger flexors or extensors from assisting during movement, instruct the individual to keep the thumb and fingers relaxed. As always, painful motions should be delayed until last. **Figure 11-19** demonstrates motions that should be tested (myotomes are listed in parentheses):

1. Elbow flexion (C_6)
2. Elbow extension (C_7)
3. Forearm supination
4. Forearm pronation
5. Wrist flexion (C_7)
6. Wrist extension (C_6)

Neurological Testing

Neurological integrity can be assessed with the use of myotomes, reflexes, and segmental dermatomes and peripheral nerve cutaneous patterns.

Myotomes

Isometric muscle testing to test the myotomes should be performed in the loose-packed position and include: scapular elevation (C_4), shoulder abduction (C_5), elbow flexion and/or wrist extension (C_6), elbow extension and/or wrist flexion (C_7), thumb extension and/or ulnar deviation (C_8), and abduction and/or adduction of the hand intrinsics (T_1).

Reflexes

Reflexes in the upper extremity include the biceps (C_5-C_6), brachioradialis (C_6), and triceps (C_7). The individual should be relaxed

---

End feels at the elbow include:
flexion—tissue approximation
extension—bone to bone
supination and pronation—tissue stretch

At the elbow and forearm test the biceps, brachioradialis, and triceps reflexes

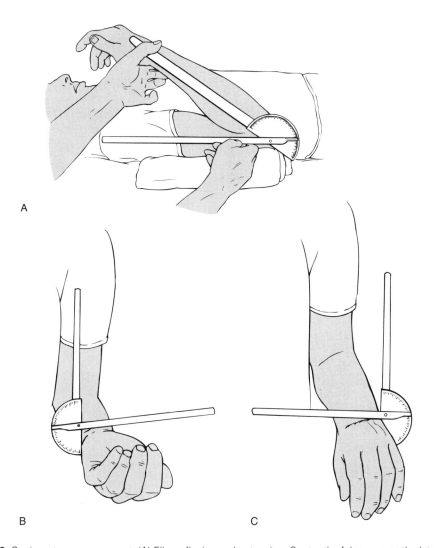

Fig. 11.18: Goniometry measurement. (A) Elbow flexion and extension. Center the fulcrum over the lateral epicondyle of the humerus. Align the proximal arm along the humerus using the acromion process for reference. The distal arm is aligned along the radius using the styloid process for reference. (B) Forearm supination. The fulcrum is centered medial to the ulnar styloid process. The proximal arm is parallel to the midline of the humerus, and the distal arm is placed across the palmar aspect of the forearm just proximal to the styloid processes of the radius and ulna. (C) Forearm pronation. The fulcrum is centered lateral to the ulnar styloid process. The arms are placed in the same position but on the dorsal aspect of the forearm.

with the elbow flexed. The biceps and triceps reflex testing was explained in Chapter 10 (**Figure 10-31**). The brachioradialis reflex is tested in a similar manner. The elbow is flexed and supported by the examiner's forearm with the wrist in slight ulnar deviation. Using a reflex hammer, strike the brachioradialis tendon at the distal end of the radius (**Figure 11-20**). In some individuals, the tap may need to be elicited two to three inches proximal to the wrist. A slight jerk in elbow flexion is a normal sign.

Cutaneous Patterns

The segmental nerve dermatome patterns for the elbow region are demonstrated in **Figure** **11-21**. The peripheral nerve cutaneous patterns are demonstrated in **Figure 11-22**. Test bilaterally for altered sensation with sharp and dull touch by running the open hand and fingernails over the neck, shoulder, anterior and posterior chest walls, and down both sides of the arms and hands.

Stress and Functional Tests

Stress tests are performed when you have a clear indication of what structures may be damaged. Use only those tests deemed relevant, and always compare the results to the uninvolved arm.

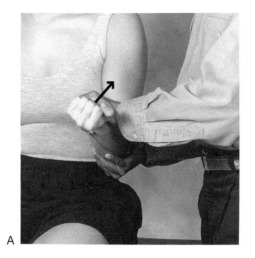
A

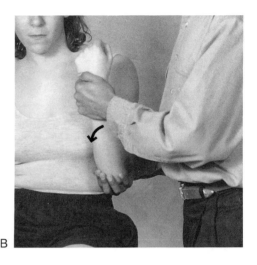
B

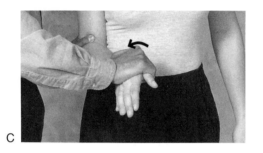
C

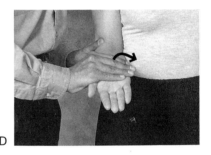
D

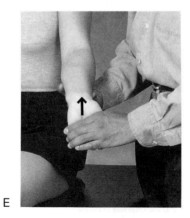
E

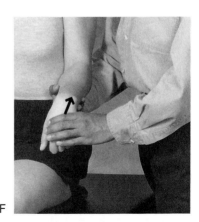
F

Fig. 11.19: Resisted manual muscle testing for the elbow. (A) Elbow flexion. (B) Elbow extension (C) Forearm supination (D) Forearm pronation. (E) Wrist flexion. (F) Wrist extension

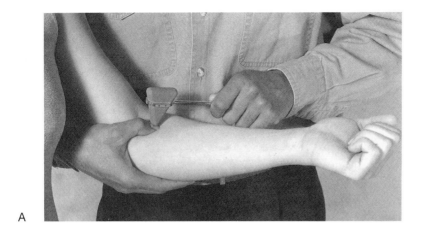

A

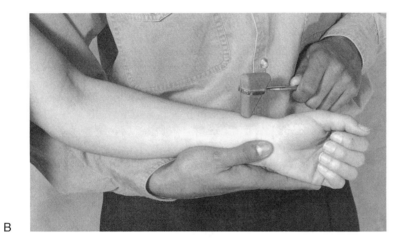

B

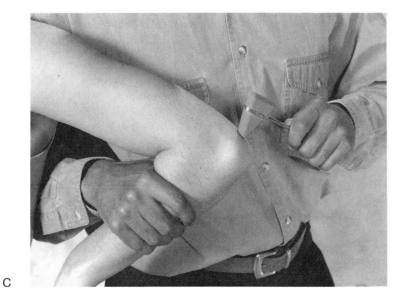

C

Fig. 11.20: Reflex testing. (A) Biceps reflex. (B) Brachioradialis reflex. (C) Triceps reflex.

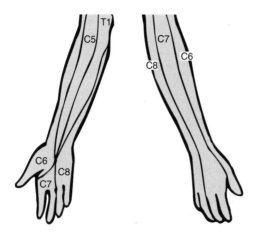

Fig. 11.21: Dermatomes around the elbow region.

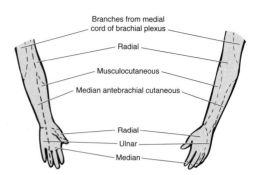

Fig. 11.22: Cutaneous sensation patterns for the peripheral nerves at the elbow region.

Ligamentous Instability Tests

Because of the amount of rotation that occurs at the shoulder, it is difficult to get an accurate valgus or varus stress at the elbow. To compensate for this, perform these tests at multiple angles from full extension to 30 to 40° of flexion. When the olecranon is "unlocked" from the olecranon fossa, the ligamentous structures are isolated. With the individual seated, stabilize the arm and apply a valgus or abduction force to the distal forearm to stress the ulnar collateral ligament (**Figure 11-23A**). A varus or adduction force is then applied at the forearm in the various angles to stress the radial collateral ligament (**Figure 11-23B**). Apply the force several times with increasing overpressure and note any pain or joint laxity.

> Perform ligament instability tests at multiple angles from full extension to 30 to 40° of flexion

Common Extensor Tendinitis Test (Lateral Epicondylitis or Tennis Elbow Test)

Stabilize the individual's flexed elbow and palpate the lateral epicondyle. Have the individual make a fist and pronate the forearm. Ask them to radially deviate and extend the wrist while you resist the motion (**Figure 11-24A**). A positive sign is indicated if severe pain is present over the lateral epicondyle of the humerus. The same results can be elicited by stretching the extensor muscles by slowly pronating the forearm, flexing the wrist, and extending the elbow simultaneously (**Figure 11-24B**). Additional discomfort can be produced by testing the extensor digitorum communis of the third digit by applying resistance distal to the proximal interphalangeal joint with the wrist extended (**Figure 11-24C**).

Medial Epicondylitis Test

Stabilize the flexed elbow and palpate the medial epicondyle. Slowly supinate the forearm, and extend the wrist and elbow while the individual resists this movement. A positive sign is indicated by pain over the medial epicondyle of the humerus.

Tinel's Sign for Ulnar Neuritis

The cubital tunnel is tapped on the posteromedial side of the elbow. A positive sign is indicated by a tingling sensation that runs down the ulnar aspect of the forearm into the medial half of the fourth and all of the fifth finger (**Figure 11-25**).

Elbow Flexion Test for Ulnar Neuritis

This test determines whether the ulnar nerve is entrapped in the cubital tunnel. Have the individual completely flex the elbow and hold it in that position for five minutes. A positive test is indicated by tingling or numbness in the ulnar nerve distribution pattern of the forearm and hand.

Functional Tests

It is necessary to remember that the elbow is in the middle of the upper extremity kinetic chain. Therefore, it must function properly to position the hand so that daily activities can be performed smoothly and efficiently. Activities such as combing the hair, throwing a ball, lifting an object, or pushing an object should be performed pain-free. Ask the individual to perform those skills needed to complete their daily living activities and sport-specific tasks. Each movement should be pain-free and fluid.

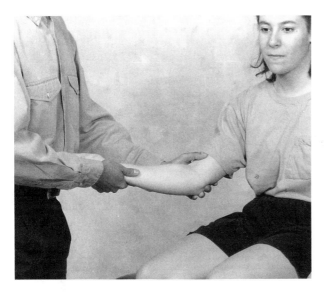

A

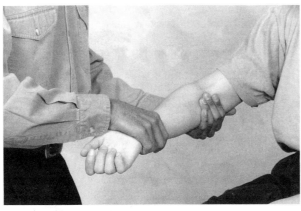

B

Fig. 11.23: Ligamentous instability tests. (A) To stress the ulnar collateral ligament apply a valgus force at multiple angles. (B) To stress the radial collateral ligament, apply a varus force at multiple angles.

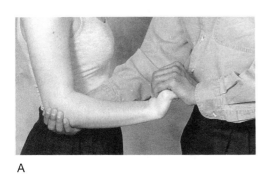

A

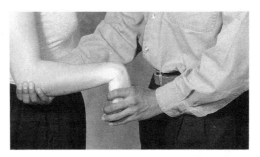

B

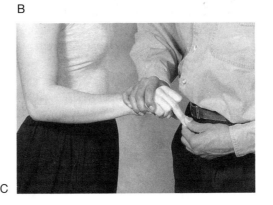

C

Fig. 11.24: Tests for common extensor tendinitis. (A) Resisted extension and radial deviation of the wrist. (B) Passive stretching of the wrist extensors. (C) Resisted extension of the extensor digitorum communis in the middle finger with the wrist extended.

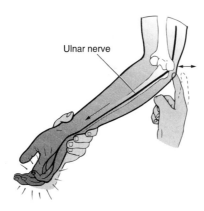

Fig. 11.25: Tapping over the cubital tunnel will produce a tingling sensation down the ulnar nerve into the forearm and hand. A positive Tinel's sign indicates ulnar nerve entrapment.

💡 *Active and passive elbow flexion is limited by about 10°, which may be due to intra-articular swelling. Passive terminal extension is painful, and increased pain and muscle weakness is evident in wrist flexion and pronation. Valgus stress produces only slight pain and no laxity. Tinel's sign is positive. This individual may have an acute impingement injury involving ulnar neuritis, posterior impingement of the olecranon process in the fossa, and a strain of the flexor-pronator group. This individual needs to be referred to a physician.*

Stepping up and down on boxes of differing heights is an excellent closed chain kinetic exercise

REHABILITATION

❓ *The wrestler has a painful elbow as a result of an impingement syndrome. After the physician assesses and treats the individual, what exercises should be included in the general rehabilitation program for this elbow injury?*

Rehabilitation of the upper arm, elbow, and forearm must involve exercises for the entire kinetic chain, since muscles in the upper arm cross the shoulder and elbow, and muscles in the forearm cross the elbow and wrist. Traumatic injuries to the elbow often require immobilization. Although the elbow is immobilized, early range of motion and strengthening exercises can be conducted at the wrist, hand, and shoulder. In overuse injuries where immobilization is usually not present, pain may be exacerbated by certain motions. The exercise program should focus on early mobilization in the available pain-free motions, and expand to the other motions once pain has subsided. Individuals who are involved in throwing-like activities should also be sure to include scapular stabilization exercises along with strengthening exercises for the shoulder. The reader should refer to Chapter 10 for appropriate shoulder exercises. This section will focus on only those exercises specifically for the upper arm, elbow, and forearm. Hand and finger exercises are discussed in Chapter 12.

Restoration of Motion

Range of motion exercises focus on elbow flexion and extension, forearm pronation and supination, wrist flexion and extension, and wrist radial and ulnar deviation. The individual can use the opposite hand to apply a low load, prolonged stretch in the various motions to minimize joint trauma and increase flexibility (**Figure 11-26**). The upper body ergometer (UBE) is also an effective range of motion tool.

Restoration of Proprioception and Balance

Closed chain exercises may be performed immediately after injury. Shifting body weight from one hand to the other may be performed on a wall, table top, or unstable surface, such as a foam mat or BAPS board. Push-ups and exercises in a frontal and sagittal plane can be performed on a ProFitter or slide board, if available. Step-ups can be completed on a box, stool, or Stair Master. This activity can progress to stepping up and down on boxes of differing heights arranged so the exercise is

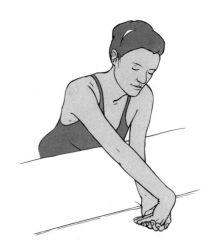

Fig. 11.26: Range of motion exercises can be facilitated by using the opposite hand to apply a sustained stretch.

performed in diagonal patterns, circles, or figure 8's.

As with the shoulder injury, the throwing motion should be rehearsed through the use of mirrors or videotape. As the motion is performed, biomechanical errors at the elbow are corrected. When motion is perfected, speed of movement and distance of throw is gradually increased. A sample throwing program was listed in **Field Strategy 10-10.**

Muscular Strength, Endurance, and Power

Gentle resisted isometric exercises can begin immediately after injury or after surgery while the arm is still immobilized. As the individual improves, a more moderate overload is applied. Once normal range of motion is achieved, apply a reistance force in an unanticipated direction to make the individual adjust to the resistance. Open kinetic chain exercises can be performed in the various motions utilizing light-weight dumbbells. Many of these exercises were demonstrated in **Field Strategy 11-1.** The individual should complete 30 to 50 repetitions with a one pound weight, and should not progress in resistance until 50 repetitions are achieved. With the forearm supported on a table, perform wrist curls, reverse wrist curls, pronation, and supination. A weighted bar or hammer can be used for radial and ulnar deviation, and for pronation and supination. Another common exercise is the wrist curl-up using a broomstick with a light weight suspended on a three to four foot rope. The individual slowly winds the rope up around the stick, then slowly unwinds the rope. PNF resisted exercises and surgical tubing are used for concentric and eccentric loading.

Plyometric exercises may involve catching a weighted ball utilizing a quick eccentric stretch of the muscle to facilitate a concentric contraction in throwing the ball. The exercise can progress through various one- and two-arm chest passes and overhead passes. A mini-tramp may also be used to do plyometric bounding push-ups.

Cardiovascular Fitness

General body conditioning should be maintained throughout the rehabilitation program. Several examples of programs were provided in **Field Strategy 5-9,** and included use of a jump rope, Stair Master, treadmill, and upper body ergometer (UBE).

The wrestler should focus on restoration of motion in elbow flexion/extension, forearm pronation/supination, wrist flexion/extension, and radial and ulnar deviation. Isometric strengthening exercises should begin immediately in pain-free motions, with active exercises beginning as soon as normal range of motion is achieved. The program should also include general body conditioning and strengthening exercises for the shoulder, elbow, and wrist.

SUMMARY

The elbow is constantly subjected to various forces and stress during normal daily activity. In sports, excessive force can lead to contusions, joint sprains, dislocations, muscle strains, fractures, or neurovascular impairment. Although attention is often focused on acute injuries, this joint is very susceptible to overuse conditions. Often these injuries result from inadequate warm-up, excessive training past the point of fatigue, inadequate rehabilitation of previous injuries, or neglect of seemingly minor conditions that progress to major complications. Because the elbow works with the shoulder and wrist to provide complex patterns of motion, an injury to one structure can affect other joints. **Field Strategy 11-8** demonstrates an assessment of the upper arm, elbow, and forearm.

Keep in mind during the assessment that pain may be referred from other areas of the body, particularly the cervical neck, shoulder, and wrist. With a significant finding, refer the individual to a physician for further evaluation. Examples of these conditions might include: obvious deformity suggesting a dislocation or fracture, significant loss of motion or weakness in a myotome, excessive joint swelling, possible epiphyseal or apophyseal injuries, gross joint instability, abnormal or absent reflexes, abnormal sensations in either the segmental dermatomes or peripheral cutaneous patterns, absent or weak pulse, or any unexplained pain.

Should a decision be made to refer an individual to a physician for care, immobilize the limb in a comfortable position. This may be accomplished by wrapping the arm to the body, or using a sling and swathe, posterior splint, vacuum splint, or a commercial product that can pad and protect the area. Apply cryotherapy to control inflammation and

A weighted bar or hammer can be used for strengthening exercises

PNF-resisted exercises and surgical tubing can be used for concentric and eccentric loading

Field Strategy 11–8. Elbow Evaluation.

History
_____

Primary complaint including:
    Description and mechanism of the current injury
    Onset of symptoms
Pain perception and discomfort
Disability and functional impairments from the injury
Previous injuries to the area
Family history

Observation and Inspection
_____

Inspect the carrying angle and position of function
Inspect the injured area for:
    Muscle symmetry   Hypertrophy or muscle atrophy
    Swelling   Visible congenital deformity
    Discoloration   Surgical incisions or scars

Palpation
_____

Bony structures to rule out fracture
Soft tissue structures to determine:
    Temperature   Deformity
    Swelling   Muscle spasm
    Point tenderness   Cutaneous sensation
    Crepitus   Vascular pulses

Special Tests
_____

Active range of motion
Passive range of motion
Resisted muscle testing
Neurologic testing
Stress and functional tests
    Ligamentous instability tests
    Common extensor tendinitis test
    Medial epicondylitis test
    Tinel's signs for ulnar neuritis
    Elbow flexion test for ulnar neuritis
    Functional tests

swelling, and transport the individual in an appropriate manner. Follow-up with the physician to obtain instructions for further care of the injury. When appropriate, protective braces or padding should be worn to prevent reinjury.

REFERENCES

1. Josefsson, PO, and Nilsson, BE. 1986. Incidence of elbow dislocation. Acta Orthopedica Scandinavica, 57(6):537–538.
2. Stanitski, CL. 1993. Combating overuse injuries: A focus on children and adolescents. Phys Sportsmed, 21(1):87–106.
3. Zuckerman, JD, and Matsen, FA. "Biomechanics of the elbow." In *Basic biomechanics of the skeletal system*, edited by M Nordin and VH Frankel. Philadelphia: Lea & Febiger, 1989.
4. De Carlo, MS, Carrell, KR, Misamore, GW, and Sell, KE. 1992. Rehabilitation of myositis ossificans in the brachialis muscle. J Ath Train, 27(1):76–79.
5. Reid, DC. *Sports injury assessment and rehabilitation.* New York: Churchill Livingstone, 1992.
6. Garrick, JG, and Webb, DR. *Sports injuries: Diagnosis and management.* Philadelphia: WB Saunders, 1990.
7. Mehlhoff, TL, and Bennett, JB. "Elbow injuries." In *The team physician's handbook*, edited by MB Mellion, WM Walsh, and GL Shelton. Philadelphia: Hanley & Belfus, 1990.
8. Hoffman, DF. 1993. Elbow Dislocations: Avoiding complications. Phys Sportsmed, 21(11):56–67.

9. Bennet, JB, and Tullos HS. "Acute injuries to the elbow." In *The upper extremity in sports medicine*, edited by JA Nicholas, EB Hershman, and MA Posner. St. Louis: CV Mosby, 1990.

10. Andrews, JR, Schemmel, SP, and Whiteside, JA. "Evaluation, treatment, and prevention of elbow injuries in throwing athletes." In *The upper extremity in sports medicine*, edited by JA Nicholas, EB Hershman, and MA Posner. St. Louis: CV Mosby, 1990.

11. Kegerreis, S, Jenkins, WL, and Malone, TR. (eds). 1989. *Throwing injuries*. Sport injury management, vol. 2, no. 4. Baltimore: Williams & Wilkins, 1990.

12. Glousman, RE. "Ulnar nerve problems in the athlete's elbow." In *Clinics in sports medicine*, edited by EB Hershman, vol. 9, no 2. Philadelphia: WB Saunders, 1990.

13. Gainor, BJ, and Allen, WE. "Injuries of the arm, elbow, and forearm." In *Clinical sports medicine*, edited by WA Grana and A Kalenak. Philadelphia: WB Saunders, 1991.

14. Weiker, GG., "Upper extremity gymnastic injuries." In *The upper extremity in sports medicine*, edited by JA Nicholas, EB Hershman, and MA Posner. St. Louis: CV Mosby, 1990.

15. Weber, J. "Gymnastics." In *The team physician's handbook*, edited by MB Mellion, WM Walsh, and GL Shelton. Philadelphia: Hanley & Belfus, 1990.

16. Watson, JT. "Fractures of the forearm and elbow." In *Clinics in sports medicine*, edited by JT Watson and JA Bergfeld, vol. 9, no. 1. Philadelphia: WB Saunders, 1990.

Wrist and Hand Injuries

After you have completed this chapter, you should be able to:

■ Locate the important bony and soft tissue structures of the wrist and hand

■ Describe the motions of the wrist and hand and identify the muscles that produce them

■ Explain what forces produce the loading patterns responsible for common injuries of the wrist and hand

■ Describe measures that can be taken to prevent injuries at the wrist and hand

■ Recognize and manage specific injuries to the wrist and hand

■ Demonstrate a thorough assessment of the wrist and hand

■ Demonstrate general rehabilitation exercises for the wrist and hand

The wrist and hand are used extensively in activities of daily living, as well as in many sport skills. Injuries to the wrist and hand often result from the natural tendency to sustain the force of a fall on the hyperextended wrist (**Figure 12-1**). Other wrist/hand injuries, such as metacarpal fractures, or "boxer's fractures," are directly related to the nature of a given sport. Golfers are prone to problems such as carpal tunnel syndrome, the impingement of the nerve supply to the hand and fingers, and de Quervain's tenosynovitis, a condition involving the extensor pollicis brevis and abductor pollicis longus tendons (1). Accidents during sports such as wrestling, football, hockey, and skiing can often result in forced abduction of the thumb and subsequent ulnar collateral ligament injury. Receivers in football and catchers in baseball/softball are subject to "mallet" deformity caused by injury to the distal interphalangeal joint (2).

This chapter begins with a review of the anatomy, kinematics, and kinetics of the wrist and hand. Discussion on prevention of injury is followed by information on common injuries to the wrist and hand and their management. Finally, assessment techniques and rehabilitation exercises are presented.

ANATOMY REVIEW OF THE WRIST AND HAND

? *A softball player has pain and swelling at the metacarpophalangeal joint of the*
middle finger. What anatomical structure(s) are likely to have been injured?

The wrist and hand are composed of numerous small bones and articulations. These function effectively to enable the dexterous movements performed by the hands during both daily living and sport activities.

Wrist Articulations

The wrist consists of a series of radiocarpal and intercarpal articulations (**Figure 12-2**). However, most wrist motion occurs at the radiocarpal joint, a condyloid joint where the radius articulates with the scaphoid, lunate,

The radiocarpal joint is the major joint of the wrist

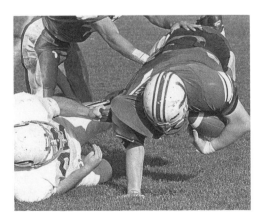

Fig. 12.1: Sustaining the force of a fall with a hyperextended wrist can result in serious injuries to the wrist and hand.

and triquetrum. The joint allows sagittal plane motions (flexion, extension, and hyper-extension) and frontal plane motions (radial deviation and ulnar deviation), as well as circumduction. The intercarpal joints are gliding joints that contribute little to wrist motion.

The distal radioulnar joint is immediately adjacent to the radiocarpal joint. A cartilaginous disc separates the distal ulna and radius from the lunate and triquetral bones. Although the two joints share the articular disk, they have separate joint capsules. The **volar** radiocarpal, **dorsal** radiocarpal, radial collateral and ulnar collateral ligaments reinforce the radiocarpal joint capsule. Its close packed position is in extension with radial deviation.

Hand Articulations

A large number of joints are required to provide the extensive motion capabilities of the hand. Included are the carpometacarpal (CM), intermetacarpal (IM), metacarpophalangeal (MP), and interphalangeal (IP) joints **(Figure 12-2)**. The fingers are numbered digits one through five, with the first digit being the thumb.

Carpometacarpal and Intermetacarpal Joints

The carpometacarpal joint of the thumb is a classic **saddle joint**. A capsule surrounding the joint serves to restrict motion. The carpometacarpal joints of the four fingers are essentially gliding joints, although some anatomists have described them as modified saddle joints (3). The carpometacarpal and intermetacarpal joints of the fingers are mutually surrounded by joint capsules that are reinforced by the dorsal, volar, and interosseous carpometacarpal ligaments.

Metacarpophalangeal Joints

The knuckles of the hand are formed by the metacarpophalangeal (MP) joints. These are condyloid joints where the rounded distal heads of the metacarpals articulate with the concave proximal ends of the phalanges. The metacarpophalangeal joints are each enclosed in a capsule reinforced by strong collateral ligaments. A dorsal ligament also merges with the metacarpophalangeal joint of the thumb. Close packed positions of the MP joints in the fingers and thumb are full flexion and opposition, respectively.

Interphalangeal Joints

The proximal interphalangeal (PIP) and distal interphalangeal (DIP) joints of the fingers and the single interphalangeal (IP) joint of the thumb are all hinge joints. An articular capsule joined by volar and collateral ligaments surrounds each interphalangeal joint. These joints are most stable in the close packed position of full extension.

Muscles of the Wrist and Hand

Given the numerous highly controlled precision movements of which the hand and fingers are capable, it is no surprise that a relatively large number of muscles are responsible. There are nine **extrinsic muscles** that cross the wrist and 10 **intrinsic muscles** that

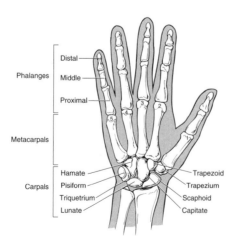
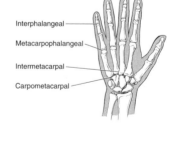

Fig. 12.2: The bones and joints of the wrist and hand.

have both of their attachments distal to the wrist. The muscles of the wrist and hand are shown in **Figures 12-3** and **12-4**, and their locations and actions are summarized in **Table 12-1**.

Nerves of the Wrist and Hand

The median, ulnar, and radial nerves are major terminal branches of the **brachial plexus** that provide motor and sensory innervation to the wrist and hand (**Figure 12-5**). The median nerve supplies the majority of the flexor muscles of the wrist and hand, as well as the intrinsic flexor muscles on the radial side of the palm (**Figure 12-3**). It also provides afferent supply to the skin on the lateral two-thirds of the palmar side of the hand and the dorsum of the second and third fingers. The ulnar nerve innervates the flexor carpi ulnaris and the ulnar portion of the flexor digitorum profundus, along with most of the intrinsic muscles of the hand. It also provides afferent nerve supply to the fifth and half of the fourth finger on both dorsal and palmar sides. The radial nerve divides into superficial and deep branches distal to the lateral epicondyle of the elbow. The superficial branch supplies the skin on the dorsum of the hand. The deep branch innervates most of the extensor muscles of the forearm (**Figure 12-4**). Specific nerve-muscle associations are presented in **Table 12-1**.

Blood Vessels of the Wrist and Hand

The major vessels supplying the muscles of the wrist and hand are the radial and ulnar arteries (**Figure 12-6**). The radial artery supplies the muscles on the radial side of the forearm, as well as the thumb and index finger. The radial artery is superficial on the anterior aspect of the wrist, where the pulse is readily palpable. The ulnar artery spawns a major branch known as the common interosseous artery, which divides into anterior and posterior interosseous arteries. The anterior branch supplies the deep extrinsic flexor muscles, and the posterior branch supplies the extensor muscles of the forearm. The radial and ulnar arteries merge in the palm to form the superficial and deep palmar

Extrinsic muscles
Muscles with attachments located both proximal and distal to the wrist

Intrinsic muscles
Muscles with attachments located distal to the wrist

Brachial plexus
Nerve plexus formed by the intertwined ventral rami of the lower four cervical and first thoracic nerves (C_5-T_1)

The radial pulse should be palpated with the fingers rather than the thumb, since a pulse can also sometimes be felt in the thumb

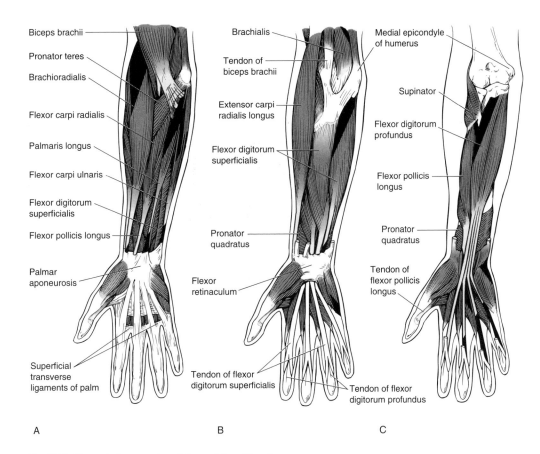

Fig. 12.3: The anterior muscles of the wrist and hand.

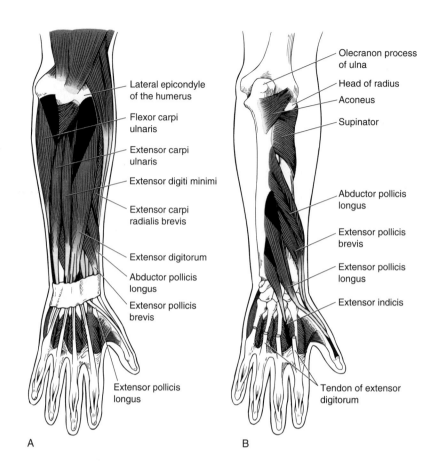

A

Lateral epicondyle of the humerus

Flexor carpi ulnaris

Extensor carpi ulnaris

Extensor digiti minimi

Extensor carpi radialis brevis

Extensor digitorum

Abductor pollicis longus

Extensor pollicis brevis

Extensor pollicis longus

B

Olecranon process of ulna

Head of radius

Aconeus

Supinator

Abductor pollicis longus

Extensor pollicis brevis

Extensor pollicis longus

Extensor indicis

Tendon of extensor digitorum

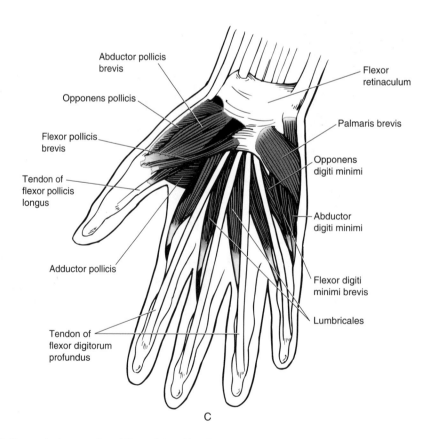

C

Abductor pollicis brevis

Opponens pollicis

Flexor pollicis brevis

Tendon of flexor pollicis longus

Adductor pollicis

Tendon of flexor digitorum profundus

Flexor retinaculum

Palmaris brevis

Opponens digiti minimi

Abductor digiti minimi

Flexor digiti minimi brevis

Lumbricales

Fig. 12.4: The posterior muscles of the wrist and hand.

Table 12–1. Major Muscles of the Hand and Fingers.

Extrinsic Muscles

Muscle	Proximal Attachment	Distal Attachment	Primary Action(s)	Nerve Innervation
Extensor pollicis longus	Middle dorsal ulna	Dorsal distal phalanx of thumb	Extension of MP and IP joints of thumb	Radial (C_7, C_8)
Extensor pollicis brevis	Middle dorsal radius	Dorsal proximal phalanx of thumb	Extension at MP and CM joints of thumb	Radial (C_7, C_8)
Flexor pollicis longus	Middle palmar radius	Palmar distal phalanx of thumb	Flexion at IP and MP joints of thumb	Median (C_8, T_1)
Abductor pollicis longus	Middle dorsal ulna and radius	Radial base of 1st metacarpal	Abduction at CM joint of thumb	Radial (C_7, C_8)
Extensor indicis	Distal dorsal ulna	Ulnar side of the extensor digitorum tendon	Extension at MP joint of 2nd digit	Radial (C_7, C_8)
Extensor digitorum	Lateral epicondyle of humerus	Base of 2nd and 3rd phalanges, digits 2–5	Extension at MP, proximal and distal IP joints, digits 2–5	Radial (C_7, C_8)
Extensor digiti minimi	Proximal tendon of extensor digitorum	Tendon of extensor digitorum distal to 5th MP joint	Extension at 5th MP joint	Radial (C_7, C_8)
Flexor digitorum profundus	Proximal 3/4 ulna	Base of distal phalanx, digits 2–5	Flexion at distal and proximal IP joints and MP joints, digits 2–5	Ulnar and Median (C_8, T_1)
Flexor digitorum superficialis	Medial epicondyle of humerus	Base of middle phalanx, digits 2–5	Flexion at proximal IP and MP joints, digits 2–5	Median (C_7, C_8, T_1)

Intrinsic Muscles

Muscle	Proximal Attachment	Distal Attachment	Primary Action(s)	Nerve Innervation
Flexor pollicis brevis	Ulnar side, 1st metacarpal	Ulnar, palmar base of proximal phalanx of the thumb	Flexion at MP joint of the thumb	Median (C_8, T_1)
Abductor pollicis brevis	Scaphoid and trapezium bones	Radial base of 1st phalanx of thumb	Abduction at 1st CM joint	Median (C_8, T_1)
Opponens pollicis	Scaphoid bone	Radial side 1st metacarpal	Opposition at CM joint of the thumb	Median (C_8, T_1)
Adductor pollicis	Capitate, distal 2nd and 3rd metacarpals	Ulnar proximal phalanx of thumb	Adduction and flexion at CM joint of thumb	Ulnar (C_8, T_1)
Abductor digiti minimi	Pisiform bone	Ulnar base of proximal phalanx, 5th digit	Abduction and flexion at 5th MP joint	Ulnar (C_8, T_1)
Flexor digiti minimi brevis	Hamate bone	Ulnar base of proximal phalanx, 5th digit	Flexion at 5th MP joint	Ulnar (C_8, T_1)
Opponens digiti minimi	Hamate bone	Ulnar metacarpal of 5th metacarpal	Opposition at 5th CM joint	Ulnar (C_8, T_1)

(continued)

Table 12–1. Major Muscles of the Hand and Fingers (*continued*)

Intrinsic Muscles

Muscle	Proximal Attachment	Distal Attachment	Primary Action(s)	Nerve Innervation
Dorsal interossei (four muscles)	Sides of metacarpals, all digits	Base of proximal phalanx, all digits	Abduction at 2nd and 4th MP joints, radial and ulnar deviation of 3rd MP joint, flexion of MP joints 2–4	Ulnar (C_8, T_1)
Palmar interossei (three muscles)	2nd, 4th, and 5th metacarpals	Base of proximal phalanx, digits 2, 4, and 5	Adduction and flexion at MP joints, digits 2, 4 and 5	Ulnar (C_8, T_1)
Lumbricales (four muscles)	Tendons of flexor digitorum profundus, digits 2–5	Tendons of extensor digitorum, digits 2–5	Flexion at MP joints of digits 2–5	Median and Ulnar (C_8, T_1)

arches. Another connecting branch from these arteries forms the carpal arch on the dorsal side of the wrist. Digital arteries branch from the palmar arches to supply the fingers, and branches from the carpal arch run distally along the metacarpal bones.

Retinacula of the Wrist

The fascial tissue surrounding the wrist is thickened into strong fibrous bands called retinacula that form protective passageways through which tendons, nerves, and blood vessels pass. On the palmar side of the wrist

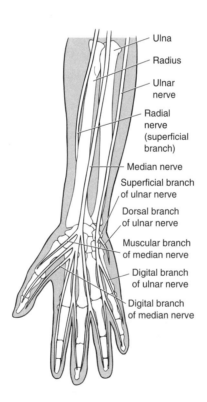

Fig. 12.5: The peripheral nerve supply to the wrist and hand.

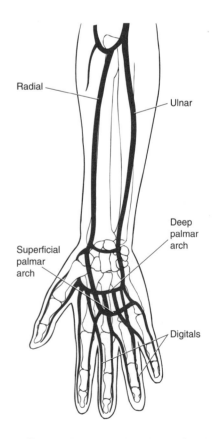

Fig. 12.6: The blood supply to the wrist and hand.

the flexor retinaculum protects the extrinsic flexor tendons and the median nerve. On the dorsal side of the wrist the extensor retinaculum provides a passageway for the extrinsic extensor tendons.

💡 *Did you determine what structures may have been damaged on the softball player's finger? If you concluded possible damage to the bones, joint capsule, collateral ligaments, or the dorsal ligament, you are correct.*

KINEMATICS AND MAJOR MUSCLE ACTIONS OF THE WRIST AND HAND

❓ *Why is the range of motion permitted by the carpometacarpal joint of the thumb so much greater than the ranges of motion allowed at the carpometacarpal joints of the second through fifth digits?*

The wrist is capable of sagittal and frontal plane movements, as well as rotary motion (**Figure 12-7**). Flexion occurs when the palmar surface of the hand is moved toward the anterior forearm. Extension involves the return of the hand to anatomical position from a position of flexion, and hyperextension occurs when the dorsal surface of the hand is brought toward the posterior forearm. Movement of the hand toward the radial side of the arm is radial deviation, with movement in the opposite direction known as ulnar deviation. Rotational movement of the hand through all four directions is termed **circumduction**.

Flexion

The major flexor muscles of the wrist are the flexor carpi radialis and flexor carpi ulnaris (**Figure 12-3**). The palmaris longus, which is often absent in one or both forearms, con-
tributes to flexion when present. The flexor digitorum superficialis and flexor digitorum profundus assist with flexion at the wrist when the fingers are completely extended, but when the fingers are in flexion these muscles cannot develop sufficient tension to assist.

Extension and Hyperextension

Extensor carpi radialis longus, extensor carpi radialis brevis, and extensor carpi ulnaris produce extension and hyperextension at the wrist (**Figure 12-4**). The other posterior wrist muscles may also assist with extension movements, particularly when the fingers are in flexion. Included are the extensor pollicis longus, extensor indicis, extensor digiti minimi, and extensor digitorum (**Figure 12-4**).

Radial and Ulnar Deviation

The flexor and extensor muscles of the wrist cooperatively develop tension to produce radial and ulnar deviation of the hand at the wrist. The flexor carpi radialis and extensor carpi radialis act to produce radial deviation, and the flexor carpi ulnaris and extensor carpi ulnaris cause ulnar deviation (**Figures 12-3, 12-4**).

Carpometacarpal Joint Motion

The carpometacarpal joint of the thumb allows a large range of movement, comparable to that of a ball and socket joint. However, the fifth carpometacarpal joint permits significantly less range of motion, and only a very small amount of motion is allowed at the second through fourth carpometacarpal joints due to the presence of restrictive ligaments.

Circumduction
Circular motion of a body segment resulting from sequential flexion, abduction, extension, and adduction or vice versa

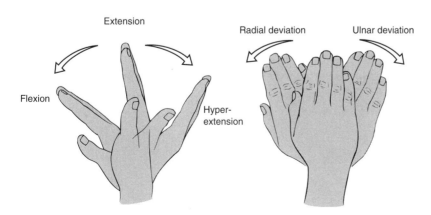

Fig. 12.7: Directional movement capabilities at the wrist.

Metacarpophalangeal Joint Motion

The metacarpophalangeal joints of the fingers allow flexion, extension, abduction, adduction, and circumduction (**Figure 12-8**). Among the fingers, abduction is defined as movement away from the middle finger and adduction is movement toward the middle finger. However, the metacarpophalangeal joint of the thumb functions more as a hinge joint, with the primary movements being flexion and extension.

Interphalangeal Joint Motion

The interphalangeal joints permit flexion and extension, and in some individuals, slight hyperextension. These are classic hinge joints.

There are actually two reasons why the thumb possesses a greater range of car-pometacarpal joint motion than the other digits. As discussed, ligaments restrict the range of motion across the carpometacarpal joints of digits two to five. Also remember that the car-pometacarpal joint of the thumb is a classic saddle joint that allows greater freedom of motion than the modified saddle joints of the other digits.

KINETICS OF THE WRIST AND HAND

In what position should the wrist be held if maximum grip strength is desired?

The extrinsic flexor muscles of the hand are more than twice as strong as the strongest extrinsic extensor muscles (4). This should come as little surprise given that the flexor muscles of the hand are used extensively in everyday activities involving gripping, grasping, or pinching movements, while the extensor muscles rarely exert much force.

Three types of hand grips are predominantly used in sport activities (**Figure 12-9**). The power grip, typified by the baseball bat grip, is one in which the fingers and thumb are used to clamp the grip of the bat against the palm of the hand. The wrist is held in a position of ulnar deviation and slight hyperexten-

> Finger flexion strength is greater when the wrist is slightly hyperextended, and finger extension strength is greater when the wrist is in flexion, because in these positions, muscle tension is increased

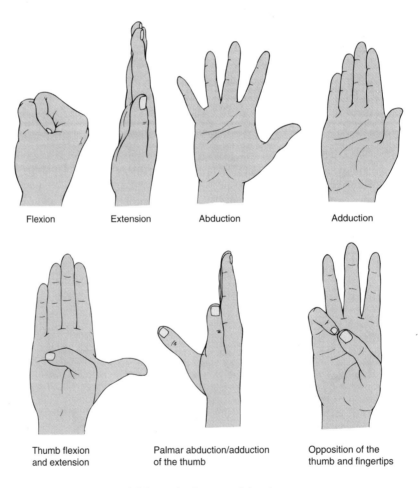

Flexion   Extension   Abduction   Adduction

Thumb flexion and extension   Palmar abduction/adduction of the thumb   Opposition of the thumb and fingertips

Fig. 12.8: Directional movement capabilities at the fingers and thumb.

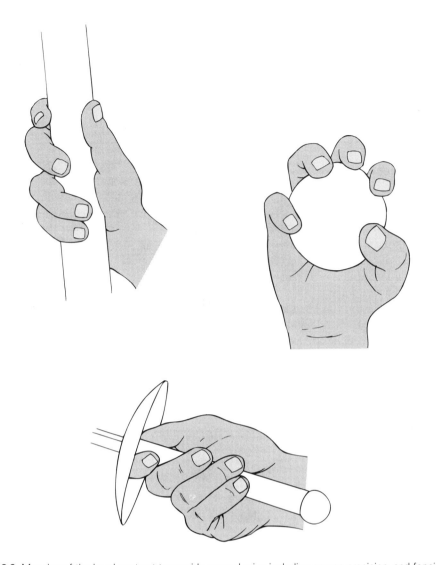

Fig. 12.9: Muscles of the hand contract to provide several grips including power, precision, and fencing grips.

sion to increase the tension in the flexor tendons. In contrast to the power grip, the precision grip, exemplified by the baseball grip, involves use of the semiflexed fingers and thumb to pinch the ball against the palm, with the wrist in slight hyperextension. A third grip that is intermediate to the two previously described might be termed a lateral pinch, also referred to as the "fencing grip." Fencing requires both power and precision. The grip on the foil is essentially a power grip, but with the thumb aligned along the long axis of the foil handle, it enables precise control of the direction of force application (5).

Maximum grip strength can be exerted when the wrist is in a position of ulnar deviation and slight hyperextension to increase tension in the flexor tendons.

PREVENTION OF WRIST AND HAND INJURIES

The wrist, hand, and fingers must be positioned to perform intricate tasks, yet must sustain tremendous loads to cushion the body during collisions, or lessen body movement during falls. What measures can be taken to protect and strengthen the region to prevent injuries?

The very nature of many contact and collision sports place the wrist and hands in an extremely vulnerable position for injury. The hands are almost always the first point of contact to cushion the body during collisions, deflect flying implements, or lessen body impact during a fall. Falling on an outstretched hand is the leading cause of fractures and dislocations at the distal forearm, wrist, and hand. Few sports require protective padding for the wrist and hand, although several pads and gloves are available. Combined with physical conditioning and proper skill technique, these three factors can prevent some injuries to the wrist and hand.

Protective Equipment

Goalies, baseball/softball catchers, and field players in many sports, such as hockey and lacrosse, are required to wear wrist and hand protection (**Figure 6-13**). The padded gloves prevent direct compression from a stick, puck, or ball. Football linemen wear padded gloves to cushion the dorsum of the hand to lessen impact should the hand be stepped on by another player. Specialized hand grips are worn by gymnasts to reduce friction between the bars and the palmar aspect of the hand. Several leather gloves are also designed for specific sport demands, and have extra padding placed at high impact areas. Gloves used in biking, rowing, and weight lifting for example, have extra padding on the palm of the hand. Other gloves are worn to protect the hand from friction, to increase grip, and to protect the hand from abrasions, particularly when playing on artificial turf, or on a baseball/softball field. Whenever possible, protective pads and gloves should always be worn during sport participation to lessen the risk of injury.

> Several leather gloves are designed for specific sport demands and have extra padding at high impact areas

Physical Conditioning

Several muscles that move the wrist and hand cross the elbow. Therefore, flexibility and strengthening exercises for the wrist and hand must also incorporate exercises for the elbow. For example, after stretching the shoulder, an individual can use the left hand to stretch the right elbow and wrist to increase flexibility. This action is reversed to stretch the left elbow and wrist.

Several strengthening exercises for the elbow and wrist were discussed in **Field Strategy 11-1**. These exercises included general strength in elbow flexion and extension, forearm pronation and supination, wrist flexion and extension, and radial and ulnar deviation. Other exercises, such as squeezing a tennis ball or a spring-loaded grip device can be used to strengthen the finger flexors.

> Always determine the possibility of an underlying fracture in a contusion or abrasion of the hand

Proper Skill Technique

Unlike the shoulder and elbow, which is subjected to excessive stress during a throwing-like motion, nearly all wrist and hand injuries result from accidental direct trauma. Although analysis of specific movements may detect improper technique, in many cases, this analysis may be incidental. An important skill technique, however, that can prevent injury to the wrist and hand is proper instruction on the shoulder roll method of falling. Here, the force of impact is dispersed over a wider area, lessening the risk for injury. Falling on an extended wrist is the leading cause of fracture and dislocation at the wrist and hand.

💡 *Physical conditioning should include exercises for the elbow, wrist, and hand. Specialized padded gloves are available for a variety of sports, and should be worn whenever possible. However, one of the key elements in preventing injury to the wrist and hand is learning how to fall properly to avoid direct impact on an extended wrist.*

CONTUSIONS AND ABRASIONS

❓ *A track athlete hit a hurdle and fell onto the cinder track and now has an abrasion on the palmar side of the hand. What immediate and long-term concerns are there in cleaning this superficial wound?*

Contusions and abrasions to the hand area can be very painful. With the vast neurovascular matrix coursing through the hand and fingers, simple injuries, if treated improperly, can lead to infections and long-term disability.

Contusions to the hand produce a soft, painful, bluish discoloration. During assessment, always determine the possibility of an underlying fracture. Initial treatment involves ice, compression, elevation, and rest. Symptoms will usually disappear in two to three days.

Abrasions must be thoroughly cleansed of all foreign matter. A soap wash for 10 minutes using surgical soap with a water-soluble iodine solution and brush can remove imbedded foreign matter. Following cleansing, an antiseptic is applied, and the wound is covered with a sterile nonadherent dressing. The dressing is changed daily, and the wound is inspected for signs of infection. These signs include a red, swollen, hot, and tender wound that may or may not have visible pus. Swollen, tender lymph nodes may be accompanied by a general feeling of malaise, and the individual may have a mild fever and headache.

After cleansing the abrasion on the palm, apply an antiseptic and a sterile nonadherent dressing. Check the wound daily for signs of infection.

SPRAINS

A gymnast is experiencing pain during vaulting and floor routines when body weight is supported on the hands. Radiographs and muscle testing did not show anything conclusive. You have determined that the wrist joint may be sprained from excessive extension, and have begun to manage the condition with ice treatments and gentle stretching. Can the individual continue to participate without making the condition worse?

Because the hands are frequently used to break a fall or block an object, the wrist and fingers are often traumatized. Ligamentous sprains in the wrist and hand are the most common injuries to the area. Most sprains also involve muscular strains caused from hyperextension or hyperflexion. Unfortunately most individuals do not allow ample time for healing due to the need to perform simple daily activities. Consequently, many sprains are neglected leading to chronic instability.

Wrist Sprains

Most wrist injuries are caused by axial loading on the proximal palm as a result of falling on an outstretched hand, although hyperflexion and torsion may also damage supporting tissues. Wrist stability is maintained by extensive, strong ligaments. Gymnasts have a high incidence of dorsal wrist pain when excessive forces are exerted on the wrist producing combined hyperextension, ulnar deviation, and intercarpal supination. These excessive forces occur during vaulting, floor exercise, or during pommel horse routines. Divers who enter the water with the hands in extension, and skaters and wrestlers who fall on an extended hand are also prone to this injury.

Assessment will reveal point tenderness on the dorsum of the radiocarpal joint. Pain increases with active or passive extension. After a fracture and joint instability has been ruled out through a radiograph, treatment involves decreasing intensity of training, cryotherapy before and after practice, nonsteroidal anti-inflammatory drugs (NSAIDs),

and the use of an appropriate bandage, taping technique, or splint to prevent excessive hyperextension. As pain decreases, range of motion exercises and wrist and hand strengthening exercises, such as those listed in **Field Strategy 11-1** and **11-8** can begin.

Gamekeeper's Thumb

The thumb is exposed to more force than the fingers by the virtue of its position on the hand. Integrity of the ulnar collateral ligament at the MP joint is critical for normal hand function, as it stabilizes the joint as the thumb is pushed against the index and middle fingers while performing many pinching, grasping, and gripping motions. **Gamekeeper's thumb** is common in football, baseball/softball, hockey, and in skiing when the individual falls on the ski pole (skier's thumb). When the MP joint is in extension and the thumb is forcefully abducted away from the hand, the ulnar collateral ligament at the MP joint is torn. With partial tears, only moderate laxity is present and a definite end feel is felt. In more severe cases, laxity greater than 35° and the absence of an end feel indicate total rupture of the ulnar collateral ligament (**Figure 12-10**).

The ulnar aspect of the joint is painful, swollen, and may have visible bruising. Instability is detected by applying a radial or abduction stress to the proximal phalanx in both extension and flexion of the thumb. Bilateral comparison, along with assessing joint laxity at other major joints, will help determine the normal joint laxity for the individual. Initial treatment includes ice, compression, and elevation with referral to a physician to rule out an undisplaced avulsion fracture. In first or second degree injuries with no instability, early mobilization accompanied with NSAIDs, contrast baths, cryotherapy, and ultrasound have had good success rates. The thumb should be protected by strapping or taping to prevent reinjury. If there is joint instability, the individual will be placed in a thumb spica cast for three to six weeks followed by further taping during risk activities for another three to six weeks. Severe cases require surgical repair.

Interphalangeal Collateral Ligament Sprains

Excessive varus and valgus stress and hyperextension can damage the collateral liga-

Wrist sprains commonly result from axial loading, although hyperflexion and torsion can also damage supporting tissues

In a wrist sprain, pain can be elicited on the dorsum of the radiocarpal joint and increases with active or passive wrist extension

Gamekeeper's thumb
Rupture of the volar ligament at the MP joint due to forceful abduction of the thumb while the thumb is extended

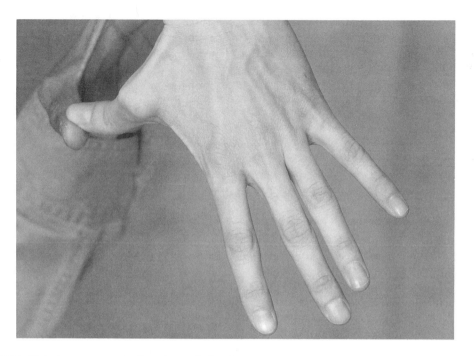

Fig. 12.10: Clinical appearance of a Gamekeeper's thumb.

ments of the fingers. Hyperextension of the proximal phalanx can stretch or rupture the volar plate on the palmar side of the joint **(Figure 12-11)**. An obvious deformity may not be present unless there is a fracture or total rupture of the supporting tissues leading to a dorsal dislocation. Rapid swelling makes assessment difficult. A radiograph is needed to rule out an associated dislocation or fracture.

Acute care involves ice and elevation. A mild sprain can be treated by taping the injured finger to an adjacent finger (buddy taping) during competition. This provides some support and mobility, but should not be used on an acute swollen, painful finger because of possible constriction to the vascular flow. If more support is needed, the involved joint can be splinted in extension with a molded polyprophylene splint to avoid flexion contractures.

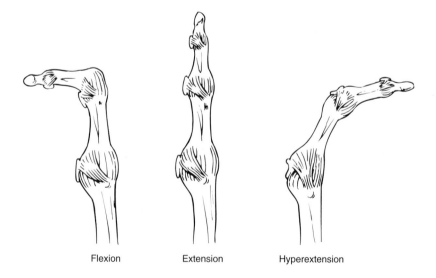

Flexion   Extension   Hyperextension

Fig. 12.11: The collateral ligaments and volar plate of the fingers can be damaged in hyperextension injuries to the fingers.

Dislocations

Axial loading at the wrist can tear ligaments at the radiocarpal joint leading to a carpal dislocation. Because of the shape of the lunate and its position between the large capitate and lower end of the radius, this carpal bone is particularly prone to dislocation. The displacement is usually in a volar direction (toward the palm), and can easily be overlooked (**Figure 12-12**). Point tenderness can be elicited on the dorsum of the hand just distal to the lower end of the radius. Palpation may also reveal a thickened area on the palmar aspect under the flexor tendons that is not bilateral. However, rapid swelling may preclude this sign. Passive and active motion may not be painful. If the bone moves into the carpal tunnel, compression of the median nerve results in pain, numbness, and tingling in the first and second fingers.

Immediate treatment involves immobilization in a wrist splint or sling, application of ice to reduce swelling and inflammation, and referral to a physician. After the dislocation is reduced by the physician, the wrist is immobilized in moderate flexion with a silicone cast for three to four weeks. The wrist is then placed into neutral position and protected from any wrist extension, particularly during sport participation (6). This condition is often overlooked until complications, such as flexor tendon contractures and median nerve palsies arise from chronic dislocations.

Metacarpophalangeal (MP) joint dislocations are rare but readily recognizable as a very serious injury demanding immediate attention by a physician (**Figure 12-13**). Hyperextension causes the anterior capsule to tear, allowing the proximal phalanx to move backward over the metacarpal to stand at a 90° angle to the metacarpal. An attempt to straighten the finger by flexing the phalanx often traps a portion of the anterior capsule between the metacarpal and phalanx. Such action should never be attempted by an untrained individual. Instead, apply ice to control hemorrhage, immobilize the area, and refer the individual to a physician.

Dislocations at the proximal interphalangeal joint are by far the most common hand joint dislocation (**Figure 12-14**). Because digital nerves and vessels run along the sides of the fingers and thumb, dislocations here can be serious. A swollen, painful finger caused by a ball striking the extended finger is frequently the initial complaint. Pain will be present at the joint line and will increase when the mechanism of injury is reproduced. If inadequately cared for, dislocations at the PIP joint can result in a painful, stiff finger with a fixed flexion deformity commonly called, "**coach's finger**."

Distal interphalangeal dislocations usually occur dorsally and may be associated with an open wound. Frequently the individual may reduce the injury themselves. As with the MP joint dislocation, injuries to the collateral ligaments at the PIP and DIP joints can involve ruptures of the volar plate. Because of this, reduction of finger dislocations should only be attempted by a physician. Acute care involves ice, immobilization, and transportation to a physician.

In a dislocation of the proximal interphalangeal joint, the finger may be splinted in about 30° of flexion with active motion started

Dislocations at the wrist commonly involve the lunate

If the lunate moves into the carpal tunnel it can compress the median nerve resulting in paresthesia in the first and second fingers

Dislocations at the PIP joint is the most common hand joint dislocation

Coach's finger
Fixed flexion deformity of the finger resulting from dislocation at the PIP joint

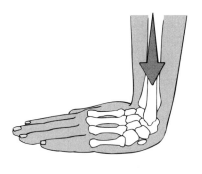

A

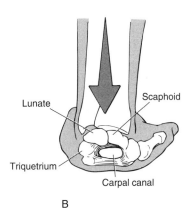

Lunate
Scaphoid
Triquetrium
Carpal canal

B

Fig. 12.12: The lunate can dislocate during a fall on an outstretched hand when the load from the radius compresses the lunate in a volar direction (A). If the bone moves into the carpal tunnel, the median nerve can become compressed leading to sensory changes in the first and second fingers (B).

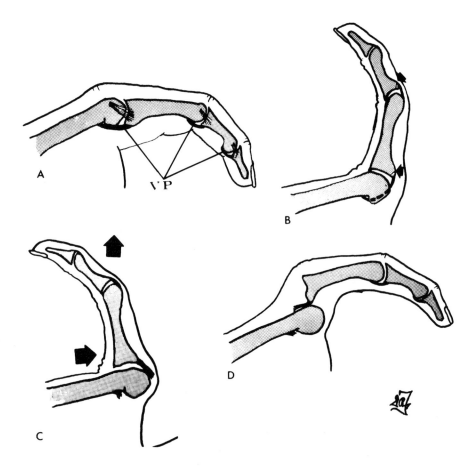

Fig. 12.13: Hyperextension of the fingers can damage the anterior capsule at the metacarpophalangeal joint. (A) The normal position of the volar plate. Notice that it is attached proximally to the head of the proximal bone. (B) Initial effects of hyperextension cause a sprain of the anterior capsule and supporting ligaments. (C) As the force continues the anterior capsule is ruptured dislocating the phalanx. The arrows indicate the direction of the forces which should be used to reduce the dislocation. (D) If improperly reduced with the phalanx merely straightened, the head of the proximal bone will protrude through a split in the capsule.

at 10 to 14 days. Immobilization for a distal interphalangeal joint dislocation involves splitting the DIP joint with a volar splint for approximately three weeks. The PIP joint can be left free so motion can continue at this joint. Protective splinting is continued for at least three weeks until the finger is pain-free.

You determined the gymnast had a first degree wrist sprain with only mild instability. The physician may prescribe NSAIDs to alleviate some of the symptoms. Applying tape or a splint to reduce excessive wrist extension can permit the individual to continue performing. Cryotherapy, thermotherapy, EMS, and interferential current may also be used to enhance optimal healing.

STRAINS

While holding a jersey tightly in one hand in an effort to stop the opposing player, a rugby player felt a sharp pain in the distal pha-lanx of the ring finger. Upon release of the jersey, the player was unable to flex the DIP joint of the ring finger. What structure(s) are responsible for motion at this joint? How would you assess which structures are damaged?

Muscular strains occur as a result of excessive overload against resistance or overstretching the tendon beyond its normal range. In mild or moderate strains, pain and

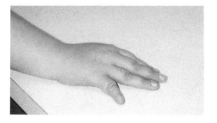

Fig. 12.14: Dislocations at the PIP joint can result in a painful, stiff finger with a fixed gross deformity.

Muscular strains occur as a result of excessive overload against resistance or overstretching the tendon beyond its normal range

restricted motion may not be a major factor. Muscular strains in the hand and wrist are common in all sports but are often neglected. For example, in overextension injuries of the fingers, both a strain of the flexor tendons and a sprain of the joint capsule and supporting ligaments may be present. The sprained joint takes precedent in priority of care, especially with an associated dislocation. As a result, tendon damage may go unrecognized and untreated leading to permanent disability and disfigurement for the unsuspecting individual. In the wrist and hand region the potential for more than one injury at a time is always present.

Jersey Finger
(Profundus Tendon Rupture)

This injury typically occurs when an individual grips an opponent's jersey while the opponent simultaneously twists and turns to get away from the grasp. This jerking motion may force the fingers to rapidly extend resulting in a rupture of the flexor digitorum profundus tendon from its attachment on the distal phalanx, hence the name "**jersey finger.**" The ring finger is more commonly involved, because this finger assumes a position of slight extension relative to the other more flexed fingers during grip. If avulsed, the individual will be unable to flex the DIP joint against resistance. With the forearm supinated, the tendon can be palpated at the proximal aspect of the involved finger, and will typically have a hematoma formation (7).

Ice should be applied immediately to control swelling and hemorrhage, and the individual referred to the physician. A radiograph can rule out an avulsion fracture. Surgical repair is usually indicated with the hand immobilized for at least five weeks. At three weeks, the splint can be removed during the exercise session to allow active range of motion exercises (7).

Mallet Finger

Mallet finger occurs when an object hits the end of the finger while the extensor tendon is taut, such as when catching a ball; hence it is sometimes called baseball finger. The resulting forceful flexion of the distal phalanx causes the extensor tendon to avulse from the attachment on the distal phalanx. With the forearm pronated and the hand palm down, the tip of the finger drops and active extension is not possible (**Figure 12-15**). Unlike the jersey finger where the flexor tendon retracts into the proximal aspect of the finger, isolated rupture of the extensor tendon usually does not retract. In nearly 25% of cases, an avulsion fracture to the proximal distal phalanx occurs (8).

With a mallet finger, the DIP joint is immobilized in extension with the PIP joint left free to move (**Figure 12-16**). This splint is applied for six to eight weeks. An alternative technique involves immobilization of the PIP joint in flexion and the DIP joint in extension. This position pulls the extensor mechanism distal, and prevents contractures from forming in the lateral ligamentous bands at the PIP joint (9,10). This splint is applied for five weeks followed by splinting only the DIP joint for another four weeks. Extended immobilization may lead to skin ulcerations. To avoid this, keep the splint dry and alternate its position between the dorsal and palmar aspect of the finger. Extreme hyperextension of the distal phalanx may also

Jersey finger
Rupture of the flexor digitorum profundus tendon from the distal phalanx due to rapid extension of the finger while actively flexed

If the flexor digitorum profundus tendon is avulsed, the individual will be unable to flex the DIP joint against resistance

Mallet finger
Rupture of the extensor tendon from the distal phalanx due to forceful flexion of the phalanx

In a mallet finger, the isolated rupture of the extensor tendon does not usually retract in the finger, and may be associated with an avulsion fracture

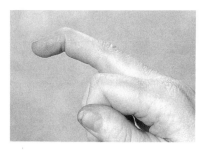

Fig. 12.15: Mallet finger is caused when the extensor tendon is avulsed from the attachment on the distal phalanx.

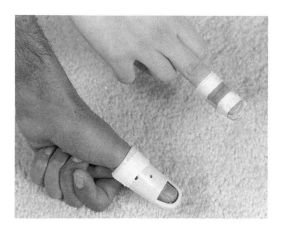

Fig. 12.16: Immobilization of the DIP joint allows the PIP joint to move freely.

Boutonniere deformity
Rupture of the central slip of the extensor tendon at the middle phalanx resulting in no active extensor mechanism at the PIP joint

Because the head of the proximal phalanx protrudes through the split in the extensor hook, this condition is sometimes referred to as a "buttonhole rupture"

Trigger finger
Condition whereby the finger flexors contract but are unable to re-extend due to a nodule within the tendon sheath or the sheath being too constricted to allow free motion

Stenosing
Narrowing of an opening or stricture of a canal; stenosis

de Quervain's tenosynovitis
An inflammatory stenosing tenosynovitis of the abductor pollicis longus and extensor pollicis brevis tendons

impair vascular supply to the tip of the finger leading to further skin damage (11). Periodic checks can prevent skin irritation and ensure proper splint alignment.

Boutonniere Deformity

A **boutonniere deformity** is caused by a rapid, forceful flexion at the PIP joint. The central slip of the extensor tendon ruptures at the middle phalanx leaving no active extensor mechanism intact over the PIP joint. The ruptured middle slip allows the lateral slips to move in a palmar direction resulting in flexion at the PIP joint and extension at the DIP joint (**Figure 12-17**). Because the head of the proximal phalanx protrudes through the split in the extensor hood, this condition is sometimes referred to as a "buttonhole rupture". Initial treatment involves splinting the PIP joint in an extended position with the DIP joint free to move. This immobilization should be maintained for six to eight weeks (12). The individual is encouraged to flex the DIP joint frequently to avoid adhesions.

Trigger Finger

Snapping flexor tendons, or **trigger finger**, may be present in individuals who have multiple, severe trauma to the palmar aspect of the hand. It more commonly occurs to the middle or ring finger, but may occur at the thumb and other fingers. Repeated trauma and inflammation results in a thickening of the tendon sheath as it passes over the proximal phalanx. A nodule can form and grow within the thickened synovium-lined tendon sheath to eventually prevent the tendon from sliding within the annular ligaments of the finger. Flexion occurs and the finger becomes

locked in flexion when the nodule becomes too thick, or the sheath too constricted to allow the finger to be actively re-extended (**Figure 12-18**). Cortisone injections into the sheath, ultrasound, friction massage, NSAIDs, and decreasing aggravating activities may relieve the obstruction. Often, however, an incision proximal to the palpable nodule is necessary to cut the annular ligament to allow the tendon to slide freely (13).

Tendinitis and Stenosing Tenosynovitis

Individuals involved in strenuous and repetitive training often inflame tendons and tendon sheaths in the wrist and hand. For example, oarsmen repeatedly extend the wrist while "feathering" the oar, leading to extensor synovitis. A prolonged tight grip on the oar may result in flexor tendinitis.

In the wrist, the abductor pollicis longus and extensor pollicis brevis are commonly affected. These two tendons share a single synovial tendon sheath that travels through a bony groove over the radiostyloid process, then turns sharply as much as 105° to enter the thumb when the wrist is in radial deviation (**Figure 12-19**). Tenosynovitis results from friction between the tendons, the **stenosing** sheath, and bony process. The tendons slide within the sheath not only during movements of the thumb but also in movements of the wrist with the thumb fixed, as in bowling or throwing. Referred to as "**de Quervain's tenosynovitis**," the individual will complain of pain over the radial styloid process that may radiate into the hand or forearm.

Palpation reveals point tenderness over the tendons, and occasionally crepitation. Movements of the thumb are painful, and snapping of the tendons during the throwing motion may be present. Pain is reproduced in two manners: (1) abduction of the thumb against resistance, and (2) flexing the thumb and cupping it under the fingers, then flexing the wrist in ulnar deviation to stretch the thumb tendons (see Finkelstein's test, **Figure 12-37**). Treatment is conservative with ice, rest, and NSAIDs as prescribed by a physician. If symptoms are not relieved, steroid injections or immobilization with a thumb spica for three weeks, or both may be helpful. In severe cases, surgical decompression may be necessary.

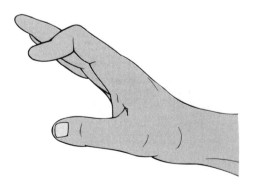

Fig. 12.17: With a boutonniere deformity, the proximal joint flexes while the distal joint hyperextends.

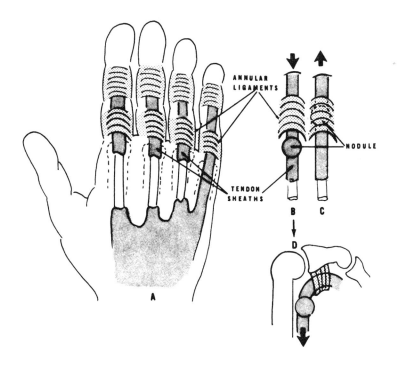

Fig. 12.18: Under normal conditions, the flexor tendons slide within the synovial sheaths under the annular ligaments at the proximal and middle phalanx (A). Repeated trauma can cause a nodule to form in the tendon sheath, or the sheath may become thickened (B). Flexion occurs and the finger becomes locked in flexion when the nodule becomes too thick or the sheath too constricted (C). The finger is then unable to reextend (D).

Ganglion Cysts

Ganglion cysts are benign tumor masses typically seen on the dorsal aspect of the wrist, although they may occur on the volar aspect (**Figure 12-20**). Associated with tissue sheath degeneration, the cyst itself contains a jelly-like colorless fluid of mucin, and is freely mobile and palpable. Occurring spontaneously, they seldom cause any pain or loss of motion. As the ganglion increases in size, discomfort from the pressure may occur. Treatment is symptomatic. Aspiration, injection, or rupture of the cyst have not proven to be successful, as the condition may recur. Surgical excision still remains the treatment of choice (6).

In assessing the rugby player, did you determine that the flexor digitorum profundus tendon was avulsed from the distal phalanx, preventing flexion of the DIP joint? When rehabilitation begins, range of motion and strength in the finger flexors must be restored.

FINGERTIP INJURIES

A water polo player pinched a finger between the pool deck and weighted base of a goal cage causing blood to accumu-

late under the fingernail. The fingertip is extremely painful from the increasing pressure. What must you keep in mind in deciding whether or not to relieve the pressure?

Ganglion cyst
Benign tumor mass commonly seen on the dorsal aspect of the wrist

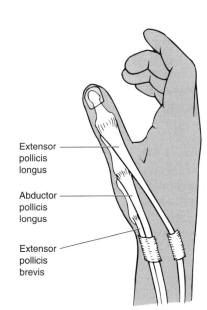

Fig. 12.19: The abductor pollicis longus and extensor pollicis brevis share the same synovial sheath. Excessive friction among the tendons, sheath, and bony process lead to tenosynovitis of the tendons.

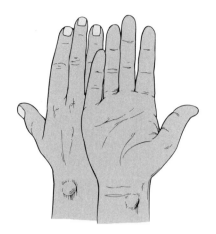

Fig. 12.20: Ganglion cysts are benign tumor masses associated with tissue sheath degeneration.

Direct trauma to the nail bed, such as when the finger is impacted by a ball, jammed into an object, or crushed when stepped on can lead to a subungual hematoma. Infections, such as paronychia and felons, may also occur at the fingertip. Open wounds were discussed in Chapter 2.

Subungual Hematomas

Direct trauma to the nail bed can result in blood forming under the fingernail, and is called a **subungual hematoma**. Increasing pressure can lead to throbbing pain. After determining the possibility of an underlying fracture, soak the finger in ice water for 10 to 15 minutes to numb the area and reduce bleeding under the nail bed. If it is not absolutely necessary to relieve the blood from the nail, do not do so, as this opens an avenue for infection. If, however, discomfort is so great the individual is unable to perform, drain the hematoma under the direction of a physician. Cut a hole through the nail with a rotary drill, a number 11 surgical blade, or melt a hole through the nail with the end of a paper clip heated to a bright red color. **Field Strategy 12-1** explains how to properly care for a subungual hematoma. After draining the blood, check the area daily for signs of infection.

Paronychia

Paronychia is an infection along the nail fold. It commonly follows a hangnail, or is seen in individuals whose hands are frequently immersed in water. The nail fold becomes red, swollen, painful, and can pro-

duce purulent drainage. The condition is treated with warm water soaks and germicide. In more severe cases, the physician may recommend systemic antibiotics and drainage of localized pus (14). The area is then protected with a dry, sterile dressing.

Felons

A **felon** is an abscess located within the fat pad of the fingertip. Because fat pads act as cushioning agents on the palmar aspect of the fingers, infection here can lead to increased pressure and pain in the septal spaces. As the abscess continues to grow unabated, the whole fingertip can become involved (**Figure 12-21**) (14). This may lead to **osteomyelitis** of the phalanx if the abscess is not drained by a physician.

The water polo player has a subungual hematoma. If it is not absolutely necessary to relieve pressure under the nail, do not do so, as this opens an avenue for infection. Any drainage of fluid should be done under the supervision of a physician, and should follow universal safety precautions.

NERVE ENTRAPMENT SYNDROMES

A long-distance cyclist is complaining of bilateral numbness in the little finger and medial half of the ring finger, and an inability to adduct the little finger. The individual can not recall an incident that could have caused this condition, but stated that training distance has significantly increased this past week. What possible factors are involved in this condition, and what suggestions can be made to alleviate the symptoms yet still allow this cyclist to continue training?

Neurovascular syndromes in the wrist and hand are seen in certain activities, such as bowling, cycling, karate, rowing, baseball/softball, field hockey, lacrosse, rugby, weight lifting, handball, and in wheelchair athletes. Nerve entrapment syndromes include carpal tunnel syndrome, ulnar entrapment (commonly associated with "cyclist's palsy"), superficial radial entrapment, and "Bowler's thumb," a digital nerve syndrome.

Carpal Tunnel Syndrome

Carpal tunnel syndrome is the most common compression syndrome of the wrist and hand, and is caused by direct trauma or repetitive overuse. Repetitive overuse of the wrist

Subungual hematoma
Collection of blood under the fingernail caused by direct trauma

Paronychia
Infection along the nail fold commonly associated with a hangnail

Felon
Abscess within the fat pad of the fingertip

Osteomyelitis
Inflammation or infection of the bone and bone marrow

Carpal tunnel syndrome
Compression of the median nerve as it passes through the carpal tunnel leading to pain and tingling in the hand

Field Strategy 12-1. Management of a Subungual Hematoma.

Under the direction of a physician:

1. Soak the finger in ice water for 10 to 15 minutes to numb the area and reduce hemorrhage
2. Cleanse your hands thoroughly with antiseptic soap and water, and apply latex gloves
3. Thoroughly cleanse the finger with antiseptic soap or an antibacterial solution
4. Use a sterile number 11 surgical blade, clean rotary drill, or melt a hole through the nail bed with the end of a paper clip heated to a bright red color

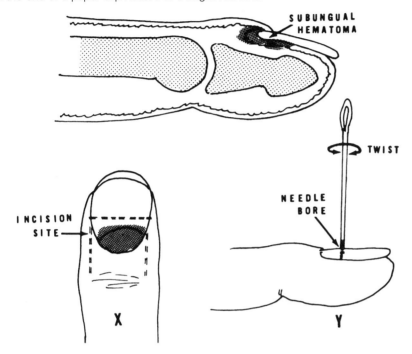

5. After the hole has been made, have the individual exert mild pressure on the distal pulp of the finger to drive excess blood through the hole
6. Watch the individual carefully for signs of shock as it sometimes occurs in minor injuries. Treat accordingly
7. Soak the finger in an iodine solution for ten minutes. Heat should not be applied for 48 hours
8. Cover the phalanx with a sterile dressing and apply a protective splint. Check the finger daily for signs of infection. If any appear, refer the individual to a physician

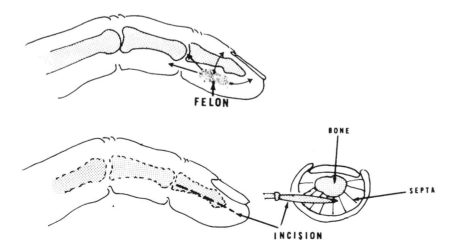

Fig. 12.21: If a felon abscess is not corrected, this can lead to osteomyelitis of the phalanx.

and finger flexors is three times more common in women, and peaks between 30 to 50 years of age with the right hand most commonly affected (15,16). The higher incidence in women may be largely due to daily occupational tasks that demand repetitive digital manipulations, such as typing or computer keyboard work.

The carpal tunnel is formed by the floor of the volar wrist capsule, with the roof formed by the transverse retinacular ligament traveling from the hook of the hamate and pisiform on the lateral side to the volar tubercle of the trapezium and tuberosity of the scaphoid on the medial side (**Figure 12-22**). This unyielding tunnel accommodates the median nerve, the tendons of the flexor digitorum profundus and superficialis in a common flexor sheath, and the tendon of the flexor pollicis longus in an independent sheath. Therefore, synovitis or thickening of the synovial covering of these tendons can produce pressure on the median nerve (**Figure 12-23**).

The individual may report initially that pain wakes them in the middle of the night and is often relieved with shaking and letting the hands dangle out of bed (17). There may be associated morning stiffness, also alleviated with activity (6). Numbness, tingling, or a burning sensation may initially be felt only in the fingertips on the palmar aspect of the thumb, index, and middle finger. As the condition progresses, sensory changes extend into the palm, or radiate into the forearm and shoulder. Symptoms are reproduced when direct compression is applied over the

median nerve in the carpal tunnel for about thirty seconds (18). Grip strength and pinch strength may be limited. Muscle strength should be bilaterally tested to determine what is normal for the individual. A positive Phalen and Tinel's sign indicates a possible carpal tunnel syndrome (see **Figures 12-39** and **12-40**). Individuals with suspected carpal tunnel syndrome should be referred to a physician for care.

Immobilization in slight wrist extension with a dorsal splint is used to rest the wrist for up to three to five weeks, particularly at night when symptoms occur (16). An ice cup or ice bag, NSAIDs, or in some situations, diuretics, can initially reduce swelling and pain in the area due to tenosynovitis. Use of a compression wrap should be avoided, since this adds additional compression on the already impinged structures. Over half of the individuals with this condition respond well to conservative treatment, although symptoms may recur, necessitating a corticosteroid injection into the canal. In cases that do not respond well to conservative treatment, surgical decompression or carpal tunnel release can be performed.

Ulnar Neuropathy

The ulnar nerve courses between the hook of the hamate and pisiform, then passes through Guyon's canal to move distally into the fingers (**Figure 12-24**). Edema and inflammation within the canal can compress the nerve. This condition is frequently seen in cycling, racquet sports, and in baseball/softball catchers

> Pain and paresthesia from a carpal tunnel syndrome commonly wakes the individual in the middle of the night

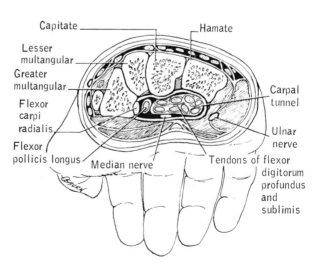

Fig. 12.22: Cross section of the wrist and carpal tunnel.

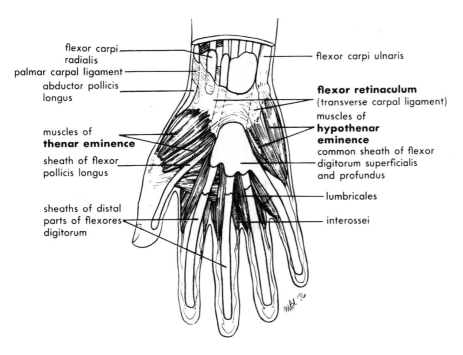

flexor carpi radialis
palmar carpal ligament
abductor pollicis longus

muscles of **thenar eminence**
sheath of flexor pollicis longus

sheaths of distal parts of flexores digitorum

flexor carpi ulnaris

flexor retinaculum (transverse carpal ligament)
muscles of **hypothenar eminence**
common sheath of flexor digitorum superficialis and profundus

lumbricales

interossei

Fig. 12.23: The flexor tendons of the fingers pass through the carpal tunnel in a single synovial sheath.

that experience repetitive trauma to the palmar aspect of the hand.

The individual will complain of numbness in the ulnar nerve distribution, particularly in the little finger, and will be unable to grasp a piece of paper between the thumb and index finger (see Froment's sign, **Figure 12-42**). Slight weakness in grip strength and atrophy of the hypothenar mass may also be present. Tapping just distal to the pisiform bone will produce a tingling sensation that radiates into

the little finger and ulnar aspect of the ring finger (positive Tinel's sign).

Cyclist's palsy, also linked to ulnar nerve entrapment, occurs when a biker leans on the handlebar an extended period of time, leading to swelling in the hypothenar area. Symptoms mimic the more serious ulnar nerve entrapment syndrome, but in this condition symptoms usually disappear rapidly after completion of the ride. Properly padding the handlebars, wearing padded gloves, varying

Ulnar neuropathy is frequently seen in activities involving repetitive trauma to the palmar aspect of the hand

Cyclist's palsy
Seen when biker's lean on the handlebar an extended period of time resulting in paresthesia in the ulnar nerve distribution

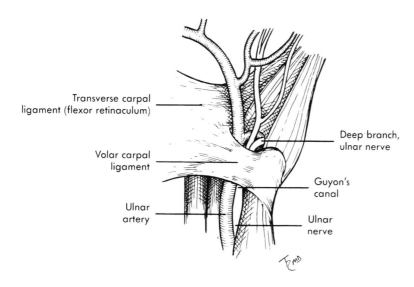

Transverse carpal ligament (flexor retinaculum)

Volar carpal ligament

Ulnar artery

Deep branch, ulnar nerve

Guyon's canal

Ulnar nerve

Fig. 12.24: The ulnar nerve can become impinged in the tunnel of Guyon as it runs under the ligament between the hamate and pisiform.

hand position, and properly fitting the bike to the rider can greatly reduce the incidence of this condition (19).

Treatment of ulnar nerve entrapment involves rest and cryotherapy to minimize pain and inflammation. NSAIDs may be prescribed, but this may not alleviate symptoms. If symptoms do not disappear within six months of conservative treatment, surgical decompression is indicated.

Superficial Radial Nerve Entrapment

The superficial branch of the radial nerve can be compressed at the wrist from gloves that are strapped too tight or from tight wrist bands, commonly seen in racquet sports. The individual will complain of burning pain, sensory changes, and night pain over the dorsoradial aspect of the hand and thumb. Treatment is conservative with ice, rest, immobilization, and referral to a physician if symptoms do not improve.

Bowler's Thumb

"**Bowler's thumb**" involves compression of the digital nerve on the medial aspect of the thumb in the webspace during gripping of a ball. Constant pressure on this spot can lead to scarring in the area. Numbness, tingling, or pain may develop on the medial aspect of the thumb. Athletic trainers develop similar symptoms from excessive use of dull scissors, or added pressure on the thumb as one cuts through thick tape jobs or pads.

The individual may have swelling or thickening over the medial palmar aspect at the base of the thumb. Treatment depends on the stage of injury. Since the predominant cause is inflammatory in nature, treatment is directed at reducing inflammation. Cryotherapy, immobilization with a molded plastic thumb guard, NSAIDs, and corticosteroid injection, if needed, are usually successful in relieving symptoms. Bowlers can prevent this condition by never completely inserting the thumb into the thumb hole, backsetting the thumb hole to increase extension and abduction of the thumb to relieve pressure, or by wearing a well-padded splint (13).

The cyclist may have compressed the ulnar nerve while leaning on the handlebars during the recent increased training. To alleviate symptoms, suggest padding the handlebars, wearing padded gloves, varying hand position, and properly fitting the bike to the rider.

FRACTURES TO THE WRIST AND HAND

A tennis player tripped and fell forward onto the outstretched hand holding the racquet, resulting in the racquet grip being driven into the hand. The individual is supporting the injured hand with the other hand. There is noticeable swelling on the dorsum of the hand. Palpation of the third metacarpal and percussion on the distal end of the third finger causes pain. What should you suspect? How will you immobilize the hand?

Fractures of the wrist and hand present a special challenge. Physicians want to immobilize the fracture to promote optimal healing, yet individuals want to continue sport participation with the least amount of material to interfere with performance. It is sometimes difficult to find a middle ground to please all parties, but the healing process should never be compromised.

The majority of wrist and hand fractures are simple and nondisplaced. With the advent and fabrication of external orthoses, many fractures can be immobilized adequately to allow individuals to continue with regular sport participation. However, specific rules governing special protective equipment require that braces, casts, or any unyielding substances on the elbow, forearm, wrist, or hand be padded on all sides so as not to endanger other players. Once the fracture has reached a stage where external support is no longer necessary during daily activities, a splint may be worn just during sport participation.

Fractures to the distal ulna and radius, and carpal bones are usually caused by axial loading when an individual falls on an outstretched hand. The scaphoid is the most commonly fractured carpal bone because it becomes impinged against the radial styloid process during wrist hyperextension. The hamate can be fractured while swinging a golf club, baseball bat, or tennis racquet, which drives the butt of the handle into the hook of the hamate. Fractures to the metacarpals, commonly seen in sport participation, result from bending of the bone, such as when someone steps on the hand or when a closed fist is driven into a solid object. Axial compression when an individual is hit on the end of the finger with a ball or object, or torsion, such as when fingers are caught in the fabric of an opponent's jersey are mechanisms that can lead to fractures of the phalanges.

The superficial radial nerve can be compressed at the wrist from gloves that are strapped too tight or from tight wrist bands

Bowler's thumb
Compression of the digital nerve on the medial aspect of the thumb leading to paresthesia in the thumb

The majority of hand and wrist fractures are simple and nondisplaced, and if properly immobilized, sport participation can continue

The scaphoid is the most commonly fractured carpal bone when it becomes impinged against the radial styloid process during hyperextension

Distal Radial and Ulnar Fractures

Fractures to the distal radius and ulna present a special problem. One or both bones may be fractured, or one bone may be fractured with the other bone dislocated at the elbow or wrist joint. A **Monteggia fracture** involves an ulnar fracture with an associated dislocation of the radial head (**Figure 12-25A**). A **Galeazzi fracture** involves a fractured radius with an associated dislocation of the ulna at the distal radial ulnar joint (**Figure 12-25B**). A **Colles fracture** involves a dorsally angulated and displaced, and a radially angulated and displaced fracture within one and a half inches of the wrist joint (**Figure 12-25C**) (6). There may also be an additional avulsion or fracture of the tip of the styloid process of the distal ulna. The deformity is classically called the "dinner-fork" deformity. A reverse of this fracture is the **Smith fracture** that tends to be either volar angulation or displacement (**Figure 12-25D**). Complications from these fractures may include circulatory impairment caused by swelling or hemorrhage, or damage to the median nerve as it passes through the forearm. In some cases, closed reduction is acceptable, but in serious fractures open reduction and internal fixation with rigid plates and screws is necessary to restore function (6,20).

Scaphoid Fracture

The scaphoid, sometimes referred to as the navicular, is a challenging fracture for even the best surgeon. Often the individual will fall on the wrist, have normal radiographs, and be discharged with a diagnosis of a wrist sprain without further care. Yet, several months later the individual will continue to experience persistent wrist pain. Radiographs at this time may reveal an established nonunion fracture of the scaphoid (**Figure 12-26**). Because of a poor blood supply to the area, **aseptic necrosis** is a common complication with this fracture.

Assessment will reveal a history of falling on an outstretched hand. Point tenderness is elicited on the radial styloid process. Severe pain will be present during palpation of the "**anatomical snuff box**" (**Figure 12-27**), or with inward pressure along the long axis of the first metacarpal bone, thereby compressing the scaphoid between the trapezium and radial styloid process. Pain will increase during wrist extension and radial deviation.

Treatment involves ice, compression, immobilization in an appropriate splint, and referral to a physician. Nondisplaced scaphoid fractures are usually handled with either a long-arm-thumb spica cast that extends above the elbow to include the humeral epicondyles, or a short-arm-thumb spica cast. The choice of immobilization will depend on the type of fracture and mechanism of injury. Follow up radiographs are taken at two, four, and six weeks. Some fractures may take several weeks or months to heal. During this time, the individual may participate with a padded short-arm-thumb cast or silicone cast (21). Dis-

Monteggia fracture
Ulnar fracture with an associated dislocation of the radial head

Galeazzi fracture
Radial fracture with an associated dislocation of the ulna at the distal radial ulnar joint

Colles fracture
Fracture involving a dorsally angulated and displaced, and a radially angulated and displaced fracture within one and a half inches of the wrist

Smith fracture
Forearm fracture with volar angulation or displacement; opposite of Colles fracture

Aseptic necrosis
The death or decay of tissue due to a poor blood supply in the area

Anatomical snuff box
Region directly over the scaphoid bone bounded by the extensor pollicis brevis medially and the extensor pollicis longus laterally

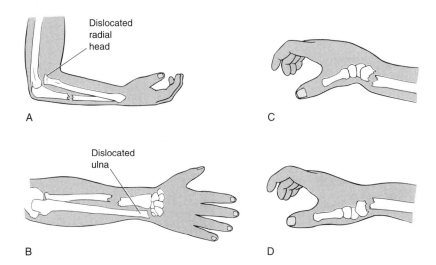

Fig. 12.25: Forearm fractures. (A) Monteggiia fracture. (B) Galeazzi fracture. (C) Colles fracture. (D) Smith fracture.

Hypothenar
Mass of intrinsic muscles of the little finger including the abductor digiti minimi, flexor digiti minimi brevis, and opponens digiti minimi

Thenar
Mass of intrinsic muscles of the thumb including the flexor pollicis brevis, abductor pollicis brevis, and opponens pollicis

Boxer's fracture
Fracture of the fifth metacarpal resulting in a flexion deformity due to rotation of the head of the metacarpal over the neck

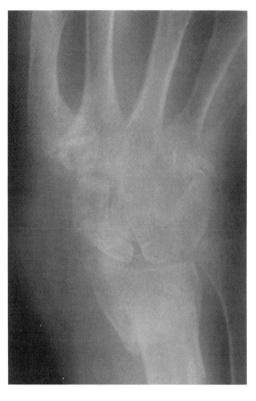

Fig. 12.26: Nonunion fractures of the scaphoid occur when there is a poor blood supply to the area. Note this individual also has a fractured radius.

placed scaphoid fractures are secured with internal fixation (22).

Hamate Fracture

Due to the close proximity of the ulnar nerve and artery to the hook of the hamate, and because of the pull of the attached muscles, fractures to the hamate may also lead to

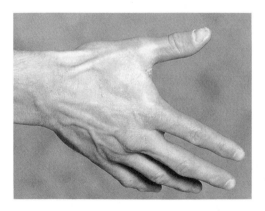

Fig. 12.27: The scaphoid forms the floor of the anatomical snuff box and is bounded by the extensor pollicis brevis medially, and the extensor pollicis longus laterally.

nonunion. Palpable pain is present in the **hypothenar** muscle mass, and the individual will have decreased grip strength. Radiographs and tomograms utilizing a carpal tunnel view with the wrist in extension will confirm the diagnosis. Care is usually symptomatic with a protective orthosis worn for four to six weeks until tenderness subsides. It may be two to three months before a racquet or bat will feel comfortable in the hand again.

Metacarpal Fractures

Uncomplicated fractures to the metacarpals result in severe pain, swelling, and deformity (**Figure 12-28**). A unique fracture involving the neck of the fifth metacarpal is called a **Boxer's fracture**. It occurs when an individual punches an object with a closed fist leading to rotation of the head of the metacarpal over the neck providing a palpable deformity in the palm of the hand.

Gentle palpation, percussion, and compression along the long axis of the bone will increase pain at the fracture site. **Field Strategy 12-2** lists how to determine a possible

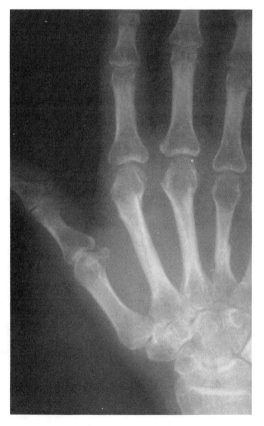

Fig. 12.28: Fractured fourth metacarpal.

Field Strategy 12–2. Determining a Possible Fracture to a Metacarpal.

PRIMARY SURVEY

• Check the ABCs. Shock may set in, particularly if there is angulation and deformity
• Determine responsiveness

SECONDARY SURVEY

History
• Determine mechanism of injury (compression, tension, shear, bending, or torsion)
• Primary complaint (pain and/or loss of motion)
• Pain perception
• Disability from injury (limited or loss of function)
Observation and Inspection
• Obvious deformity or angulation
• Swelling or discoloration directly over the bone
Palpation
• Pain along the shaft of the bone
• Pain on compression of soft tissue around the bone
Stress tests for fracture
• Compression along the long axis of the bone (A)
• Percussion at the end of the bone (B)
• Use of a tuning fork over the bone
  Positive sign occurs if pain is felt at the fracture site
• Distraction at the end of the bone (C)
  Positive sign occurs if pain is decreased. (Increased pain may indicate a ligamentous injury)

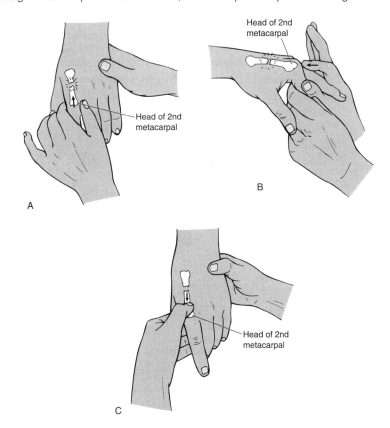

MANAGEMENT

If any positive signs are noted, immobilize the joint above and below the fracture site with a wrist splint, apply ice to reduce hemorrhage and swelling, and refer the individual to a physician

metacarpal fracture. These techniques can also be used to detect possible fractures in the carpals and phalanges. Fractures should be immobilized in the position of function with the palm face down and fingers slightly flexed. Ice is applied to reduce hemorrhage and swelling, however, an elastic compression bandage should not be applied to a swollen hand, as it may lead to increased distal swelling in the fingers.

Bennett's Fracture

Bennett's fracture
Fracture-dislocation to the proximal end of the first metacarpal at the carpal-metacarpal joint

A **Bennett's fracture** is an articular fracture to the proximal end of the first metacarpal. It is typically due to axial compression, such as when a punch is thrown with a closed fist or the individual falls on a closed fist. The pull of the abductor pollicis longus tendon at the base of the metacarpal displaces the shaft proximally. However, a small medial fragment is held in place by the deep volar ligament leading to a fracture-dislocation (**Figure 12-29**). Pain and swelling is localized, but deformity may or may not be present. Inward pressure exerted along the long axis of the first metacarpal will elicit pain at the fracture site. Acute care consists of ice, compression, immobilization in a wrist splint, and referral to a physician. The preferred treatment for this fracture is closed reduction with a short-arm-thumb spica cast worn for about four weeks (23–25). In cases where soft tissues may block reduction, surgery may be necessary.

Failure to maintain the longitudinal and rotational alignments of the fingers can led to long-term disability in grasping or manipulating small objects in the palm of the hand

Fig. 12.29: A Bennett's fracture involves the first metacarpal, and is usually associated with a dislocation of the MP joint of the thumb.

Phalangeal Fractures

Fractures of the phalanges are very common in sport participation and difficult to manage. They may be caused by having the fingers stepped on, impinged between two hard objects such as a football helmet and the ground, or through hyperextension which may lead to a fracture-dislocation (**Figure 12-30**). Particular attention should be given to a possible fracture of the middle and proximal phalanx. These fractures tend to have marked deformity due to the strong pull of the flexor and extensor tendons. The four fingers move as a unit. Failure to maintain the longitudinal and rotational alignments of the fingers can lead to long-term disability in grasping or manipulating small objects in the palm of the hand (26). This deformity often results in a finger overlapping another when a fist is made.

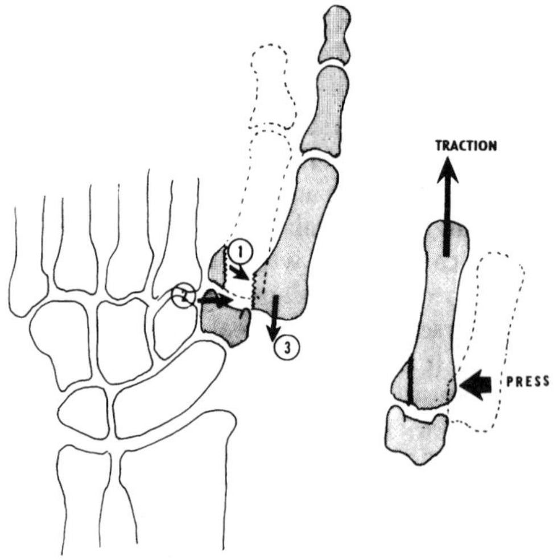

Acute care involves ice to reduce pain and swelling. With the hand immobilized in a full wrist splint, place gauze pads or a gauze roll under the fingers to produce about 30° finger flexion to reduce the pull of the flexor tendons. Refer the individual to a physician for care. Immobilization will depend upon the type of fracture and its location, and may vary from two to four weeks.

The tennis player probably has a metacarpal fracture caused when the racquet grip was driven into the palm of the hand during the fall. Immobilize the hand in the position of function with a wrist splint, apply ice to reduce swelling, and transport the individual to the physician.

ASSESSMENT OF THE WRIST AND HAND

A diver has pain on the anterior wrist during entry. Pain increases with resisted wrist and finger flexion, and passive wrist

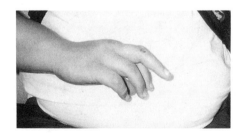

Fig. 12.30: This fractured phalanx was caused when the finger was compressed between two football helmets during a tackle.

and finger extension. How will you assess this injury?

The upper extremity acts as a functional unit. As such, an injury anywhere along the kinetic chain can impact the ability to perform simple daily activities or sport skills. The wrist and hand are difficult to evaluate because of the number of anatomical structures providing motor and sensory function to the region. Furthermore, without both motor and sensory acuity, it would be nearly impossible to accurately assess any sports injury. Sensitivity to touch, feeling crepitus, sensing temperature or texture of one's skin, and denoting the quantity and quality of swelling or edema are all perceived through skin receptors. The intricate muscles of the wrist and hand place the fingers in such a position to ascertain the shape of structures, and determine muscle strength and joint laxity. Although uncommon, pain at the wrist and hand may be referred from the cervical spine, shoulder, and elbow. As such, an injury at an isolated joint may necessitate a full functional assessment of the upper extremity.

HISTORY

What information must be gathered from the diver to identify the primary complaint and ascertain if other factors, such as sport-specific skills contributed to this injury?

Questions about a wrist injury should focus on the primary complaint, past injuries, and other factors that may have contributed to the current problem (referred pain, changes in technique, overuse, or occupational requirements). For example, ask how the injury occurred. Determine what symptoms are currently present, and how they progressed. Is the pain localized, general, or does it radiate into the forearm? What activities increase or decrease pain? What recent

Field Strategy 12–3. Developing a History of the Injury.

Current Injury Status

1. *If you have an acute problem identify the mechanism of injury. Ask:* What were you doing at the time of the injury? How did the injury occur? Did you hear any sounds during the incident, such as snaps, cracks, or pops? *If the injury came on gradually ask:* What different activities have you been doing in the last week? (*Look for changes in the training frequency, duration, intensity, type, or method*)
2. Where is the pain (or weakness) located? Can you point to the most painful area? Is the pain constant or intermittent? Does the pain come on gradually or suddenly? How long has it been a problem?
3. What actions bring on the pain? Is it worse in the morning, during activity, after activity, or at night? Does it wake you up at night? (*Remember that carpal tunnel syndrome often wakes the person up at night*). What actions relieve the pain? Are there any activities that you are unable to perform because of the pain or weakness? Which activities?
4. Did you notice any swelling or discoloration at the time of the injury? How soon did it occur? What did you do for the swelling? Have you had any muscle spasms, numbness, tingling, or burning sensations in your forearm or hand?
5. What have you done for the condition? Has there been any improvement in the injury?
6. How old are you? (*Remember that neurovascular problems often occur in older individuals*)

Past Injury Status

1. Have you ever injured your wrist and hand before? Who evaluated and cared for the injury? What was the diagnosis? What was done to treat the injury? Did you have any difficulty returning to your full functional status?
2. Does this injury appear to be the same or similar to the previous injury? In what ways is it different?
3. Have you had any medical problems recently that might contribute to this? (*Referred pain?*)

changes, if any, have occurred in the training program? In addition to general questions discussed in Chapter 4, specific questions for the wrist and hand region are listed in **Field Strategy 12-3**.

🔆 *The nineteen year old diver has been working quite extensively on several new dives on the 3-meter board in preparation for an upcoming competition. Pain on the anterior wrist started three weeks ago when both wrists were hyperextended during entry on a dive. Pain has continued to persist, increasing as the practice session progresses. It now hurts to pick up a book bag or hook an object with the fingers.*

OBSERVATION AND INSPECTION

❓ *What specific factors should be observed at the injury site? Since pain is present in both wrists, can you still do bilateral comparison?*

The entire arm should be exposed for observation and inspection. Although the individual may have a wrist injury, the elbow and shoulder region may also need to be evaluated, depending on the mechanism of injury. With an acute injury, it is critical early in the assessment to recognize possible fractures and dislocations. If the individual is in great pain, unable or unwilling to move the wrist or hand, complete the assessment in a position most comfortable for the individual. First observe the position of the wrist, hand, and fingers. Is there a noticeable deformity? How is the individual holding the wrist and hand? If swelling is present in a specific joint, the individual may be unable to fully extend that joint, supporting it in a slightly flexed position. Perform the fracture tests listed in **Field Strategy 12-2**. Any positive sign that indicates a possible fracture should be treated accordingly. Immobilize the wrist and hand in a vacuum splint, wrist splint, or sling, apply ice to control pain and inflammation, and transport the individual to a physician.

When a possible fracture or dislocation is not present, observe the individual's willingness and ability to place the hand in the various positions requested. The position of rest for the hand is with the wrist in 20 to 35° of extension and 10 to 15° of ulnar deviation. This position allows for the greatest amount of flexion of the fingers. With bilateral comparison, the dominant hand tends to be slightly larger than the nondominant hand.

Inspect the specific injury site for obvious abrasions, deformity, swelling, discoloration, symmetry, hypertrophy, muscle atrophy, or previous surgical incisions. **Field Strategy 12-4** summarizes observations at the wrist and hand from a dorsal and palmar view.

🔆 *Bilateral comparison reveals slight swelling over the carpal tunnel on both hands, however it is greater on the right hand. Erythema is present on the palmar aspect of the carpal tunnel on the right hand. No bilateral differences are visible in the thenar or hypothenar muscle masses. The fingers appear to be normal with no discoloration or swelling present.*

PALPATIONS

❓ *Pain and swelling are confined over the carpal tunnel on both wrists. Where will you begin palpations? What specific factors are you looking for?*

Palpate the wrist and hand proximal to distal beginning on the dorsal aspect, then move to the palmar aspect. Support the individual's hand throughout the palpations. Bilateral palpations can determine temperature, swelling, point tenderness, crepitus, deformity, muscle spasm, and cutaneous sensation. Temperature changes may indicate inflammation, infection, or a reduction in circulation. Crepitus may indicate tenosynovitis, an irregular articular surface, or possible fracture. Circulation can be assessed by blanching the fingernails. Squeeze the nail. Initially the nail should turn white, but color should return immediately upon release of pressure. Vascular pulses can also be taken at the radial and ulnar arteries in the wrist.

Dorsal Aspect

1. Radial styloid process and tubercle of the radius
2. Styloid process of the ulna
3. Finger and thumb extensors and thumb abductor
4. Carpal bones can be palpated on the dorsal and palmar aspect at the same time
   Scaphoid. It lies distal to the radial styloid process and forms the floor of the anatomic snuff box. *Tenderness is indicative of a possible fracture*
   Lunate. It can be palpated just distal to the radial tubercle, particularly during wrist flexion

The position of rest for the hand is with the wrist in 20 to 35° of extension and 10 to 15° of ulnar deviation, which allows for the greatest amount of finger flexion

Field Strategy 12–4. Observation and Inspection of the Wrist and Hand.

Dorsal View

1. Check bilateral posture, shape, and smooth contours of the bony and soft tissue structures at the wrist and hand. Note the use of the hand as the individual moves it into the requested positions
2. Note skin color. Do the hands appear healthy? Many vascular problems, such as peripheral vascular disorders, Raynaud's disease, or diabetes mellitus, may be indicated by changes in skin color and temperature
3. Note any ganglions. They often appear on the dorsum of the wrist region
4. Observe any muscle wasting
5. Note any localized swelling, effusion, or synovial thickening at the metacarpophalangeal and interphalangeal joints
6. Observe for any hypertrophy of one or more fingers and take note of any angular deformities of the fingers that may have resulted from a previous fracture or dislocation
7. With the forearm in pronation, note whether or not the distal phalanx fails to remain in an extended position. *This may indicate a mallet finger*
8. Observe the fingernails for any abnormality or change in color. Many systemic diseases, cardiac, or respiratory problems are manifested in the fingernails

Palmar View

1. Check the smooth contours of the bony and soft tissue structures of the forearm, wrist, and hand
2. Look for muscle wasting in the thenar eminence (median nerve) and hypothenar eminence (ulnar nerve) that may indicate a nerve injury
3. Have the individual flex the MP and PIP joints, and keep the DIP joint extended. Note any angular deformity of the fingers that may indicate a previous fracture
4. Note any localized swelling, effusion, or synovial thickening at the MP, PIP, and DIP joints. (This may be more visible on the dorsal view)
5. Check the color of the skin and presence of any abrasions or scars. Scars may decrease the mobility of a joint because of the formation of scar tissue around the tendons and joint

---

Triquetrum. It lies distal to the ulnar styloid process
Pisiform. Slightly flex the wrist and palpate on the medial palmar side
Trapezium. A radial pulse can be taken at this time in the anatomical snuff box
Trapezoid
Capitate (distal to lunate)
Hamate (distal to Triquetrum; the hook of the hamate is more easily palpated on the palmar aspect)

5. Metacarpal bones and phalanges. Palpate the MP, PIP, and DIP joints for synovial thickening, swelling, and tenderness

Palmar Aspect

1. Flexor tendons
2. Carpal transverse arch that forms the carpal tunnel, and the longitudinal arch comprised of the carpal bones, metacarpals, and phalanges **(Figure 12-31)**

3. Palmar fascia and intrinsic muscles within the thenar and hypothenar muscle masses

Swelling and exquisite point tenderness was apparent over the flexor tendons and carpal tunnel on both hands, particularly the right hand. Slight crepitation was felt during flexion and extension of the wrist flexors on the right hand. Circulation was normal.

SPECIAL TESTS

Although the right hand appears to be more seriously injured, it is imperative that both hands continue to be assessed. What specific tests should be performed to determine the extent and seriousness of this injury?

Perform special tests in a comfortable position and begin with gentle stress. Note what range of motion is the most painful. Do not force the wrist or hand through any sudden motions, nor cause undue pain. Proceed cautiously through the assessment.

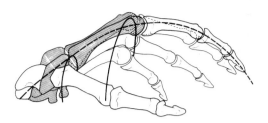

Fig. 12.31: Longitudinal and transverse arches of the hand should be palpated and observed for any abnormality.

Normal end feel for the wrist and finger joints is tissue stretch

Active Movements

In determining active movements at the wrist and hand, perform the most painful movements last. Finger active motion is usually done in a continuous pattern of flexion and extension. Ask the individual to: (a) make a tight fist (flexion), (b) straighten the fingers (extension), (c) spread the fingers (abduction), and (d) bring the fingers together (adduction). Note how fluid each digit moves throughout the range of motion. If one finger does not move through the full ROM, that finger can be evaluated separately. The following movements at the wrist and hand should be assessed:

1. Pronation/supination of the forearm (85 to 90°)
2. Wrist flexion (80 to 90°)
3. Wrist extension (70 to 90°)
4. Radial deviation (15°)
5. Ulnar deviation (30 to 45°)
6. Finger flexion and extension
7. Finger abduction and adduction
8. Thumb flexion, extension, abduction, and adduction
9. Opposition of the thumb and little finger (tip to tip)

Technique for taking goniometry measurements of wrist flexion and extension, and radial and ulnar deviation are listed in **Figure 12-32**.

Passive Range of Motion

If the individual is unable to perform active movements in all ranges, assess passive movements. Slight overpressure at the end of each motion can test the end feel of each joint. Normal end feel for the wrist and finger joints is tissue stretch, however in thin individuals, end feel for pronation may be bone-to-bone. Passive movements tested are the same as the active movements listed above.

Resisted Muscle Testing

Active movements are tested using resisted movements throughout the full range of motion. The individual can be standing or seated. The proximal joint is stabilized and a mild resistance is applied to the distal joint. The following movements should be tested **(Figure 12-33)**:

A. Forearm supination and pronation
B. Wrist flexion and extension
C. Ulnar and radial deviation
D. Finger flexion and extension

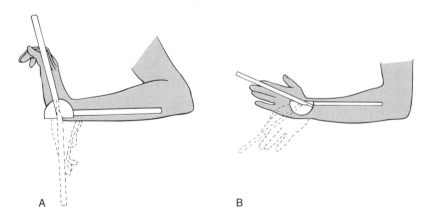

A   B

Fig. 12.32: Goniometry measurement. (A) Wrist flexion and extension. The fulcrum is centered over the lateral aspect of the wrist close to the triquetrium. Align the proximal arm along the lateral aspect of the ulna using the olecranon process as reference. Align the distal arm along the midline of the fifth metacarpal. (B) Radial and ulnar deviation. Center the fulcrum over the middle of the dorsum of the wrist close to the capitate. Align the proximal arm with the midline of the forearm using the lateral epicondyle as reference. Align the distal arm along the midline of the third metacarpal.

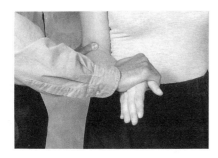

Fig. 12.33A: Resisted manual muscle testing. Supination and pronation.

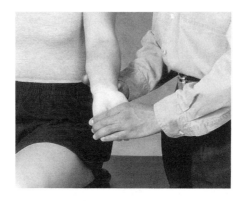

Fig. 12.33B: Wrist flexion and extension.

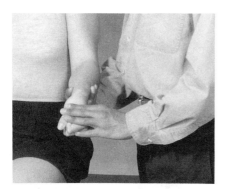

Fig. 12.33C: Ulnar and radial deviation.

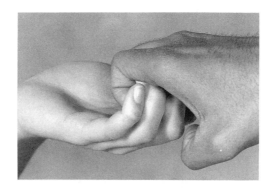

Fig. 12.33D: Finger flexion and extension.

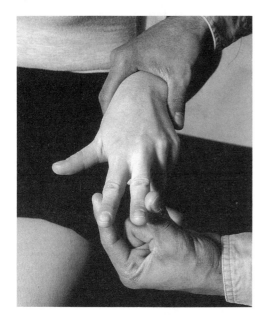

Fig. 12.33E: Finger abduction and adduction.

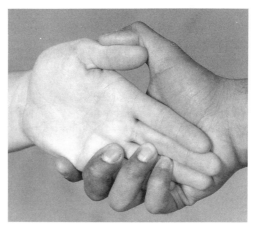

Fig. 12.33F: Thumb flexion and extension.

E. Finger abduction and adduction
F. Thumb flexion and extension
G. Thumb abduction and adduction
H. Opposition of the thumb and little finger

Neurological Testing

Neurological integrity can be assessed with the use of myotomes, reflexes, and segmental dermatomes and peripheral nerve cutaneous patterns.

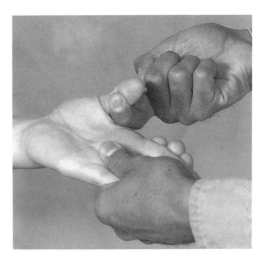

Fig. 12.33G: Thumb abduction and adduction.

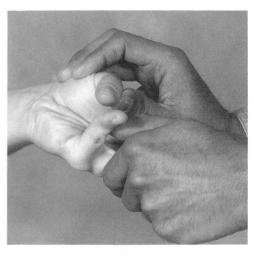

Fig. 12.33H: Opposition.

Myotomes

Isometric muscle testing to test the myotomes should be performed in the loose-packed position and include: scapular elevation (C_4), shoulder abduction (C_5), elbow flexion and/or wrist extension (C_6), elbow extension and/or wrist flexion (C_7), thumb extension and/or ulnar deviation (C^8), and abduction and/or adduction of the hand intrinsics (T_1).

Reflexes

Reflexes in the upper extremity include the biceps (C_5-C_6), brachioradialis (C_6), and triceps (C_7). These were discussed and demonstrated in Chapter 11.

Cutaneous Patterns

The segmental nerve dermatome patterns for the wrist and hand region are demonstrated

in **Figure 12-34**. The peripheral nerve cutaneous patterns are demonstrated in **Figure 12-35**. Test bilaterally for altered sensation with sharp and dull touch by running the open hand and fingernails over the shoulder and down both sides of the arms and hands.

Stress and Functional Tests

Stress tests are performed when you have a clear indication of what structures may be damaged. Use only those tests deemed relevant, and always compare the results to the uninvolved arm.

Ligamentous Instability Tests

Stabilize the thumb or finger with one hand proximal to the joint being tested. Apply a valgus and varus stress to the joint to test the integrity of the collateral ligaments (**Figure 12-36**). Do bilateral comparison with the

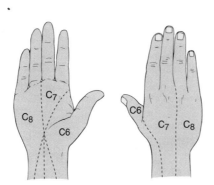

Fig. 12.34: Segmental dermatomes for the wrist and hand.

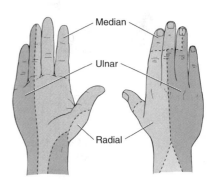

Fig. 12.35: Cutaneous nerve distribution patterns for the wrist and hand.

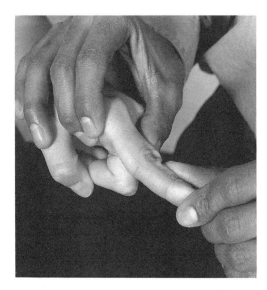

Fig. 12.36: To stress the ligamentous structures around the joints, apply a varus and valgus force at the specific joint.

uninvolved hand. This test is used for game-keeper's thumb or joint sprains of the fingers.

Finkelstein Test

Have the individual make a fist with the thumb inside the fingers (**Figure 12-37**). Stabilize the forearm and flex the wrist in an ulnar direction. A positive test, indicating de

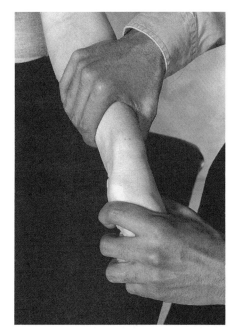

Fig. 12.37: Have the individual make a fist with the thumb inside the fingers. Flex the wrist in an ulnar direction. A positive Finkelstein's test indicates tenosynovitis of the thumb tendons.

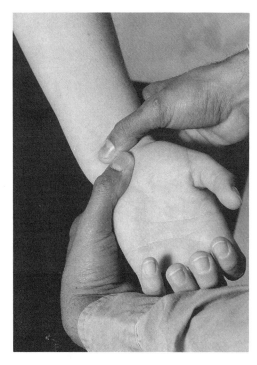

Fig. 12.38: Compression over the carpal tunnel may lead to tingling into the palmar aspect of the thumb, index finger, and middle finger, and indicates a carpal tunnel syndrome.

Quervain's tenosynovitis, produces pain over the abductor pollicis longus and extensor pollicis brevis tendons at the wrist. Because the test may be uncomfortable for even a healthy individual, all positive tests should be compared bilaterally to the uninvolved wrist.

Carpal Tunnel Compression Test

Exert even pressure with both thumbs directly over the carpal tunnel and hold for at least 30 seconds (**Figure 12-38**). A positive test produces numbness or tingling into the palmar aspect of the thumb, index finger, and middle finger.

Phalen's (Wrist Flexion) Test

Place the dorsum of the hands together to maximally flex the wrists. Hold this position for one minute by gently pushing the wrists together (**Figure 12-39**). A positive test, indicating either median nerve or ulnar nerve compression, produces numbness or tingling into the specific nerve distribution pattern. If the median nerve is compressed, sensory changes will be evident in the thumb, index finger, third finger, and lateral half of the ring finger. If the ulnar nerve is compressed, sen-

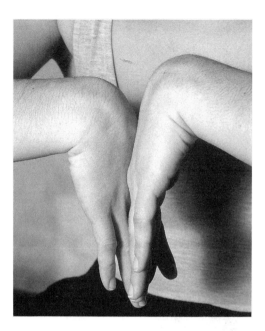

Fig. 12.39: Phalen's (wrist flexion) test indicates if the median or ulnar nerve is compressed by producing numbness or tingling into the specific nerve distribution pattern.

sory changes will occur in the fifth finger and medial half of the ring finger.

Tinel's Sign (at the wrist)

To test for median nerve compression, tap over the carpal tunnel at the wrist (**Figure 12-40**). A positive test produces numbness or

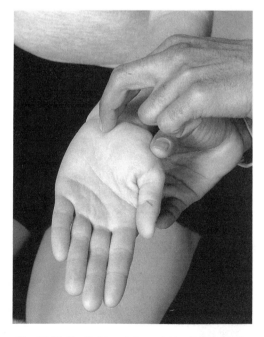

Fig. 12.40: Tinel's Sign at the wrist is also used to indicate median nerve compression.

tingling in the median nerve distribution. This test can also be adapted for ulnar nerve compression in the hypothenar mass and radial nerve compression on the dorsoradial aspect of the wrist.

Pinch Grip Test for Entrapment of the Anterior Interosseous Nerve

Ask the individual to pinch the tip of the index finger and thumb together (**Figure 12-41**). If an abnormal pulp to pulp pinch is performed, the anterior interosseous nerve, an extension of the median nerve, may be entrapped at the elbow as it passes between the two heads of the pronator teres.

Froment's Sign for Ulnar Nerve Paralysis

The patient grasps a piece of paper between the thumb and forefinger (**Figure 12-42**). The examiner attempts to pull the paper away. If the distal phalanx of the thumb flexes to hold the paper, it indicates paralysis of the adductor pollicis muscle indicative of ulnar nerve damage.

Functional Tests

Because the wrist, hand, and fingers are vital to perform activities of daily living, the individual should be assessed for manual dexterity and coordination. Can they hook, pinch, and grasp an object? Can they comb their hair, hold a fork, brush their teeth, or pick up a briefcase? Prior to return to sport, the individual should be able to perform these simple functional skills in addition to having bilateral range of motion and strength in the wrist and fingers.

The diver had pain on active and resisted wrist and finger flexion, particularly with the right hand. There was a slight sensory change on the palmar aspect of the thumb, second, and third fingers that was reproduced with the carpal tunnel compression test, Phalen's test, and the Tinel's sign. This individual has strained the flexor muscles of the wrist and fingers. The resulting inflammation has added compression to the median nerve in the carpal tunnel. How will you manage this condition?

REHABILITATION

The diver has a flexor wrist strain and mild carpal tunnel syndrome. After the physician assesses and treats the individual,

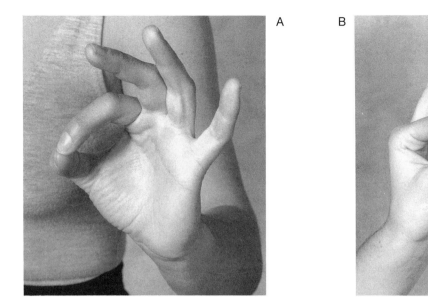

Fig. 12–41: Pinch Grip Test. Ask the individual to make an O with the thumb and forefinger. (A) Normal tip to tip. (B) Abnormal pulp to pulp signifies entrapment of the interior interosseous nerve.

what exercises should be included in the general rehabilitation program for this wrist injury?

Rehabilitation of the wrist and hand must involve exercises for the entire kinetic chain. Traumatic injuries to the wrist and hand often require immobilization, however, early range

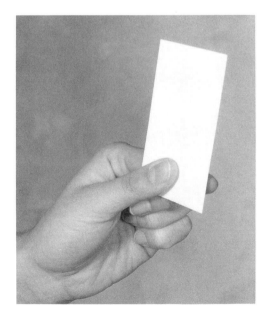

Fig. 12.42: If the individual flexes the distal phalanx of the thumb to prevent a piece of paper from being pulled away, the positive Froment's test indicates paralysis of the adductor pollicis muscle resulting from possible ulnar nerve damage.

of motion and strengthening exercises should be conducted at the elbow and shoulder. Many of the exercises for the wrist and hand were discussed and demonstrated in Chapter 11, because they are often combined with rehabilitation of the elbow.

Restoration of Motion

Immobilization typically results in joint contractures and stiffness in the fingers, therefore active range of motion exercises should begin as soon as possible. Exercises should focus on forearm pronation and supination, wrist flexion and extension, wrist radial and ulnar deviation, and finger and thumb flexion, extension, abduction, adduction, and opposition of the thumb. In the acute phase, exercises can be performed using cryokinetic techniques. Ice immersion is alternated with active range of motion exercises. The individual can use the opposite hand to apply a low load, prolonged stretch in the various motions to minimize joint trauma and increase flexibility. As inflammation decreases, a warm whirlpool or paraffin bath may be used to facilitate motion.

Restoration of Proprioception and Balance

Closed chain exercises involve those used in the elbow and shoulder, such as shifting body weight from one hand to the other on a wall, table top, or unstable surface, such as a foam mat or BAPS board. Push-ups and step-ups on a box, stool, or Stair Master can also be used.

Precision techniques to restore dexterity can be performed by picking up and manipulating the following objects: (a) coins of different thickness, (b) playing cards, (c) small objects of differing shapes, (d) large, light objects, and (e) large, heavy objects. In addition, the individual can tear tape, use scissors to cut paper, or juggle balls of different sizes.

Muscular Strength, Endurance, and Power

Once range of motion approximates normal for the individual, open chain kinetic exercises are performed in the various motions utilizing light-weight dumbbells. Many of these exercises were listed and explained in **Field Strategy 11-1**. The individual should

---

 Field Strategy 12–5. Wrist and Hand Evaluation.

History

Primary complaint including:
    Description and mechanism of current injury
    Onset of symptoms
Pain perception and discomfort
Disability and functional impairments from the injury
Previous injuries to the area
Family history

Observation and Inspection

Shape, contour, and posture of the hand
Inspection of the injured area for:

Muscle symmetry	Hypertrophy or muscle atrophy
Swelling	Visible congenital deformity
Discoloration	Surgical incisions or scars

Palpation

Bony structures to rule out fracture
Soft tissue structures to determine

Temperature	Deformity
Swelling	Muscle spasm
Point tenderness	Cutaneous sensation
Crepitus	Vascular pulses

Special Tests

Active range of motion
Passive range of motion
Resisted manual muscle testing
Neurologic testing
Stress tests and functional tests
    Ligamentous instability tests
    Finkelstein test for de Quervain's tenosynovitis
    Carpal tunnel compression test
    Phalen's wrist flexion test
    Tinel's signs for nerve entrapment
    Pinch grip test for anterior interosseus nerve entrapment
    Froment's sign for ulnar nerve paralysis
    Functional tests

---

complete 30 to 50 repetitions with a one pound weight, and should not progress in resistance until 50 repetitions are achieved. With the forearm supported on a table, perform wrist curls, reverse wrist curls, pronation, and supination. Wrist curl-ups using a light weight suspended from a broomstick on a three to four foot rope can be used to increase strength in the wrist flexors and extensors. A weighted bar or hammer can be used for radial and ulnar deviation, and pronation and supination. PNF resisted exercises, surgical tubing, or strong rubber bands can be used in all motions for concentric and eccentric loading. Gripping exercises using a tennis ball or putty can be combined with pinching small and large objects.

Plyometric exercises may involve catching a weighted ball in a single hand and throwing it straight up and down. A mini-tramp may be used to do bounding push-ups.

Cardiovascular Fitness

General body conditioning should be maintained throughout the rehabilitation program. Several examples of programs were provided in **Field Strategy 5-9,** and included use of a jump rope, Stair Master, treadmill, and upper body ergometer (UBE). *The diver should restore motion at the wrist and fingers, and begin early concentric and eccentric strengthening exercises using light resistance. Gripping exercises, PNF resisted exercises, and surgical tubing can be incorporated early in the program. Precision skills can be done to improve dexterity. The program should also include general body conditioning and strengthening exercises for the shoulder and elbow.*

SUMMARY

The hands of sport participants have special requirements for strength and dexterity, and can ill afford casual assessment and misdiagnosis. Failure to adequately assess the extent and seriousness of injury can lead to long-term deformity and disability. Although many injuries can be managed without seeking medical assistance, any injury that does not show an improvement within a week should be seen by a physician. Hand and wrist injuries that demand immediate attention by a physician include those with a suspected fracture or dislocation, significant pain, excessive swelling in soft tissues or around joints, joint instability,

loss of motion, or the presence of sensory changes. **Field Strategy 12-5** outlines a full wrist and hand assessment.

If a decision is made to refer the individual to a physician, immobilize the area in a wrist splint or sling to prevent further damage, apply ice to control hemorrhage and swelling, and transport the individual in an appropriate manner. Follow-up with the physician to obtain instructions for further care of the injury. When appropriate, protective braces or padding should be worn to prevent reinjury.

REFERENCES

1. Duda, M. 1987. Golf injuries: They really do happen. Phys Sportsmed, 15(6):191–196.
2. Johnson, RE, and Rust, RJ. 1985. Sports related injury: An anatomic approach, part 2. Minn Med, 68(11):829–831.
3. Shafer, JP (ed.). *Morris' human anatomy.* New York: Hafner, 1967.
4. Von Lanz, T, and Wachsmuth, W. "Functional anatomy." In *Bunnell's surgery of the hand,* edited by JH Boyes. Philadelphia: JB Lippincott, 1970.
5. Benjjani, FJ, and Landsmeer, JMF. *Basic biomechanics of the musculoskeletal system.* Philadelphia: Lea & Febiger, 1989.
6. Reid, DC. *Sports injury assessment and rehabilitation.* New York: Churchill Livingstone, 1992.
7. Ferlic, TP. "Hand and wrist injuries." In *The team physician's handbook* edited by MB Mellion, WM Walsh, and GL Shelton. Philadelphia: Hanley & Belfus, Inc, 1990.
8. Garrick, JG, and Webb, DR. *Sports injuries: Diagnosis and management.* Philadelphia: WB Saunders, 1990.
9. Evans, D, and Weightman, B. 1988. "The pipflex splint for treatment of mallet finger." J Hand Surg, Br. 13(2):156–158.
10. Warren, RA, Norris, SH, and Ferguson, DG. 1988. "Mallet finger: A trial of two splints." J Hand Surg, Br. 13(2):151–153.
11. Ryan, GM, and Mullins, PT. 1987. "Skin necrosis complicating mallet finger splinting and vascularity of the distal interphalangeal joint overlying skin." J Hand Surg, Am. 12A(4):548–552.
12. Souter, WA. 1974. "The problem of the boutonniere deformity." Clin Orthop Rel Res 104:116–133.
13. Posner, MA, Langa, V, and Green, SM. 1986. "The locked metacarpophalangeal joint: Diagnosis and treatment." J Hand Surg, Am. 11A(2):249–253.
14. Canales, FL, Newmeyer, WL, and Kilgore, ES. 1989. "The treatment of felons and paronychias." Hand Clin 5(4):515–523.
15. Bravaccio, F, Trabucco, M, Ammendola, A, and Cantore, R. 1990. "Carpal tunnel syndrome: A clinical electrophysiological study of 84 cases." Neurophysio Clin 20(4):269–281.
16. Pecina, MM, Krmpotic-Nemanic, J, and Markiewitz, AD. *Tunnel syndromes.* Boca Raton: CRC Press, 1991.
17. Murtagh, J. 1990. "The painful arm." Aust Fam Phys 19(9):1423–1426.

18. Durkan, JA. 1991. A new diagnostic test for carpal tunnel syndrome. J Bone Joint Surg, Am. 73A(4): 535–538.

19. Mellion, MB. 1991. Common cycling injuries: Management and prevention. Sports Med 11(1): 52–70.

20. Watson, JT. Fractures of the forearm and elbow. In *Clinics in sports medicine*, edited by JT Watson and JA Bergfeld, vol. 9, no. 1. Philadelphia: WB Saunders, 1990.

21. Riester, JN, Baker, BE, Mosther, JF, and Lowe, D. 1985. A review of scaphoid fracture healing in competitive athletes. Am J of Sports Med, 13(3):159–161.

22. Nakamura, P, Imaeda, T, and Miura. T, 1991. Scaphoid malunion. J Bone Joint Surg, Br., 73(1):134–137.

23. Howard, FM. 1987. Fractures of the basal joint of the thumb. Clin Orthop, 220(7):46–51.

24. Opgrande, JD, and Westphal, SA. 1983. Fractures of the hand. Orthop Clin North Am, 14(4):779–792.

25. Pollen, AG. 1968. The conservative treatment of Bennett's fracture: Subluxation of the thumb metacarpal. J Bone Joint Surg 50B:91–101.

26. Coonrad, RW, and Pholman, MH. 1969. Impacted fractures in the proximal portion of the proximal phalanx of the finger. J Bone Joint Surg 51A:1291–1296.

Injuries to the Axial Region

Injuries to the Axial Region

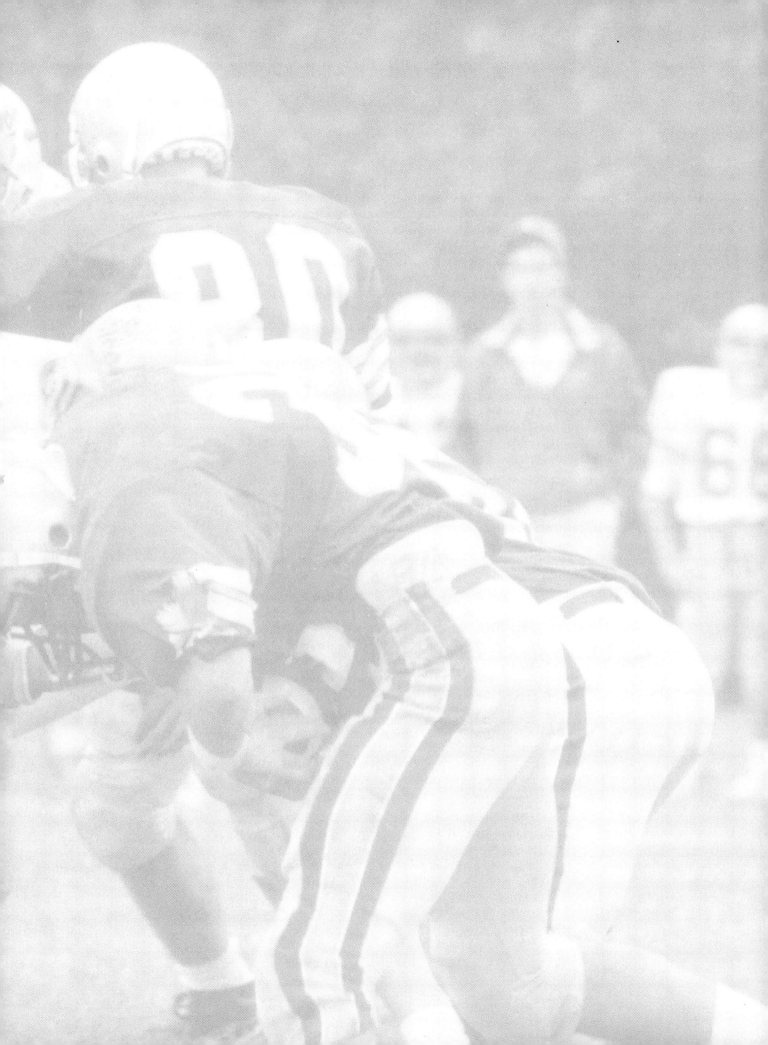

Maria Hutsick, M.S., L.A.T.,C.

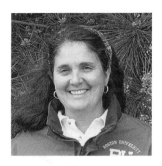

Maria Hutsick is the Head Athletic Trainer at Boston University in Boston, Massachusetts. As one of the few women who serve as the head athletic trainer at a Division I institution, Maria has established herself as an outstanding role model and professional in the field of athletic training.

I went to Ithaca College in New York to become a teacher. After fracturing my ankle in competition and observing what went on in the training room, however, I immediately switched over to the athletic training program. I did my Master's work at Indiana University, but in the early 1970s, women did not work with many of the men's sports. After coaching a year at Cortland, I landed my first training job at Yale University, and worked there for three years with Daphne Benas. She was great and helped me perfect many of my evaluation skills. Boston University hired me in 1980 as the Women's Athletic Trainer, and I eventually moved into the head athletic training position. Today, we take care of over 500 athletes with four staff trainers and one graduate assistant. Because of our NATA curriculum program, thankfully we also have the assistance of 25 student athletic trainers. We could not provide the quality care without these students.

As the Head Athletic Trainer, I am directly responsible for administering the budget, ordering all the protective equipment, hiring, supervising, and evaluating personnel, developing policies and procedures for the training room, doing physical exams, drug testing, supervising the treatment plans for rehabilitation and use of the modalities, assessing the clinical supervision of the student athletic trainers, and doing individual referrals to other medical professionals on campus.

I require the staff and student athletic trainers to wear a designated uniform and follow a strict conduct code, which includes not dating an athlete. I think this diminishes the professional standards we must maintain to carry out our role as part of the medical staff. Every time an athlete walks in the door, that visit is logged in and recorded in the athlete's S.O.A.P. notes in their permanent medical files. We have an excellent medical staff that respects the work the trainers do. The physicians and specialists contact me daily to discuss specific cases and treatment of the athletes.

When I was first appointed head trainer, the hardest thing to deal with was getting the football coaches and officials to recognize that I was the boss and they had to communicate with me. The players never blinked twice about having women in the locker room. They always respected and appreciated the care we provided, but the old football staff just couldn't accept it. Needless to say, they aren't with us anymore. Our current staff is excellent, but it's really a shame that women have to continually prove themselves in football, despite the fact that we are fully qualified.

Another realization about working at a big-time Division I school is the long hours. You have to be prepared to work ten hours a day, seven days a week, and no time off between seasons. For a woman, that means a limited social or personal life, especially if you are thinking of having a family. It's real tough, but it can be done. I require my staff to take one morning off a week just to get their errands done. Hopefully, this will avoid some burnout. All of us work out regularly, and recognize the need to stay healthy and fit.

Working on the university level is personally gratifying when you see these young women and men achieve success in their sport. But to be a trainer at this level, you have to be sharp, professional, and a cut above the next person. A master's degree in athletic training is almost essential. The job is exciting because you're always meeting new people and facing new challenges. You see people at their worst and most vulnerable state, yet you are the one to work with them and help them return safely to their sport. It's just neat to have that kind of positive impact on a person's well-being, and I love it. You just can't find a more challenging and satisfying career.

Head And Facial Injuries

After you have completed this chapter, you should be able to:

■ Locate the important bony and soft tissue structures of the head and facial region

■ Recognize the importance of wearing protective equipment to prevent injury to the head and facial region

■ Identify forces responsible for cranial injuries

■ Recognize important signs and symptoms that indicate a cranial injury

■ Demonstrate a thorough assessment of a cranial injury

■ Identify common facial injuries, their assessment and management

The head and facial areas are frequent sites for minor injuries including lacerations, contusions, and mild concussions. Although intracranial injuries have been a key factor in sport-associated fatalities—particularly in football and auto racing—the number of these fatalities has significantly decreased since the mid-1970s (1). Several factors account for this decrease including: (a) a conscious effort to establish standards for quality and protective properties of helmets used in competitive and recreational sports; (b) rule changes in football that prohibit leading with the head for contact; and (c) the development and use of the face mask (1). A significant decrease has also been seen in eye, ear, and dental injuries when protective equipment is worn.

This chapter begins with a review of the anatomy of the head and facial region. Discussion on prevention of injuries is followed by information on cranial injuries and their management, including a thorough assessment of a head injury. The final section discusses common injuries to the facial area and their management.

ANATOMY REVIEW OF THE HEAD AND FACIAL REGION

A basketball player has fallen and sustained what appears to be a superficial cut on the back of the head. The cut is bleed-ing profusely. What anatomical structure(s) are likely to have been damaged? How serious is this injury?

The review of anatomy focuses on bony structure, the brain and its coverings, and the nerve and blood supply to the region. Although the numerous muscles of the face and jaw enable speaking, chewing, and facial expression, because these muscles are not commonly involved in sport injuries they will not be discussed.

Bones of the Skull

The skull is primarily composed of flat bones that interlock at immovable joints called sutures **(Figure 13-1).** The cranial bones form the portion of the skull referred to as the cranium, the protective encasement for the brain. The thin bones of the cranium include the frontal, occipital, sphenoid, and ethmoid bones, as well as two parietal bones and two temporal bones. Material properties and thickness of the cranial bones vary. The facial bones provide the structure of the face and form the sinuses, orbits of the eyes, nasal cavity, and the mouth. The facial bones include paired maxilla, zygomatic, palatine, nasal, lacrimal, and inferior nasal concha bones, along with the bridge and mandible. The large opening at the base of the skull that sits atop the spinal column is called the foramen magnum.

> The cranium is divided from the face by an imaginary line that runs above the eyes and around the back of the ears

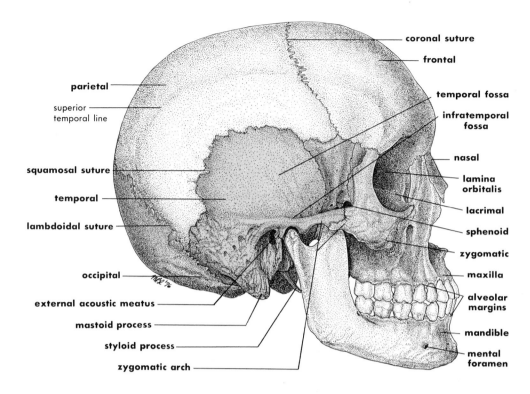

Fig. 13.1: The bones of the skull.

parietal
superior temporal line
squamosal suture
temporal
lambdoidal suture
occipital
external acoustic meatus
mastoid process
styloid process
zygomatic arch

coronal suture
frontal
temporal fossa
infratemporal fossa
nasal
lamina orbitalis
lacrimal
sphenoid
zygomatic
maxilla
alveolar margins
mandible
mental foramen

When a glancing blow to the head is sustained the scalp displaces, thereby dissipating force

White matter
Composed of myelinated nerve axons; it is the myelin sheaths that give the tissue its characteristic white coloring

Gray matter
Composed of neuron cell bodies, dendrites, and short unmyelinated axons

The Scalp

The scalp is composed of three layers: the skin, subcutaneous connective tissue, and the pericranium. The protective function of these tissues is enhanced by the hair as well as by the fact that the looseness of the scalp enables some dissipation of force when the head sustains a glancing blow. The scalp and face have an extensive blood supply, which is why superficial lacerations tend to bleed profusely.

The Brain

The four major regions of the brain are the cerebral hemispheres, diencephalon, brain stem, and cerebellum **(Figure 13-2)**. The left and right cerebral hemispheres form the major portion of the brain, accounting for 83% of total brain mass (2). Each hemisphere contains frontal, parietal, temporal and occipital lobes **(Figure 13-3).** The interior of the cerebral hemispheres is composed primarily of cerebral **white matter**, which is composed of myelinated nerve axons. The cerebral cortex, or outer layer of the brain, is composed of gray cells, including neuron cell bodies, dendrites, and short unmyelinated axons. It is the **gray matter** of the cerebral cortex that is responsible for motor and sensory function,

as well as consciousness, understanding, and memory.

The other major components of the brain lie interior to or beneath the cerebral hemispheres. The diencephalon, consisting of the thalamus, hypothalamus, and epithalamus, sits at the uppermost end of the brain stem. The brain stem itself includes the midbrain, pons, and medulla oblongata. The cerebellum, located on the inferior posterior aspect of the cerebrum, contributes to control of motor function.

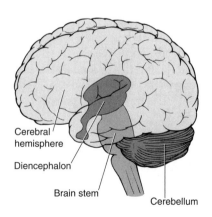

Cerebral hemisphere
Diencephalon
Brain stem
Cerebellum

Fig. 13.2: The four regions of the brain.

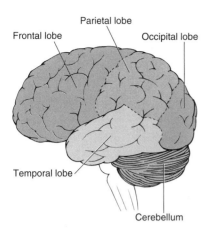

Parietal lobe
Frontal lobe
Occipital lobe

Temporal lobe

Cerebellum

Fig. 13.3: The lobes of the cerebral hemispheres.

The brain and spinal cord are enclosed in three layers of protective tissue known collectively as the **meninges (Figure 13-4)**. The outermost membrane is the dura mater, a thick, fibrous tissue containing **dural sinuses** that act as veins to transport blood from the brain to the jugular veins of the neck. The arachnoid mater is a thin membrane internal to the dura mater that is separated from the dura mater by the subdural space. Beneath the arachnoid mater is the subarachnoid space, which is filled with cerebrospinal fluid and contains the largest of the blood vessels supplying the brain. The arachnoid mater is connected to the inner pia mater by web-like strands of connective tissue. Whereas the dura mater and arachnoid mater are rather loose membranes, the pia mater is in direct contact with the cerebral cortex. The pia mater contains numerous small blood vessels.

The Eyes

The eye is a hollow sphere of approximately 2.5 cm (1 in) diameter in adults **(Figure 13-5)**. The anterior surface of the eye receives protection from the eyelids, eyelashes, and the attached conjunctiva. The conjunctiva is a membrane that lines the eyelids and the external surface of the eye. It secretes mucus that lubricates the external eye, reducing friction between the eyelids and external surface of the eye. The meibomian and ciliary glands, respectively located around the eyelash follicles and posterior to the eyelashes, also produce lubrication for the region. The lacrimal glands, located above the lateral ends of the eyes, continually release tears across the sur-

Menges
Three protective membranes that surround the brain and spinal cord

Dural sinuses
Formed by tubular separations in the inner and outer layers of the dura mater, these sinuses function as small veins for the brain

The meninges include the:
   Dura mater
   Arachnoid mater
   Pia mater

The anterior eye receives protection from the eyelids, eyelashes, and the attached conjunctiva

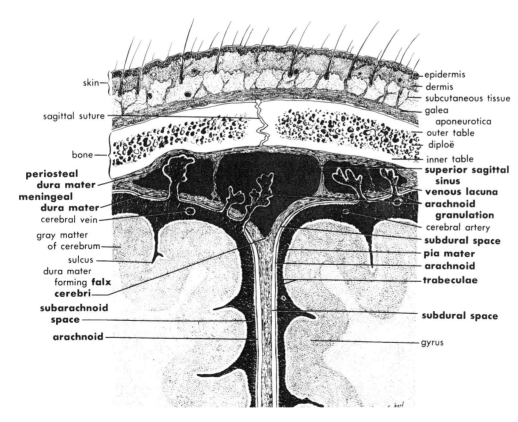

skin
sagittal suture
bone
periosteal dura mater
meningeal dura mater
cerebral vein
gray matter of cerebrum
sulcus
dura mater forming **falx cerebri**
subarachnoid space
arachnoid

epidermis
dermis
subcutaneous tissue
galea aponeurotica
outer table
diploë
inner table
superior sagittal sinus
venous lacuna
arachnoid granulation
cerebral artery
subdural space
pia mater
arachnoid
trabeculae
subdural space
gyrus

Fig. 13.4: The meninges.

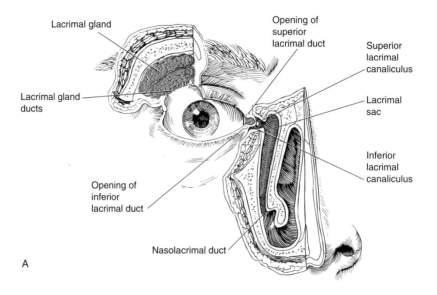

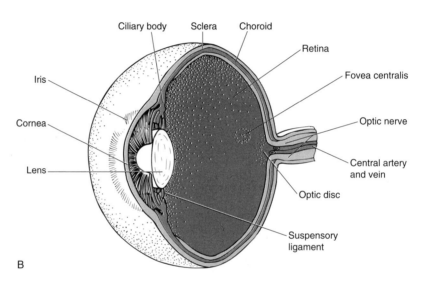

Fig. 13.5: The eye.

Tunics

Three layers of protective tissues that surround the eye

face of the eye through several small ducts. The lacrimal ducts, located at the medial corners of the eyes, serve as drains for moisture from the eye. These ducts funnel moisture from each eye into the lacrimal sac, then into the nasolacrimal duct that drains into the nasal cavity.

Like the brain, the eye is surrounded by three protective tissue layers, which in the eye are known as **tunics**. The outer tunic is a thick white connective tissue called the sclera, or fibrous tunic. It is the sclera that forms the "white of the eye." The central anterior sclera, however, is clear to permit passage of light into the eye. This transparent region of the sclera is known as the cornea. The choroid, the middle covering of the eye, is a highly vascularized tissue. The anterior choroid is continuous with the ciliary body and iris, which usually appears to be blue or brown, and has a central circular opening called the pupil. The iris controls the size of the pupil, regulating the amount of light that enters the eye. The internal tunic of the eye is the retina, which extends posteriorly from the ciliary body. It is the retina that contains light-sensitive photoreceptor cells that stimulate nerve endings to provide sight.

Nerves of the Head and Face

Twelve pairs of cranial nerves emerge from the brain, some with motor functions, some with sensory functions, and some with both (**Figure 13-6**). The cranial nerves are numbered and named in accordance with their

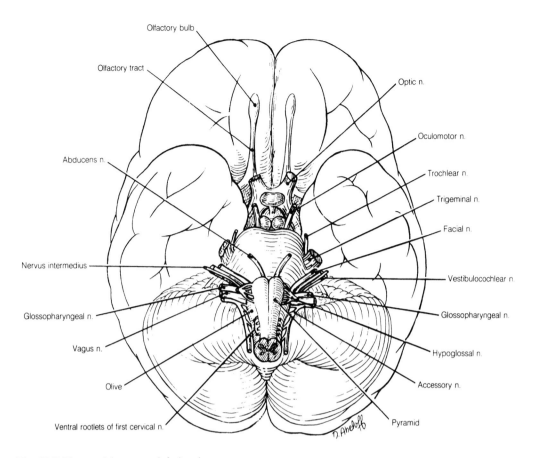

Fig. 13.6: The cranial nerves—inferior view.

functions, as listed in **Table 13-1**. Cranial nerves with purely sensory functions include the olfactory (smell), optic (vision), vestibulo-cochlear (hearing and equilibrium), and vagus (taste and sensation to the throat region). Those with purely motor functions

Table 13–1. The Cranial Nerves.

Number	Name	Sensory	Motor	Function
I	Olfactory	X		Sense of smell
II	Optic	X		Vision
III	Oculomotor		X	Control of some of the extrinsic eye muscles
IV	Trochlear		X	Control of other of the extrinsic eye muscles
V	Trigeminal	X	X	Sensation of the facial region and movement of the jaw muscles
VI	Abducens		X	Control of lateral eye movement
VII	Facial	X	X	Control of facial movement, taste, and secretion of tears and saliva
VIII	Vestibulocochlear	X		Hearing and equilibrium
IX	Glossopharyngeal	X	X	Taste, control of the tongue and pharynx, secretion of saliva
X	Vagus	X		Taste, sensation to the pharynx, larynx, trachea, and bronchioles
XI	Accessory		X	Control of movements of the pharynx, larynx, head, and shoulders
XII	Hypoglossal		X	Control of tongue movements

are the oculomotor and trochlear (extrinsic eye muscles), abducens (muscles responsible for lateral eye movement), accessory (selected muscles of the head and shoulder regions), and hypoglossal (muscles of the tongue). The remaining cranial nerves have both sensory and motor functions; the trigeminal nerve provides sensation in the facial region and motor supply to the jaw muscles, the facial nerve contributes to taste, the secretion of tears and saliva, and motor supply to some of the facial muscles, and the glossopharyngeal nerve contributes to taste, the secretion of saliva, and motor supply to the tongue and pharynx.

Blood Vessels of the Head and Face

The major vessels supplying the head and face are the common carotid and vertebral arteries (**Figure 13-7**). The common carotid artery ascends through the neck on either side, dividing into the external and internal carotid arteries just below the level of the jaw. The left and right vertebral arteries and their branches furnish blood supply to the posterior region of the brain.

The external carotid arteries send off numerous branches to supply most regions of the head external to the brain. Included are the superior thyroid arteries, which supply the thyroid and larynx, the facial arteries to the muscles and skin of the anterior portion of the face, the lingual arteries to the tongue, and the occipital arteries to the posterior aspect of the scalp. At about the level of the ear the external carotid artery divides into the superficial temporal artery, which supplies the majority of the scalp, and the maxillary artery, which supplies the muscles of the jaw and lower face, as well as the teeth and the nasal cavity. The middle meningeal artery branches upward from the maxillary artery through the floor of the cranium to supply the skull and dura mater. If this artery is damaged, serious epidural bleeding can result.

The internal carotid arteries send off the ophthalmic arteries to the eyes, and then divide to form the anterior and middle cerebral arteries. The left and right anterior cere-

> The common carotid artery is superficial on the lateral anterior aspect of the neck just below the jaw, where it may be readily palpated. Severance of this major artery can result in death in a matter of minutes

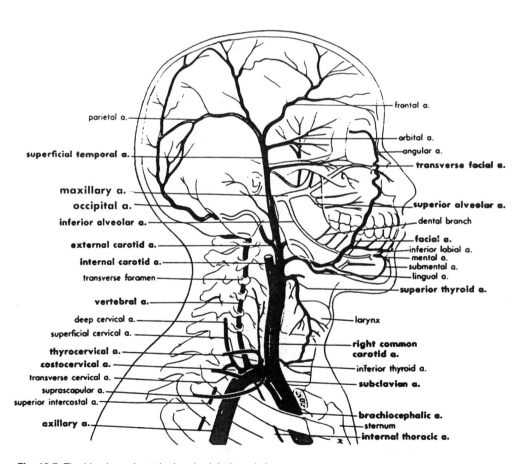

Fig. 13.7: The blood supply to the head—right lateral view.

bral arteries interconnect through the anterior communicating artery, providing blood supply to the medial surfaces of the cerebral hemispheres. The middle cerebral arteries supply the lateral aspects of the parietal and temporal lobes of the cerebrum.

💡 *Because the scalp and face have an extensive blood supply, superficial lacerations of the head tend to bleed profusely. If there are no signs of a concussion or other more serious injury, (discussed later in the Chapter), the injury is probably a superficial cut of the scalp.*

PREVENTION OF HEAD AND FACIAL INJURIES

❓ *What steps can a football player take to prevent head and facial injuries?*

The head and facial area is constantly subjected to impact forces during sport participation. In reviewing measures normally taken to prevent injuries at the other joints, i.e., protective equipment, physical conditioning, and proper skill technique, by far, the most important preventative measure for the head and facial area is use of protective equipment. Many sports, such as baseball/softball, competitive bicycling, fencing, field hockey, football, hockey, lacrosse, and wrestling require some type of head or facial protective equipment for participation. Protective equipment, when properly used, can protect the head and facial area from accidental or routine injuries. However, even regular use cannot prevent all injuries. To be effective, equipment must be properly fitted, clean, in good condition, utilized regularly, and used in the manner for which it was designed.

Protective equipment includes the helmet, face guard, mouth guard, eye wear, ear wear, and throat protector. Helmets protect the cranial portion of the skull by absorbing and dispersing impact forces, thereby reducing cerebral trauma. Face guards protect and shield the facial region from flying projectiles. Mouth guards have been shown to reduce dental and oral soft tissue injuries, as well as reduce cerebral concussions, jaw fractures, and temporomandibular joint injuries. Eye wear, ear wear, and throat protectors reduce injuries to their respective regions. Refer to Chapter 6 to review head and facial protection.

💡 *A football player can protect the head and facial region by wearing a face guard and helmet that is approved by the* National Operating Committee for Athletic Equipment (NOCSAE). In addition, protective eye wear and a mouth guard can be worn to protect the eyes and oral region.

CRANIAL INJURY MECHANISMS

❓ *Think about what happens to the skull and brain during impact from a solid object. Will damage be limited to the area directly under the point of impact? Why or why not?*

Impact forces to the cranial area may be sustained locally by direct impact or transmitted through other structures. Direct impact causes two phenomena to occur. First, local elements beneath the site of impact cause deformation of the skull, and shock waves pass through the skull to the brain. The occurrence of a skull fracture or intracranial injury is dependent on the material properties of the skull, thickness of the skull in the specific area, magnitude and direction of impact, and size of the impact area (3).

Mechanical failure in bone typically results from an overload of tensile stress rather than compression. For example, when a blow impacts the skull the bone deforms and bends inward, placing the inner border of the skull under tensile strain, whereas the outer border is placed in compression (**Figure 13-8A**). If impact is of sufficient magnitude and the skull is thin in the region of impact, a skull fracture will occur at the site where tensile loading occurs. In contrast, if the skull is thick and dense enough at the area of impact, it may sustain inward bending without fracture. However, fracture may occur some distance from the impact zone in a region where the skull is thinner (**Figure 13-8B**). Protective equipment is designed to disperse these forces over a larger area, thus reducing mechanical load on a specific site.

Secondly, impact causes acceleration; whether the head is directly impacted or set in motion by forces exerted elsewhere in the body, the result is the same. Acceleration causes shear, tensile, and compression strains within the brain substance, with shear being the most serious (3). Axial rotation coupled with acceleration can lead to injuries away from the actual injury site, referred to as a **contrecoup injury (Figure 13-9)**.

Intracranial cerebral trauma can be focal or diffuse. **Focal injuries** involve local damage and account for over two thirds of all

To be effective, equipment must be properly fitted, clean, in good condition, utilized regularly, and used in a manner in which it was designed to be used

Impact forces to the cranial area may be sustained locally or transmitted through other structures

Skull fractures are dependent on:
    material properties of the skull
    thickness of the skull in various areas
    magnitude and direction of impact
    size of the impact area

Acceleration forces cause shear, tensile, and compression strains within the brain substance, with shear being the most serious

Contrecoup injuries
Injuries away from the actual injury site due to axial rotation and acceleration

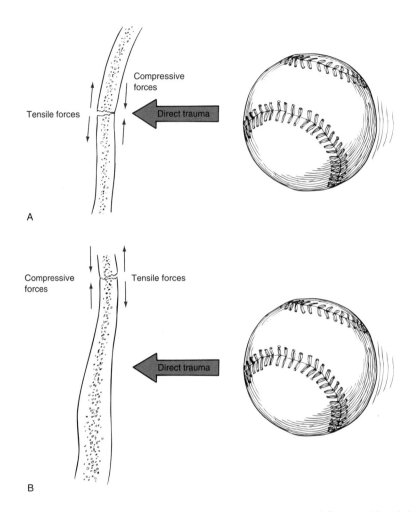

Fig. 13.8: Mechanical failure in bone. When a blow impacts the skull, the bone deforms and bends inward placing tensile stress on the inner border of the skull. (A) If impact is of sufficient magnitude and the skull is thin in the region of impact, a skull fracture occurs at the impact site. (B) If the skull is thick and dense enough at the area of impact, it may sustain bending inward without fracture. However, the fracture may occur some distance from the impact zone in another region where the skull is thinner.

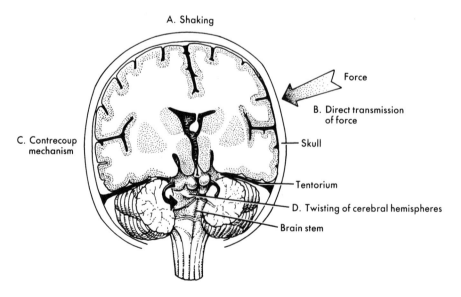

Fig. 13.9: Axial rotation coupled with acceleration can lead to injuries away from the actual injury site, called a contrecoup injury.

head injury deaths (3,4). Injuries such as an epidural hematoma, subdural hematoma, and intracerebral hematoma fall into this category. **Diffuse injuries**, typically caused by acceleration, can involve widespread disruption and damage to the function and/or structure of the brain (5). Cerebral concussions fall into this category. Although diffuse injuries account for only one quarter of the fatalities due to head trauma, they are the most prevalent cause of long-term neurological deficits in individuals (3).

If cerebral injuries are recognized and treated immediately, the severity is limited to the initial structural damage. If other factors, however, such as ischemia, hypoxia, cerebral swelling, and hemorrhaging around the brain occur, additional damage and possible neurological dysfunction result (3). It is important, therefore, to accurately assess head injuries, and initiate prompt medical attention to rule out serious underlying problems that may complicate the original injury. A conscious, ambulatory individual should not be considered to have only a minor injury, but rather should be continually assessed to determine if post-traumatic signs or symptoms indicate a more serious underlying condition.

Impact forces cause skull deformation and shock waves to pass through the skull to the brain. Rotation coupled with acceleration causes shear, tensile, and compression strains elsewhere in the brain. As such, the probability exists that damage will occur at the point of impact and/or at a point away from the site of impact as a contrecoup injury.

SKULL FRACTURES

During hitting practice a foul tip struck the head of another baseball player standing near the dugout. The skin is not broken but the individual is complaining of an intense headache, disorientation, blurred vision, and cannot recall what happened. What signs might indicate that a skull fracture is present?

Skull fractures may be *linear* (in a line), *comminuted* (in multiple pieces), *depressed* (fragments are driven internally toward the brain), or *basilar* (involving the base of the skull (**Figure 13-10**) (6,7). They may also be classified as closed (simple), not involving a break in the skin or underlying membrane; compound, which implies a superficial skin laceration adjacent to the fracture site; and

Focal injuries
Localized cerebral damage

Diffuse injuries
Widespread disruption to the function and/or structure of the brain

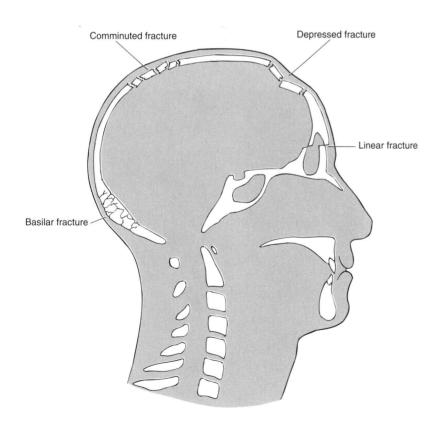

Fig. 13.10: Fractures of the skull are categorized as linear, comminuted, depressed, or basilar.

Meningitis
Inflammation of the meninges of the brain and spinal column

Raccoon eyes
Delayed discoloration around the eyes from anterior cranial fossa fracture

Battle's sign
Delayed discoloration behind the ear due to basilar skull fracture

open, which implies a skin laceration adjacent to the fracture site and a tear to the underlying dura mater are present. A danger with open fractures is the greater risk of bacterial infection through the fracture site into the intracranial cavity, which can result in septic **meningitis**. Whenever a severe blow to the head occurs, a skull fracture should be suspected. Blows may occur as a result of hitting one's head on a diving board or floor, being struck with a bat or ball, or in a collision with another player. Skull fractures are often difficult to detect and may be overlooked when a deep scalp hematoma is present.

Depending on the fracture site, different signs may appear. For example, a fracture at eyebrow level may travel into the anterior cranial fossa and sinuses leading to discoloration around the eyes (**raccoon eyes**). Blood or cerebrospinal fluid (CSF) may leak from the nose. Bony fragments may damage the optic or olfactory cranial nerves leading to blindness or loss of smell. A basilar fracture above and behind the ear may lead to **Battle's sign**, a discoloration that can appear within a matter of minutes behind the ear (**Figure 13-11**). With this fracture, blood or cerebrospinal fluid may leak from the ear canal. Basilar skull fractures are critical because of possible laceration to the dura mater, arachnoid mater, or cranial nerves leading to a hearing loss or facial paralysis. A fracture to

either side of the temple region may damage the meningeal arteries causing an epidural hemorrhage between the dura mater and skull (epidural hematoma). Intracranial hemorrhaging can be life-threatening and will be discussed in more detail in the section on cerebral injuries. **Table 13-2** summarizes signs and symptoms that indicate a possible skull fracture.

A skull fracture requires immediate action. Fluids from the ears or nose indicate serious danger. To determine if cerebrospinal fluid is present, gently absorb some of the fluid onto a gauze pad and watch the clear fluid separate from the blood. This is called "targeting" or the "halo test," but may not always be reliable (8). Do not apply any pressure bandage or attempt to restrict the flow of fluid as it may increase intracranial pressure complicating a brain injury. Immediately initiate the emergency care plan and summon an ambulance. Monitor vital signs and initiate any emergency procedures (artificial ventilation or CPR) if necessary. Cover open wounds with a sterile dressing but do not apply pressure. Stabilize the neck region, as it may also be injured. Periodically recheck vital signs and treat for shock until help arrives. **Field Strategy 13-1** suggests management of a suspected skull fracture.

Signs that indicate a possible skull fracture include deformity, unequal pupils,

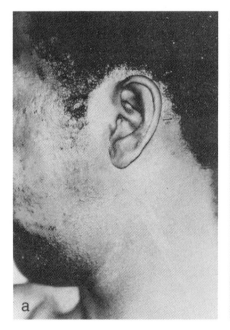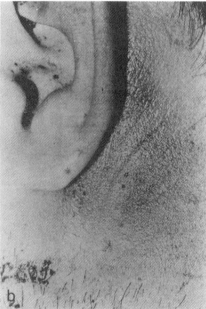

Fig. 13.11: Signs of a skull fracture include: (A) cerebrospinal fluid from the ear or nose, and (B) mastoid ecchymosis (Battle's sign), a discoloration that appears within minutes behind the ear.

Table 13–2. Identifying Possible Skull Fractures.

Suspect a skull fracture if any of the following are present:
- Visible deformity can be seen
  Do not be misled by a "goose egg." A fracture may be under the site
- Deep laceration or severe bruise to the scalp
  Do not probe into the wound or separate the skin edges
- Palpable depression or crepitus
- Unequal pupils
- Discoloration under both eyes (raccoon eyes) or behind the ear (Battle's sign)
  This may be a delayed finding
- Bleeding or clear fluid (CSF) from the nose and/or ear
- Loss of smell
- Loss of sight or major vision disturbances
- Individual is unconscious after direct trauma to the head for more than 2 minutes

discoloration around both eyes or behind the ears, bleeding or cerebrospinal fluid leaking from the nose and/or ear, and any loss of sight or smell. If any of these signs are present summon an ambulance immediately.

CEREBRAL HEMATOMAS

(?) *A softball player collided with the shortstop accidentally taking an elbow to the side of the head. The individual is dazed and is removed from the game. After 15 minutes of icing the region the individual has an increasing headache and is feeling nauseous. The player appears lethargic, disoriented, and sensitive to sunlight. What might be happening? How will you manage this injury?*

A hematoma is a collection of blood, or a blood clot, in a localized area. Within the skull there is no room for additional accumulation of blood or fluid. Any additional foreign matter within the cranial cavity increases pressure on the brain, leading to significant alterations in neurological function. Depending on the location of the blood clot relative to the dura mater, these hematomas are classified as epidural (outside the dura mater), or subdural (deep to the dura mater).

Epidural Hematoma

An epidural hematoma, typically caused by a direct blow to the side of the head, is almost always associated with a skull fracture (**Figure 13-12A**) (9). If the middle meningeal

Hematomas within the skull are classified in relation to the dura mater, and include epidural (outside the dura mater), or subdural (inside the dura mater)

Epidural hematomas frequently invoke tearing of the middle meningeal artery leading to a "high pressure" hematoma

 Field Strategy 13–1. Management of a Suspected Skull Fracture.

- Stabilize the head and neck
- Check the ABCs
- Initiate emergency care plan and summon EMS
- Take vital signs
- Observe for:
  Swelling or discoloration around the eyes or behind the ears
  Blood or CSF leaking from the nose or ears
  Pupil size, pupillary response to light, and eye movement
- Palpate for depressions, blood, and crepitus. Palpate cervical vertebrae for associated neck injury
- Cover any open wounds with a sterile dressing but do not apply pressure
- Elevate the upper body and head if there is no evidence of shock, neck, or spinal injury. If present, keep the individual lying flat
- Recheck vital signs and symptoms every five minutes until ambulance arrives
- Treat for shock and monitor ABCs

artery or its branches are severed, the subsequent arterial bleeding will lead to a "high-pressure" epidural hematoma. The individual may appear fine for a short time, but within 10 to 20 minutes will show signs and symptoms of neurological deterioration. This deterioration may include increased headache, drowsiness, nausea, vomiting, decreased level of consciousness, and a dilated pupil on the side of the hematoma coupled with muscular weakness on the side opposite the hematoma (5,9). Immediate surgery is needed to **decompress** the hematoma and control arterial bleeding.

Subdural Hematoma

A subdural hematoma occurs deep to the dura mater and involves bleeding from a cerebral vein rather than an artery (**Figure 13-12B**). As impact occurs to the side of the head, the brain is thrust against the point of impact, tearing veins on the opposite side (6). This contrecoup, or rotational acceleration injury, tears the bridging veins, leading to low-pressure venous bleeding. The hematoma usually forms very slowly. Signs and symptoms may not become apparent for hours, days, or even weeks after injury when the clot absorbs fluid and expands (6,10).

In an acute subdural hematoma, the blood clot generally accompanies simultaneous

brain injury. Blood accumulates rapidly. The individual is typically knocked out and remains unconscious. Signs of rapidly increasing intracranial pressure include a dilated pupil on the affected side, reduced pulse, vomiting, and **dyspnea**. In general, approximately three times as many acute subdural hematomas occur as compared to epidural hematomas (5,9).

In a subacute, or simple subdural hematoma, there may or may not be a loss of consciousness. Signs and symptoms may not be present for 24 hours or more after injury. Brain injury is usually not substantial; otherwise, the hematoma would be identified much earlier. Because of delayed signs and symptoms, this subacute injury is the most prevalent cause of death from trauma in contact sports.

Chronic subdural hematomas are rare and more commonly seen in the elderly, partially due to atrophy of the brain with aging (7). These hematomas result in a small amount of bleeding that becomes surrounded by a semipermeable membrane. As osmotic pressure changes, fluid moves into the capsule, increasing the size of the hematoma. Initially, signs and symptoms are nonexistent to mild. Two or more weeks later, however, an increasing persistent headache, vomiting, or change in behavior may progress to loss of appetite, blurred vision, drowsiness, and gait disturbances.

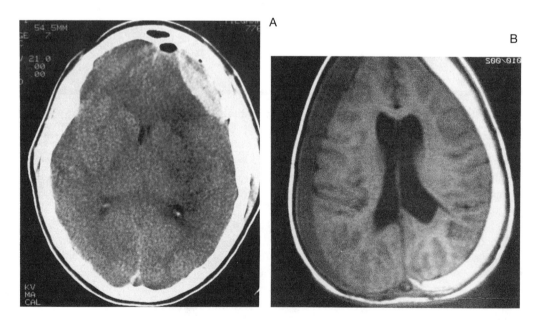

Fig. 13.12: Cerebral hematomas. (A) This epidural hematoma resulted from a fracture that extended into the orbital roof and sinus area leading to rapid hemorrhage in the right frontal lobe of the brain. (B) The subdural hematoma on the right side of the brain is fairly evident, however, note the darkened area on the far left side of the brain. This indicates bilateral subdural hematomas of different ages.

Once identified, the hematomas require surgical drainage. Acute subdural hematomas have a poorer prognosis because of the associated brain injury. Subacute and chronic subdural hematomas respond better to treatment without associated or prolonged brain dysfunction (7). Thus, the coach, athletic trainer, or sport supervisor must be suspicious of a blow to the head and carefully watch the person for complications. In addition, long-term observation should be continued. **Table 13-3** is an example of an information sheet that can be given to parents of minor children who have sustained a head injury. This information should inform parents of danger signs that indicate a serious underlying problem, and can alert parents to seek immediate medical treatment for the child, should the condition deteriorate.

💡 *The softball player is experiencing an increase in intracranial pressure, possibly due to an epidural hematoma. Disorientation, headache, and nausea are red flags indicating serious intracranial hemorrhage. Summon EMS to transport this individual to the nearest medical facility.*

CONCUSSIONS

❓ *A swimmer misjudged the distance to the wall and collided head-first into the wall. The individual was momentarily stunned, "saw stars," and had blurred vision for about 30 seconds. After three or four minutes the individual reports feeling much better except for a slight headache. What signs and symptoms indicate a progressive serious problem that needs immediate care?*

A "**concussion**" literally means a violent shaking or jarring action that can result in immediate or transient impairment of neurological function. Under normal conditions the brain balances a series of electrochemical

Concussion
Violent shaking or jarring action of the brain resulting in immediate or transient impairment of neurologic function

---

Table 13–3. Information Sheet on Follow-up Care for a Head Injury.

_____ has recently received a head injury during interscholastic athletic practice. Often many signs and symptoms from a head injury do not become apparent until hours after the initial trauma. As such, we want to alert you to possible signs and symptoms that may indicate a significant head injury. If you observe any of these symptoms, please seek medical help immediately.

- Persistent or increasing headache, particularly if it becomes localized
- Restless, irritable, or drastic changes in emotional control
- Mental confusion or disorientation that gets progressively worse
- Loss of appetite
- Drowsiness, lethargy, or sleepiness
- Unequal pupils or dilated pupils
- Bleeding and/or clear fluid from the nose or ears
- Persistent or increasing nausea and/or vomiting
- Progressive or sudden impairment of consciousness
- Alterations in breathing pattern
- Dizziness or unsteady gait
- Difficulty speaking or slurring of speech

For the rest of the day _____ should:

- Rest quietly
- Not consume any medication except Tylenol as prescribed
- Not consume alcohol
- Not drive a vehicle

She/He should not participate or play again without medical clearance by a doctor.

Emergency Phone Numbers:
Ambulance   911
Hospital_____

Remember: If any of the symptoms or signs listed above become apparent, do not delay seeking medical treatment.

events in billions of brain cells. With shaking or jarring of even the slightest magnitude, brain function can be disrupted, at least temporarily, without causing anatomical or structural damage to brain tissue. Therefore, physiologic cerebral dysfunction can occur in the absence of damage to brain tissue (11). For example, with mild trauma, cerebral function is first interrupted. Signs and symptoms will fall in the mild or moderate range, and are transient and reversible since damage to soft tissue structures is minimal. As impact magnitude increases with an acceleration injury, both cerebral function and cerebral structural damage occurs, resulting in more serious signs and symptoms. These include varying degrees of consciousness, headache, memory loss, nausea, tinnitus, pupillary changes, confusion, dizziness, and loss of coordination. Concussions are graded by the length of mental impairment and loss of memory before and after injury. Signs and symptoms for the various grades of concussions are summarized in **Table 13-4.** Grades I and II are ranked as mild concussions, grade III is a moderate concussion, and grades IV and V are severe concussions. Grade VI concussions are associated with death.

Grade I Concussion

A grade I concussion involves no loss of consciousness. The force of impact may lead to slight alterations in neurological function, such as slight mental confusion, dizziness, minimal unsteadiness, and a brief loss of judgment. The individual may simply report "I had my bell rung." Usually the state of confusion is over within 5 to 15 minutes and the individual can return to sport participation, but should be carefully watched for any signs of deterioration. Symptoms such as unsteady balance (**vertigo**), headache, nausea, **photophobia**, mood swings or anxiety should preclude the individual from returning to activity (4,5,9). A second mild concussion during the same game, or within a few days should mandate removal from activity for about two weeks (12). All symptoms should be absent for one week before being allowed to return to participation.

Grade II Concussion

With a grade II concussion, there is a transitory loss of consciousness lasting from a few

seconds up to three to four minutes. This stage is followed by mental confusion, moderate dizziness and unsteady gait, blurred vision, **tinnitus**, and headache. **Post-traumatic memory loss** develops after 5 to 15 minutes, and is a very common symptom. This memory loss may diminish somewhat, but the player will always have some degree of permanent, although short memory loss about the injury (11). This individual should not be allowed to continue play that day. They may develop "**postconcussion syndrome**" which can last for several weeks (4). This condition is characterized by persistent headaches, blurred vision, irritability, and inability to concentrate even on the simplest task. This individual should be thoroughly evaluated by a physician. Return to play may occur one week after being asymptomatic during rest and exercise. After a second grade II concussion, return to play may be delayed for at least one month. Three concussions should necessitate further neurological assessment and termination of activity for the season.

Grade III Concussion

With a grade III concussion the individual will experience many of the symptoms in a grade II concussion. Unconsciousness will last more than two minutes and can extend up to five minutes. If examined immediately after injury, the individual may have total recall of events prior to the injury. As the condition deteriorates, however, **retrograde amnesia** develops (5,9). This individual may be conscious, disoriented, and have marked unsteadiness for more than 10 minutes. One or both eyes may appear dilated or irregular, be sensitive to light, and exhibit involuntary eye movement (**nystagmus**). Later, the individual may appear fine and ready to re-enter the game, then suddenly collapse (4). An individual who is unable to remember events leading up to the injury, or events following the injury should not be permitted to continue play, and should be referred immediately to a physician. The individual should be excluded from participation for one month, including at least two weeks without symptoms. Two grade III concussions in the same season mandates removal from participation for the rest of the season. If asymptomatic at the start of the next season, the individual may be allowed to participate.

Table 13–4. Signs and Symptoms of Concussions.

Degree of Concussion	Mild		Moderate	Severe	
	Grade I	Grade II	Grade III	Grade IV	Grade V
Loss of Consciousness	None	Few seconds up to 3 to 4 minutes	Unconscious for 2 to 5 minutes, or may appear normal, then suddenly collapse	Involves being "knocked-out." May appear in paralytic coma and pass through stages of stupor	Person in paralytic coma. May need CPR
Headache	None	Mild	Moderate	Severe	Convulsions may occur
Confusion	Slight/ temporary	Mild	Moderate	Severe	Initially severe with or without delirium; then may become alert
Dizziness	Slight/ temporary	Moderate	Moderate	Severe	Severe
Memory loss	None	Post-traumatic amnesia present after injury. Transient and reversible	Post-traumatic amnesia for 5 to 15 minutes Memory usually returns within 6 hours	Post-traumatic amnesia and retrograde amnesia present	Post-traumatic amnesia, retrograde amnesia and post-concussion syndrome present
Nausea	None	Slight	Present	Present	Present
Tinnitus	None	Slight	Moderate	Severe	Severe
Pupils/Vision	Normal	Normal pupils Blurred vision	One or both dilated. Nystagmus and photophobia present	One or both dilated. Nystagmus and photophobia present	Both dilated initially but may appear unequal later
Balance problems	Minimal	Mild + Romberg as are other special tests	May appear normal, then collapse Moderate + Romberg as are other tests	Severe + Romberg as are other special tests	

An individual who cannot remember events leading up to the injury or after the injury should be referred immediately to a physician

Grade IV Concussion

A grade IV concussion is characterized by being "knocked out", and is sometimes referred to as a diffuse axonal injury associated with a cerebral contusion. An inability to stimulate movement, or paralytic coma, can last a few seconds to several minutes, followed by progression through the stages of stupor (4). They appear confused with or without delirium, then pass through a lucid state before becoming fully alert and oriented to the surroundings. Post-traumatic memory loss, retrograde amnesia, and post-concussion syndrome may be present. Convulsions may be triggered by the concussion (12). If unconsciousness lasts for more than five minutes or if other signs of neurological deficits become apparent, this individual should be placed on a spineboard or stretcher, removed from the field, and transported to the nearest medical facility (5,9).

Grade V Concussion

Impact, acceleration, and shearing forces can lead to severe diffuse axonal injuries. At impact, shearing causes blood vessels to rupture within the brain, the diencephalon, and/or the brainstem leading to severe bleeding within the cranial cavity. The resulting coma may be associated with altered vital signs, unequal pupils, and partial paralysis of one side of the body. As bleeding continues, intracranial pressure rises, leading to further cerebral structural damage.

Decortication (extension of the legs with flexion of the elbows, wrists, and fingers) or decerebration (extension of all four extremities) are often present (See **Figure 3-10**). Collapse of the cardiorespiratory system may require that CPR be implemented (4). Immediate recognition and transportation to the nearest medical facility permits a prompt diagnosis. Surgical decompression is usually not required unless damage is extensive.

Grade VI Concussion

Severe head trauma in a grade V concussion can lead to massive intracranial bleeding, total cardiorespiratory collapse, and death.

The individual was momentarily stunned, "saw stars," and had blurred vision. This is not uncommon in a grade I concussion. However, a lingering headache should signal caution. This individual should be carefully watched for increases in headache, an unsteady gait, nausea, photophobia, or mood swings, which dictate immediate referral to a physician.

SCALP INJURIES

An individual has a scalp laceration that is bleeding freely. How will you care for this injury? What concerns must be kept in mind when dealing with an open head wound?

The scalp is the outermost anatomical structure of the cranium and is the first area of contact to receive trauma. For example, in most contact sports when facing an opponent, the shoulder is frequently lowered to ward off a block, or dodge the opponent. Hence, the shoulder and head receive the initial impact. The scalp is highly vascular and bleeds freely, making it a frequent site for abrasions, lacerations, contusions, or hematomas between the layers of tissue.

The primary concern with any scalp laceration is to control bleeding, prevent contamination, and determine a possible skull fracture. As with any open wound, latex gloves should be worn as part of universal precautions. Apply mild direct pressure with sterile gauze until bleeding has stopped. Inspect the wound for any foreign bodies or signs of a skull fracture. Once a skull fracture is ruled out, cleanse the wound with surgical soap or saline solution, and cover the wound with a sterile dressing until it can be sutured (**Figure 13-13**).

Abrasions and contusions can be treated with gentle cleansing, topical antiseptics, and ice to control hemorrhage. Hematomas, or "goose eggs," require a more thorough assessment. These injuries involve a collection of blood between the layers of the scalp and skull. Treatment with ice and a pressure bandage to control hemorrhage is usually sufficient to care for the injury. With a possible skull fracture, use of a pressure bandage is contraindicated. The individual should be referred to a physician for examination.

In caring for the laceration, did you put on latex gloves, control hemorrhage, inspect the wound for foreign material, palpate for possible fracture, cleanse and cover the wound, and refer the individual to a physician for possible sutures? If so, you did the correct procedure.

ASSESSMENT OF CRANIAL INJURIES

A skater fell on the ice, landed flat on the back, and bumped the head on the ice. The individual is somewhat disoriented, dizzy, has a slight headache, but vision appears to be normal. How will you assess the severity of this injury? What danger signs indicate the condition is deteriorating and immediate medical care is warranted?

Head trauma demands immediate assessment for life-threatening conditions. In Chapter 3, primary and secondary assessment included establishing and maintaining the ABCs and determining the level of con-

---

At impact, shearing causes blood vessels to rupture within the brain leading to severe bleeding within the cranial cavity

---

With lacerations of the scalp, control bleeding, prevent contamination, and rule out a possible skull fracture

---

If a skull fracture is suspected, do not apply pressure over a "goose egg" or hematoma.

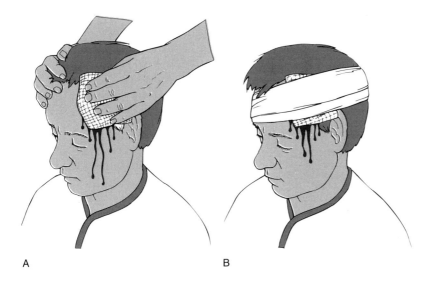

Fig. 13.13: To treat a scalp wound, cleanse the wound with a saline solution (A). Cover the wound with a sterile dressing and transport the individual to a physician for further examination and suturing (B).

sciousness. In head injuries, this encompasses gathering a history, observing and inspecting the head and facial area, and assessing motor control. These components are not separate and distinct, but rather occur simultaneously. For matters of clarity these components are presented in separate parts of this section.

Because significant head trauma may also cause cervical injury, always assume a cervical neck injury is present until one is ruled out. As you approach the individual, gather a brief history of the mechanism of injury, duration of unconsciousness, and any other pertinent information from individuals at the scene. Never place ammonia capsules under the nose to arouse the person, as they may jerk the head and neck, which can lead to serious complications if a spinal injury is present. Establish and maintain an open airway. If the individual is face down, stabilize the head and neck, and log roll the individual to a supine position. Stabilize the cervical spine if the individual is unconscious or confused. A face mask should be removed but do not remove the helmet or chin strap. Begin rescue breathing and CPR as needed. If breathing, remove any mouth guard, dentures, or partial plates that may occlude the airway. If alert, establish the duration of post-traumatic amnesia as a guide to severity.

Vital signs, history of the injury, observation, inspection, and general assessment are then used to judge the magnitude of a cerebral injury. A practical measure commonly used to quantify the level of consciousness in head trauma is the Glasgow Coma Scale **(Table 13-5)** (5). This coma scale measures the individual's response to stimulation by eye opening, motor response, and verbal response. A numerical score is given for the best response. For example, eyes that open spontaneously are given a score of 4; to a verbal command, a 3; to pain, a 2; and no response with the eyes remaining closed, a score of 1 is given. Motor response is given a 6 if the individual responds to a verbal command. Otherwise, values are assessed depending on how the individual responds to painful stimuli (e.g., pinching under the arms or knuckle to the sternum). Verbal response that is coherent and clear is given a 5, with the remaining values dependent on quality of speech or sentence structure. Total scores range from 3 to 15. A score of 12 or more is considered to be a mild injury, 9 to 11 is a moderate injury, and 8 or less is considered a serious head injury.

Vital Signs

Vital signs should be taken early in the assessment to establish a baseline of information that can be periodically rechecked to determine if the individual's status is improving or deteriorating. Vital signs include pulse, respiration, blood pressure, and body temperature, however, with head trauma, body temperature is not as critical as the others. In addition, skin color, pupillary response to

Always assume a cervical neck injury is present until one is ruled out

Vital signs, history of the injury, observation, inspection, and general assessment are used to judge the magnitude of a cerebral injury

The Glasgow Coma Scale measures the individual's response to stimulation of eye opening, motor response, and verbal response

Table 13–5. Glasgow Coma Scale.*

Eyes	Open	Spontaneously	4
		To verbal command	3
		To pain	2
		No response	1
Best motor response	To verbal commands	Obeys	6
	To painful stimulus+	Localizes pain	5
		Flexion-withdrawal	4
		Flexion-abnormal (decorticate rigidity)	3
		Extension (decerebrate rigidity)	2
		No response	1
Best verbal response++		Oriented and converses	5
		Disoriented and converses	4
		Inappropriate words	3
		Incomprehensible sounds	2
		No response	1
Total			3–15

* The Glasgow Coma Scale is based on eye opening, motor, and verbal response, and is used to monitor changes in level of consciousness. If response on the scale is given a number, then responsiveness of the injured party can be expressed by totalling the figures. Lowest score is 3; highest is 15. A score of 12 or greater is considered to be a mild injury, 9–11 is a moderate injury, and 8 or less is a severe head injury.
+ Squeeze trapezius, pinch soft tissue between thumb and forefinger or in the axilla, knuckle to sternum; observe arms.
++ Arouse injured party with painful stimulus if necessary.

light, and eye movement should also be documented and will be discussed in the following sections. Normal response for vital signs was discussed in Chapter 3.

1. **Pulse**. A slow, bounding pulse may indicate increasing intracranial pressure or a possible skull fracture. A rapid, weak pulse indicates shock.
2. **Respiration**. Slowed breathing indicates a head injury. Rapid, shallow breathing indicates shock. If the individual shows signs of respiratory difficulty, or collapses into respiratory arrest, immediate action is necessary to initiate and maintain respiratory function.
3. **Blood pressure**. An increase in the systolic blood pressure or a decrease in the diastolic blood pressure indicates increasing intracranial pressure. Low blood pressure rarely occurs in a head injury. It may, however, indicate a possible cervical injury or serious blood loss from an injury elsewhere in the body.

Any of these signs should indicate a serious injury is present. Summon EMS and proceed with the secondary assessment.

History

Determine the level of consciousness by arousing the individual through verbal and/or painful stimuli. While gathering the history of the mechanism of injury and symptoms, assess the level of consciousness, ability to recall events (amnesia), and pupil abnormalities. Remember that a possible neck injury may also be present. Therefore, stabilize the head and neck throughout the assessment. Call the person's name, gently tap them on the cheek, or touch the arm. You may have to shout loudly to get a response.

1. **Mechanism of injury**. Ask the individual what happened. Can the individual remember what position they were in and the direction of impact? If the individual is unable to respond or is confused, ask others who might have seen the impact.
2. **Loss of consciousness**. Did the individual lose consciousness? Did it occur immediately on direct impact or did the person progress to unconsciousness? How long were they unconscious? Was the individual totally unresponsive, confused, or disoriented? Do they respond to painful stimuli (e.g. squeezing the trapezius, pinching soft tissue between the thumb and index finger in the axilla, knuckle to the sternum, or squeezing the Achilles tendon)? Was there a seizure? Has the individual ever had a head injury before? When? How bad was it?
3. **Amnesia**. Start with simple questions then progress to more difficult questions (e.g.,

date, time, what they had for breakfast, or what play was called before the injury). Confusion or transient memory loss indicates a mild or grade I concussion. Loss of memory for events immediately after the injury (post-traumatic amnesia) indicates a grade II concussion. Loss of memory for events prior to (retrograde amnesia) and immediately after the injury indicate a grade III concussion. Amnesia may not become apparent until 5 to 15 minutes after trauma, so continually ask questions and reassess the status of the individual.

4. **Pupil abnormalities**. Note pupil size and accommodation to light; both should be equal. A one-sided dilated pupil may indicate a subdural or epidural hematoma. Dilated pupils on both sides indicate severe cranial injury with death imminent. Ask the individual to look up, down, and sideways (six cardinal planes of vision). Determine the coordinated and fluid motion of both eyes. Can the individual focus on your face? Is there blurred or double vision? Did she or he see "stars" or flashes of light on impact? Blurred or double vision, abnormal oscillating movements of the eye (nystagmus), or uncoordinated gross movement through the cardinal planes indicate disturbance to the cranial nerves that innervate the eye and eye muscles.

5. **Headache**. Does the individual have a headache or ringing in the ears? Headaches are common symptoms that follow head trauma. Progressive headaches indicate increasing intracranial pressure and signal danger.

6. **Nausea and/or vomiting**. Does the individual feel nauseous? Intracranial pressure can stimulate the reflex onset of nausea and vomiting. If this symptom is present, it indicates a fairly serious intracranial injury.

7. **Associated neck injury**. Is there pain, numbness or weakness elsewhere in the body? Is grip strength bilaterally equal? Can sharp and dull sensations be distinguished?

Observation and Inspection

Observe facial expression and function, as this can indicate cerebral damage (**Table 13-1**). Cranial nerve integrity can be assessed quickly by sense of smell, vision, eye tracking, smiling, clenching the jaw, hearing, balance, sense of taste, speaking, and strength of shoulder shrugs. Watch the face and listen to the responses. Note any slurred speech, difficulty in constructing sentences, or inability to understand commands. Continue to watch the eyes for neurological signs indicating increasing intracranial pressure.

1. **Leakage of cerebrospinal fluid.** Cerebrospinal fluid (CSF) is a clear, colorless fluid that protects and cushions the brain and spinal cord. A basilar fracture may result in bleeding and CSF leaking from the ear. A fracture to the cribriform plate in the anterior cranial area may result in bleeding and CSF leaking from the nose.

2. **Signs of trauma**. Look for discoloration around the eyes (raccoon's eyes) and behind the ears (Battle's sign) that may indicate a skull fracture. Note any depressions, elevations, or bleeding that may indicate skull fractures, lacerations, or hematomas. Listen for snoring which may occur as a result of a fracture to the anterior cranial floor (8).

3. **Skin color**. Note skin color and presence of moisture. If shock is setting in, the skin may appear ashen or pale, and may be moist and cool.

4. **Loss of emotional control**. Irritability, aggressive behavior, or uncontrolled crying for no apparent reason indicates cerebral dysfunction and should signal immediate referral to a physician.

Palpation

Most of the vital information will be gained in the vital signs, history, and observation portion of the assessment. Palpations can help pinpoint possible skull or facial fractures. Palpate for point tenderness, crepitus, depressions, elevations, swelling, blood, or changes in skin temperature. The following sites can be palpated:

1. Scalp and hair
2. Cervical spinous process
3. Base of the skull and around the external ear
4. Frontal bone, eye orbit, and bridge of the nose
5. Zygomatic arch (cheek)
6. Upper and lower jaw

Special Tests

Use of myotomes and dermatomes are not an effective technique in assessing cranial

> Blurred or double vision, nystagmus, or uncoordinated gross movement through the cardinal planes indicates disturbance to the cranial nerves that innervate the eye and eye muscles

injuries because they assess lower motor neuron function associated with the spinal column and spinal nerves. Tests listed in this section directly assess upper motor neuron function of the brain through coordination, balance, depth perception, and logical thought processes in responding to simple commands. If the assessment has already determined a possible intracranial or spinal injury, do not subject the individual to these tests. Immobilize the head and neck and transport the individual to the nearest medical facility. The following tests can be performed:

1. **100 minus 7 test**. This tests one's ability to concentrate and critically think about the response. The individual is asked to start at 100 and subtract 7, then subtract 7 from that number, and so on. This can be adapted to other mathematical problems. Start with 3 and multiply by factors of 3, or start at 100 and subtract by 5 each time.

2. **Finger to nose test**. This tests depth perception and ability to focus on an object. Hold a finger in front of the injured individual. Ask the person to reach out and touch it while alternating between the right and left hand **(Figure 13-14)**. Change the position of your finger after two or three touches. A variation is to ask the individual to touch their nose between each touch of your finger. Progressively

increase the speed of touch between their nose and your finger.

3. **Romberg test**. The individual is asked to stand with the feet together, arms at the side, and eyes closed while maintaining balance **(Figure 13-15)**. Variations include raising the arms at 90°, standing on the toes, or touching the nose with the hand while the eyes are closed. From an anterior view, observe if a body sway occurs, indicating a positive test.

4. **Stork stand**. With the eyes closed, have the individual place the foot of one leg on the opposite knee **(Figure 13-16)**. A variation is to have the individual stand on one leg while placing the foot on the opposite knee while maintaining balance.

5. **Heel/toe walking**. Ask the individual to walk on the toes, then the heels. Note any swaying or inability to walk in a straight line.

Determination of Findings

If the individual is not in a crisis situation, vital signs and special tests should be completed every five to seven minutes to determine progress of the condition. If physical signs and symptoms improve or appear normal, the individual may be returned to play. If signs and symptoms linger but appear minor, an individual close to the injured party, such as a parent or roommate, should be informed of the injury and told to look for changes in

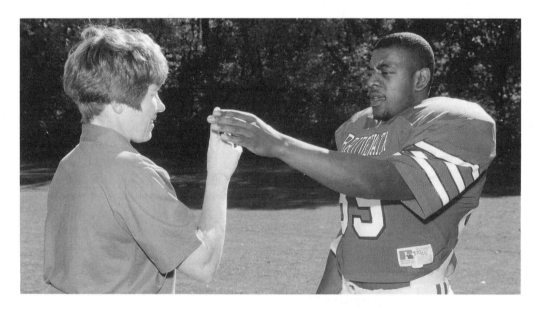

Fig. 13.14: Finger-to-nose test. Ask the person to alternately touch their nose and touch your finger. Progressively increase the speed of touch and the placement of your finger.

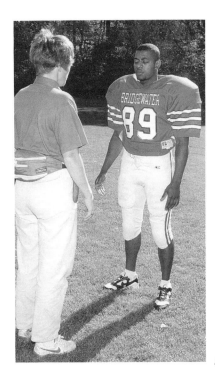

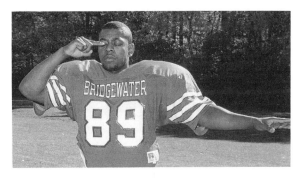

B

Fig. 13.15: To perform the Romberg test, the person should be able to maintain balance while standing with the eyes closed (A). Variations may include raising the arms to the side, standing on the toes, or touching the nose with a finger (B). A tendency to sway is a positive sign.

A

behavior, unsteady gait, slurring of speech, a progressive headache or nausea, restlessness, mental confusion, or drowsiness. These danger signs should be fully explained to the observer orally and provided on an information sheet, such as the one demonstrated in **Table 13-2**. **Field Strategy 13-2** summarizes an assessment of a cranial injury and lists danger signs indicative of a serious underlying cerebral injury. The individual must be transported immediately to the nearest medical facility. **Table 13-6** lists criteria used to determine when a player can return to play following intracranial injury.

Did you determine how to assess the skater with the head injury? Danger signs include progressive headache, disorientation, amnesia, or unsteady gait. Refer to Field Strategy 13-2 for more danger signs.

JAW INJURIES

A lacrosse player stepped in front of an opposing player who was taking a shot on goal and was struck on the jaw by the ball. Although the player was wearing a mouth guard, bleeding from the mouth is apparent and they are unable to close the jaw. What

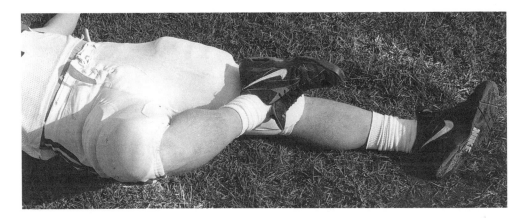

Fig. 13.16: The stork stand can initially be performed while the individual is lying down. With the eyes closed, place the foot of one leg on the opposite knee. It may also be performed in a standing position.

Field Strategy 13–2. Cranial Injury Evaluation.

PRIMARY SURVEY
- Stabilize head and neck
- Check ABCs
- If a helmet is worn, remove the face mask but do not remove the helmet or chin strap
- Determine initial level of consciousness

SECONDARY SURVEY
Vital signs. Check pulse, respiration, and blood pressure
History
- Mechanism of injury
- Loss of consciousness (dizziness, disorientation, confusion)
- Presence of post-traumatic and/or retrograde amnesia
- Pupil abnormalities (pupil size, pupillary response to light, eye movement, nystagmus, blurred or double vision)
- Headache or tinnitis
- Nausea and/or vomiting
Observation and Inspection
- Obvious deformities and body posturing
- Discoloration around the eyes and behind the ears, bleeding and/or CSF from ears or nose, depressions or elevations, and skin color
- Observe facial expression and behavior of the individual (irritability, aggressiveness, or uncontrolled crying)
- Listen for snoring, slurred speech, or inability to organize thoughts
- Observe voluntary or involuntary movements of the extremities
Palpation
- Bony and soft tissue structures for point tenderness, crepitus, depressions, elevations, swelling, blood, or changes in skin temperature
Special Tests
- 100 minus 7 test or multiply by factors of 3
- Perform the finger/nose coordination test, Romberg test, stork stand, and heel/toe walking
- Check for spinal injury
  (Response to verbal commands, painful stimuli, grip strength, sensory ability)
- Take vital signs and recheck every five minutes

Danger Signs that Indicate Emergency Action

- Signs about the head indicating possible skull fracture:
  Bleeding and/or CSF from the ears or nose
  Raccoon eyes
  Battle's sign
- Persistent or increasing headache, particularly if it becomes localized
- Unequal pupils or bilateral dilated pupils that fail to react to light
- Mental confusion or disorientation that gets progressively worse
- Progressive or sudden impairment of consciousness
- Prolonged amnesia
- Drastic changes in emotional control
- Persistent or increasing nausea and/or vomiting
- Alterations in breathing pattern
- Difficulty speaking or slurring of speech
- Gradual increase in systolic blood pressure or a decrease in diastolic blood pressure
- Decrease in pulse rate
- Any suspicions regarding the presence of an intracranial injury

Table 13–6. Criteria for Return to Play.

	1st Episode	2nd Episode	3rd Episode
Grade I Concussion	May return to play if asymptomatic*	Return to play in 2 wks if asymptomatic at that time for at least 1 wk	Terminate season; may return to play next season if asymptomatic
Grade II Concussion	Return to play after asymptomatic for 1 wk	Minimum of 1 mo; may return to play then if asymptomatic for 1 wk; consider terminating season	Terminate season; may return to play next season if asymptomatic
Grade III Concussion	Minimum of 1 mo; may then return to play if asymptomatic for 2 wks	Terminate season; may return to play next season if asymptomatic	Terminate season; consider other sport activity
Grade IV/V Concussion	Terminate season; further neurologic tests should be conducted with suggestions made to select another sport activity to participate in		

*No headache, dizziness, or impaired orientation, concentration, or memory during rest or exertion.

injury might you expect to find? How will you manage this traumatic injury?

Injuries to the cheek, nose, lips, and jaw are very common in sports with moving projectiles (sticks, balls, bats, racquets), in contact sports (football, rugby, or ice hockey), or in sports where collisions with objects occur (diving, skiing, hockey, swimming). Many of these injuries can be prevented by wearing properly fitted face masks and mouth guards. Because the facial area has a vast expansive arterial system, lacerations bleed freely and rapid swelling often hides the true extent of injury. Contusions, abrasions, and lacerations are managed the same as elsewhere on the body. Always remember, however, if the magnitude of force is great enough to cause soft tissue damage, the possibility exists for underlying bony tissue damage. Therefore, after hemorrhage is controlled, inspect the area for possible fracture.

Fractures to the upper and lower jaw occur from direct impact. For example, a player may be struck with an opponent's shoulder or elbow, by a hockey stick, ball, or thrown punch. The bony fragments may be pushed internally, resulting in severe deformity, bleed-

ing, and possible occlusion of the airway. Normally the priority would be to apply direct pressure to control bleeding, but in a fracture to the upper jaw, extreme caution must be exercised in applying pressure over a fracture site. Common sites for fractures include the mandible, maxilla, and zygomatic arch. Fractures to the nose and eye orbit will be discussed in their respective sections.

Mandibular Fractures

Fracture to the mandible is the third most common facial bone fracture associated with sports participation behind nasal and zygomatic fractures, respectively (12). They seldom occur as an isolated single fracture, but rather occur as a double fracture or fracture-dislocation. The most common fracture site is near the angle of the lower jaw (**Figure 13-17**). Signs and symptoms include an immediate change in bite, called malocclusion. **Malocclusion** occurs when the mouth is closed and the teeth do not fit together because the integrity of the lower jaw is lost. This leads to changes in speech patterns because articulation of words is nearly impossible. Bleeding

Many jaw injuries can be prevented by wearing properly fitted face masks and mouth guards

Fractures to the mandible often involve a double fracture or a fracture-dislocation

Malocclusion
Inability to bring the teeth together in a normal bite

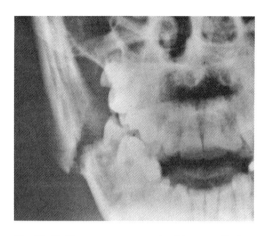

Fig. 13.17: The most common site for a mandibular fracture is near the angle of the jaw which leads to malocclusion of the teeth.

may occur around the teeth even though a mouth guard is properly fitted and worn. Pain, discoloration, swelling, and facial distortion may be present.

It is important to maintain an open airway with this fracture, as the tongue may occlude the airway. Dress any open wounds and immobilize the jaw in a temporary Barton bandage (**Figure 13-18**), or elastic wrap from under the chin around the occiput. Repair will involve internal fixation (wiring the jaw closed) or using bone plates, which may allow some individuals to return to sport participation.

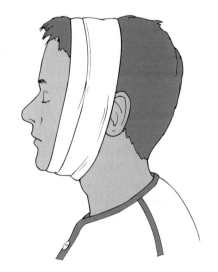

Fig. 13.18: A Barton bandage is used to restrict jaw movement and minimize pain with a mandibular fracture.

Maxillary Fractures

Fractures to the maxilla, or midface fractures (LeFort fractures), involve the upper jaw and associated bony structures (**Figure 13-19**). With displaced fractures, the face appears longer than usual. Stabilize the nasal bones and apply gentle pressure to the upper jaw. If fractured, the upper jaw may be mobile (**Figure 13-20**). Slight ecchymosis can be seen in the cheek or buccal region. This fracture is often associated with nasal bleeding and deformity. An inability to close the jaw (malocclusion) also indicates a possible fracture. Treatment will involve maintaining the airway, and immediate transportation to the nearest medical facility. A forward sitting position will allow for adequate drainage of saliva and blood.

Zygomatic Fractures

A fracture to the zygomatic arch (cheek bone) is the most common facial bone fracture to the upper jaw (12). With direct impact forces, the cheek will appear flat or depressed. Swelling and ecchymosis about the eye may occlude vision and hide damage to the eye orbit. Occasionally the eye on the side of the fracture may appear sunken in, or the eye opposite the fracture may appear to be raised. Double vision is common, and paresthesia or anesthesia (numbness) may be present on the affected cheek.

In most cases the condition can be easily reduced surgically and may not require internal fixation. An exception occurs when the fracture involves the eye orbit, and surgical repair becomes more extensive. Healing usually occurs within six to eight weeks. Special facial protection should be worn for three to four months. A complication may involve blurred vision over an extended period. As such, individuals in activities requiring eye-hand coordination may not return to their previous level of participation for some time.

Temporomandibular Dislocation

Dislocation of the temporomandibular joint (TMJ) results from excessive opening of the mouth during eating or yawning, and seldom occurs during trauma. The condyle of the mandible slips forward and cannot return to its normal position without assistance. The individual is unable to close the mouth, and will have severe pain due to muscle fatigue

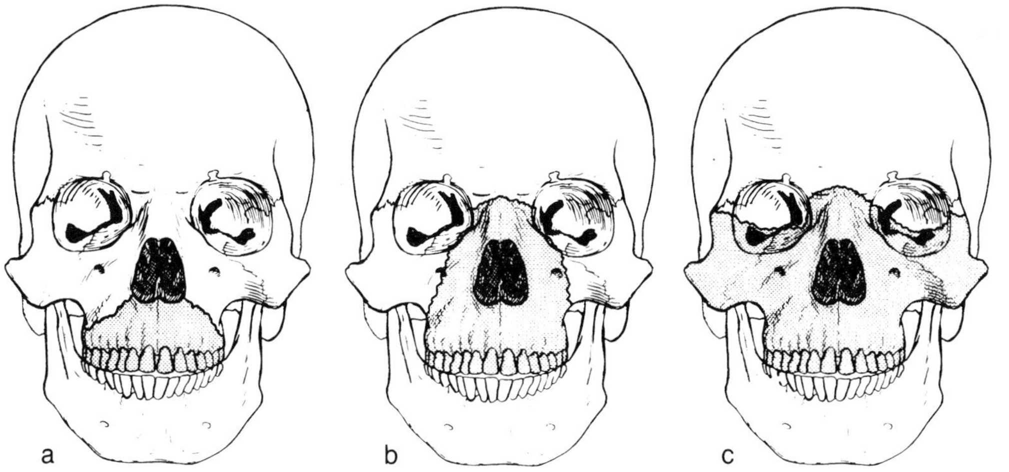

Fig. 13.19: Fractures to the maxilla may involve separation of the palate (A), may extend into the nasal region (B), or may involve complete craniofacial dissociation (C).

and ligamentous stretch (13). Refer the individual to a physician who will reposition the jaw. Recurrence of this condition is common.

Facial Soft Tissue Injuries

Soft tissue injuries commonly occur with direct impact. Facial contusions, abrasions, and lacerations are managed the same as elsewhere on the body. Contusions are treated with ice to control swelling and hemorrhage. With abrasions and lacerations, cleanse the wound with a saline solution, apply an antibiotic ointment, and cover with a sterile gauze dressing. In minor lacerations (less than one inch long and an eighth of an inch deep), application of butterfly bandages or Steri-strips can facilitate wound closure (see **Field Strategy 13-3**). Protect the area with sterile gauze and tape. The individual can return to sport participation, but at the conclusion of the event refer the individual to a physician to determine if sutures are needed. Larger and more complicated injuries, such as those with jagged edges or damage to nerves, veins, or bony structures, should be immediately referred to a physician.

The individual may have a fractured jaw due to the apparent malocclusion and inability to close the jaw. Apply a Barton bandage and refer this person to a physician.

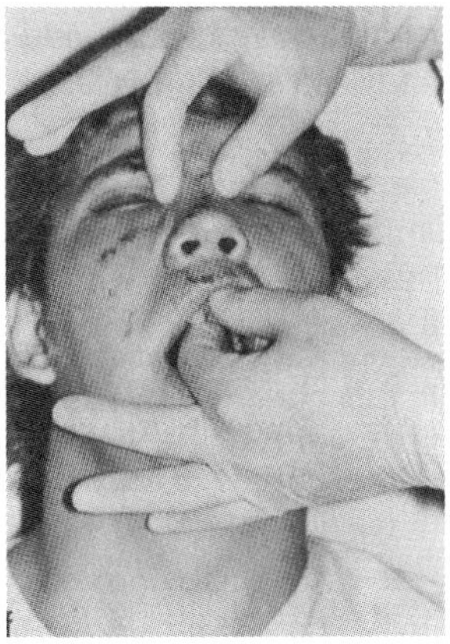

Fig. 13.20: To assess a possible maxillary fracture, stabilize the nasal bones and forehead and apply gentle pressure to the upper jaw. A positive sign is increased pain or a mobile jaw. Malocclusion may also be present.

NASAL INJURIES

A third baseman covering a hit was struck on the side of the nose when the ball bounced unexpectedly. The nose is bleeding and appears to be swollen at the top. What assessment and management protocol will you follow?

Nasal injuries are common in sports where protective face guards are not worn. Nosebleeds (epistaxis) and nasal fractures are traumatic injuries frequently seen.

Epistaxis

Epistaxis, or nosebleeds, occur when superficial blood vessels on the anterior septum are lacerated. This is a frequent occurrence in sports like wrestling or boxing. In most cases bleeding will stop spontaneously. After ruling out a possible fracture, application of a

Epistaxis
Profuse bleeding from the nose; nosebleed

1. Put on latex gloves
2. Control bleeding with direct compression using a sterile gauze pad
3. Carefully clean the wound with a saline solution and antiseptic, such as Betadine
4. Spray tape adherent on a cotton-tipped applicator and dab below and above the wound. Be careful not to get the adherent in the wound
5. Beginning in the middle of the wound, bring the edges together and secure the Steri-Strip below the wound. Lift up against gravity and secure above the wound. Make sure the edges of the wound are approximated

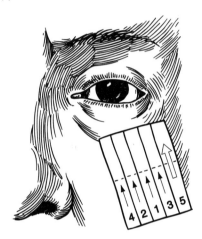

6. Apply the second Steri-Strip in a similar manner immediately adjacent to one side of the original strip. Apply the third strip on the other side. Alternate sides until the entire wound is covered
7. Cover the wound with a sterile dressing and secure in place
8. After the contest, refer the athlete to a physician for medical care if the wound is greater than one inch long or one-eighth inch deep
9. Check the wound daily for signs of infection. Keep it clean and protected for at least one week

squeezing pressure at the nasal bone junction and application of ice can stop persistent bleeding. A nasal plug or pledget may be used, although this is seldom needed. If used, the plug should protrude from the nostrils at least one half inch to facilitate removal. If bleeding persists, topical astringents or vasoconstrictors, such as tannic acid or 0.5% phenylephrine hydrochloride solution can be applied if the individual is not allergic to them (14). If bleeding continues for more than five minutes in spite of manual pressure and ice, refer the individual to a physician.

> After ruling out fracture, apply gentle pressure at the nasal bone junction and apply ice to stop persistent bleeding

Nasal Fractures

Fractures to the nasal bone are the most common facial fractures in sport. Because of its prominence, the nose is particularly susceptible to lateral displacement. Severity can range

> The nose is particularly susceptible to lateral displacement in a fracture

from a slightly depressed greenstick fracture (seen in adolescents) to total displacement and/or disruption in the bony and cartilaginous parts of the nose **(Figure 13-21A)** (12). With direct impact, epistaxis is almost always seen. The nasal airway can be obstructed with bony fragments or the fracture can extend into the cranial region leading to a loss of cerebrospinal fluid. Therefore, always check for signs of concussion.

The nose may appear flattened and lose its symmetry. Deformity is usually present, particularly with a lateral force. Stand behind and above the individual, and look down an imaginary line to determine if the nose is centered **(Figure 13-21B).** Hand a small mirror to the injured individual and have them look at the nose to determine if it appears normal to them. There may be crepitus over the nasal bridge and ecchymosis under the eyes. Con-

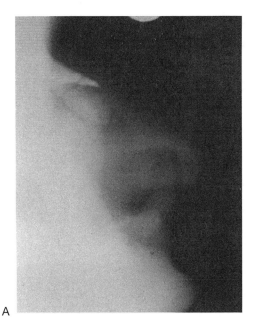

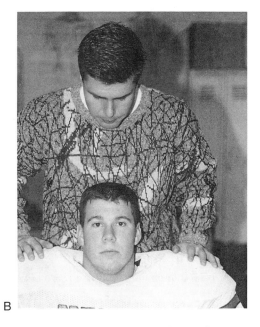

Fig. 13.21: (A) Nasal deformity from a nasal fracture. (B) A nasal deformity can best be seen by standing behind the injured person and looking down an imaginary line to determine if the nose is centered.

trol bleeding, apply ice to limit swelling and hemorrhage, and refer the individual to a doctor for further examination. A nose guard can be worn after a few days to protect the area from additional injury. **Field Strategy 13-4** suggests assessment and care of a fractured nose.

After assessing the injury for a possible fracture, apply ice to control bleeding and swelling, and transport this individual to a physician.

ORAL AND DENTAL INJURIES

A basketball player was struck in the mouth by an elbow. The inside of the upper lip is bleeding. At least three teeth are loose and one tooth appears to be broken in half. How will you manage this injury? Can the top part of the tooth be reattached?

Approximately 15% of school-aged children will have significant dental injuries before the age of 18 (15). For those who participate in sport, nearly all are preventable through regular use of mouth protectors. Mouth protectors provide protection to the lips, teeth, and gums by absorbing shock, spreading impact, cushioning the contact between the upper and lower jaw, and keeping the upper lip away from the incisal edges of teeth (13). Not only do mouth protectors

reduce the incidence of oral injuries, but have also been shown to reduce head concussions by reducing force transmitted to the brain during sudden jaw closure and direct impact to the jaw (16). Although certain sports (football, boxing, field hockey, and lacrosse) require mouth guards, few coaches or league officials require wearing mouth guards in other contact and collision sports. Oral injuries include lacerations to the mouth, and loose, fractured, and dislocated teeth.

Lacerations of the Mouth

Mouth lacerations result from the tooth edge being driven into the lip or tongue. Lacerations that extend completely through the lip or involve the outer border of the lip require special suturing for cosmetic effect. In minor lacerations, treatment is the same as in other lacerations. Apply direct pressure to stop bleeding, cleanse the area with a saline solution, apply Steri-strips if needed, and cover the wound with a dry sterile dressing. Large tongue lacerations should also be sutured. A badly scarred tongue can affect taste and interfere with speech patterns. With tongue lacerations, cleanse the wound with water or mouthwash gargle and refer for possible suturing. The individual should not be

Mouth guards protect the lips, teeth, and gums by absorbing shock, spreading impact, cushioning the contact between the upper and lower jaw, and keeping the upper lip away from the incisal edges of teeth

Field Strategy 13–4. Management of a Nasal Injury.

PRIMARY SURVEY
- Check ABCs. Bony fragments may occlude the airway
- Determine responsiveness
- Check for signs of a concussion and/or skull fracture

SECONDARY SURVEY
History
- Determine mechanism of injury
- Primary complaint
  (dizziness, disorientation, nausea, vision disturbances, tinnitis)
- Presence of post-traumatic and/or retrograde amnesia
- Pain perception
- Disability from injury
  (inability to breathe through one side of nose)

Observation and Inspection
- Obvious deformity or abnormal deviation
- Bleeding and/or CSF from the nose
- Check pupil size, pupillary response to light, eye movement, nystagmus, blurred or double vision that may indicate an associated cranial injury
- Abnormal breathing rate and pattern
- Stand behind the individual and look down an imaginary line to see if the nose is deviated

Palpation
- Palpate the two nasal bones with the forefinger and thumb
  (swelling, depressions, crepitus, mobility, etc.)
- Check the internal structures of the nasal area for any abnormalities
- Control any bleeding

After bleeding is controlled, inspect the internal structures for any abnormalities
Apply ice to control hemorrhage and refer the individual for medical care

---

Intruded
Tooth driven in an inwardly direction

Extruded
Tooth driven in an outwardly direction

When a loose tooth is displaced outwardly or laterally displaced, try to place the tooth back into its normal position

Teeth that are intruded should be left alone

returned to participation until the wound is healed. If sutures are applied, protection is continued for at least seven days.

Loose Teeth

A loosened tooth may be partially displaced, **intruded, extruded**, or avulsed (**Figure 13-22**). When the tooth has been displaced outwardly or is laterally displaced, try to place the tooth back into its normal position. Immediately transport the individual to the dentist for follow-up treatment. A dental radiograph can rule out damage under the gum line and ensure the tooth is properly replaced. The damaged tooth is then splinted to surrounding teeth for two to three weeks. Teeth that are intruded should be left alone. Any attempt to move the tooth may result in permanent loss of the tooth or damage to any underlying permanent teeth. The individual should be referred to a dentist immediately (13).

Fractured Tooth

Fractures may occur through the enamel, dentin, pulp, or root of the tooth (**Figure 13-23**). Fractures involving the enamel cause no symptoms and can be smoothed by the dentist to prevent further injury to the lips and inner lining of the oral cavity. Fractures extending into the dentin cause pain and increased sensitivity to cold and heat. The individual should be referred to a dentist who will apply a sedative dressing over the exposed area. The tooth can then have a permanent composite resin crown attached.

Fractures exposing the pulp lead to severe pain and sensitivity, and involve more extensive dental work. If the pulp exposure is small, a pulp capping procedure placing calcium hydroxide on the area can bridge the exposed area. If successful, it eliminates the need for a root canal (13). Another treatment involves removing a portion of the pulp in the root

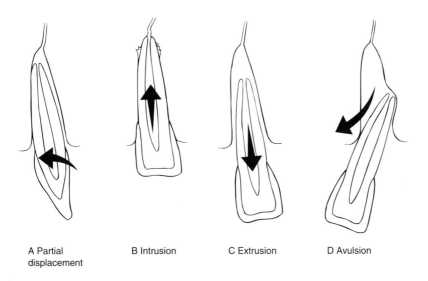

A Partial
displacement

B Intrusion

C Extrusion

D Avulsion

Fig. 13.22: Loose teeth may involve partial displacement (A), intrusion (B), extrusion (C), or avulsion (D).

canal, leaving uninjured pulp in the root. This has been successful in younger patients whose roots have not yet fully formed. The final method of treatment involves a total root canal.

Root fractures are commonly seen in male athletes in contact and collision sports. The predominant sign is a mobile tooth. Radi-

ographs are needed to verify the condition, but initial radiographs may not show the fracture clearly. Additional films taken one to two days later will show the separation. A tooth with a horizontal fracture can be successfully splinted to the surrounding teeth for six weeks (13). Vertical fractures involving the length of the crown and root require extraction.

Fractures extending into the dentin cause pain and sensitivity to heat and cold

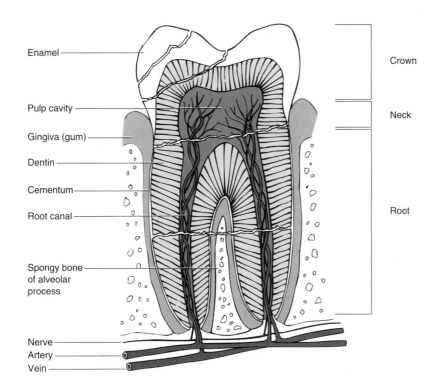

Enamel

Pulp cavity

Gingiva (gum)

Dentin

Cementum

Root canal

Spongy bone
of alveolar
process

Nerve

Artery

Vein

Crown

Neck

Root

Fig. 13.23: Tooth fractures may occur through the enamel, dentine, pulp, or root of the tooth.

Dislocated Tooth

Teeth that have been totally avulsed from their socket can often be located in the individual's mouth or on the ground. These teeth can be saved, but speed is of the essence. Do not touch the root of the tooth or brush the tooth off. Rinse the tooth with cool saline solution and attempt to replace it in its normal position in the socket. If it is properly placed, the individual should be able to close the jaw normally. If the tooth can not be replaced by gentle pressure, place it under the individual's tongue and transport the individual to a dentist. Successful reimplantation can occur if the tooth is implanted within two hours of the injury.

💡 *With the basketball player, you should: (a) put on latex gloves, (b) stop the bleeding with a sterile gauze pad and compression, (c) cleanse the mouth with a saline solution, and (d) refer the individual immediately to a dentist. The dentist may be able to apply a permanent composite resin crown to the tooth.*

EAR INJURIES

❓ *A wrestler was not wearing protective headgear during practice. He is now complaining about a burning, aching sensation on the outer ear. It appears to be somewhat inflamed and sensitive to touch, but no swelling is apparent. How will you manage this injury? What signs might indicate a more serious problem?*

Several conditions may affect the ear. Foreign bodies in the ear are usually harmless and easily removed with a speculum. Trauma to the external ear can lead to auricular hematoma or "cauliflower ear," rupture of the eardrum, localized inflammation of the auditory canal, and swimmer's ear.

External Ear Injury

Auricular hematoma, or "**cauliflower ear**," is a relatively minor injury, but if left untreated, can cause permanent cosmetic alterations to the outer ear. Direct blunt trauma causes a shearing force to pull the cartilage away from the pinna or perichondrium. A hematoma forms between the perichondrium and cartilage of the ear, and compromises blood supply to the cartilage. The hematoma must be drained or aspirated by a physician to avoid pressure and permanent cartilage damage. Once aspirated, a contoured compression

bandage is applied to force the perichondrium against the underlying cartilage to prevent recurrence of the hematoma. If left untreated, blood begins to organize and forms a fibrosis in the overlying skin, leading to pressure necrosis of the auricular cartilage (14). The result is the characteristic "cauliflower ear" appearance (**Figure 13-24**). Protective headgear in sports such as boxing, wrestling, water polo, baseball, and softball is designed to prevent major trauma to the ear, but must be worn regularly to be effective.

Internal Ear Injury

A blow to the ear, pressure changes (seen in diving and scuba diving), and infection may injure the eardrum. Although typically seen in water sports, damage to the internal ear may occur in any sport, such as in soccer when a player is hit on the ear by a ball. Any individual with intense pain in the ear, a feeling of fullness, nausea, tinnitis, dizziness, or a hearing loss should be evaluated immediately by a physician. If the eardrum is ruptured, most minor ruptures heal spontaneously. Larger ruptures may necessitate surgical repair.

Bleeding or cerebrospinal fluid leaking from the ear may indicate a basilar skull fracture behind the tympanic membrane or auditory canal (6). Any bleeding from the ear should be presumed to have originated from a skull fracture and the individual treated accordingly.

Localized infections of the middle ear (**otitis media**) are often secondary to upper respiratory infections. Swelling of the mucous membranes may cause a partial or complete

Cauliflower ear
Hematoma between the perichondrium and cartilage of the outer ear; auricular hematoma

An individual with intense pain in the ear, a feeling of fullness, nausea, tinnitis, dizziness, or a hearing loss should be evaluated by a physician

Otitis media
Localized infection in the middle ear secondary to upper respiratory infection

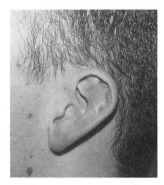

Fig. 13.24: Cauliflower ear deformity. Note how the hematoma has pulled the skin away from the ear cartilage.

block of the eustachian tube (the connection between the middle ear and pharynx). When the mastoid area is pressed, the individual will complain of pain and a sense of fullness in the ear. The tympanic membrane may appear red and bulging. **Serous otitis** is often associated with otitis media and upper respiratory infection. An amber-colored or bloody fluid is seen through the eardrum and is associated with complaints of "ears popping." The supervising physician may prescribe an antibiotic for both conditions if there is an infection, or decongestants may be used to shrink the swollen mucous membranes.

Swimmer's Ear

Swimmer's ear (**otitis externa**) is a bacterial infection involving the lining of the auditory canal. It frequently occurs in individuals who fail to dry the canal after being in water, thereby changing the pH of the ear canal's skin. The individual will feel itching and intense pain in the ear. There may or may not be a discharge of pus. Gentle pressure around the external auditory opening and pulling on the pinna will cause increased pain. If left untreated, the infection can spread to the middle ear, causing balance disturbances or hearing loss.

Commercial ear plugs may not be helpful in preventing the condition. Custom ear plugs from an audiologist or otolaryngologist may be necessary. The condition can also be prevented by using ear drops to dry the canal. A weak solution of either 2% vinegar (acetic acid), 70% alcohol, or 3% boric acid in isopropyl alcohol will re-establish the proper pH (17). If no improvement is seen, refer the individual to a physician.

Place ice on the wrestler's ear to control swelling. If you notice any hemorrhage or edema between the perichondrium and cartilage that appears to flatten the wrinkles or creases of the ear, refer the individual to a physician for follow-up care. Protective eye wear should be worn by this wrestler at every practice and competition.

EYE INJURIES

A basketball player going up for a rebound was struck in the eye by an opponent's finger. The eye is swollen and closed. Attempts to open the eye produce excessive tearing and discomfort for the individual. How will you assess this injury and rule out a serious underlying condition?

The eyes are exposed daily to potential trauma and injury, yet are one of the most valuable sense organs. Many eye injuries could be prevented if protective eyewear is worn. This is especially true in racquetball and squash when players are confined to a limited space with swinging racquets and balls traveling at high speeds. No individual should be allowed to participate in racquetball or squash without wearing eye protectors. Individuals who wear corrective lenses should use strong plastic or semirigid rubber frames, and impact-resistant lenses (18). If glasses are not required, protective eyewear and/or face masks should be worn in sports where risk of injury is high.

Sport participants with only one good eye are at particular risk, since a serious injury to the good eye could result in serious visual disturbance or blindness. Therefore, it is suggested that an ophthalmologist be consulted to determine if this individual should participate in a specific activity, and if so, what protective eyewear can be worn to prevent injury.

Periorbital Ecchymosis (Black eye)

Impact forces can cause significant swelling and hemorrhage into the surrounding eyelids leading to **periorbital ecchymosis**. The eye quickly swells **(Figure 13-25)**. Examine the surrounding eye orbit and function of the eye to determine a possible underlying orbital fracture. Have the individual lie down in a comfortable position and slowly retract the eyelid. Inspect the eye for obvious abnormalities. Check for pupillary response to light by shining a concentrated light beam into the eye and note the bilateral rate of constriction. Ask the individual if they can focus clearly on an object. Have the individual sit up. Inspect the anterior chamber of the eye for any obvious bleeding (refer to hemorrhage into the anterior chamber). If present, it will appear as a pool of blood with a meniscus. Control swelling and hemorrhage by using crushed ice or ice water in a latex surgical glove. Make sure the glove does not have rosin or other powdered substances on it. Do not use chemical ice bags, as they may leak. Refer the individual to an ophthalmologist for further examination and x-rays to rule out an underlying fracture or injury to the globe.

Serous otitis
Fluid build-up behind the eardrum, association with otitis media and upper respiratory infections

Otitis externa
Bacterial infection involving the lining of the auditory canal; swimmer's ear

No individual should be allowed to participate in racquetball or squash without wearing eye protectors

Periorbital ecchymosis
Swelling and hemorrhage into the surrounding eyelids; black eye

Examine the condition and function of the eye to rule out an underlying orbital fracture

Control swelling and hemorrhage by using crushed ice or ice water in a latex surgical glove. Make sure the glove does not have rosin or other powdered substances on it

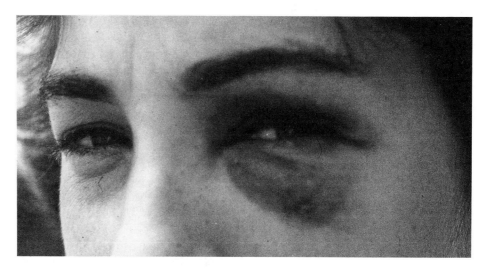

Fig. 13.25: Periorbital ecchymosis caused by direct trauma to the eye.

Foreign Bodies

Dust in the eyes can lead to intense pain and tearing. In sport participation dirt, gravel, cinder, or a fingertip from an opposing player can easily cause more serious damage. Often there is excessive eye movement and spasm in the muscles around the eye to complicate the evaluation. The foreign body, if not imbedded or on the cornea, should be removed and the eye inspected for any scratches, abrasions, or lacerations.

To remove a foreign object, have the person sit in an upright position and open the eye as wide as possible. Begin by gently pulling down on the lower lid and inspect the lower conjunctiva. Have the individual move the eye in all directions while you try to locate the foreign body. Next, grasp the upper lid and ask the individual to move the eye again in the various directions. When located, the foreign object can sometimes be irrigated out of the eye with a sterile saline solution or commercial irrigating solution, such as Dacriose. If this does not work, it should be carefully removed with a sterile gauze pad. **Field Strategy 13-5** describes the procedure to remove a foreign body in the eye.

Sty

A **sty** is an infection of the sebaceous gland of an eyelash or eyelash follicle. The condition starts as a red nodule that progresses into a painful pustule within a few days. Treatment involves hot, moist compresses. If the pustule does not improve within two days, a physician may need to prescribe a topical ointment.

Conjunctivitis (Pinkeye)

Conjunctivitis is an inflammation or bacterial infection of the conjuctiva, the membrane between the inner lining of the eyelid and anterior eyeball. The infection leads to itching, burning, and watering of the eye, causing the conjunctiva to become inflamed and red, giving a pinkeye appearance. This condition can be highly infectious, and therefore, the individual should be referred immediately to a physician for medical treatment.

Corneal Abrasion

Occasionally a foreign body will scratch the cornea, resulting in a sudden onset of pain, tearing, and photophobia. Blinking and movement of the eye only aggravate the condition. Examination may not reveal a foreign object, but the individual continues to complain that something is in the eye. A corneal abrasion is best seen by using a fluorescein dye strip. The orange color of the dye is augmented by using a blue light, changing the orange dye to a bright green, illuminating the abrasion (18). Treatment usually involves a topical ointment to reduce pain and relax ciliary muscle spasms, and an antibiotic ointment to prevent secondary bacterial infection. An eye patch may be worn for 24 to 48 hours. If used, the patch must be tight enough to ensure that the lids are closed beneath the patch, and firm enough to prevent the lids from opening and closing (18). Make sure soft contacts are removed before applying the dye, as they will absorb the dye and can be ruined.

Field Strategy 13–5. Removing a Foreign Body from the Eye.

1. Have the individual sit in an upright position. Examine the lower lid by gently pulling the skin down below the eye. Ask the individual to look up and inspect the lower portion of the globe and eyelid for any foreign object
2. Examine the upper lid by asking the individual to look downward
3. Grasp the eyelashes and pull downward
4. Place a cotton-tipped applicator on the outside portion of the upper lid
5. Pull the lid over the applicator and hold the rolled lid against the upper bony ridge of the orbit

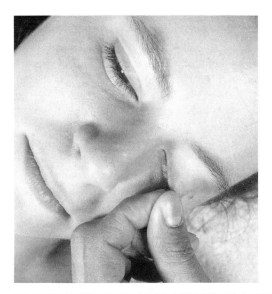
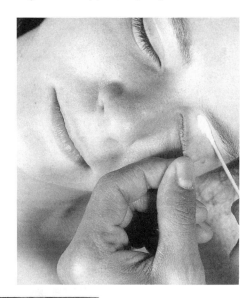
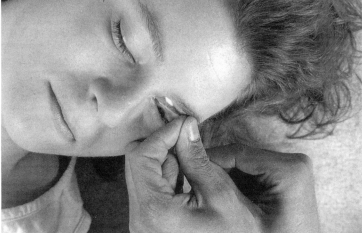

6. Remove the foreign body with a sterile, moist gauze pad. If you are unable to successfully remove the foreign object, patch both eyes with a sterile, nonpressure oval gauze pad and refer the individual to a physician

Corneal Laceration

Lacerations to the cornea are caused by sharp objects, such as a fingernail, darts, skate blades, or broken glass. Any pressure on the globe should be avoided to prevent extrusion of the intraocular contents. If a laceration is suspected, the eye should be covered immediately with a protective shield. The pressure should be on the bony orbit, not the soft tissue. Transport the individual to the nearest medical facility.

Any pressure on the globe should be avoided to prevent extrusion of the intraocular contents

Imbedded Object

If the foreign object is impaled or embedded, do not attempt to remove the object, as serious damage can occur. Summon an ambulance. Medically-trained technicians will place gauze bandages on either side to stabilize the object, and will provide rigid protection for the orbit. Do not touch the object.

Subconjunctival Hemorrhage

A blow to the eye can lead to **subconjunctival hemorrhage**. Several small capillaries rupture, making it look much worse than it is. This relatively harmless condition requires no treatment and resolves spontaneously in one to three weeks. If symptoms, such as blurred vision, pain, limited eye movement, or blood in the anterior chamber are present, immediate referral to an ophthalmologist is warranted.

Hemorrhage into the Anterior Chamber

Hemorrhage into the anterior chamber (**hyphema**) usually results from blunt trauma from a small ball (squash or racquetball), hockey puck, stick (field hockey or ice hockey), or swinging racquet (squash or racquetball). The small size of the object can fit within the confines of the eye orbit, thereby inflicting direct damage to the eye. Initially, a red tinge in the anterior chamber may be present but within a few hours, blood will begin to settle into the anterior chamber, giving a characteristic meniscus appearance (**Figure 13-26**).

Drowsiness, particularly in children, is also seen with this condition although the cause is not fully understood (18). Treatment involves

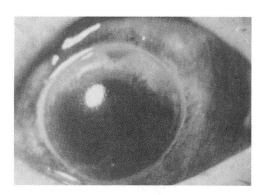

Fig. 13.26: Blood in the anterior chamber of the eye signals a serious eye injury.

hospitalization, bed rest, bilateral patching of the eyes and sedation. Non-aspirin analgesics are frequently required. The initial hemorrhage usually resolves in a few days with good prognosis for full recovery. In about 20% of the cases, a rebleed occurs between three to five days after the initial trauma. These cases are more difficult to handle and have a higher incidence of poor visual recovery (18).

Detached Retina

Damage to the posterior segment of the eye can occur with or without trauma to the anterior segment. A **detached retina** occurs when fluid seeps into the retinal break and separates the neurosensory retina from the retinal epithelium. This can occur days or even weeks after the initial trauma. The individual frequently describes the condition with phrases like, "a curtain fell over my eye," or "I keep seeing flashes of light going on and off." Floaters and light flashes are early signs that the retina is damaged. Be alert to these symptoms and immediately refer this person to an ophthalmologist. A retinal detachment often requires surgical correction.

Orbital "Blowout" Fracture

A blowout fracture is caused by impact from a blunt object, usually larger than the eye orbit, to the anterior portion of the orbit. Upon impact, forces drive the orbital contents posteriorly against the orbital walls. This sudden increase in intraorbital pressure is released in the area of least resistance, typically the orbital floor. The globe descends into the defect in the floor.

Careful examination may reveal **diplopia**, absent eye movement, impaired sensation on the side of fracture below the eye, upper lip, gum line above the teeth, and a recessed, downward displacement of the globe. The lack of eye movement becomes evident when the individual is asked to look up, and only one eye is able to move (**Figure 13-27**). The loss of sensation is due to damage of the infraorbital nerve as it courses through the orbital floor. Tomograms or radiographs are necessary to confirm a fracture. Surgery is indicated to repair the defect in the orbital floor.

Displaced Contact Lens

The increased use of contact lenses by sport participants presents a special problem to the athletic trainer or coach who must assess and

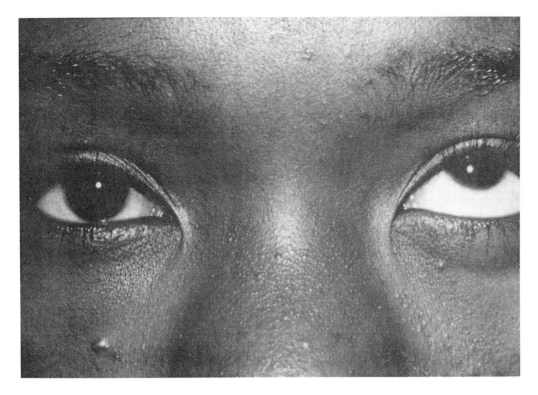

Fig. 13.27: An orbital fracture can entrap the inferior rectus muscle leading to an inability to elevate the eye.

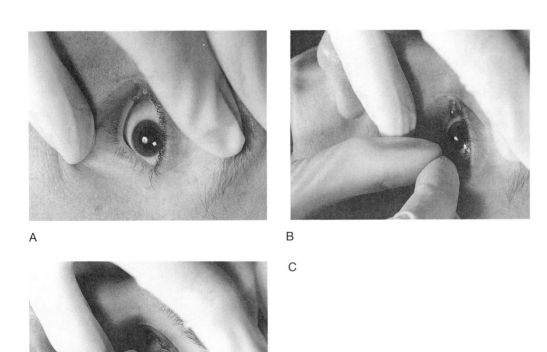

A

B

C

Fig. 13.28: Removal of a soft contact lens. (A) Open the upper and lower eye lids to view the contact lens. (B) Ask the person to look up while you maneuver the lens below the pupil. (C) Remove the lens by pinching it between your thumb and forefinger. Place the lens in contact lens solution.

Field Strategy 13–6. Eye Evaluation.

PRIMARY SURVEY
- Check ABCs
- Determine responsiveness

SECONDARY SURVEY
History
- Determine mechanism of injury. Objects larger than the eye orbit may lead to orbital fracture; objects smaller than the eye orbit may lead to direct trauma to the eye globe. Did the trauma result from blunt trauma, a sharp object, or projectile?
- Primary complaint and disability from injury. Ask about level of pain, discomfort, extent of voluntary eye lid movement, and vision
- Eye irritation from a foreign body and blurring vision that clears quickly with blinking can be managed on-site

Observation and Inspection
- Look for obvious deformity or abnormal deviation in the surrounding eye orbit
- Observe ecchymosis and extent of swelling in the eyelids and surrounding tissue. If the eyelid is swollen shut and the individual cannot voluntarily open it, do not force it open as it may cause further damage
- Observe any bleeding from deep lacerations of the eyelid
- Observe the level of both pupils and the eye globe for anterior or posterior displacement, presence of any corneal lacerations, and bleeding in the anterior chamber
- Inspect pupil size, accommodation to light, and sensitivity to light with a penlight

Palpation
- Carefully palpate the bony rim of the eye orbit and cheek bone for any swelling, depressions, crepitus, or mobility
- Control any bleeding

Special tests
- Determine eye vision. Compare the vision of the uninjured eye to the injured eye. Is it blurred, sensitive to light, or does the individual have double vision? Can the individual distinguish how many fingers you are holding up in all four quadrants of vision? Can the individual distinguish close objects and objects far away?
- Determine eye movement. Move your finger through the six cardinal planes of vision. Do the eyes move in a coordinated manner? If one eye moves upward and the other remains in a stationary position, the inferior rectus muscle may be entrapped due to an orbital fracture

Vision disturbances, such as persistent blurred vision, diplopia, sensitivity to light, loss of all or part of a field of vision, dilated pupils, any abnormal eye movement, and throbbing pain or headache indicate a serious eye injury that warrants immediate referral.

Myopia
Nearsightedness

manage an eye injury. Hard contact lenses frequently are involved in corneal abrasions. Foreign objects may get underneath the lens and damage the cornea, or the cornea may be injured while putting in or taking out the lens. If irritation is present, the lens should be removed and cleaned. Hard contact lenses can slow the progression of **myopia,** however in sports, soft contact lenses are preferred. This is because eye accommodation and adjustment time is less, they can be easily replaced, and can be worn for longer periods of time. In an eye injury, individuals may be

able to remove the lens themselves. However, pain or photophobia (sensitivity to light) may preclude them from doing this, and it may become necessary to assist them. **Figure 13-28** demonstrates how to remove a soft contact lens so an evaluation can proceed. **Field Strategy 13-6** demonstrates a full assessment of an eye injury.

With the basketball player, did you rule out an orbital fracture, check pupillary response to light, vision acuity, and look for possible blood in the anterior chamber? If not, you should have. Reread this section.

Table 13–7. Signs and Symptoms that Indicate Immediate Medical Referral.

Facial bones
- Obvious deformity or crepitus
- Increased pain on palpation
- Malocclusion of the teeth

Nasal region
- Bleeding or CSF from the nose
- Loss of smell
- Nasal deformity or fractures
- Nosebleeds that do not stop within 5 minutes
- Foreign objects that cannot be easily removed

Oral and dental region
- Lacerations involving the lip, outer border of the lip, or tongue
- Loose teeth either laterally displaced, intruded, or extruded
- Chipped, cracked, fractured, or dislodged teeth
- Any individual complaining of persistent toothache or sensitivity to heat and cold
- Inability to close the jaw
- Malocclusion of the teeth

Ear
- Bleeding or CSF from the ear canal
- Bleeding or swelling behind the ear (Battle's sign)
- Hematoma or swelling that removes the creases of the outer ear
- Tinnitis or hearing impairment
- Feeling of fullness in the ear or vertigo
- Foreign body in ear that cannot be easily removed
- "Popping" or itching in the ear
- Pain when the ear lobe is pulled

Eye
- Visual disturbances or loss of vision
- Unequal pupils or bilateral dilated pupils
- Irregular eye movement or failure to accommodate to light
- Severe ecchymosis and swelling (raccoon eyes)
- Imbedded foreign body
- Suspected corneal abrasion or corneal laceration
- Blood in the anterior chamber
- Individual complaining of floaters, light flashes, or a "curtain falling over the eye"
- Itching, burning, watery eye that appears pink
- Lost contact lens that cannot be easily removed

Skin
- Lacerations longer than one inch or deeper than one-eighth inch

SUMMARY

The head and facial region are frequent sites for injury. Wearing protective equipment can significantly reduce the incidence and severity of head and facial injuries. Minor injuries, such as nosebleeds, contusions, abrasions, lacerations, and grade I concussions can easily be handled on the field by the coach, athletic trainer, or sport supervisor. Injuries that require referral to a physician are listed in **Table 13-7**. In evaluating any head or facial injury, it is always best to err on the conservative side and refer questionable injuries to a physician or appropriate specialist. If a decision is made to refer an individual for medical care, control any bleeding, cover the area with a sterile gauze pad, maintain an open airway, and treat for shock.

REFERENCES

1. Clarke, KS. "An epidemiologic view." In *Athletic injuries to the head, neck, and face,* edited by JS Torg. St. Louis: Mosby-Year Book, 1991.

2. Marieb, EN, and Mallatt, J. *Human anatomy.* Redwood City, CA: Benjamin/Cummings Publishing, 1992.

3. Gennarelli, TA. "Head injury mechanisms." In *Athletic injuries to the head, neck, and face,* edited by JS Torg. St. Louis: Mosby-Year Book, 1991.

4. Vegso, JJ, and Lehman, RC. "Field evaluation and management of head and neck injuries." In *Clinics in sports medicine,* edited by JS Torg, vol. 6, no. 1. Philadelphia: WB Saunders, 1987.

5. Bruno, LA, Gennarelli, TA, and Torg, JS., "Management guidelines for head injuries in athletics." In *Clinics in sports medicine,* edited by JS Torg, vol. 6, no. 1. Philadelphia: WB Saunders, 1987.

6. American Academy of Orthopaedic Surgeons. 1991. *Athletic Training and Sports Medicine.* Park Ridge, IL.

7. Carter, RL, and Day, AL. "Head and neck injuries." In *The team physician's handbook,* edited by MB Mellion, WM Walsh, and GL Shelton. Philadelphia: Hanley and Belfus, 1990.

8. Grant, HD, Murray, RH, and Bergeron, JD. *Brady emergency care.* Englewood Cliffs: Prentice Hall, 1990.

9. Bruno, LA. "Focal intracranial hematoma." In *Athletic injuries to the head, neck, and face,* edited by JS Torg. St. Louis: Mosby-Year Book, 1991.

10. Vegso, JJ, and Torg, JS. "Field evaluation and management of intracranial injuries." In *Athletic injuries to the head, neck, and face,* edited by JS Torg. St. Louis: Mosby-Year Book, 1991.

11. Gennarelli, TA. "Cerebral concussions and diffuse brain injuries." In *Athletic injuries to the head, neck, and face,* edited by JS Torg. St. Louis: Mosby-Year Book, 1991.

12. Tu, HK, Davis, LF, and Nique, TA. "Maxillofacial injuries." In *The team physician's handbook,* edited by MB Mellion, WM Walsh, and GL Shelton. Philadelphia: Hanley and Belfus, 1990.

13. Greenberg, MS, and Springer, PS. "Diagnosis and management of oral injuries." In *Athletic injuries to the head, neck, and face,* edited by JS Torg. St. Louis: Mosby-Year Book, 1991.

14. Handler, SD, "Diagnosis and management of maxillofacial injuries." In *Athletic injuries to the head, neck, and face,* edited by JS Torg. St. Louis: Mosby-Year Book, 1991.

15. Bishop BM, Davies, EH, and von Fraunhofer, JA. 1985. Materials for mouth protectors. J Prosthet Dent, 53:256–261.

16. Hickey, JC, et al. 1967. The relation of mouth protectors to cranial pressure and deformation. J Am Dent Assoc, 74:735–739.

17. Hammer, RW, "Swimming and diving." In *The team physician's handbook,* edited by MB Mellion, WM Walsh, and GL Shelton. Philadelphia: Hanley and Belfus, 1990.

18. Brucker, AJ, Kozart, DM, Nichols, CW, and Raber, IM. "Diagnosis and management of injuries to the eye and orbit." In *Athletic injuries to the head, neck, and face,* edited by JS Torg. St. Louis: Mosby-Year Book, 1991.

Chapter 14

Injuries to the Spine

After you have completed this chapter, you should be able to:

- Locate and explain the functional significance of the important bony and soft tissue structures of the spine
- Describe the motion capabilities in the different regions of the spine
- Explain what factors contribute to mechanical loads on the spine
- Specify strategies in activities of daily living to reduce spinal stress
- Identify anatomical variations that may predispose individuals to spine injuries
- Explain important measures used to prevent injury to the spinal region
- Recognize and describe common sports injuries to the spine and back
- Demonstrate a thorough assessment of the spine
- Demonstrate rehabilitative exercises for the region

The spine is a complex linkage system that transfers loads between the upper and lower extremities, enables motion of the trunk in all three planes, and protects the delicate spinal cord. The most common sports injuries to the back are relatively minor, consisting of contusions, muscle strains, and ligament sprains. Acute spinal fractures and dislocations, however, are extremely serious and can lead to paralysis or death. Unfortunately, with the increasing prevalence of leisure time in recent years there has been a concomitant increase in the incidence of spinal injuries and low back pain (1). Low back problems are especially common among certain sport participants, such as female gymnasts and male football linemen (2–4). Sports consistently associated with back injuries include gymnastics, ice hockey, springboard and platform diving, football, wrestling, and rugby (5–9).

This chapter begins with a review of the intricate anatomical structures that make up the spine, followed by a discussion of the kinematics and kinetics of the spine. Identification of anatomical variations that may predispose individuals to spine injuries lead into strategies used to prevent injury. Information on common injuries sustained within the various regions of the spinal column during sport participation is followed by a presentation of techniques used in spinal injury assessment. Finally, examples of general rehabilitation exercises are provided.

ANATOMY REVIEW OF THE SPINE

How is vertebral structure related to the function of the cervical, thoracic, and lumbar regions of the spine?

The five regions of the spine—cervical, thoracic, lumbar, sacral, and coccygeal—are all structurally and functionally distinct. These differences translate to differences in the likelihood of certain injuries.

Spinal Column

The vertebral column consists of thirty-three vertebrae, most of which are separated and cushioned by discs composed of fibrocartilage (**Figure 14-1**). There are five regions of the spine based on vertebral structure and function. These regions include seven cervical vertebrae, twelve thoracic vertebrae, five lumbar vertebrae, five fused sacral vertebrae, and four small, fused coccygeal vertebrae. The bony structures of the vertebrae and ribs govern the varying amounts of spinal motion permitted throughout the cervical, thoracic, and lumbar regions. Within these regions,

> The bony structures of the vertebrae and ribs govern the amount of motion allowed at each motion segment

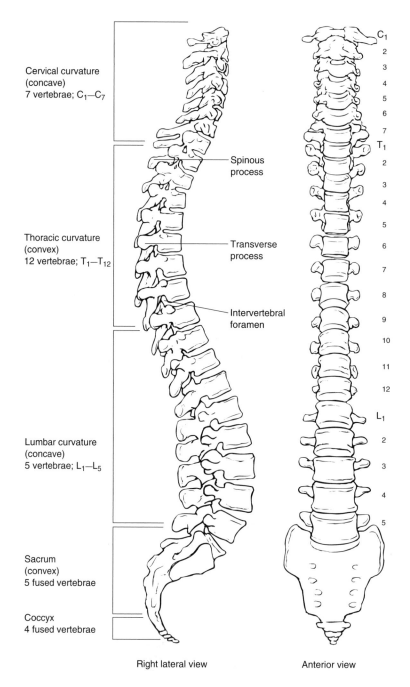

Cervical curvature
(concave)
7 vertebrae; C$_1$—C$_7$

Thoracic curvature
(convex)
12 vertebrae; T$_1$—T$_{12}$

Lumbar curvature
(concave)
5 vertebrae; L$_1$—L$_5$

Sacrum
(convex)
5 fused vertebrae

Coccyx
4 fused vertebrae

Spinous
process

Transverse
process

Intervertebral
foramen

C$_1$
2
3
4
5
6
7
T$_1$
2
3
4
5
6
7
8
9
10
11
12
L$_1$
2
3
4
5

Right lateral view

Anterior view

Fig. 14.1: The vertebral column has four characteristic curves of the spine viewed from the lateral aspect.

Motion segment
Two adjacent vertebrae and the intervening soft tissues; the functional unit of the spine

The articulating surfaces of the spinous processes are called facets ("little faces"), giving the joints their names

any two adjacent vertebrae and the soft tissues between them are collectively referred to as a **motion segment**. The motion segment is the functional unit of the spine (**Figure 14-2**).

Vertebrae

A typical vertebra consists of a body, a hollow ring known as the vertebral arch, and several bony processes (**Figure 14-3**). Forming a stacked column, the neural arches, posterior sides of the bodies, and the intervertebral discs form a protective passageway for the spinal cord and associated blood vessels known as the vertebral canal. The thinnest part of the neural arch is called the pars interarticularis. It is the pars region of the vertebrae that is most susceptible to stress fractures. The superior and inferior articular processes mate with the articular processes of adjacent vertebrae to form the facet joints. The right and left pedicles have notches on

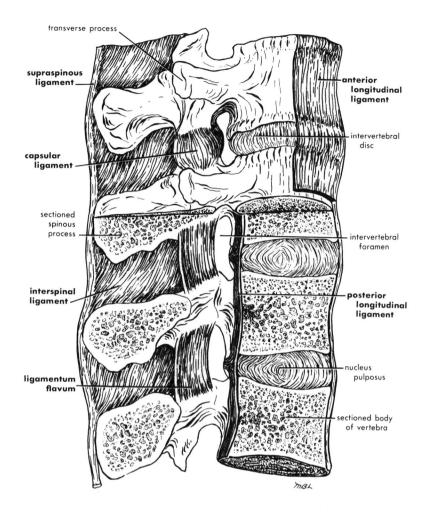

transverse process

supraspinous ligament

anterior longitudinal ligament

intervertebral disc

capsular ligament

sectioned spinous process

intervertebral foramen

interspinal ligament

posterior longitudinal ligament

nucleus pulposus

ligamentum flavum

sectioned body of vertebra

Fig. 14.2: A motion segment of the spine, including two adjacent vertebra and the intervening soft tissues. The motion segment is considered to be the functional unit of the spine.

their superior and inferior borders, providing openings between adjacent pedicles, called intervertebral foramina **(Figure 14-2)**. The spinal nerves pass through these foramina. The spinous and transverse processes serve as handles for muscle attachments.

There is a progressive increase in vertebral size from the cervical region down through the lumbar region **(Figure 14-1)**. The bodies of the lumbar vertebrae, in particular, are both larger and thicker than those in the more superior regions of the spine. This serves a

The spinal nerves exit the spinal canal through the intervertebral foramina

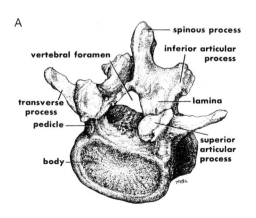

A

spinous process

vertebral foramen

inferior articular process

transverse process

pedicle

lamina

superior articular process

body

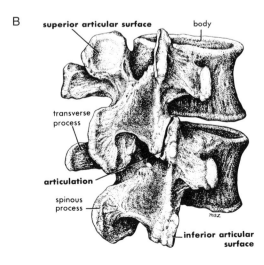

B

superior articular surface   body

transverse process

articulation

spinous process

inferior articular surface

Fig. 14.3: The structure of a typical vertebra. (A) Superior view. (B) Lateral view.

Atlas
The first cervical vertebra; so-named because it supports the skull

Axis
The second cervical vertebra; named after its bony prominence around which the atlas rotates

Annulus fibrosus
Tough outer covering of the intervertebral disc composed of fibrocartilage

Nucleus pulposus
Gelatinous-like material comprising the inner portion of the intervertebral disc

functional purpose, because when the body is in an upright position, each vertebra must support the weight of all of the trunk positioned above it, in addition to the arms and head.

The size and angulation of the vertebral processes also vary throughout the spinal column. This changes the orientation of the facet joints, which limit range of motion in the different spinal regions **(Figure 14-4)**.

Although all vertebrae differ at least slightly in size and shape, the structural adaptations of the first two cervical vertebrae are particularly of note **(Figure 14-5)**. The first, known as the **atlas**, consists of a bony ring with large, flat, superior articular facets upon which the skull rests. The second cervical vertebra is called the **axis** after its most prominent special feature, the dens, a superiorly directed bony protrusion that serves as an axis of rotation for the atlas.

Intervertebral Discs

Fibrocartilaginous discs provide cushioning between the articulating vertebral bodies. In the intervertebral disc, a thick ring of fibrous cartilage, the **annulus fibrosus**, surrounds a gelatinous material known as the **nucleus pulposus (Figure 14-2)**. The discs serve as shock absorbers and also allow the spine to bend.

Because the discs are avascular, they receive no blood supply. Instead, the discs must rely upon changes in posture and body position to produce a pumping action to bring in nutrients and flush out metabolic waste products with an influx and outflux of fluid (10). Because maintaining a fixed body position curtails this pumping action, sitting in one position for a long period of time can negatively affect disc health.

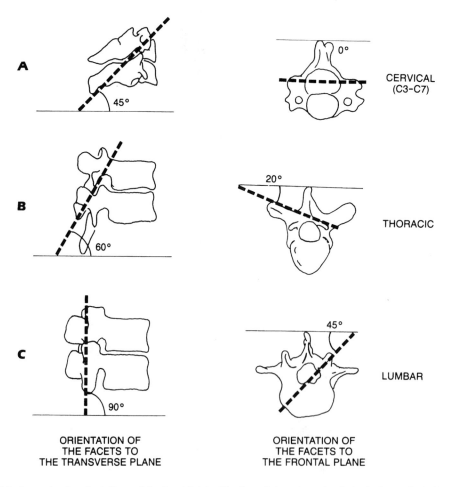

Fig. 14.4: Approximate orientations of the facet joints. The facet joint orientation in both the sagittal plane (lateral view) and transverse plane (superior view) shifts progressively throughout the length of the spinal column.

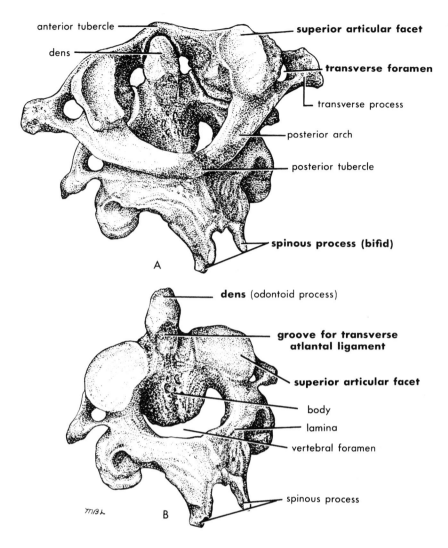

anterior tubercle

dens

superior articular facet

transverse foramen

transverse process

posterior arch

posterior tubercle

spinous process (bifid)

A

dens (odontoid process)

groove for transverse atlantal ligament

superior articular facet

body

lamina

vertebral foramen

spinous process

B

Fig. 14.5: The first and second vertebrae are referred to respectively as the atlas and axis.

Ligaments of the Spine

A number of ligaments support the spine (**Figure 14-2**). Anterior and posterior longitudinal ligaments connect the vertebral bodies of motion segments in the cervical, thoracic, and lumbar regions. The supraspinous ligament attaches to the spinous processes throughout the length of the spine. The supraspinous ligament is enlarged in the cervical region, where it is known as the ligamentum nuchae or "ligament of the neck." Another major ligament, the ligamentum flavum, connects the pedicles of adjacent vertebrae. This ligament contains a high proportion of elastic fibers that keep it constantly in tension, contributing to spinal stability. The interspinous ligaments, intertransverse ligaments, and ligamenta flava respectively link the spinous processes, transverse processes, and laminae of adjacent vertebrae.

Spinal Curves

There are four normal spinal curves (**Figure 14-1**). As viewed from the side, the thoracic and sacral curves are convex posteriorly, and the lumbar and cervical curves are concave posteriorly. These normal spinal curves constitute posture. The curves can be modified by a host of factors, including heredity, pathological conditions, and forces acting on the spine. Abnormal spinal curves are referred to as **curvatures** and are discussed later in the chapter.

Muscles of the Spine and Trunk

Muscles of the neck and trunk are paired, with one on the left and one on the right side of the body. These muscles can cause lateral flexion and/or rotation of the trunk when they act unilaterally, and trunk flexion or extension

The ligament flavum is constantly in tension, thereby serving as a major contributor to spinal stability

Normal spinal curves can be affected by heredity, pathological conditions, and forces acting on the spine

Curvature
An overdeveloped spinal curve that inhibits proper mechanical functioning

Cauda equina

Lower spinal nerves that
course through the lumbar
spinal canal, resembling a
horse's tail

Reflex

Action involving stimulation
of a motor neuron by a sensory neuron in the spinal cord
without involvement of the
brain

Deep tendon reflexes are
used consistently in injury
assessment to determine
possible spinal nerve damage

when acting bilaterally. Collectively, the primary movers for back extension are called the
erector spinae muscles **(Figure 14-6)**. The
attachments, actions, and innervations of the
major muscles of the trunk are summarized in
Table 14-1.

The Spinal Cord and Spinal Nerves

The brain and spinal cord make up the central
nervous system. The spinal cord extends from
the brain stem to the level of the first or second lumbar vertebrae **(Figure 14-7)**. Like
the brain, the spinal cord is encased in the
three meninges. Thirty-one pairs of spinal
nerves emanate from the cord, including
eight cervical, twelve thoracic, five lumbar,
five sacral, and one coccygeal. A bundle of
spinal nerves extends downward through the
vertebral canal from the end of the spinal
cord at the L_1-L_2 level. This nerve bundle is

known collectively as the **cauda equina** after
its resemblance to a horse's tail.

The spinal cord serves as the major neural
pathway for conducting sensory impulses to
the brain and motor impulses from the brain.
It also provides direct connections between
sensory and motor nerves inside the cord,
enabling **reflex** activity. Reflex actions occur
very quickly, before there is time for the brain
to process a sensory input and respond with
an appropriate motor signal. An example is
removing a hand from a source of extreme
heat through reflex action before the sensory
information that the hand is being burned
even reaches the brain. Deep tendon reflexes
are used consistently in injury assessment to
determine possible spinal nerve damage.
Exaggerated, distorted, or absent reflexes
indicate damage to the nervous system, often
before other signs are apparent.

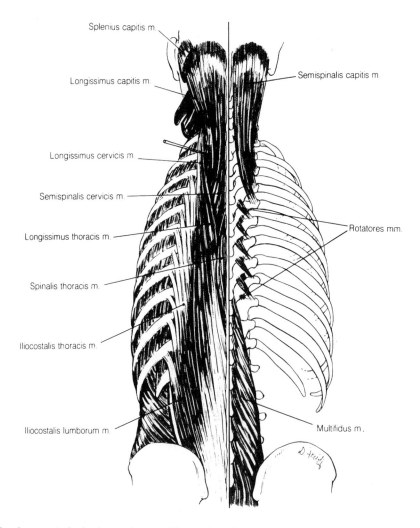

Splenius capitis m.

Longissimus capitis m.

Longissimus cervicis m.

Semispinalis cervicis m.

Longissimus thoracis m.

Spinalis thoracis m.

Iliocostalis thoracis m.

Iliocostalis lumborum m.

Semispinalis capitis m.

Rotatores mm.

Multifidus m.

Fig. 14.6: The deep posterior back muscles attaching to the spine.

Table 14–1. Muscles of the Spine.

Muscle	Proximal Attachment	Distal Attachment	Primary Action(s)	Nerve Innervation
Prevertebral muscles (Rectus capitis anterior, rectus capitis lateralis, longus capitis, longus coli)	Anterior aspect of occipital bone and cervical vertebrae	Anterior surfaces cervical and first three thoracic vertebrae	Flexion, lateral flexion, rotation to opposite side	Cervical nerves (C_1-C_6)
Rectus abdominis	Costal cartilage of ribs 5–7	Pubic crest	Flexion, lateral flexion	Intercostal nerves (T_6-T_{12})
External oblique	External surface of lower eight ribs	Linea alba and anterior iliac crest	Flexion, lateral flexion, rotation to opposite side	Intercostal nerves (T_7-T_{12})
Internal oblique	Linea alba and the lower four ribs	Inguinal ligament, iliac crest, and the lumbodorsal fascia	Flexion, lateral flexion, rotation to same side	Intercostal nerves (T_7-T_{12}, L_1)
Splenius (Capitis and Cervicis)	Mastoid process of the temporal bone, transverse processes of C1-C3 vertebrae	Lower half of the ligamentum nuchae, spinous processes of C7-T6 vertebrae	Extension, lateral flexion, rotation to same side	Middle and lower cervical nerves (C_4-C_8)
The suboccipitals (Obliquus capitus superior and inferior, rectus capitis posterior major and minor)	Occipital bone, transverse process of C1 vertebra	Posterior surfaces, C1-C2 vertebrae	Extension, lateral flexion, rotation to same side	Suboccipital nerve (C_1)
Erector spinae (Spinalis, longissimus, and iliocostalis)	Lower part of the ligamentum nuchae, posterior cervical, thoracic, and lumbar spine, lower 9 ribs, iliac crest, posterior sacrum	Mastoid process of the temporal bone, posterior cervical, thoracic, and lumbar spine, twelve ribs	Extension, lateral flexion, rotation to opposite side	Spinal nerves (T_1-T_{12})
Semispinalis (Capitis, cervicis, and thoracis)	Occipital bone, spinous processes of T2-T4 vertebrae	Transverse process, C7-T12 vertebrae	Extension, lateral flexion, rotation to opposite side	Cervical and thoracic spinal nerves (C_1-T_{12})
The deep spinal muscles (Multifidi, rotators, interspinales intertransversarii, levatores costarum)	Posterior processes of all vertebrae, posterior sacrum	Spinous and transverse processes and laminae of vertebrae below those of the proximal attachment	Extension, lateral flexion, rotation to opposite side	Spinal and intercostal nerves (T_1-T_{12})
Sternocleido-mastoid	Mastoid process of the temporal bone	Superior sternum, inner third of the clavicle	Flexion of the neck, extension of the head, lateral flexion, rotation to opposite side	Accessory nerve and C_2 spinal nerve

(continued)

Table 14–1. Muscles of the Spine. (*continued*)

Muscle	Proximal Attachment	Distal Attachment	Primary Action(s)	Nerve Innervation
Levator scapulae	Transverse process of the first four cervical vertebrae	Vertebral border of the scapula	Lateral flexion	C_3-C_4 spinal nerves, dorsal scapular nerve (C_3-C_5)
The scaleni (Scalenus anterior, medius, and posterior)	Transverse processes, C1-C7 vertebrae	Upper two ribs	Flexion, lateral flexion	Cervical nerves (C_3-C_8)
Quadratus lumborum	Last rib, transverse processes of L1-L4 vertebrae	Iliolumbar ligament, adjacent lumbar iliac crest	Lateral flexion	T_{12}-L_4 spinal nerves
Psoas major	Sides of twelfth thoracic and all lumbar vertebrae	Lesser trochanter of the femur	Flexion	Femoral nerve (L_1-L_3)

💡 *Structure and function are intimately related in the spinal column. The size of each vertebral body is proportional to the amount of weight that it must support. The orientations of the facet joints also vary throughout the spinal column, governing range of motion. Finally, the first two cervical vertebrae are uniquely designed for their special functions.*

Spinal movements always involve a number of motion segments

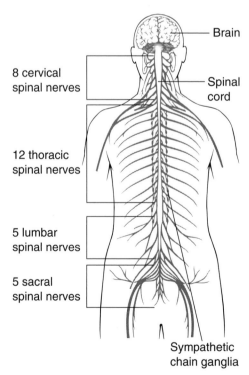

8 cervical spinal nerves

12 thoracic spinal nerves

5 lumbar spinal nerves

5 sacral spinal nerves

Brain

Spinal cord

Sympathetic chain ganglia

Fig. 14.7: The spinal cord and spinal nerves

KINEMATICS AND MAJOR MUSCLE ACTIONS OF THE SPINE

❓ *Which regions of the spine allow the freest motion? Can you speculate as to what implications this might have for injury potential?*

The vertebral joints enable motion in all planes of movement, as well as circumduction (**Figure 14-8**). Because the motion allowed between any two adjacent vertebrae is small, however, spinal movements always involve a number of motion segments. The range of motion allowed at each motion segment is governed by anatomical constraints that vary though the cervical, thoracic, and lumbar regions of the spine (**Figure 14-4**).

Flexion, Extension, and Hyperextension

Spinal flexion is anterior bending of the spine in the sagittal plane, with extension being the return to anatomical position from a position of flexion. As shown in **Table 14-2**, the flexion/extension capability of the motion segments at all levels of the spine is relatively small, with a maximum range of 5° at T1-T2. The thoracic region permits the largest cumulative range of motion in flexion/extension with 46°, compared to only 16° for both the cervical and lumbar regions (11).

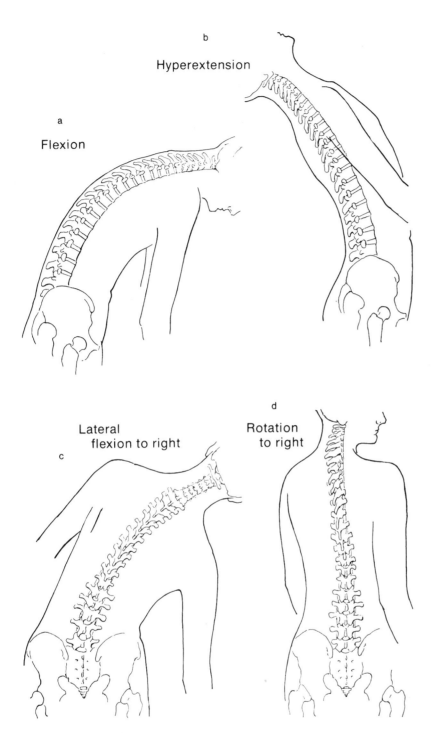

b

Hyperextension

a

Flexion

c

Lateral
flexion to right

d

Rotation
to right

Fig. 14.8: Motions of the trunk. (A) Flexion. (B) Hyperextension in the sagittal plane. (C) Lateral flexion in the frontal plane. (D) Rotation in the transverse plan. Extension, the return to anatomical position from a position of flexion, and circumduction, a sequence of movements in which the head traces a circular path, are not shown.

It is important not to confuse spinal flexion with hip flexion or forward pelvic tilt, although all three motions occur during an activity such as touching the toes. As discussed in Chapter 9, hip flexion consists of anteriorly directed sagittal plane rotation of the femur with respect to the pelvic girdle (or vice versa) and forward pelvic tilt is anteriorly directed movement of the anterior superior iliac spine with respect to the pubic symphysis.

When the spine is extended backward past anatomical position in the sagittal plane, the motion is termed hyperextension. The range

Table 14–2. Spinal Range of Motion.[a,b]

Movement	Cervical	Thoracic	Lumbar
Flexion/extension			
Most mobile segment	C5-C6	T1-T2	L5-S1
ROM for that segment	4°	5°	2°
ROM for total region	16°	46°	16°
Hyperextension			
Most mobile segment	C5-C6	T1-T2	L5-S1
ROM for that segment	17°	5°	21°
ROM for total region	64°	22°	54°
Lateral Flexion			
Most mobile segment(s)	C3-C5	all	L2-L5
ROM for that segment	6°	3°	8°
ROM for total region	23°	31°	24°
Rotation			
Most mobile segment	C1-C2	T1-T2	L5-S1
ROM for that segment	50°	7°	5°
ROM for total region	80°	52°	9°

[a]Schultz, A.B. 1974. Mechanics of the human spine. *Applied Mechanics Review*, 27:1487–1497.
[b] White, A. A., and Panjabi, M. M. *Clinical Biomechanics of the Spine*. Philadelphia: J.B. Lippincott, 1978.

of motion for spinal hyperextension is considerable in the cervical and lumbar regions, ranging as high as 17° at the C5-C6 level and 21° at L5-S1. As shown in **Table 14-2**, cumulative range of motion for hyperextension is greatest in the cervical region with 64°, followed by the lumbar region with 54°, followed by the thoracic region with 22° (11). Lumbar hyperextension is required in the execution of many sport skills, including several swimming strokes, the high jump and pole vault, wrestling, and numerous gymnastic skills. It has been reported that during a back handspring the lumbar curvature may be increased to as much as twenty times that present during relaxed standing (12).

Lateral Flexion and Rotation

Movement of the spine away from anatomical position in a lateral direction in the frontal plane is termed lateral flexion. In the thoracic region, the cumulative range of motion for lateral flexion is approximately 31°, with 23° and 24° permitted in the cervical and lumbar regions, respectively (11).

Spinal rotation capability is greatest in the cervical region, with up to 50° of motion allowed at C1-C2. In the thoracic region, approximately 9° of rotation is permitted among the upper six motion segments. From T7-T8 downward, however, the range of motion in rotation progressively decreases, with only about 2° of motion allowed in the lumbar spine because of the interlocking of the articular processes there. At the lumbosacral joint about 5° of rotation is allowed (13).

Motion capability of the cervical, thoracic, and lumbar regions varies with the direction of movement. Mobility often translates to greater activity in the surrounding muscles and subsequently to higher intra-joint forces, which increase the potential for injury.

KINETICS OF THE SPINE

Why is it important to maintain the spine in an erect posture during weight-training exercises?

Forces acting on the spine include body weight, tension in the spinal ligaments and paraspinal muscles, intra-abdominal pressure and any applied external loads. When the body is in an upright position, the major form of loading on the spine is axial. In this position, body weight, the weight of any load held in the hands, and tension in the surrounding ligaments and muscles all contribute to spinal compression. Intra-abdominal pressure, on the other hand, works like a balloon inside the abdominal cavity to support the adjacent lumbar spine by creating a tensile force that partially offsets the compressive load. Intra-abdominal pressure has been observed to increase just prior to the lifting of a heavy load, although the mechanism

Spinal rotation is greatest in the cervical region, with up to 50° of motion at C1-C2

Forces acting on the spine include body weight, tension in the spinal ligaments and paraspinal muscles, intra-abdominal pressure, and any applied external loads through which this is accomplished is not well understood (14).

Although most of the axial compressional load on the spine is borne by the vertebral bodies and discs, the facet joints also assist with load bearing. When the spine is in hyperextension the facet joints may bear up to approximately 30% of the load (11,15).

Effect of Body Position

One factor that can dramatically affect the load on the spine is body position. When the body is in an upright position the line of gravity passes anterior to the spinal column (**Figure 14-9**). As a result, the spine is under a constant forward bending moment. As the trunk is progressively flexed, the line of gravity shifts farther away from the spine. The farther the line of gravity from the spine, the larger the moment arm for body weight and the greater the bending moment generated. To maintain body position, this moment must be counteracted by tension in the back muscles. The more tension required of these muscles to maintain body position, the greater the compressional load on the spine. In comparison to the load present during upright standing, compression on the lumbar spine increases with sitting, increases more with spinal flexion, and increases still further with a slouched sitting position (**Figure 14-10**). During lifting and carrying, holding the load as close to the trunk as possible minimizes the load on the back. **Field Strategy 14-1** provides guidelines to reduce spinal

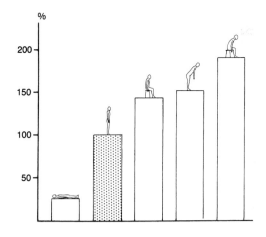

Fig. 14.10: The relative loads on the 3rd lumbar disc with various body positions. Adapted with permission from Nachemson, A. 1975. Towards a better understanding of back pain; A review of the mechanics of the lumbar disc. *Rheumatol Rehabil,* 14(3):129–143.

stress in daily activities to prevent low back injuries.

Effect of Movement Speed and Impact

Another factor affecting spinal loading is body movement speed. It has been shown that executing a lift in a very rapid, jerking fashion dramatically increases compression and shear forces on the spine, as well as tension in the paraspinal muscles (14). This is one of the reasons that isotonic resistance training exercises should always be performed in a slow, controlled fashion.

For individuals participating in high-speed and contact sports, impact forces are also potential causes of spinal injuries. Axial compressional loading has been implicated as the leading mechanism of injury for severe cervical spine injuries (6–8). Because the range of motion in the cervical spine is greatest in flexion, a head position of extreme flexion generates the largest bending moment. When a tackle in football is executed with the head in a flexed position, the cervical spine is subject to both large compressional forces generated by the cervical muscles and to axial impact forces (**Figure 14-11**). With the head in flexion the cervical vertebrae are aligned in a segmented column (**Figure 14-12A**). Impact causes loading along the longitudinal axis of the cervical vertebrae, leading to compression deformation (**Figure 14-12B**). Initially the intervertebral discs absorb the energy (**Figure 14-12C**). However, as continued

When the trunk is erect the back muscles must develop tension to balance the spinal moment—the product of weight and distance from the spine. Thus, the heavier an object or the farther it is held from the body, the more the back muscles must work

Axial loading is the leading mechanism of injury for severe cervical spine injuries

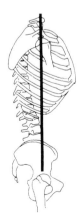

Fig. 14.9: The line of gravity for the head and trunk passes anterior to the spinal column during upright standing. The moment arm for head/trunk weight at any given vertebral joint is the perpendicular distance between the line of gravity and the spinal column.

Sitting
- Sit on a firm, straight-back chair
- Avoid slouching in the chair by placing the buttocks as far back into the chair as possible
- Sit with the feet flat on the floor
- Avoid sitting for long periods of time, particularly with the knees fully extended

Driving
- Place the seat forward so the knees are level with the hips and you do not have to reach for the pedals
- If the left foot is not working the pedals, place it flat on the floor
- Avoid leaning forward or slouching
- Keep the back of the seat in a nearly upright position

Standing
- If you must stand in one area for an extended time:
  Shift position from one foot to the other.
  Place one foot on an elevated piece of furniture to keep the knees slightly bent.
  Do toe flexion and extension inside the shoes
- Concentrate on holding the chin up, keeping the shoulders back and relaxing the knees

Lifting and carrying
- Avoid lifting heavy objects without a lumbosacral belt or assistance
- To lift an object:
  Place the object close to the body.
  Bend at the knees, not the waist, and keep the back erect.
  Tighten the abdominal muscles and inhale while lifting the object. Exhale at the end of the lift.
  Do not hold your breath.
  Do not twist while lifting
- To carry a heavy object:
  Hold the object close to the body at waist level
  Carry the object in the middle of the body not to one side

Sleeping
- Sleep on a firm mattress. If needed, a sheet of 3/4 inch plywood can be placed under the mattress
- Sleep on your side and place pillows between the legs
- If you sleep supine, place pillows under the knees. Avoid sleeping in the prone position
- Waterbeds may relieve low back pain since they support the body curves evenly

Fig. 14.11: In a normally erect position, the cervical spine is slightly extended. When a tackle in football is executed with the head flexed at about 30°, the cervical vertebrae are straightened into a column and subject to compressional forces generated by the cervical muscles and to axial loading.

B

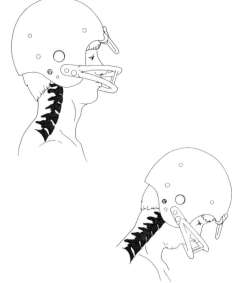

A

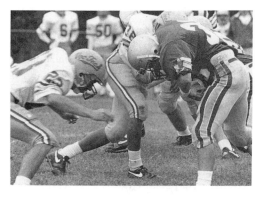

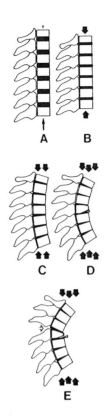

Fig. 14.12: Axial loading on the vertebral column causes compressive deformation of the intervertebral discs (A,B). As load continues and maximum compression deformation is reached, angular deformation and buckling occurs (C,D). Continued force results in an anterior compression fracture, subluxation, or dislocation (E).

force is absorbed by the cervical region, further deformation and buckling occurs, leading to failure of the intervertebral discs, cervical vertebrae, or both (**Figure 14-12D**). This results in subluxation, disc herniation, facet dislocation, or fracture-dislocation at one or more spinal levels (**Figure 14-12E**) (6).

💡 *Lifting with the trunk erect minimizes the tension requirement for the lumbar muscles because the moment arm for body weight is minimized. Exercises involving trunk flexion should be performed in a slow, controlled manner to progressively strengthen the lumbar extensors.*

ANATOMICAL VARIATIONS PREDISPOSING INDIVIDUALS TO SPINE INJURIES

❓ *The normal anatomical curves of the spine vary in size among individuals. Can extreme variations in these curves predispose an individual to a back injury?*

Mechanical stress derived from lateral spinal muscle imbalances or from sustaining repeated impact forces can cause back pain and/or injury. Excessive spinal curvatures can be congenital or acquired through weight training or sport participation. Defects in the pars interarticularis of the neural arch can be caused by mechanical stress, also placing an individual at risk for serious spinal injury.

Kyphosis

Accentuation of the thoracic curve is called **kyphosis (Figure 14-13)**. **Scheuermann's disease**, or osteochondritis of the spine,

Kyphosis
Excessive curve in the thoracic region of the spine

Scheuermann's disease
Osteochondrosis of the spine due to abnormal epiphyseal plate behavior that allows herniation of the disc into the vertebral body, giving a characteristic wedge-shaped appearance

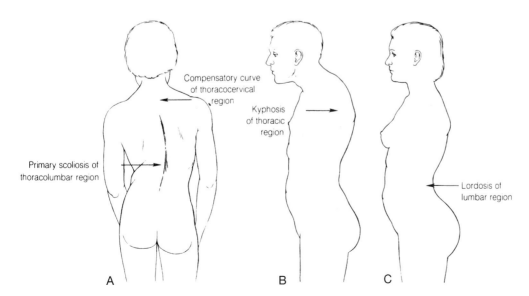

Fig. 14.13: Spinal anomalies. (A) Scoliosis. (B) Thoracic kyphosis. (C) Lordosis.

involves the development of one or more wedge-shaped vertebrae through abnormal epiphyseal plate behavior and is a common cause of kyphosis (**See Figure 14-18B**). This condition has been called "rounded back" or "swimmer's back" because it can be caused by overtraining with the butterfly stroke, particularly among adolescents. Athletes such as weight lifters, gymnasts, and football linemen, who may over-develop the pectoral muscles, are also prone to this condition.

Scoliosis
Lateral rotational spinal curvature

Scoliosis

Lateral curvature of the spine is known as **scoliosis (Figure 14-13)**. The lateral deformity is coupled with rotational deformity of the involved vertebrae, with the condition ranging from mild to severe. Scoliosis may appear as either a "C" or an "S" curve involving the thoracic spine, the lumbar spine, or both.

Scoliosis can be structural or nonstructural. Structural scoliosis involves inflexible curvature that persists even with lateral bending of the spine. Nonstructural scoliotic curves are flexible and are corrected with lateral bending.

Lordosis
Excessive curve in the lumbar region of the spine

Scoliosis results from a variety of causes. Congenital abnormalities and selected cancers can contribute to the development of structural scoliosis. Nonstructural scoliosis may occur secondary to a leg length discrepancy or local inflammation. Approximately 70 to 90% of all scoliosis cases, however, are termed idiopathic, which means that the cause is unknown (16,17). Idiopathic scoliosis is most commonly diagnosed between the ages of 10 and 13 years, but can be seen at any age, and is more common in females.

Spondylolysis
A stress fracture of the pars interarticularis

Symptoms associated with scoliosis vary with the severity of the condition. Mild cases may be asymptomatic and may self-correct with time. Although mild to moderate cases can be treated with appropriate strengthening exercises, severe scoliosis, characterized by extreme lateral deviation and localized rotation of the spine, can be painful and deforming and is treated with bracing and/or surgery.

Lordosis

Abnormal exaggeration of the lumbar curve, or **lordosis** is often associated with weakened abdominal muscles and forward pelvic tilt (**Figure 14-13**). Causes of lordosis include congenital spinal deformity, weakness of the abdominal muscles, poor postural habits, and overtraining in sports requiring repeated lumbar hyperextension such as gymnastics, figure skating, football (linemen), javelin throwing, or swimming the butterfly stroke.

Symptoms of lordosis vary with the severity of the condition. Because lordosis places added compressive stress on the posterior elements of the spine, low back pain is a common symptom. Lordosis is a problem for many adolescent athletes, predisposing them to low back injuries (18).

Pars Interarticularis Fractures

The pars interarticularis is the weakest bony portion of the vertebral neural arch, the region between the superior and inferior articular facets. A fracture in this region is termed **spondylolysis (Figure 14-14)**. Although some pars defects may be congenital, they are also known to be caused by mechanical stress.

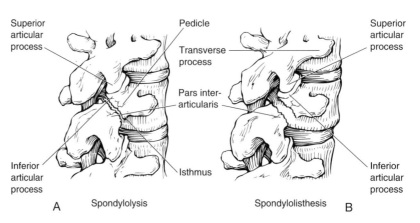

Fig. 14.14: Spondylolysis is a stress fracture of the pars interarticularis (A). Spondylolisthesis is a bilateral fracture of the pars interarticularis accompanied by anterior slippage of the involved vertebra (B).

One mechanism of injury appears to involve repeated axial loading of the lumbar spine when it is hyperextended. Fractures of the pars interarticularis may range from hairline to complete separation of the bone. A bony defect in spondylolysis tends to occur at an earlier age, typically before age eight, yet often does not produce symptoms at that age. Furthermore, the pars fracture may heal with less periosteal callus and tends to form a fibrous union more often than fractures at other sites. The condition also has a strong genetic component with prevalence as high as 33% among those with family members who also have the condition (19).

A bilateral separation in the pars interarticularis, called **spondylolisthesis**, results in the anterior displacement of a vertebra with respect to the vertebra below it **(Figure 14-15)**. The most common site for this injury is the lumbosacral joint, with 90% of the slips occurring at this level. Spondylolisthesis is often initially diagnosed in children between the ages of 10 and 15 years, and is more common in boys (20). Whereas 2% of the general population have spondylolysis, 5% of those with spondylolysis also have spondylolisthesis (21).

Unlike most stress fractures, spondylolysis and spondylolisthesis do not typically heal with time, but tend to persist, particularly when there is no interruption in sport participation. Individuals whose sports or positions require repeated hyperextension of the lumbar spine are prime candidates for stress-related spondylolysis **(Figure 14-16)**. Those particularly susceptible are female gymnasts, interior football linemen, weight lifters, volleyball players, pole vaulters, wrestlers, and rowers (21).

Although most spondylitic conditions are asymptomatic, when the underlying cause is repeated mechanical stress, low back pain and associated neurological symptoms are likely to occur. The individual may complain of unilateral low back pain at the level of the belt aggravated by activity, usually extension and rotation (19). Pain may radiate into the buttock region or down the sciatic nerve if the L_5 nerve root is compressed. Muscle spasm may occur in the erector spinae muscles or hamstrings. This individual should be referred to a physician. In mild cases, modifications in training and technique can permit the individual to continue to participate. However, in moderate cases, most physicians will not begin active rehabilitation until the individual is asymptomatic for four weeks. At that time, flexibility in the hamstrings and gluteal muscles is combined with strengthening the abdomen and back extensors. If the slip is greater than 25%, the individual may be excluded from participation in contact sports unless the person is asymptomatic and absence of continued slippage has been documented (20).

Spina Bifida Occulta

Spina bifida occulta is a congenital defect in the vertebral canal characterized by absence of the laminae and spinous process. It typically involves the lumbosacral region but manifests no neural deficits. Individuals frequently complain of low back discomfort, and a small dimple or tuft of hair can be seen over the site of the involved vertebra. The condition is confirmed only by radiograph, and unless it is severe, the individual can continue to participate in sport. In fact, many athletes with spina bifida are unaware that they have the condition.

💡 *Spine anomalies can predispose an individual to injury, however, training modifications, correction of technique, and muscle strengthening can permit individuals to continue participating in sport. Each case must be evaluated by a physician on an individual basis.*

Spondylolisthesis
Anterior slippage of a vertebrae resulting from a complete bilateral fracture of the pars interarticularis

Most spondylitic conditions are asymptomatic; however, repeated mechanical stress can lead to low back pain and associated neurological symptoms

Spina bifida occulata
Congenital defect in the vertebral canal characterized by absence of the laminae and spinous process

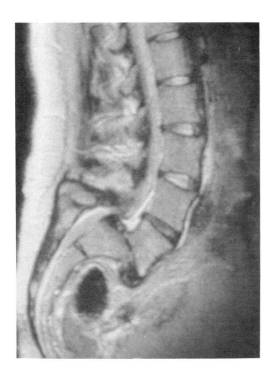
Fig. 14.15: In this MRI scan of spondylolisthesis, note the anterior shift of the L5 vertebra.

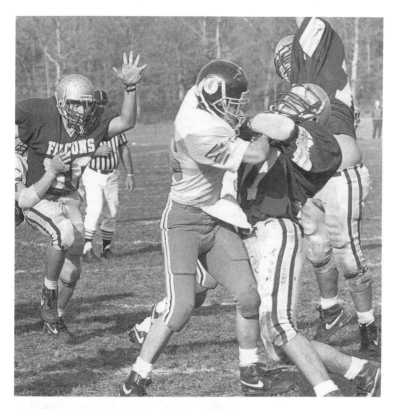

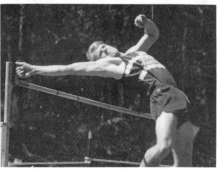

Fig. 14.16: The bodies of football linemen, female gymnasts, pole vaulters, and high jumpers are often forced into trunk hyperextension, predisposing them to low back conditions.

PREVENTION OF SPINAL INJURIES

❓ *The spine is a complex linkage system that transfers loads between the upper and lower extremities, enables motion of the trunk in all three planes, and protects the delicate spinal cord. What measures can be taken to protect this vulnerable region?*

The most common injuries to the back are minor in nature, however, serious injuries can occur. As with other joint regions, protective equipment can prevent some injuries from occurring, particularly at the cervical, sacrum, and coccyx. However, even use of protective equipment cannot prevent accidental catastrophic injuries from occurring. Physical conditioning, including flexibility and strengthening exercises, and proper skill technique play a more important role in preventing injuries to the region.

Protective Equipment

Several pieces of equipment can be used to protect the spinal region. In the cervical region, a neck roll or a posterolateral pad made of a high, thick, and stiff material can be attached to shoulder pads to limit motion of the cervical spine, and has been shown to be effective in reducing the incidence of repetitive burners and stingers. In the upper body, shoulder pads extend over the upper thoracic region to absorb and disperse shock from impact forces, thus protecting soft and bony tissue structures in the thoracic region. Rib protectors composed of air-inflated, interconnected cylinders can protect a limited region of the thoracic spine. Weight-training belts, abdominal binders, and other similar lumbar/sacral supportive devices support the abdominal contents, stabilize the trunk, and prevent spinal deformity and damage. These devices place the low back in a more vertical lifting posture, and significantly increase intra-abdominal pressure to reduce compressive forces in the vertebral bodies. Many of these protective devices were discussed and demonstrated in Chapter 6.

Physical Conditioning

Flexibility and strengthening of the back muscles is imperative to stabilize the spinal column. Although stretching exercises for the low back region and hip flexors are commonly done prior to sport participation, range of motion exercises for the cervical and thoracic regions should also be performed. In the cervical region, the hands are used to provide a slow, prolonged stretch in the various motions. Exercises, such as those shown in **Field Strategy 14-2** can be used to stretch the thoracic and lumbar regions.

Strengthening exercises for the cervical region may involve isometric contractions,

---

 Field Strategy 14–2. Prevention of Spinal Injuries.

Flexibility Exercises

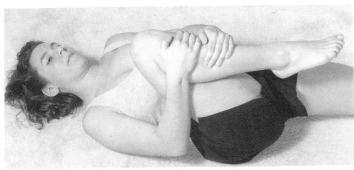

A. *Single knee to chest stretch.* In a supine position, pull one knee toward the chest with the hands. Keep the back flat. Switch to the opposite leg and repeat.

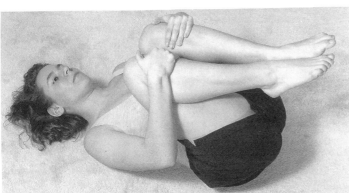

B. *Double knee to the chest stretch.* In a supine position, pull both knees to the chest with the hands. Keep the back flat.

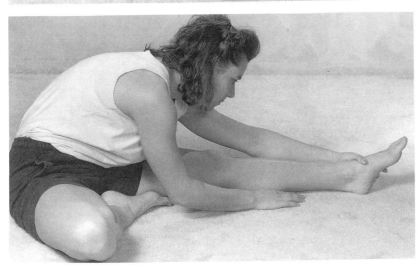

C. *Hamstring stretch.* See Field Strategy 8–1.

(*continued*)

Field Strategy 14–2. Prevention of Spinal Injuries. (*continued*)

Flexibility Exercises

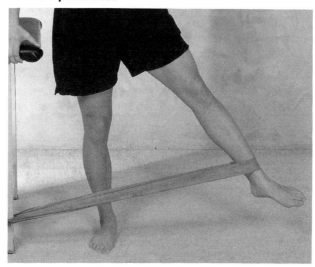

D. *Hip flexor stretch.* See Field Strategy 9–1.

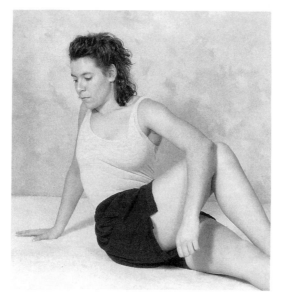

E. *Lateral rotator stretch.* See Field Strategy 9–1.

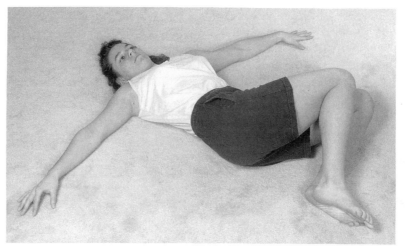

F. *Lower trunk rotation stretch.* In a supine position, rotate the flexed knees to one side, keeping the back flat and the feet together.

Flexibility Exercises

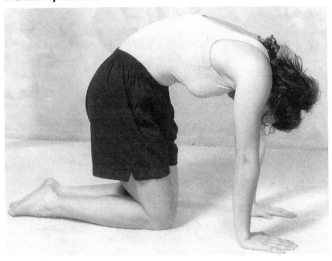

G. *Angry cat stretch (posterior pelvic tilt).* Kneel on all fours with knees hip-width apart. Tighten the buttocks and arch the back upward while lowering the chin and tilting the pelvis backwards. Relax the buttocks and allow the pelvis to drop downward and forward.

Strengthening exercises

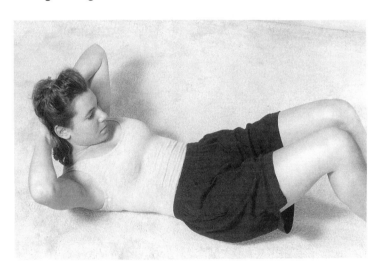

H. *Crunch curl-up.* In a supine position with the knees flexed, flatten the back, and curl up to elevate the head and shoulders from the floor. Alternate exercises include diagonal crunch curl-ups and hip crunches.

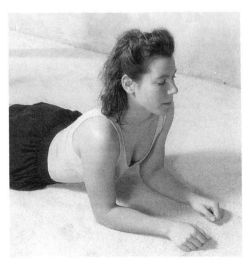

I. *Prone extension.* In a prone position, raise up on the elbows. Progress to raising up onto the hands.

(continued)

Strengthening exercises

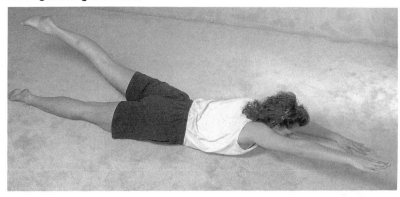

J. *Alternate arm and leg lift.* In a fully extended prone position, lift one arm and the opposite leg off the surface at least three inches. Repeat with the opposite arm and leg.

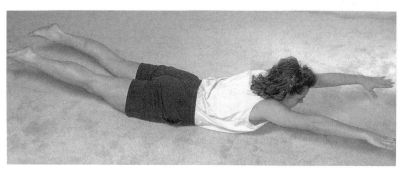

K. *Double arm and leg lift.* In a fully extended prone position, lift both arms and legs off the surface at least three inches. Hold and return to starting position.

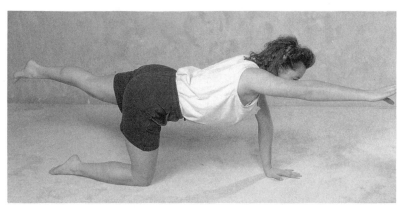

L. *Alternate arm and leg extension on all fours.* Kneel on all fours, raise one leg behind the body while raising the opposite arm in front of the body. Ankle and wrist weights may be added for additional resistance.

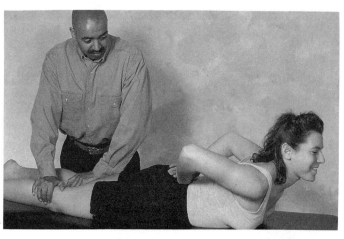

M. *Back extension.* Using a back extension machine or having another individual stabilize the feet and legs, raise the trunk into a slightly hyperextended position.

manual resistance, use of surgical tubing, or weight training with free weights or specialized machines. Exercises should include neck flexion, extension, lateral flexion and rotation, as well as scapular elevation. Stabilization of the cervical spine is of particular importance to wrestlers and football lineman who are consistently subjected to the extremes of motion at the neck.

Exercises to strengthen the thoracic and low back area should involve back extension, lateral flexion and rotation, abdominal strengthening, and exercises for the lower trapezius and latissimus dorsi. Many of these exercises are also demonstrated in **Field Strategy 14-2**.

Proper Skill Technique

Proper skill technique is vital to prevent spinal injuries. Helmets are designed to protect the cranial region from injury. However, some players develop a false sense of security and may use the helmet as a point of impact, thereby increasing the risk of injury to the cervical spine. For example, when a tackle in football is executed with the head in a flexed position, the cervical vertebrae are aligned in a segmented column, and subjected to both large compressional forces generated by the cervical muscles, and to axial impact forces **(Figures 14-11, 14-12)**. If magnitude is sufficient, deformation and buckling occur, leading to a possible subluxation, disc herniation, dislocation, or fracture-dislocation.

Proper lifting technique and use of a supportive weight-training belt can prevent injury to the lumbar region. During strength training, observe proper breathing procedures to fix the stabilizing musculature of the trunk. Inhale deeply as the lift is initiated, and exhale forcefully and smoothly at the end of the lift. A spotter can assist in taking the barbell from the lifter and returning it to the supports during squats, bench presses, and incline presses, and should always be present when lifting heavy weights.

Proper body position and posture can also prevent injuries to the spinal region. Poor posture during walking, sitting, standing, lying, and running can subject bony and soft tissue structures to abnormal compressive and shearing forces that may lead to chronic low back strain or ligamentous sprains. All cases of postural deformity should be assessed to determine the cause. Then,

appropriate flexibility and strengthening exercises should be added to the conditioning program to address the deficits.

Although protective equipment can protect limited portions of the spine, its use cannot prevent accidental catastrophic injuries. Improved flexibility and strength in the spinal musculature, and proper technique can, however, prevent or limit severity of injury.

CERVICAL SPINE INJURIES

After practice, a wrestler is complaining of a sore neck. He is most comfortable with the head slightly rotated to the right. Point tenderness is present in the muscle mass on the left side of the neck. There is full range of motion, although it is somewhat painful. Resisted neck lateral flexion to the left and rotation to the right increase the pain. No change in sensation or grip strength is evident. What injury might you suspect? How would you manage this injury?

The relatively small size of the cervical vertebrae combined with the nearly horizontal orientation of the cervical facet joints make the cervical spine the most mobile region of the spinal column. This, combined with the small mass of the neck as compared to the trunk, makes the cervical spine especially vulnerable to injury.

The National Football Head and Neck Injury Registry, established in 1975, documented head and neck injuries retrospectively during 1971–1975 and compared them with an earlier study by Schneider and Kahn during 1959–1963 (22). A 204% increase in cervical spine fractures, subluxations, and dislocations, and a 116% increase in the rate of cervical spine injuries associated with permanent quadriplegia were documented (8). Axial loading was identified as the predominant mechanism of injury. In an effort to reduce head and neck injuries, the National Collegiate Athletic Association (NCAA) and National Federation of High School Athletic Associations (NFHSAA) adopted rule changes in 1976 to prohibit the use of the head in tackling or spearing an opponent. The goal was to prevent use of the head as the initial point of contact in blocking and tackling. As a result of the rule changes, fractures, subluxations, and dislocations of the cervical spine have progressively decreased since 1976–1987 (8). In 1984, injury rates had

In an effort to reduce head and neck injuries in football, rule changes were adopted in 1976 to prohibit the use of the head in tackling or spearing an opponent

decreased 82% in high schools and 100% in colleges (6). Although some cervical injuries continue to occur, a recent study in 1989 showed an overall injury rate for two seasons of collegiate football to be only .3 overall neck injuries/1000 participants (23). Great strides have been made in reducing head and spinal injuries, however, the potential still exists for catastrophic injuries.

Cervical Strains and Sprains

Cervical strains usually involve the sternocleidomastoid or upper trapezius, although the scalenes, levator scapulae, and splenius muscles may also be involved. They typically occur at the extremes of motion, such as hyperflexion, hyperextension, or excessive rotation, or in association with a violent muscle contraction or external force. Symptoms include pain, stiffness, and restricted range of motion. Muscle spasms may be palpated with increased pain elicited during active contraction or passive stretching of the involved muscle. Generally, symptoms subside within three to seven days.

Sprains can occur to major ligaments traversing the cervical spine, as well as to the capsular ligaments surrounding the facet joints. The same mechanisms that cause cervical strains also cause cervical sprains. Both injuries often occur simultaneously. Minor activity, such as maintaining the head in an uncomfortable posture or sleeping position, can also produce sprains of the neck. Symptoms mirror those seen in cervical strains, however, with severe sprains, symptoms tend to persist longer. In severe cases when pain or numbness radiates into the back of the head or extremities, referral to a physician is warranted to rule out a possible spinal fracture, dislocation, or disc injury.

Initial treatment includes rest, cryotherapy, prescribed non-steroidal anti-inflammatory drugs (NSAIDs), and use of a cervical collar for support. Follow-up treatment may involve continued cryotherapy or use of superficial heat, gentle stretching, and isometric exercises. Individuals participating in contact sports should strengthen the neck muscles through appropriate resistance exercise.

Cervical Spinal Stenosis

Spinal stenosis is defined as a loss of cerebrospinal fluid around the spinal cord, or in more extreme cases, deformation of the spinal cord (24). The condition may involve a narrowing of the neural canal which can impinge the spinal cord leading to quadriplegia or transient quadriplegia. Stenosis may also occur in the lumbar region impinging neural segments of the cauda equina. The National Center for Catastrophic Sports Injury Research reported that 22 cases of quadriplegia and three cases of transient quadriplegia occurred between the years 1989–1991. Of these cases, 62% involved some degree of spinal stenosis (24).

Individuals may remain asymptomatic. However, the condition becomes apparent after an acute injury leads to neurological deficits. The individual may have sensory changes, or motor deficits in both arms, both legs, or all four extremities, following forced hyperextension, hyperflexion, or axial loading of the cervical spine (25,26). Sensory changes may include burning pain, numbness, tingling, or total loss or sensation. Motor changes may include weakness or complete paralysis. The changes are always bilateral, differentiating this condition from a nerve root injury which is always unilateral (26). The episode may be transient with full recovery in 10 to 15 minutes; although in some cases complete recovery does not occur for 36 to 38 hours (25). This condition is often called a **neurapraxia**, since neural changes are only temporary.

The condition may be discovered during routine radiographs, but often an MRI is needed. An individual who has had an episode of cervical spinal neurapraxia, with or without transient quadriplegia, is not necessarily predisposed to permanent neurological injury. Individuals with developing spinal stenosis or spinal stenosis associated with congenital abnormalities have returned safely to participation. However, a growing number of physicians have concluded that individuals with stenosis of the cervical spine with associated cervical spine instability, or acute or chronic intervertebral disc disease should be advised to discontinue participation in contact sports (24–26).

Cervical Fractures and Dislocations

Unsafe practices involving axial loading with violent flexion of the neck, such as diving into shallow water, spearing in football, or landing on the posterior neck during gymnastics or trampoline activities, can lead to cervical fractures. Cervical dislocations occur more frequently than cervical fractures, yet are equally as serious. Cervical dislocations involve flexion and rotation, and are more common than dislocations in the thoracic or lumbar region (7,8,27–29).

In sports, fractures and dislocations commonly occur at the fourth, fifth, and sixth cervical vertebrae. Since neural damage resulting from a fracture or dislocation can range from none to complete severance of the spinal cord, there is a range of accompanying symptoms. Painful palpation over the spinous processes, undue muscle spasm, or a defect indicates a possible fracture or dislocation. Radiating pain, numbness, weakness in a myotome, paralysis in the limbs and trunk, or loss of bladder or bowel control are all serious signs of neural damage. **Table 14-3** summarizes key signs that indicate the presence of a cervical fracture or dislocation. If a unilateral cervical dislocation is present, the neck will be visibly tilted toward the dislocated side, with muscle tightness due to stretch on the convex side and muscle slack on the concave side.

Because fractures and dislocations of the cervical spine can damage the spinal cord leading to paralysis or death, any suspected injury should be treated as a medical emergency. Although a radiograph is required to confirm the presence or absence of a fracture-dislocation, always assume one is present and treat accordingly. A primary survey should be conducted to recognize and manage a life-threatening situation. If cardiopulmonary resuscitation is required, the jaw-thrust maneuver should be used to open the airway. The head and neck should not be moved. Immobilize the neck in the position the injured party is in. Since improper movement of the cervical region can cause additional soft tissue and nerve damage, trans-

portation should be carried out only by trained personnel.

💡 *Did you determine the wrestler had a muscle strain of the sternocleidomastoid muscle? If so, you are correct. Cryotherapy and support from a cervical collar will alleviate some of the discomfort. A mild stretching program and isometric strengthening should be initiated immediately.*

BRACHIAL PLEXUS INJURIES

❓ *A defensive lineman charged the quarterback preparing to throw a pass, and struck the throwing arm, forcing it into excessive external rotation, abduction, and extension. An immediate burning sensation traveled down the length of the quarterback's arm and now his thumb is tingling. What might have happened here? Is this a serious injury?*

The brachial plexus is a complex neural structure that innervates the upper extremity. Damage to the plexus may involve a stretch-injury, or compression of the fixed plexus between the football shoulder pad and the superior medial scapula where the brachial plexus is most superficial (30). One method of tensile force involves forceful downward distraction over the clavicle while the head is distracted to the opposite side (**Figure 14-17**). This commonly occurs in football when an individual is tackled and subsequently rolls forward onto the shoulder with the head turned to the opposite side. Damage may also occur when the arm is forced into excessive external rotation, abduction, and extension. The injury usually affects the upper trunk (C_5, C_6) of the brachial plexus, with subsequent sensory loss or paresthesia in the thumb and index finger (31).

Acute symptoms consist of a burning or stinging pain radiating from the supraclavicu-

> If a unilateral cervical dislocation is present, the neck will be visibly tilted toward the dislocated side

> Brachial plexus injuries usually affect the upper trunk (C_5, C_6) leading to sensory loss or paresthesia in the thumb and index finger

---

Table 14–3. Danger Signs Indicating a Possible Cervical Spine Injury.

- Pain over the spinous process with or without deformity
- Unrelenting neck pain or muscle spasm in the cervical region
- Presence of muscular weakness in the extremities
- Loss of coordinated movement
- Paralysis or inability to move a body part
- Abnormal sensations on the head, neck, trunk, or extremities
- Absent or weak reflexes
- Loss of bladder or bowel control
- Suspect this condition in any injury involving violent axial loading, flexion, or rotation of the neck

Burner

Burning or stinging sensation characteristic of a brachial plexus injury

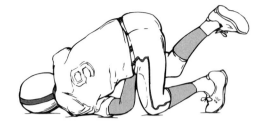

Fig. 14.17: Common mechanism of a brachial plexus stretch.

Pain is usually transient and resolves itself in five to ten minutes, but local tenderness over the supraclavicular area remain

The suprascapular nerve innervates the supraspinatus, infraspinatus, and glenohumeral joint capsule

Thoracic strains result from either overstretching or overloading muscles in the region

lar area down the arm into the hand, hence the nickname "**burner**" or "stinger." Muscle weakness is evident in actions involving the deltoid, external rotators, and biceps brachii. Pain is usually transient and resolves itself in 5 to 10 minutes, but local tenderness over the supraclavicular area remain. Often the individual will try to shake the arm to "get the feeling back." In contrast, chronic episodes are characterized by acute episodes of increasing frequency, no area of numbness, and muscle weakness in the shoulder muscles. Weakness may develop hours or days following the initial injury, and may become apparent as a dropped shoulder, or visible atrophy in the shoulder muscles (30). Therefore, continued neurological assessment days after the injury can help determine the full scope of injury.

If neck mobility and pain are present, the individual should be removed from competition and referred to a physician for a more thorough examination (31). In most instances, full resolution will occur and the individual can return to competition. Re-examine the individual after the game, during the week, and again the following week since weakness may not become apparent until days after the initial injury. Additional padding around the neck opening of the shoulder pads may reduce compressive forces on the supraclavicular region.

The suprascapular nerve may be damaged with the same mechanisms. This nerve innervates the supraspinatus, infraspinatus, and glenohumeral joint capsule. Damage to the suprascapular nerve is often overlooked in chronic shoulder injuries, but has been reported in volleyball players and pitchers (32). During rotational motion seen in pitching, spiking, or overhead serving, extreme velocity and torque forces generated during the cocking, acceleration, and release phases subject this nerve and its adjoining artery, to

rapid stretching. Both muscles may appear weak and atrophied, but infraspinatus wasting is usually more apparent because it is not hidden under the trapezius muscle. Because the supraspinatus and infraspinatus are not functioning properly, other problems, such as rotator cuff tendonitis, impingement syndrome, bicipital tenosynovitis, or bursitis of the shoulder may be present and overshadow this condition. Once identified, this condition responds well to a flexibility and strengthening program.

Did you determine the quarterback experienced a brachial plexus stretch injury? The pain and tingling in the thumb should resolve in a few minutes. If it lingers and/or muscular weakness becomes evident in the deltoid, external rotators, or biceps brachii, this person should be referred to a physician for further examination.

THORACIC SPINE INJURIES

A 15-year old butterfly stroker is complaining of localized pain and tenderness in the mid-back region over the thoracic spine. The pain came on gradually and only hurts during the execution of the stroke. Fracture tests are negative. What other condition(s) might be suspected?

The protective rib cage serves to limit movement in the thoracic motion segments. The thoracolumbar junction, however, is a region of potentially high stress during flexion-extension movements of the trunk. Injuries here may involve contusions, strains, sprains, and fractures and apophysitis.

Thoracic Contusions, Strains, and Sprains

Direct blows to the back during contact sports frequently yield contusions to the muscles in the thoracic region. Such injuries range in severity but are generally characterized by pain, ecchymosis, and limited swelling. Palpation may reveal spasm and increased pain.

Thoracic strains result from either overstretching or overloading muscles in the region. Overstretching can be caused by a forceful reaching motion with the outstretched arm in combination with rotation of the trunk. Violent or sustained muscle contractions can also result in strain, although strains in the lumbar muscles are much more common with this mechanism. Pain may be significant during the first two or three weeks but resolves rapidly with rest and activity modification.

Motions involving overstretching can also produce thoracic sprains. Painful spasms and knot-like contractions of the back muscles may develop as a sympathetic response to sprains. These sympathetic muscle spasms serve as a protective mechanism to immobilize the injured area (33). The presence of such spasms, however, make it difficult to determine whether the injury is actually a sprain or strain. Severe strains in the thoracic region may require three or four weeks to heal, whereas thoracic sprains may improve within a couple of days (21).

Initial treatment for soft tissue injuries consist of cryotherapy, prescribed NSAIDs, and activity modification. Follow-up management may include application of superficial heat, ultrasound, massage, and appropriate stretching and resistance exercise as needed to recondition the individual.

Thoracic Spinal Fractures and Apophysitis

The attached rib cage acts to stabilize and limit range of motion in the thoracic spine, thereby lessening the likelihood of injury to this area. Thoracic fractures subsequently tend to be concentrated at the lower end of the thoracic spine in the transition region between the thoracic and lumbar curvatures.

Thoracic fractures most commonly result from compression resulting in a **wedge fracture**, named after the shape of the deformed vertebral body (**Figure 14-18A**). Large compressive loads, such as those sustained during heavy weight lifting can cause fractures of the vertebral end plates. In addition, severe impact forces result in anterior compression fractures of the vertebral bodies. Although this type of injury is more commonly associated with automobile accidents, it can also result from hitting the boards during ice hockey, head-on contacts in football or rugby, or impacts during tobogganing or snowmobiling when an individual lands directly on the buttock area (34,35). For example, it has been shown that when a snowmobile drops a distance of four feet, the force on an occupant's spine is far greater than that needed to cause a compression fracture (26). Females with **osteopenia**, a condition of reduced bone mineralization, are particularly susceptible to compression fractures. The causal mechanism is typically compressive stress from small, repetitive loads in an activity such

Wedge fracture
A crushing compression fracture that leaves a vertebra narrowed anteriorly

Large compressive loads, such as those sustained during heavy weight lifting can cause fractures of the vertebral end plates

Osteopenia
Condition of reduced bone mineralization or density of a bone

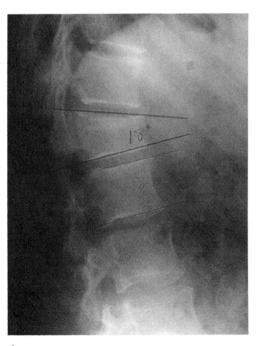

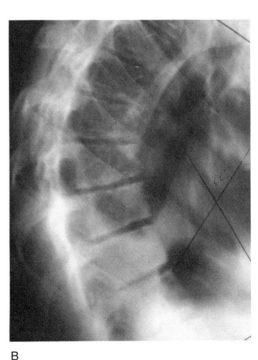

A   B

Fig. 14.18: (A) Radiograph of a compression wedge fracture in the thoracic region. (B) Scheuermann's disease occurs when endplate changes lead to erosion in the anterior vertebral body, which drives a herniated disc forward into the body.

as running, causing a progressive compression fracture of a weakened vertebral body.

Another cause of thoracic fractures among adolescents is Scheuermann's disease, discussed earlier. This condition, which appears to be related to mechanical stress, involves degeneration of the epiphyseal endplates of the vertebral bodies and typically involves at least three adjacent motion segments. Once the endplate is sufficiently compromised, additional compression from axial and flexion overload forces cause prolapse of the intervertebral disc into the vertebral body (**Figure 14-18B**). The result is a decrease in spinal height and an accentuation of the thoracic curve leading to kyphosis. Onset typically occurs at 12 or 13 years of age with the condition twice as common in girls as in boys (20). A high incidence of Scheuermann's disease has been documented among gymnasts, trampolinists, wrestlers, and rowers. Treatment involves modification of activity proportional to the pain. Stretching exercises for the shoulder, neck and back muscles should be coupled with strengthening the abdominal and spinal extensor muscles. If the kyphosis continues to progress, bracing may be included with the exercise program.

Repeated flexion-extension of the thoracic spine, such as occurs during the butterfly and breast strokes, and several gymnastic skills can cause inflammation of the apophyses, the growth centers of the vertebral bodies. Like Scheuermann's disease, apophysitis is a progressive condition characterized by local pain and tenderness. Treatment for apophysitis includes elimination of the flexion-extension stress and strengthening abdominal and other trunk muscles.

Did you determine that the swimmer had possible Scheuermann's disease or apophysitis because of the repeated flexion-extension motions executed during the butterfly stroke? This individual should be referred to a physician for follow-up examination.

LUMBAR SPINE INJURIES

A weight lifter is experiencing chronic low back pain during the dead lift. What advice would you provide the individual concerning proper lifting technique?

The lumbar spine must support the weight of the head, trunk, and arms, plus any load held in the hands. In addition, the two lower lumbar motion segments (L4-L5, L5-S1) provide a large range of motion in flexion-extension. It is not surprising then, that mechanical abuse often results in episodes of low back pain, leading to the lower lumbar discs being injured more frequently than any others in the spine.

Low Back Pain

An estimated 60 to 80% of the population experiences low back pain (LBP) at some time. Although LBP typically strikes individuals between the ages of 25 and 60 years, with frequency peaking at about age 40, it also occurs in as many as 25% of adolescents and children, ranging down to age 10 (36–38). Males and females appear to be equally susceptible (39,40).

The LBP syndrome has become an increasingly serious medical and socioeconomic problem. It is second only to the common cold as the leading cause of lost work time (41). Back injuries dominate claims for worker's compensation (42). LBP also accounts for 10% of all chronic health problems, and is ranked 11th among causes for hospitalization in the United States (43,44).

Although several known pathologies may cause LBP, most cases are idiopathic, or of unknown origin. Because it is difficult to identify anatomical structures that are the source of pain, it is also difficult to determine what biomechanical factors may be contributing to the development of pain (10). There is general agreement, however, that mechanical stress is the primary causal mechanism in most LBP cases.

Low back pain is common in runners and in individuals who participate in activities involving running, such as soccer, field hockey, or lacrosse. There is a tendency for many runners to have muscle tightness in the hip flexors and hamstrings. Tight hip flexors tend to produce a forward body lean leading to anterior pelvic tilt and hyperlordosis of the lumbar spine. This, coupled with tight hamstrings can lead to a shorter stride. An excessive sway or tight abductors may also place an additional stress on the lumbosacral region (20). To decrease the incidence of LBP, training techniques should allow for adequate progression of distance, speed, and hill work and include extensive flexibility exercises for the hip and thigh region. **Field Strategy 14-3** outlines suggestions for reducing the incidence of LBP in runners.

Field Strategy 14–3. Reducing Low Back Pain in Runners.

- Wear properly fitted shoes that control heel motion and provide maximum shock-absorption. Discard worn shoes that have lost their impact dissipation
- Increase flexibility in the iliotibial tract, hip flexors, hip abductors, hip internal and external rotators, hamstrings, ankle plantar flexors, and the trunk extensors
- Increase strength in the abdominal and trunk extensor muscles
- Avoid excessive body weight
- Warm up and stretch thoroughly before running, and stretch after running
- Run with an upright stance rather than a forward lean
- Avoid excessive side-to-side sway
- Run on even terrain and limit hill work. Avoid running on concrete
- Avoid overstriding to increase speed, as it increases leg shock
- Gradually increase distance, intensity, and duration. Do not increase more than 10% in one week, and increase only one parameter at a time
- If orthosis is worn and pain persists, check for wear and rigidity
- Assess leg length discrepancies and make appropriate adjustments
- Consider alternatives to running, such as cycling, rowing, or swimming

Lumbar Contusions, Strains, and Sprains

Soft tissue injuries are the most frequent injuries in the lumbar region. The injuries and mechanisms are the same as those described in the thoracic region. Because the lumbar muscles develop tension to counteract the forward bending moment of the entire trunk when the trunk is in flexion, these muscles are particularly susceptible to strain. Strategies for minimizing loads on the lumbar muscles during lifting and carrying activities were discussed in **Field Strategy 14-1**, and included maintaining the trunk in an erect posture and positioning the load close to the body. Use of improper technique during activities such as weight training and rowing can lead to lumbar strain. Runners who tend to over-stride are also at increased risk for lumbar muscle strains, since over-striding forces the lumbar spine into hyperextension (45).

Symptoms include localized pain, increasing with active and resisted motion. Radiating pain and neurological deficits are not present. Treatment includes rest, cryotherapy, and prescribed NSAIDs. A lumbar support brace may help alleviate some stress on the region **(Figure 6-19)**. If symptoms do not improve within a week, refer the individual to a physician to rule out a more serious underlying condition.

Sciatica

Sciatica is an inflammatory condition of the sciatic nerve that may result from a herniated disc, annular tear, myogenic or muscle-related disease, spinal stenosis, facet joint arthropathy, or compression between the two parts of the piriformis muscle (46). If related to a herniated disc, radiating leg pain is greater than back pain, and increases with sitting and leaning forward, coughing, sneezing, and straining. Pain is reproduced during an **ipsilateral** straight leg raising test (See **Figure 14-30**). With annular tears, back pain is more prevalent and exacerbated with straight leg raising. Morning pain and muscular stiffness that worsens if chilled or when weather changes (arthritis-like symptoms), or increases when subjected to prolonged use is characteristic of myogenic or muscle-related disease. Pain typically radiates into the buttock and thigh region. If lumbar spinal stenosis is present, back and leg pain develops after the individual walks a limited distance and concomitantly increases as distance increases. Pain is not reproduced with a straight leg raising test, but can be reproduced with prolonged spine extension, which is relieved with spine flexion. Facet-joint arthropathy produces localized pain over the joint on spinal extension, and is exacerbated with ipsilateral lateral flexion. If compressed between the two parts of the piriformis muscle, pain increases during internal rotation of the thigh (46).

Referral to a physician is necessary to determine the presence of a serious underlying condition. **Table 14-4** lists four stages of sciatica, the accompanying signs and symptoms, and an estimated time needed away

Sciatica
Compression of a spinal nerve due to a herniated disc, annular tear, myogenic or muscle-related disease, spinal stenosis, facet joint arthropathy, or compression from the piriformis muscle

Ipsilateral
Situated on, pertaining to, or affecting the same side, as opposed to contralateral

Table 14–4. Signs and Symptoms of Sciatica.

Causes	Signs and Symptoms
Herniated disc	Radiating leg pain is greater than back pain. Pain increases with sitting and leaning forward, coughing, sneezing, and straining. Neurologic deficits are usually present. +ipsilateral straight leg raising test
Annular tears	Back pain is more prevalent than leg pain. Pain increases with sitting and leaning forward, coughing, sneezing, and straining. May have muscle spasm and loss of lordosis. +ipsilateral straight leg raising test
Myogenic or muscle-related disease	Morning pain and muscle stiffness that worsens if chilled or when weather changes. Pain is unilateral or bilateral, not midline. Pain extends into the buttock and thigh region only. Pain is reproduced with resisted prolonged muscle contraction and passive stretching of the muscle. Contralateral pain with side bending
Spinal stenosis	Back and leg pain develop after walking a limited distance, and increases as distance increases. Leg weakness or numbness is present, with or without sciatica −straight leg-raising test +pain on prolonged spine extension, relieved with spine flexion
Facet joint arthropathy	Pain over joint on spinal extension exacerbated with ipsilateral trunk lateral flexion
Compression from piriformis	Symptoms mimic lumbar disc conditions, except for the absence of true neurologic findings. Pain increases with medial rotation of the thigh

Classification of Sciatica:

- *Sciatica only:* no sensory or muscle weakness. Modify activity appropriately and develop rehabilitation and prevention program. Any increased pain requires immediate re-evaluation
- *Sciatica with soft signs:* some sensory changes, mild or no reflex change, normal muscle strength, normal bowel and bladder function. Remove from sport participation for 6 to 12 weeks
- *Sciatica with hard signs:* sensory and reflex changes, and muscle weakness due to repeated, chronic, or acute condition. Normal bowel and bladder function. Remove from participation 12 to 24 weeks
- *Sciatica with severe signs:* sensory and reflex changes, muscle weakness, and bladder function altered. Consider immediate surgical decompression

from sport participation for adequate resolution of the condition. Under normal circumstances, bed rest is usually not indicated, although side-lying with the knees flexed may relieve symptoms. Lifting, bending, twisting, and prolonged sitting and standing aggravate the condition by increasing intradiscal pressure, and therefore should be avoided. When asymptomatic, abdominal and extensor muscle-strengthening exercises can begin with gradual return to activity. If symptoms resume, stop activity and refer the individual back to the physician. Occasionally, extended rest is needed for symptoms to totally resolve, or if a significant disc protrusion is present, surgery may be indicated.

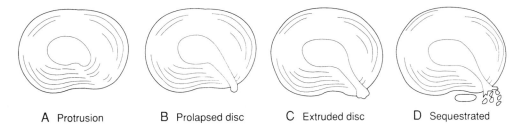

Fig. 14.19: Herniated discs are categorized by severity as an eccentrically loaded nucleus progressively moves from (A) protruded, (B) prolapsed, (C) extrusion, and culminates in (D) sequestrated when the nuclear material moves into the canal to impinge the adjacent spinal nerves.

Lumbar Disc Injuries

Mechanical loading of the spine for some time can develop microruptures in the annulus fibrosus leading to degeneration of the disc (**Figure 14-19**). Bulging or protruded discs refer to some eccentric accumulation of the nucleus with slight deformity of the annulus. When the eccentric nucleus produces a definite deformity as it works its way through the fibers of the annulus, it is called a **prolapsed disc**. An **extruded disc** refers to a condition in which the nuclear material comes into the spinal canal and runs the risk of impinging adjacent nerve roots. Finally, with a sequestrated disc, the nuclear material has separated from the disc itself and potentially migrates (20). Disc herniations can be either acute or stress-related, although the involved disc typically shows signs of previous degeneration (20,47). The most commonly herniated discs are the lower two lumbar discs between L4-L5 and L5-S1, followed by the lower two cervical discs (48,49). Most ruptures occur on the posterior or posterolateral aspect of the disc.

Because the intervertebral discs are not innervated, damage to the disc does not, in and of itself, result in the sensation of pain. Sensory nerves supply the anterior and posterior longitudinal ligaments, the vertebral bodies, and articular cartilage in the facet joints, however, and impingement on one of these structures, the spinal cord, or a spinal nerve can produce both sensory and motor symptoms (20,50). When compression is placed on a spinal nerve of the sciatic nerve complex (L_4-S_3), sensory and motor deficits are reflected in the myotome and dermatome patterns associated with the nerve root (**Figure 14-20**). A disc need not be completely herniated to give symptoms.

Prolapsed disc
Condition when the eccentric nucleus produces a definite deformity as it works its way through the fibers of the annulus fibrosus

Extruded disc
Condition in which the nuclear material come into the spinal canal and runs the risk of impinging adjacent nerve roots

The most commonly herniated discs are the lower two lumbar discs between L4-L5 and L5-S1, followed in injury frequency by the lower two cervical discs

Impingement of the ligaments, bony structures, spinal cord, or spinal nerves can produce both sensory and motor symptoms

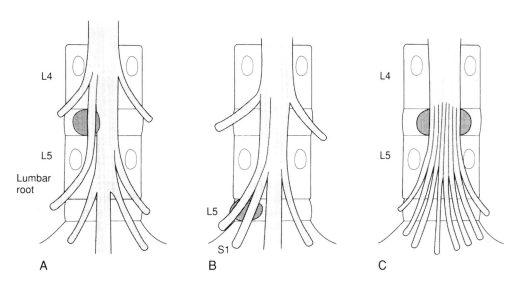

Fig. 14.20: Possible effects according to the level of herniation. (A) Herniation between L4 and L5 compresses the L_5 nerve root. (B) Herniation between L5 and S1 can compress the nerve root crossing the disc (S_1) and the nerve root emerging through the intervertebral foramina (L_5). (C) A posterior herniation at the L4–L5 level can compress the dura mater of the entire cauda equina leading to bowel and bladder paralysis.

Symptoms of a disc herniation may include severe local pain and sympathetic muscle spasms at the site of the herniation, as well as radiating pain or numbness down the sciatic nerve into the lower extremity. The individual may walk in a slightly crouched position leaning away from the side of the lesion. Forward trunk flexion or a straight leg raising test (see **Figure 14-30**) may exacerbate pain and increase distal symptoms. Significant signs indicating the need for immediate referral to a physician include muscle weakness, sensory changes, diminished reflexes in the lower extremity, and abnormal bladder or bowel function. **Table 14-5** outlines physical findings associated with disc herniation in the low back region.

Treatment depends on the severity of symptoms, type of activity in which the individual is involved, occupation, and normal daily activities. In mild cases, treatment consists of minimizing load on the spine. This includes avoiding activities that involve impact, lifting, bending, twisting, and prolonged sitting and standing, since these increase pressure on the discs. Running is allowed if it does not increase the symptoms. Since sympathetic contraction of the muscles at the site of a back injury is a common occurrence, painful muscle spasm, knots, and tightness must be eliminated. A variety of approaches can be used including ice and/or heat, administration of prescribed NSAIDs and/or muscle relaxants, ultrasound, transcutaneous electrical nerve stimulation (TENS), passive exercise, and gentle stretching. Depending on severity, the back should also be rested with strenuous activity prohibited.

Although recovery from symptoms may take several months, surgery is generally not warranted except in severe cases when significant neurological deficits are noted.

Following resolution of spasm and acute pain, rehabilitation should be initiated that focuses on restoring or improving spine and hamstring flexibility, and abdominal and trunk extensor strength. More often than not, one or more of these areas of function is below average in an individual with low back pain. An educational component on proper back mechanics should be included in the program to instruct the individual not to assume body positions or undertake movements during daily living activities that are potentially injurious.

Lumbar Fractures and Dislocations

Lumbar fractures differ in accordance with differences in the causal mechanism. Since the spinal cord ends at about L1 or L2 level, fractures of the lumbar vertebrae below this point do not pose as serious a threat as do superiorly located vertebral fractures. However, the cauda equina extends down the spinal canal in the lumbar region and suspected fractures should be handled with care to minimize potential nerve damage.

Transverse or spinous process fractures may result from extreme forceful tension development in the attached muscles, or from a hard blow to the low back during participation in contact sports, such as football, rugby, soccer, basketball, hockey, and lacrosse (33). These fractures often lead to additional injury to surrounding soft tissues but are not as seri-

Table 14–5. Physical Findings Associated with a Herniated Disc.

Signs and Symptoms	L3-L4 (L_4 root)	L4-L5 (L_5 root)	L5-S1 (S_1 root)
Pain	Lumbar region and buttocks	Lumbar region, groin, and sacroiliac area	Lumbar region, groin, and sacroiliac area
Dermatome and sensory loss	Anterior mid-thigh over patella, medial lower leg to great toe	Lateral thigh, anterior leg, top of foot, middle three toes	Posterior lateral thigh and lower leg to lateral foot and 5th toe
Myotome weakness	Ankle dorsiflexion	Toe extension (Extensor hallux)	Ankle plantar flexion (Gastrocnemius)
Reduced deep tendon reflex	Quadriceps	Medial hamstrings	Achilles tendon
Straight leg-raising test	Normal	Reduced	Reduced

ous as compression fractures. Conservative treatment consists of initial bed rest, cryotherapy, and minimizing mechanical loads on the low back until symptoms subside. This may take three to six weeks (20).

Compression fractures occur more commonly at the thoracolumbar junction, and typically involve the L1 vertebra, as discussed in the section on thoracic fractures. The mechanism of injury is generally violent hyperflexion, or jack-knifing of the trunk, resulting in crushing the anterior aspect of the vertebral body. The primary danger with this type of injury is the possibility for invasion of bone fragments into the spinal canal with subsequent damage to the spinal cord or spinal nerves. Symptoms will include localized, palpable pain that may radiate down the nerve root if a bony fragment compresses a spinal nerve. Confirmation of a fracture is made with a radiograph or CT scan.

Because of the facet joint orientation in the lumbar region, dislocations occur only when a fracture is present. Fracture-dislocations resulting from sport participation are rare.

💡 *In supervising the individual doing the dead lift, make sure the individual is using proper technique. The weight may need to be reduced to allow this. Furthermore, make sure the person is wearing a weight belt to help stabilize the low back area.*

SACRUM AND COCCYX INJURIES

❓ *An individual is complaining of sharp pain in the sacral region when running on uneven terrain. After sitting for an extended time the pain begins to ache in the low back region. What might you suspect is injured? What would you recommend for this person?*

Because the sacrum and coccyx are essentially immobile, the potential for mechanical injury to these regions is dramatically reduced. Injuries from direct blows and stress of the sacroiliac (SI) joint can result from sports participation.

Sacroiliac Joint Immobility

Sprains of the sacroiliac (SI) joint can lead to local pain and stiffness. Causes range from a single traumatic episode involving bending and/or twisting, to repetitive stress from lifting, or excessive side-to-side or up-and-down motion during running and jogging. Other contributing factors include running on

uneven terrain, suddenly slipping or stumbling forward, and wearing new shoes or orthotics (20).

During activity the individual will usually experience one-sided pain in the sacral area that may extend into the buttock and posterior thigh, but does not usually extend to the knee. When sitting for an extended time a dull aching pain may be present in the low back (20). Treatment for sacroiliac sprains includes cryotherapy, prescribed NSAIDs, and gentle stretching to alleviate stiffness. Flexibility and strengthening exercises for the low back can then be initiated.

Coccygeal Injuries

Direct blows sustained during sport participation can produce contusions and fractures of the coccyx. Pain resulting from a fracture may last for several months. Prolonged or chronic pain in the region may also result from irritation of the coccygeal nerve plexus. This condition is termed **coccygodynia**. Treatment for coccygeal pain includes analgesics and use of padding for protection and a ring seat to alleviate compression during sitting.

💡 *The runner has probably irritated the sacroiliac joint from repeated stress while running on uneven terrain. This individual should ice the region to control inflammation and pain, stretch the low back and buttock region, and run on more even terrain. If conditions do not improve, refer the individual to a physician for further assessment.*

ASSESSMENT OF SPINAL INJURIES

❓ *A seventeen-year-old male high jumper is complaining of pain in the low back and sacroiliac region, aggravated by flexion and hyperextension of the trunk during jumping. He has come to you asking for help. How will you progress through the assessment to determine the extent and severity of injury?*

Injury assessment of the spine is a complex, inclusive process that cannot be rushed. In most instances, an individual will present a spinal injury in either of two scenarios. In one, the individual will be injured in a traumatic episode leaving the individual lying on the field or court. It is uncommon, although not impossible, for a conscious individual to have a significant spinal injury without severe pain, spasm, or tenderness. It is very common, however, for an individual with a minor

Compression fractures at the thoracolumbar junction are typically caused by violent hyperflexion, or jack-knifing of the trunk, resulting in crushing the anterior aspect of the vertebral body

Sacroiliac sprains may be caused by a single traumatic episode involving bending and/or twisting, repetitive stress from lifting, or excessive side-to-side or up-and-down motion during running and jogging

Initial treatment for sacroiliac sprains includes cryotherapy, prescribed anti-inflammatory medication, and gentle stretching to alleviate the stiffness

Coccygodynia
Prolonged or chronic pain in the coccygeal region due to irritation of the coccygeal nerve plexus

injury, such as a muscular strain, to have only mild to moderate pain and tenderness. The severity of pain and presence or absence of neurological symptoms, neck spasm, and tenderness can indicate when a backboard and neck stabilization is needed (51). In this instance, assume a severe spinal injury has occurred. Determine the presence of a possible fracture and neurological involvement after completing the primary survey and initiate the emergency care plan. Do not remove the helmet or move the individual's head, neck, or spine. Once a significant physical finding indicates possible nerve involvement, immediate transportation to the nearest medical facility is warranted, regardless of whether a total assessment is completed. For example, if the individual reports no sensory perception or ability to move the extremities, it is unnecessary to complete special tests to determine the level of spinal involvement. It is clear the individual has a severe spinal injury and delay in treatment could be devastating. Immobilization of the individual should be completed under the direction of trained personnel.

The other scenario typically involves an individual who walks into the training room or clinic complaining of neck or back pain. The person is ambulatory but has pain, discomfort, or some disability. In this instance, it is relatively safe to assume that a serious spinal injury is not present and a thorough assessment should be completed to determine the extent and severity of injury. Because of the high incidence of referred pain, a scan exam should be performed during observation to determine the probable site of the lesion. A more complete assessment of that site can then be performed.

This section will focus on a spinal assessment in a conscious individual. Specific information related to an acute injury is included where appropriate. To review assessment procedures for the primary survey and an unconscious individual with a suspected spinal injury, refer to Chapter 3.

HISTORY

? *The high jumper complained of pain in the low back and sacroiliac region, aggravated by flexion and hyperextension of the trunk during jumping. What questions need to be asked to identify the cause and extent of injury?*

A history of the injury should include information on the mechanism of injury, extent of pain or disability due to the injury, previous injuries to the area, and family history which may have some bearing on this specific condition. In a spinal injury specific information must be gathered on the location of pain (localized or radiating); type of pain (dull, aching, sharp, burning); presence of sensory changes (numbness, tingling, or absence of sensation); and possible muscle weakness or paralysis. Ask questions to determine both long-term and short-term memory that may be indicative of an associated concussion or subdural hematoma. Note how long it takes to respond to the questions. If the individual is unconscious, assume that a serious neck injury is present and stabilize the neck and summon EMS.

Questions related to the spine can be seen in **Field Strategy 14-4**.

? *The seventeen-year-old jumper has been a competitive athlete since seventh grade. His primary complaint is an aching pain when bending over, aggravated with hyperextension and prolonged sitting that produces sharp radiating pains into the low back and sacroiliac region. The condition has been present for four weeks and is not getting better. He cannot recall any traumatic episode that led to the condition.*

OBSERVATION AND INSPECTION

? *Would it be appropriate to do a scan exam to determine neuromuscular capability? What specific factors should be observed to identify the extent of injury?*

Initial observation can begin immediately as the individual enters the room. Body language can signal such factors as pain, disability, and muscle weakness. Note the individual's willingness or ability to move, general posture, consistency in limitations of motion, ease in motion, and general attitude. Clothing and protective equipment may prevent visually noting abnormalities in spinal alignment. As such, the individual should be suitably dressed so the back is exposed as much as possible. For girls and women, a bra, halter top, or swim suit should be worn. Begin with a postural assessment and progress through a scan exam, gait analysis, and inspection of the injury site.

Once a significant physical finding indicates probable nerve involvement, immediate transportation to the nearest medical facility is warranted, regardless of whether a total assessment is completed

In a spinal injury, ask specific information on the location of pain, type of pain, presence of sensory changes, and possible muscle weakness or paralysis

Body language can signal such factors as pain, disability, and muscle weakness

Field Strategy 14–4. Developing a History for a Spinal Injury.

Determine (a) primary complaint including location, onset, and current nature of the problem; (b) mechanism of injury; (c) characteristics of the symptoms including the nature, location, severity, frequency, and duration of pain or disability; (d) functional deficits relative to ADLs (Activity of Daily Living), occupation, and recreational/athletic pursuits; and (e) related medical history. ASK:

- Why are you here? Where is the pain or weakness located? On a scale of one to ten with ten being very severe, how would you rate your pain or weakness? Can you describe the pain (dull ache, throbbing, sharp, shooting, burning, deep, or superficial)?
- Is there any change in sensation anywhere on your body? Any pins and needles or loss of sensation? Is there any muscle spasm present?
- In what activity were you participating when the injury occurred? Do you remember the position of the trunk? Was twisting of the trunk involved? What different activities have you been doing in the last week? (Look for activities such as lifting or carrying heavy objects, or positions involving bending over for long periods of time.)
- Have you had any recent changes in equipment or shoes in the past three weeks? Has your training program intensified or changed recently?
- Did the pain come on gradually or suddenly? How long has it been a problem? Does the pain radiate into the buttocks or leg?
- What activities aggravate or alleviate the symptoms (sitting for long periods of time, bending over, rotating the trunk)? Are there any occupational tasks that aggravate the condition? Does the severity of symptoms change when you change position?
- In what position do you sleep? What type of mattress do you have (waterbed, hard, soft)?
- Have you ever injured your back before? What did you do for it? Have you seen a physician about this condition? What was the diagnosis? What have you done since then to strengthen the area to prevent reinjury?
- Are there certain activities you are unable to perform because of the pain? Which ones? How old are you? Note the gender. Females have a higher incidence of low back pain.
- Have you had any medical problems recently? (Look for problems that may refer pain to the area from visceral organs, heart, and lungs.) Do you have any musculoskeletal problems elsewhere in the body? (These may result in changes in gait or technique that transfer abnormal forces to the spinal region.) Are you on any medication?
- Has anyone in your family had a similar problem?

Posture

Posture assessment can detect congenital or functional problems that may be contributing to the injury. Ask the individual to sit down to begin the exam; then stand. Note the head and neck posture. Is the head held erect or carried in a forward position? Are any abnormal spinal curvatures present? Are there any noticeable asymmetries, such as discrepancies in shoulder or scapula height, hip height, or patella height? Is the trunk rotated so one shoulder is forward? Are the ribs more prominent on one side? Specific factors to observe in the head and spinal region are listed in **Field Strategy 14-5**.

Scan Exam

A scan exam assesses general motor function and can rule out injury at other joints that may be overlooked due to intense pain or discomfort at the primary injury site. Active movement of the spine may be included in this step prior to palpation and need not be repeated with special tests. Note if there is any hesitation to move a body part, or if the individual prefers to use one side over another. Examples of gross motor movements for the spine are listed in **Field Strategy 14-6**. Additional gross motor movements for the upper and lower extremities should also be performed.

Gait Assessment

Ask the individual to walk several yards while observing normal body movement. Stand behind, in front, and to the side of the individual to observe from all angles. Note subtle posture abnormalities, such as kyphosis, scol-

> Active movement of the spine may be included in this step prior to palpation and need not be repeated with special tests

Field Strategy 14–5. Postural Assessment.

Anterior View
- Is the head and neck in the midline of the body? Is the nose centered?
- The slope of the shoulder muscles should appear bilaterally equal. However, the level of the shoulder on the dominant side will usually be lower than the non-dominant side
- Both shoulders should have a well-rounded musculature with no prominent bony structures
- Is the space between the arms and body the same on both sides?
- Are both hands held in the same position
- Does the rib cage look symmetrical with no rotation?
- Are the folds of the waist at the same height?

Side View
- Can you draw an imaginary straight plum line from the ear through the middle of the shoulder, hip, knee, and ankle?
- Does the neck or back have any excessive curves?
- Are the elbows held near full extension?
- Note that the chest, back, and abdominal muscles have good tone with no obvious chest deformities
- Does the pelvis appear to be level?
- Are the knees straight, flexed, or hyperextended. Normally they should be slightly flexed

Posterior View
- Is the head and neck centered? Note any abnormal prominence of bony structures or muscle atrophy
- Does the spine appear to be straight? Have the individual lean over and perform a skyline view (Adam's position) to detect possible scoliosis
- Are the scapula at the same height and resting at the same angle? Are both scapula lying flat against the rib cage?
- Is there any atrophy in the muscle groups of the shoulder and arm?
- Is the posterior side of the elbow at the same height bilaterally? Is the space between the body and elbow the same on both sides?
- Do the ribs protrude?
- Are the waist folds level? Are the posterior gluteal folds level?
- Are the skin creases on the posterior knee level?

 Field Strategy 14–6. Scan Exam for a Spinal Injury.

Ask the individual to perform the following actions:
1. Touch the chin to the chest
2. Look up at the ceiling keeping the back straight
3. Turn the head sideways in both directions
4. Try to touch the ear to the shoulder
5. Rotate the trunk sideways keeping the hips stabilized
6. Lean forward and touch the toes
7. Look up at the ceiling with hyperextension of the trunk
8. Lean sideways and do lateral flexion of the trunk
9. While placing a hand on a table for support, do a straight leg raise forward, backward, and sideways

iosis, lordosis, or pelvic tilt. A low back injury may produce a forward lean, a lean to one side, or a noticeable limp.

Inspection of the Injury Site

Local inspection at the injury site should denote deformities, swelling, discoloration, muscle spasm, scars that might indicate previous surgery, and general skin condition. A step deformity in the lumbar spine may indicate a spondylolisthesis.

Gross Neuromuscular Assessment

In an acute injury, a posture and scan exam is not possible. However, it would be beneficial to do a brief gross neuromuscular assessment prior to palpations to detect any motor and/or sensory deficits. Without moving the individual, ask them to perform a submaximal bilateral hand-squeeze test and ankle dorsiflexion. These two actions assess the cervical and lumbar spinal nerves, respectively. Muscle weakness and/or diminished sensation over the hands and feet indicate a serious injury. If a positive sign is apparent, careful attention should be taken when palpating and assessing the appropriate spinal region.

Slight lordosis and anterior pelvic tilt is present. During the scan exam, trunk flexion and extension produced a dull pain. Lateral flexion to the right caused sharp pain to radiate into the right buttock and posterior leg. A forward straight leg raise with the right leg was limited and could not be performed without bending the knee. Gait analysis showed a shortened stride on the right side. Visual inspection showed no abnormalities.

PALPATIONS

The injury is confined to the low back region. What specific structures need to be palpated to determine if the injury is bony or soft tissue in origin? Can neural involvement be ruled out during palpations? Why or why not?

In an acute injury, the submaximal hand-squeeze test and ankle dorsiflexion should have identified any motor or sensory deficits. If any deficits were noted, initiate the emergency care plan, and summon EMS. If no deficits were noted, it does not rule out possible neurological involvement or fracture. Therefore, proceed with palpations in the position in which the individual is. Abnormal alignment and/or tenderness of the spinous

processes is a significant finding, and the assessment need not proceed. The individual should be immobilized on a backboard under the direction of trained personnel and transported to the nearest medical facility.

In injuries that do not involve neural damage, fracture, or dislocation, palpations can proceed in the following manner. Palpate bony and soft tissue structures to detect temperature, swelling, point tenderness, deformity, crepitus, muscle spasm, and cutaneous sensation. Palpations may be done in a seated, standing, or lying-down position. To relax the neck and spinal muscles, the individual should lie on a table. To palpate posterior neck structures, have the individual supine. Reach around the neck with both hands and palpate either side of the spine with the fingertips. Muscle spasms in the erector spinae, sternocleidomastoid muscles, scalene muscles, and/or the upper trapezius may indicate dysfunction of the cervical spine (52). In the thoracic and low back region, have the individual prone. Place a pillow or blanket under the hip region to tilt the pelvis back and relax the lumbar curvature. Muscle spasm in the lower erector spinae, lower trapezius, serratus posterior, quadratus lumborum, latissimus dorsi, or gluteus maximus may indicate dysfunction of the thoracic or lumbar spine. **Table 14-6** lists surface landmarks on the back relative to the vertebral level at which they can be found. Palpate the following structures:

Anterior Aspect

1. Hyoid bone, thyroid cartilage, trachea, and carotid arteries (**Figure 14-21**)
2. Sternocleidomastoid muscle, manubrium, clavicle, supraclavicular fossa
3. Sternum, ribs, and costicartilage
4. Abdomen and inguinal area. Note any abnormal tenderness or masses indicating internal pathology that is referring pain to the spinal region
5. Iliac crest, anterior superior iliac spine, symphysis pubis

Posterior Aspect

1. External protuberance of the occiput
2. Spinous and transverse processes of all vertebrae. Note any tenderness, crepitus, or deviation from the norm. A noticeable discrepancy can indicate a fracture or vertebral subluxation. Pain and tenderness

Without moving the individual, ask them to do a submaximal bilateral hand-squeeze test and ankle dorsiflexion test

Place a pillow or blanket under the hip region to tilt the pelvis back and relax the lumbar curvature

Table 14–6. Surface Landmarks on the Back.

Vertebra	Surface landmark
C7 and T1	Prominent spinous process in neck
T2	Top of scapula
T4	Base of spine of scapula
T7	Inferior angle of scapula
T12	Lowest floating rib
L4	Top of iliac crest
S1-S2	Dimples marking the posterosuperior iliac spines

without positive findings on muscle movement may indicate the problem is not musculoskeletal in origin. C7 and T1 spinous processes are larger than those above them. T4 spinous process lies at the same level as the base of the spine of the scapula

3. Interspinous and supraspinous ligaments, ligamentum flavum, paraspinal muscles, and quadratus lumborum
4. Scapula, trapezius, and latissimus dorsi
5. Iliac crest, posterior superior iliac spine, and sacrum. The interspace between L4-

L5 lies at the same level as the top of the iliac crest. The S2 spinous process lies in the middle of a line drawn between the posterior superior iliac spines
6. Ischial tuberosity, sciatic nerve, and greater trochanter (**Figure 14-22**)

Point tenderness was palpated between L3-S1 vertebrae with increased pain in the L4-L5 region. Muscle spasm was present on either side of the lumbar region. Pain was also elicited with palpation midway between the ischial tuberosity and greater trochanter.

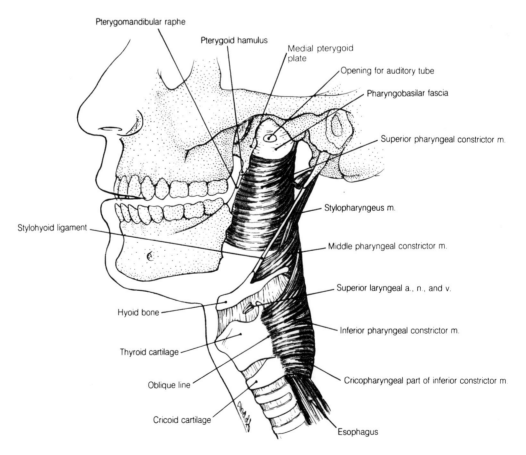

Fig. 14.21: Anatomy of the cervical spine and anterior throat structures.

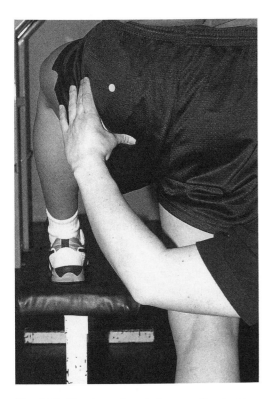

Fig. 14.22: To palpate the sciatic nerve, flex the hip and locate the ischial tuberosity and greater trochanter. The sciatic nerve may be palpated at the midpoint. It is designated here by the dot.

SPECIAL TESTS

❓ *The high jumper has concentrated palpable pain in the L4-L5 region with associated muscle spasm and pain over the sciatic nerve as it passes into the posterior thigh. How will you proceed to determine bony versus soft tissue involvement?*

Injuries to the spinal region can be very complex. As such, it is imperative to work slowly through the different tests. If at anytime, movement leads to increased acute pain or change in sensation, or the individual resists moving the spine, assume that a significant injury is present and take appropriate measures to refer this individual to a physician for further evaluation.

Active Movement

Prior to any active movement in an acute injury, the individual should demonstrate no motor or sensory deficits, nor have any point tenderness of the spinous processes. If present, the individual should have been immobilized on a backboard and transported to the nearest medical facility. In cases where these deficits are not a concern, active movement

in the spine may be conducted during the scan exam and need not be repeated here. Look for the individual's willingness to perform the movement. Is the movement fluid and complete? Does pain, spasm, or stiffness block the full range of motion? As mentioned earlier, immediate, severe pain and spasm are danger signs that indicate possible spinal injury. Remember to perform movements that cause pain last to avoid any carry-over of pain from one movement to the next. With movements to the left and right, always compare bilaterally. Cervical movements assessed include:

1. Flexion (80 to 90°)
2. Extension (70°)
3. Lateral flexion (left and right) (20 to 45°)
4. Rotation (left and right) (70 to 90°)

Movement in the thoracic and lumbar region are assessed together. Stand behind the individual and observe the thoracic region for signs of scoliosis. Ask the individual to lean forward and touch the toes while keeping the knees straight (Adam's position). Observe the vertebrae and contour of the back **(Figure 14-23)**. If a lateral curve is present while standing but disappears on flexion,

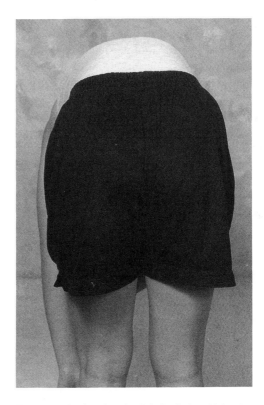

Fig. 14.23: Performing the "skyline" view (Adam's position) of the spine can assess the presence of scoliosis.

a nonstructural scoliosis curve is present. With structural scoliosis, the curve remains. Look for a hump or raised scapula on one side (convex side of curve), and a hollow (concave side of curve) on the other. The combination of the hump and hollow is due to vertebral rotation.

Thoracic and lumbar movements should also be tested, and include the motions listed below. The range of motion listed with each movement is lumbar movement and does not include thoracic movement.

1. Forward flexion (40 to 60°)
2. Extension (20 to 35°)
3. Lateral flexion (left and right) (15 to 20°)
4. Rotation (left and right) (35 to 50°)

Goniometry measurements of the spine are not typically taken due to the difficulty of measuring individual regional motions. Completion of gross movement patterns is adequate enough to determine normal ranges of motion. If motion is limited, further assessment can be conducted.

Passive Range of Motion

Passive movement should not be performed in an acute injury where motor and sensory deficits are present. These deficits indicate a spinal injury, and any movement could be catastrophic. In other injuries where motor and sensory deficits are not present, passive range of motion can be performed if the individual does not have full range of motion. To per-

form passive motion, place the individual in a supine position. Passively move the cervical region through the various movements. Normal end feels for the cervical spine are tissue stretch in all four movements. Thoracic and lumbar passive movement is seldom performed. End feels can be determined at the extremes of active movement. Like cervical movements, normal end feels for thoracic and lumbar movements are tissue stretch.

Resisted Muscle Testing

Resisted movement is done throughout the full range of motion in the same movements as active muscle testing. It is important to stabilize the hip and trunk during cervical testing to avoid muscle substitution. This can be accomplished by having the individual seated and using one hand to stabilize the shoulder or thorax while the other hand applies manual overpressure. When testing the thoracic and lumbar region, the weight of the trunk will stabilize the hips in a seated or lying down position. Inform the individual not to allow you to move the body part being tested. Cervical movements assessed are demonstrated in **Figure 14-24**. Thoracic and lumbar movements to be tested are demonstrated in **Figure 14-25**.

Neurological Assessment

Neurological integrity can be assessed with the use of myotomes, reflexes, and segmental

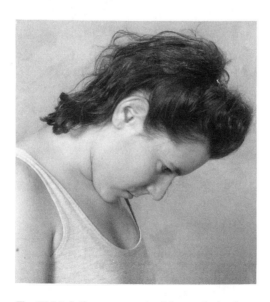

Fig. 14.24: Active movements of the cervical spine. (A) Flexion.

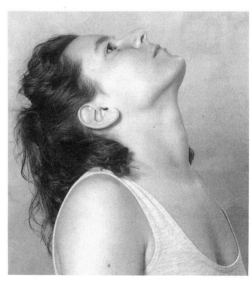

(B) Extension.

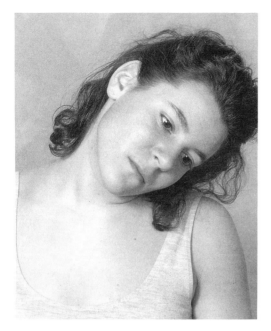

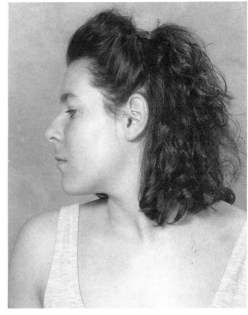

(C) Lateral flexion.

(D) Rotation.

dermatomes and peripheral nerve cutaneous patterns.

Myotomes

Isometric muscle testing is performed in the upper and lower extremities to test specific myotomes. Each has been discussed in preceding chapters. The myotomes are listed in **Table 14-7**.

Reflexes

Reflexes in the upper extremity include the biceps (C_5-C_6), brachialis (C_6), and triceps (C_7). In the lower extemity, the two major reflexes are the patella (L_3, L_4) and Achilles tendon reflex (S_1). **Table 14-8** lists the reflexes in the upper and lower extremities.

Cutaneous Patterns

The segmental nerve dermatome patterns and peripheral nerve cutaneous patterns are

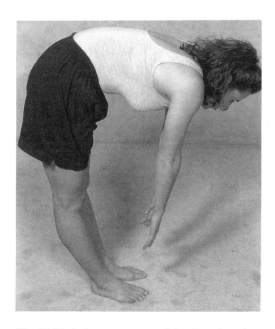

Fig. 14.25: Active movements of the thoracic and lumbar regions. (A) Flexion.

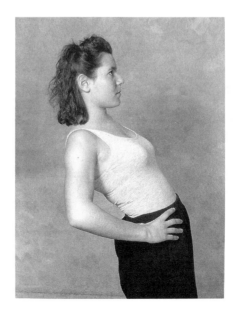

(B) Extension.

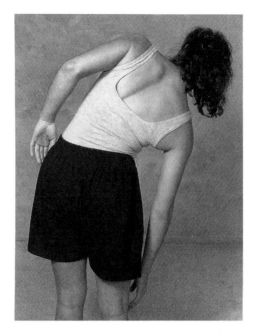

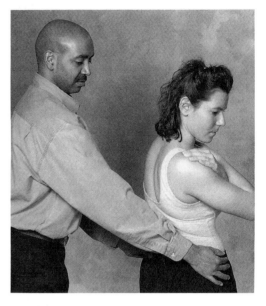

(D) Rotation.

Fig. 14.25:(C) Lateral flexion.

Table 14–7. Myotomes Used to Test Selected Nerve Root Segments.

Nerve root segment	Action tested
C1-2	Neck flexion*
C3	Neck lateral flexion*
C4	Shoulder elevation
C5	Shoulder abduction
C6	Elbow flexion and wrist extension
C7	Elbow extension and wrist flexion
C8	Thumb extension and ulnar deviation
T1	Intrinsic muscles of the hand (finger abduction and adduction)
L1-2	Hip flexion
L3	Knee extension
L4	Ankle dorsiflexion
L5	Toe extension
S1	Ankle plantar flexion, foot eversion, hip extension
S2	Knee flexion

*These myotomes should not be performed in an individual with a suspected cervical fracture or dislocation, as they may cause serious damage or possible death

Table 14–8. Deep Tendon Reflexes.

Deep tendon reflexes	Segmental levels
Biceps	Cervical **5**, 6
Brachioradialis	Cervical 5, **6**
Triceps	Cervical **7**, 8
Patellar	Lumbar 2, **3**, 4
Achilles	Sacral **1**

demonstrated in **Figure 14-26.** Test bilaterally for altered sensation with sharp and dull touch by running the open hand and fingernails over the head, neck, back, thorax, abdomen, and upper and lower extremities (front, back, and sides). Ask the person if the sensation feels the same on one body segment as compared to another.

Referred Pain

Pain can be referred to the thoracic spine from various abdominal organs. **Figure 14-27** demonstrates where pain is commonly referred to the torso.

Stress and Functional Tests

There are several stress tests that can be used in spinal assessment. Only those deemed relevant should be performed. If any increased pain or change of sensation occurs, the individual should be referred to a physician.

Cervical Compression Test

The individual slightly flexes the neck toward one side. Carefully compress straight down on the individual's head while the person is sitting on a stable chair or table (**Figure 14-28**). Increased pain or altered sensation is a positive sign, indicating pressure on a nerve root. The distribution of the pain and altered sensation can indicate which nerve root is involved.

Cervical Distraction Test

Place one hand under the individual's chin and the other around the occiput. Slowly lift

> The distribution of the pain and altered sensation can indicate which nerve root is involved

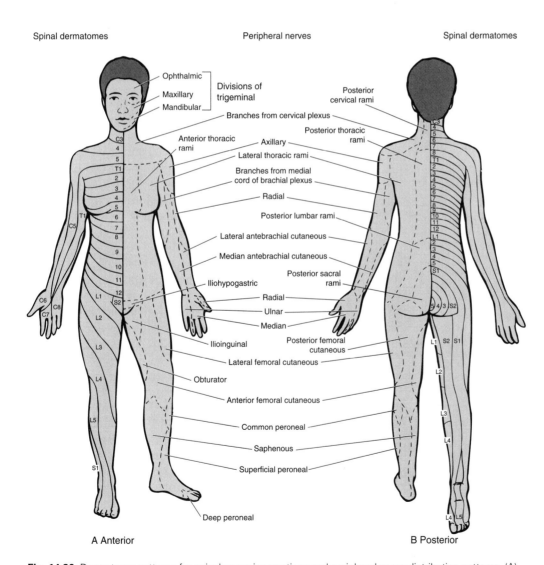

Fig. 14.26: Dermatome patterns for spinal nerve innervations and peripheral nerve distribution patterns. (A) Anterior view. (B) Posterior view.

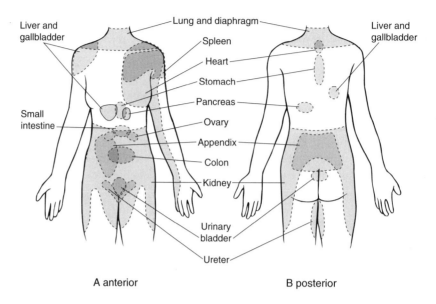

Fig. 14.27: Referred pain. Cutaneous patterns to which pain from visceral organs can be referred.

the head (**Figure 14-29**). The test is positive if pain is decreased or relieved as the head is lifted, indicating that pressure on the nerve root is relieved. If pain increases with distraction, it indicates ligamentous injury.

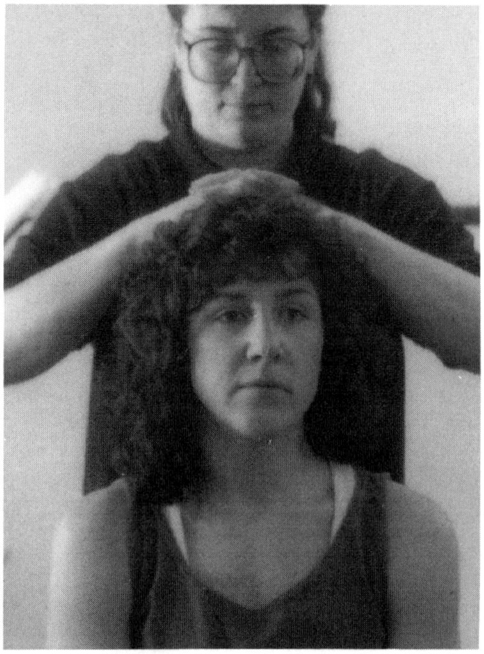

> Pain that increases with neck flexion or dorsiflexion indicates stretching of the dura mater of the spinal cord. Pain that does not increase with neck flexion or dorsiflexion indicates tight hamstrings

Fig. 14.28: To perform the compression test, carefully push straight down on the individual's head. Increased pain or altered sensation is a positive sign indicating pressure on a nerve root.

Straight Leg Raising Test

Also known as *Lasègue's test*, this test indicates stretching of the dura mater of the spinal cord and can be used to assess sacroiliac joint pain or tight hamstrings. The individual is placed in a relaxed supine position with the hip medially rotated and knee extended. Grasp the individual's heel with one hand and place the other on top of the patella to prevent the knee from flexing. Slowly raise the leg until the individual complains of pain or tightness. Lower the leg slightly until pain is relieved. The individual is then asked to flex the neck onto the chest, or dorsiflex the foot, or do both actions simultaneously (**Figure 14-30**). The neck flexion movement is called *Hyndman's sign* or *Brudzinski's sign*.

Normal hip flexion is between 80 and 90° of motion. Straight-leg raising may be limited and painful because of tight hamstrings, lumbosacral or sacroiliac joint injury, or irritation to the sciatic nerve. Pain that increases with neck flexion or dorsiflexion indicates stretching of the dura mater of the spinal cord. Pain that does not increase with neck flexion or dorsiflexion indicates tight hamstrings. The sciatic nerve is fully stretched at about 70° of flexion. Hence, pain after 70° usually indicates pain from the sacroiliac joints (**Figure 14-31**). Pain that occurs opposite the leg lifted indicates a herniated disc. Always compare both legs for any difference.

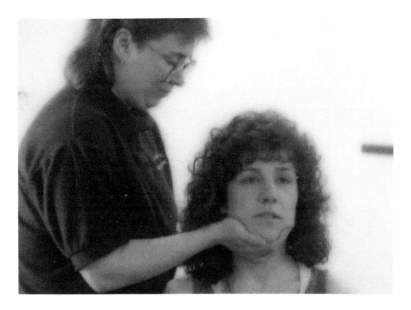

Fig. 14.29: To perform the distraction test, lift the head slowly. The test is positive if pain is decreased or relieved as the head is lifted, indicating that pressure on the nerve root is relieved. If pain increases with distraction, it indicates ligamentous injury.

Prone Knee-Bending Test

This test is used to indicate an L_2 or L_3 nerve root lesion, and also stretches the femoral nerve. Place the individual prone and passively flex the knee until the foot rests against the buttock. Maintain this position for 45 to 60 seconds (**Figure 14-32**). Do not allow the hip to rotate during this motion. If the knee cannot be flexed beyond 90° because of a pathological condition, do passive extension

of the hip with the knee flexed as much as possible. Unilateral pain in the lumbar region indicates an L_2 or L_3 nerve root lesion. Pain in the anterior thigh indicates tight quadriceps.

Sacroiliac Tests

In Chapter 9, several stress tests at the hip can also be used to stress the sacroiliac joints. These tests include the gapping test, squish

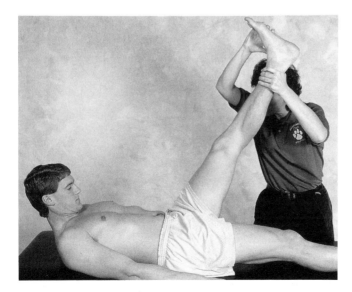

Fig. 14.30: Passively flex the individual's hip while keeping the knee extended until pain or tension is felt in the hamstrings. Slowly lower the leg until the pain or tension disappears. Then, dorsiflex the foot, have the individual flex the neck, or do both simultaneously. If pain does not increase with dorsiflexion of the ankle or flexion of the neck, it indicates tight hamstrings.

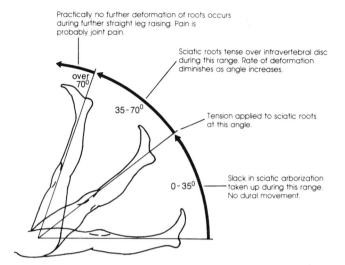

Practically no further deformation of roots occurs during further straight leg raising. Pain is probably joint pain.

Sciatic roots tense over intravertebral disc during this range. Rate of deformation diminishes as angle increases.

over 70°

35-70°

Tension applied to sciatic roots at this angle.

0-35°

Slack in sciatic arborization taken up during this range. No dural movement.

Fig. 14.31: Dynamics of a single leg raise.

test, sacroiliac rocking (knee-to-shoulder) test, and the approximation test (See **Figures 9-18, 9-19, 9-20**). The reader shoulder review these tests.

Functional Testing

Prior to return to play, the individual must have a normal neurological exam with pain-free range of motion (active and resisted), normal bilateral muscle strength in the myotomes, cutaneous sensation, and reflexes. Axial head compression can be performed on the sideline as an additional safety check. If pain is present, the individual should not return to competition (51). Other functional tests include walking, bending, lifting, jogging, running, figure-8 running, karioka running, and sport-specific skills. All must be performed pain-free and with unlimited movement.

Pain increases in the right lumbar region on resisted trunk extension, lateral flexion and rotation to the right. The quadriceps reflex is diminished on the right side and muscle weakness is apparent with knee extension and ankle dorsiflexion. Pain is elicited down the right leg during a straight leg raising test. If you determined a possible sciatica due to an extruded disc at the L_4 level, or spondylolysis

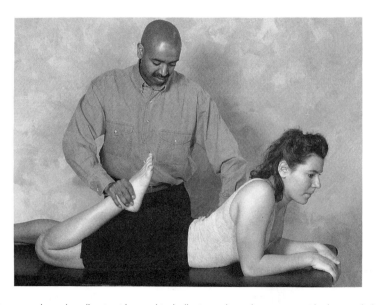

Fig. 14.32: The prone knee bending test is used to indicate an L_2 or L_3 nerve root lesion, and also stretches the femoral nerve.

is present, you are correct. What is your course of action?

REHABILITATION

❓ *The individual was seen by a physician who prescribed NSAIDs, muscle relaxants, and rest until symptoms subside. When the individual begins rehabilitation, what exercises should be included in the general program?*

Rehabilitation of back pain must follow an accurate and complete assessment of the history and clinical signs to determine the presence of an acute injury involving disc herniation or degeneration. Most injuries, however, do not have disc involvement, and can follow the regular rehabilitation phases. The exercise program, developed on an individual basis, must address the specific needs of the patient. Exercises to relieve pain related to postural problems may not address pain emanating from sciatica. Therefore, a variety of exercises are listed in this section, allowing you to select those appropriate for the patient. The program should relieve pain and muscle tension, restore motion and balance, develop strength, endurance, and power, and maintain cardiovascular fitness. Patient education is also critical in teaching skills and techniques needed to prevent recurrence. Many of these points were listed in **Field Strategy 14-1**.

Relief of Pain and Muscle Tension

Maintaining a prolonged posture or sustaining muscle contractions for a long time can lead to discomfort. Avoiding painful positions and doing active range of motion exercises in the opposite direction can relieve stress on supporting structures, promote circulation, and maintain flexibility (53). For example, to relieve tension in the cervical and upper thoracic region, do neck flexion, extension, lateral flexion, and rotation, shoulder rolls, and glenohumeral circumduction. In the lower thoracic and lumbar region, exercises such as back extension, side bending in each direction, spinal flexion (avoiding hip flexion), trunk rotation, and walking a short distance can relieve discomfort. With nerve root compression injuries, however, extension exercises may increase discomfort and may be contraindicated. Conscious relaxation training utilizing Jacobson's progressive relaxation exercises **(Field Strategy 5-3)** can relax an individual who is generally tense, or release tension in specific muscle groups, such as the upper trapezius.

Restoration of Motion

Mobilization exercises can be initiated early in the program to relieve pain and stretch tight structures that may limit range of motion. In **Field Strategy 14-2** the lower trunk rotation stretch and angry cat stretch were demonstrated. Other exercises include bringing both knees to the chest and gently rocking back and forth in a cranial/caudal direction, and in a standing position, shifting the hips from one side to another, lateral trunk flexion and rotation exercises.

Flexion exercises stretch the lumbar fascia and back extensors, open the intervertebral foramen and facet joints to reduce nerve compression, relieve tension on lumbar vertebrae due to tight hip flexors, and increase intra-abdominal pressure by strengthening the abdominals. Examples of flexion exercises in **Field Strategy 14-2** included the single knee and double knee to the chest stretch, hamstring stretch, hip flexor stretch, lateral rotator stretch, crunch curl-ups, and diagonal crunch curl-ups. Exercises to stretch the upper thoracic and pectoral region, trunk rotators and lateral flexors, and the hip adductors, abductors, extensors, and medial and lateral rotators should also be added to improve flexibility.

Extension exercises improve spinal mobility, reduce load on the intervertebral discs, strengthen the back extensors, and allow for self-mobilization of the motion segments. Back extension exercises in **Field Strategy 14-2** included prone extension exercises beginning with raising to the elbows then to the hands, the alternate arm and leg lift, double arm and leg lift, and alternate arm and leg extension on all fours. Other extension exercises may include single leg hip extension and double leg hip extension while holding onto a table, beginning with the knee(s) flexed, then with the knee(s) extended.

Pelvic and abdominal stabilizing exercises are used to teach an individual to place the hip in a neutral position to maintain the spine in the most comfortable position to control the forces exerted during repetitive microtrauma. During each exercise, the individual concentrates on maintaining the hip in a neutral position by contracting and relaxing the abdominal muscles. During functional activities, the individual can initiate stabilization contractions before starting any movement. This presets the posture and can reduce stress on the back. Many of these exercises are demonstrated in **Field Strategy 14-7.**

 Field Strategy 14–7. Stabilization and Abdominal Strengthening Exercises.

Stabilization Exercises, Quadruped Position

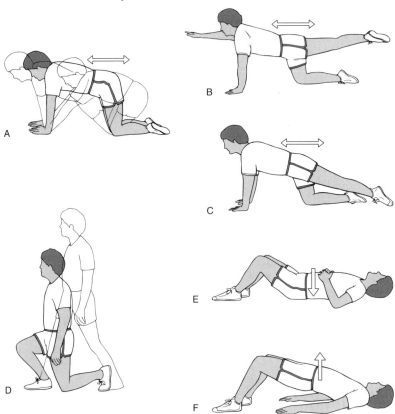

A. *Stabilization in neutral position.* With the back in a neutral position, slowly shift forward over the arms, adjusting pelvic position as you move. There will be a tendency to "sag" the back, so progressively tighten and relax the abdominal muscles during forward movement and backward movement, respectively

B. *Stabilization in "two point" position.* Balance on the right leg and left arm. Slowly move forward and back without losing neutral position. Switch to the opposite arm and leg

C. *Leg exercise.* Without arching the back, lift one leg out behind you. Do not lift the foot more than a few inches from the floor. A variation is to move a flexed knee sideways away from the body, then back to the original position

D. *Half-knee to stand (lunges).* Move to a standing position while maintaining neutral hip position. Push evenly with both legs. Repeat several times then switch the forward leg

E. *Pelvic tilt.* With the hips and knees bent and feet on the floor, do an isometric contraction of the abdominal muscles (posterior pelvic tilt) and hold. Using the phrase "tuck the stomach in" may convey the correct motion. Then, arch the back doing an anterior pelvic tilt. Alternate between the two motions until the individual can control pelvic motion

F. *Bridging.* Keeping the back in neutral position, raise the hips and back off the floor (contract the abdominal muscles to hold the position). Hold for five to ten seconds, drop down and relax. Repeat. Variations include (a) adding pelvic tilt exercises, (b) lifting one leg off the floor (keep the back in neutral position), and (c) combining pelvic tilts and one leg lift with bridging

---

Restoration of Proprioception and Balance

Proprioception and balance are regained through upper and lower extremity closed chain exercises. For example, the upper thoracic region can benefit from push-ups, press-ups, and balancing on a wobble board, ball, ProFitter, or slide board while weight bearing on the hands. Squats, the leg press, lunges, or exercises on a Stair Master, Pro-Fitter, or slide board can restore proprioception and balance in the hip and lower extremity. Stabilization exercises on all fours, and use of surgical tubing through functional patterns can also restore proprioception and balance. If available, these exercises should be performed in front of a mirror or videotaped, so the individual can observe proper posture and mechanics. Constant verbal reinforcement from the supervising therapist can also maximize feedback.

Muscular Strength, Endurance, and Power

Isometric contractions to strengthen the neck musculature can progress to manual resistance, surgical tubing, and use commercially available machines, as tolerated. Neck strength is particularly important for wrestlers and football linemen who need added stability and strength in the cervical region. Abdominal strengthening exercises, such as those listed in **Field Strategy 14-7** should precede crunch curl-ups and diagonal crunch curl-ups to maintain proper pelvic positioning and reduce functional lordosis. Progressive prone extension exercises and resisted back extension exercises can increase strength in the erector spinae.

Cardiovascular Fitness

Exercises to maintain cardiovascular fitness will depend on the extent of pain and limited motion present. Aquatic exercises are very beneficial because buoyancy can relieve load on sensitive structures. Deep water allows the individual to exercise all muscle groups through a full range of motion without the pain associated with gravity. Performing sport specific skills against water resistance can apply an equal and uniform force to the muscles similar to isokinetic strengthening. With low back pain, an upper body ergometer, stationary bicycle, Stair Master, or slide board

may be incorporated as tolerated. Jogging can begin when all symptoms have subsided.

After acute symptoms subside, pain and muscle tension should be relieved. Stretching the piriformis, gluteals, and hamstrings should be combined with flexion exercises to stretch the lumbar musculature and open the intervertebral foramen and facet joints to reduce nerve compression. Stabilization exercises, abdominal strengthening, and strengthening the medial rotators of the hip through proprioceptive neuromuscular facilitation (PNF) and Theraband exercises should be major components of the program. As strength is regained, functional activities can be incorporated with gradual return to full activity.

SUMMARY

The spine is a linkage system that transfers loads between the upper and lower extremities, enables motion in all three planes, and serves to protect the delicate spinal cord. Although most injuries to the back are relatively minor and can be successfully managed using the PRICE principles, spinal fractures and dislocations can occur.

In assessing a spinal injury always begin with a thorough history of the injury, and include neurological tests to determine possible nerve involvement. The severity of pain and presence or absence of neurological symptoms, neck spasm, and tenderness can indicate when a backboard and neck stabilization is needed. A full assessment of a spinal injury can be seen in **Field Strategy 14-8**.

If at anytime, an individual complains of acute pain in the spine, change in sensation anywhere on the body, or the individual resists moving the spine, assume that a significant injury is present and take appropriate measures to immobilize the spinal region and refer this individual to a physician for further evaluation. Conditions that warrant special attention and should be referred to a physician are listed in **Table 14-9**.

REFERENCES

1. Silver, JS. 1987. Spinal injuries as a result of sporting accidents. Paraplegia, 25(1):16–17.
2. McCarroll, JR, Miller, JM, and Ritter, MA. 1986. Lumbar spondylolysis and spondylolisthesis in college football players. Am J Sports Med, 14(5):404–406.
3. Jackson, DW, Wiltse, LL, and Cirincione, RJ. 1976. Spondylolysis in the female gymnast. Clin Orthop & Rel Res, 117:68–73.

Field Strategy 14–8. Assessment for a Spinal Injury.

HISTORY
- Primary complaint including:
  - Description and mechanism of current injury
- Onset of symptoms
- Pain perception and discomfort
- Disability and functional impairments from the injury
- Previous injuries to the area
- Family history

OBSERVATION AND INSPECTION
- Observation should analyze:
  - Overall appearance
  - Posture and body symmetry
  - General motor function through a scan exam
  - Gait analysis
- Inspection at the injury site for:

Muscle symmetry	Hypertrophy or muscle atrophy
Swelling	Visible congenital deformity
Discoloration	Surgical incisions or scars

PALPATION
- Bony structures to rule out fracture.
- Soft tissue structures to determine:

Temperature	Deformity
Swelling	Muscle spasm
Point tenderness	Cutaneous sensation
Crepitus	Vascular pulses

SPECIAL TESTS
- Active movement
- Passive movement and end feels
- Resisted movement
- Neurological testing
  - Myotomes
  - Reflexes
  - Dermatomes
- Stress and functional tests
  - Cervical compression test
  - Cervical distraction test
  - Straight leg raising test
  - Prone knee bending test
  - Sacroiliac tests
  - Functional testing

Table 14–9. Conditions that Warrant Immediate Referral to a Physician.
- Severe pain, point tenderness, or deformity along the vertebral column
- Loss or change in sensation anywhere in the body
- Paralysis or inability to move a body part
- Diminished or absent reflexes
- Muscle weakness in a myotome
- Radiating pain into the extremities
- Trunk or abdominal pain that may be referred from the visceral organs
- Any injury about which you have doubts regarding the severity or nature

4. Day, AL, Friedman, WA, and Indelicato, PA. 1987. Observations on the treatment of lumbar disc disease in college football players. Am J Sports Med, 15(1):72–75.
5. Clarke, KS. "An epidemiologic view." In *Athletic injuries to the head, neck, and face*, edited by JS Torg. St. Louis: Mosby Year Book, 1991.
6. Torg, JS, Vegso, JJ, O'Neil, MJ, and Sennett, B. 1990. The epidemiologic, pathologic, biomechanical and cinematographic analysis of football-induced cervical spine trauma. Am J Sports Med, 18(1):50–57.
7. Tator, CH, and Edmonds, VE. 1986. Sports and recreation are a rising cause of spinal cord injury. Phys Sportsmed, 14(5):157–167.
8. Torg, JS, Vegso, JJ, Sennett, B, and Das, M. 1984. The national football head and neck injury registry. Fourteen-year report on cervical quadriplegia, 1971–1984. JAMA, 254(24):3439–3443.
9. Tator, CH, and Edmonds, VE. 1984. National survey of spinal injuries in hockey players. Can Med Assoc J, 130(7):875–880.
10. Mooney, V. 1987. Where is the pain coming from? Spine, 12(8):754–759.
11. Schultz, AB. 1974. Mechanics of the human spine. App Mech Rev, 27:1487–1497.
12. Hall, SJ. 1986. Mechanical contribution to lumbar stress injuries in female gymnasts. Med Sci Sports Exerc, 18(6):599–602.
13. Lindh, M. "Biomechanics of the lumbar spine." In *Basic biomechanics of the musculoskeletal system*, edited by M Nordin and VH Frankel. Philadelphia: Lea & Febiger, 1989.
14. Hall, SJ. 1985. Effect of attempted lifting speed on forces and torque exerted on the lumbar spine. Med & Sci Spts & Exer, 17(4):440–444.
15. Shirazi-Adl, A, and Drouin, G. 1987. Load bearing role of facets in a lumbar segment under sagittal plane loadings. J Biomech, 20(6):610–614.
16. Patwardhan, AG, Bunch, WH, Victoria, VM, Gavin, TM, and Goel, VK. "Biomechanics of adolescent idiopathic scoliosis—Natural history and treatment." In *Biomechanics of the Spine: Clinical and Surgical*

Perspective, edited by VK Goel and JN Weinstein. Boca Raton: CRC Press, 1990.

17. Mercier, LR. *Practical Orthopedics.* Chicago: Year Book Medical Publishers, 1987.

18. Goldberg, B, and Boiardo, R. 1984. Profiling children for sports participation. Clin in Sports Med, 3(1):153–169.

19. Johnson, RJ. 1993. Low-back pain in sports: Managing spondylolysis in young patients. Phys Sportsmed, 21(4):53-59.

20. Reid, DC. *Sports injury assessment and rehabilitation.* New York: Churchill Livingstone, 1992.

21. American Academy of Orthopedic Surgeons. 1991. *Athletic training and sports medicine.* Park Ridge, IL.

22. Schneider, RC. 1966. Serious and fatal neurosurgical football injuries. Clin Neurosurg, 12:226–236.

23. Zemper, ED. 1989. Injury rates in a national sample of college football teams: A 2-year prospective study. Phys Sportsmed, 17(11):100–113.

24. Cantu, RC. 1993. Functional cervical spinal stenosis: A contraindication to participation in contact sports. Med Sci Sports Exer, 25(3):316–317.

25. Torg, JS. 1990. Cervical spine stenosis with cord neurapraxia and transient quadriplegia. Ath Train, 25(2):138–146.

26. Torg, JS, Pavlov H, Genuario, SE, et al. 1986. Neurapraxia of the cervical spinal cord with transient quadriplegia. J Bone Joint Surg [Am], 68A(0): 1354–1370.

27. Silver, JR, Silver, DD, and Godfrey, JJ. 1986. Injuries of the spine sustained during gymnastic activities. British Med J, 293(6551):861–863.

28. Silver, JR, Silver, DD, and Godfrey, JJ. 1986. Trampolining injuries of the spine. Injury, 17(2):117–124.

29. Byun, HS, Cantos, EL, and Patel, PP. 1986. Severe cervical injury due to break dancing: A case report. Orthop, 9(4):550–551.

30. Markey, KL, Benedetto, MD, and Curl, WW. 1993. Upper trunk brachial plexopathy: The stinger syndrome. Am J Sports Med, 21(5):650–655.

31. Hershman, EB. "Brachial plexus injuries." In *Clinics in sports medicine,* edited by EB Hershman, vol. 9, no. 2. Philadelphia: WB Saunders, 1990.

32. Ringel, SP, Treihaft, M, Carry, M, Fisher, R, and Jacobs, P. 1990. Suprascapular neuropathy in pitchers. Am J of Spts Med, 18(1):80–86.

33. Rovere, GD. 1987. Low back pain in athletes. Phys Sportsmed, 15(1):105–117.

34. Alexander, MJL. 1985. Biomechanical aspects of lumbar spine injuries in athletes: A review. Can J Applied Sport Sci, 10:1–20.

35. Keene, JS. 1987. Thoracolumbar fractures in winter sports. Clin Orthop & Rel Res, 216(Mar):39–49.

36. Spengler, DM, Bigos, SJ, Martin, NA, Zeh, J, Fisher, L, and Nachemson, A. 1986. Back injuries in industry: A retrospective study: Overview and cost analysis. Spine, 11(3):241–245.

37. Fairbank, JC, Pynsent, PB, Van Poortvliet, JA, and Phillips, H. 1984. Influence of anthropometric factors and joint laxity in the incidence of adolescent back pain. Spine, 9(4):461–464.

38. Salminen, JJ. 1984. The adolescent back: a field survey of 370 Finnish school children. Acta Paediatr Scand Suppl, 315:1–122.

39. Frymoyer, JW. 1988. Back pain and sciatica. N Engl J Med, 318(5):291–300.

40. Helliovaara, M. 1989. Risk factors for low back pain and sciatica. Ann Med, 21:257–264.

41. Frymoyer, W, and Mooney, V. 1986. Current concepts review: Occupational orthopedics. J Bone & Joint Surg, 68A(3):469–474.

42. Kelsey, J, and White, A, 1980. Epidemiology and impact of low back pain. Spine, 5(2):133–142.

43. Snook, S, Fine, L, and Silverstein, B. "Musculoskeletal disorders." In *Occupational health: Recognizing and preventing work-related disease,* edited by B Levy and D Wegman. Boston: Little, Brown and Co, 1988.

44. Cypress, B. 1983. Characteristics of physician visits for back symptoms; a national perspective. Am J Pub Health, 73(4):389–395.

45. Roncarati, A, Bucciarelli, J, and English, D. 1986. The incidence of low back pain in runners: A descriptive study. Corporate Fitness & Recreation, Feb/Mar:33–36.

46. Cox, JM. "Diagnosis of the patient with low back pain." In *Low back pain: Mechanism, diagnosis and treatment,* edited by JM Cox. Baltimore: Williams and Wilkins, 1990.

47. Adams, MA, and Hutton, WC. 1985. Gradual disc prolapse. Spine, 10(5):524–531.

48. Kelsey, JL, et al. 1984. Acute prolapsed lumbar intervertebral disc. An epidemiological study with special reference to driving automobiles and cigarette smoking. Spine, 9(6):608–613.

49. Kelsey, JL, et al. 1984. An epidemiological study of acute prolapsed cervical intervertebral disc. J Bone & Joint Surg, 66A(6): 907–914.

50. Plowman, SA. "Physical activity, physical fitness, and low back pain." In *Exercise and Sport Sciences Reviews,* edited by JO Holloszy, vol. 20. Champaign, IL: Human Kinetics, 1992.

51. Anderson, C. 1993. Neck injuries: Backboard, bench, or return to play? Phys Sportsmed, 21(8):23–34.

52. Ryan, MD. 1993. On the field assessment for the cervical spine. Current Con Spts Med, 1:4–5.

53. Kisner, C, and Colby, LA. Therapeutic exercise: Foundations and techniques. Philadelphia: FA Davis, 1990.

Throat, Thorax, and Visceral Injuries

After you have completed this chapter, you should be able to:

■ Locate the important bony and soft tissue structures of the throat, thorax, and viscera

■ Identify measures to prevent injuries to the throat, thorax and viscera

■ Recognize and manage specific injuries of the throat, thorax, and viscera

■ Describe life-threatening conditions that can occur spontaneously or as a result of direct trauma to the throat, thorax, and viscera

■ Demonstrate an assessment of the throat, thorax, and visceral regions

■ Discuss the types of altered sensation that can result from nerve injury

Torso injuries occur in nearly every sport, particularly those involving sudden deceleration and impact. Although protective equipment and padding is available to protect the anterior throat, thorax, and viscera, only football, lacrosse, hockey, fencing, baseball, and softball require specific safety equipment for this vital region. Compression, shearing and tensile forces lead to contusions, muscular strains, costochondral separations, and rib fractures. Although most injuries are superficial and easily recognized and managed, certain injuries can involve the respiratory and circulatory system leading to life-threatening situations. Trauma to the abdomen can rupture an internal organ causing hemorrhage that can also become life-threatening.

This chapter begins with a review of the anatomy of the anterior throat, thorax, and viscera, followed by a brief discussion on prevention of injuries. Common injuries are then presented, followed by internal complications that may occur as a result of significant trauma or spontaneous rupture. Finally, a step-by-step injury assessment procedure is presented beginning with a primary survey, then moves through the HOPS format to determine the extent and seriousness of injury. Because rehabilitation of the region is usually included with hip, shoulder, and spinal exercise programs, specific exercises for the thorax and visceral region will not be discussed in this chapter. The reader should refer to the chapters on the hip, shoulder, and spinal regions for suggested exercises.

ANATOMY REVIEW OF THE THROAT

Why is a blow to the throat potentially dangerous? Could respiratory arrest be a potential outcome?

The throat is an important region of the body and includes the pharynx, larynx, trachea, esophagus, a number of glands, and several major blood vessels (**Figure 15-1**). Injuries to the throat are of particular concern because of the life-dependent functions of the trachea and carotid arteries.

Pharynx

The pharynx, commonly known as the throat, connects the nasal cavity and mouth to the larynx and esophagus below. The pharynx lies between the base of the skull and sixth cervical vertebra.

Larynx

The larynx, commonly referred to as the voice box, is a cartilaginous tube connecting the throat and trachea. The laryngeal prominence on the thyroid cartilage that shields the front of the larynx is known as the "Adam's apple." A specialized spoon-shaped cartilage, the epiglottis, covers the superior opening of

> The epiglottis covers the superior opening of the larynx during swallowing to prevent food and liquids from entering the larynx

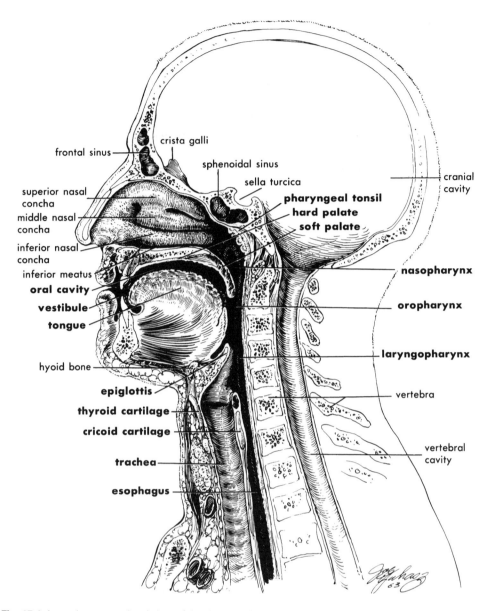

Fig. 15.1: Lateral cross-sectional view of the throat region.

crista galli

frontal sinus

sphenoidal sinus

sella turcica

pharyngeal tonsil
hard palate
soft palate

cranial cavity

superior nasal concha

middle nasal concha

inferior nasal concha

inferior meatus

oral cavity

vestibule

tongue

hyoid bone

epiglottis

thyroid cartilage

cricoid cartilage

trachea

esophagus

nasopharynx

oropharynx

laryngopharynx

vertebra

vertebral cavity

Vocal cords
Bands of elastic connective tissue encased in mucosal folds that enable the voice to make sound

The trachealis muscle allows the trachea to expand and allow food in the adjacent esophagus to pass through to the stomach

the larynx during swallowing to prevent food and liquids from entering. If a foreign body does slip past the epiglottis, the cough reflex is initiated and the foreign body is normally ejected back into the pharynx. Since the cough reflex cannot be elicited when a person is unconscious, fluids should never be administered to an unconscious individual.

The larynx also contains the **vocal cords**, two bands of elastic connective tissue surrounded by mucosal folds. The vocal cords are separated by an opening called the glottis. When expired air from the lungs pass over the vocal cords they are capable of producing sound. The laryngeal muscles manipulate the length of the vocal cords and size of the glot-

tis to produce sounds that vary in pitch and loudness.

Trachea

The trachea, commonly known as the windpipe, extends inferiorly from the larynx through the neck down into the mid-thorax, where it divides into the two major bronchial tubes. The tracheal tube is formed by C-shaped rings of hyaline cartilage joined by fibroelastic connective tissue. The open side of the C, formed by the smooth muscle fibers of the trachealis muscle, allows expansion of the posteriorly adjacent esophagus as swallowed food passes through. Contraction of the trachealis muscle during coughing can dramatically reduce the size of the airway, thus increasing pressure inside the trachea to promote expulsion of mucous.

Esophagus

The esophagus carries food and liquids from the throat to the stomach. It is a muscle-walled tube that originates from the pharynx in the mid-neck and follows the anterior side of the spine. When the esophagus is empty the tube is collapsed.

Blood Vessels of the Throat

The largest blood vessels coursing through the neck are the common carotid arteries (**Figure 15-2**). At the level of the "Adam's apple" the common carotid arteries divide into external and internal carotid arteries, which provide the major blood supply to the brain, head, and face. Branches from the carotid arteries include the superior thyroid arteries, which supply the thyroid and larynx, facial artery to the face and sinuses, and lingual artery to the mouth and tongue. Several arteries also branch from the left and right subclavian arteries and course upward through the posterior side of the neck. Included are the costocervical trunk, thyrocervical trunk, and vertebral artery.

A blow to the throat can lead to acute coughing, spasm, and an inability to catch one's breath. Because the trachea and superficial carotid arteries course through the neck, severe blows can disrupt the function of one or both of these structures, becoming life-threatening.

ANATOMY REVIEW OF THE THORAX

What anatomical structures protect the heart and lungs?

The thoracic cavity, or chest cavity, lies anterior to the spinal column and extends from the level of the clavicle down to the diaphragm. The major organs of the thorax are the heart and lungs. Although these

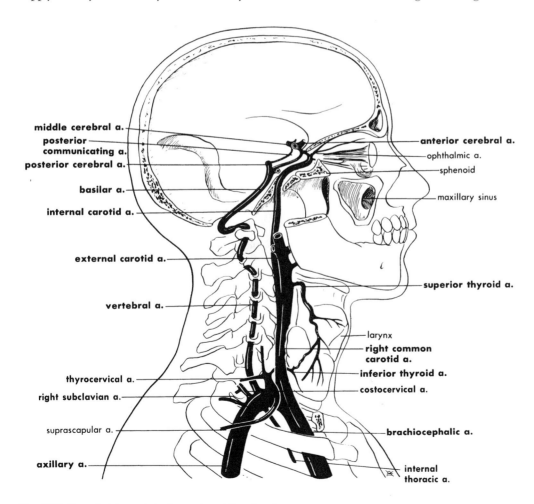

Fig. 15.2: The arterial supply to the neck and throat region.

organs are not commonly injured, internal complications due to direct trauma or spontaneous damage can necessitate emergency action during sport participation.

Thoracic Cage and Pleura

The bones of the thorax form a protective cage around the internal organs. The thoracic cage includes the sternum, ribs and costal cartilages, and thoracic vertebrae (**Figure 15-3**). The sternum consists of the manubrium, which articulates with the first and second ribs, the body, which articulates with the second through seventh ribs, and the xiphoid process, a trapezoidal projection composed of hyaline cartilage that ossifies around age 40. There are twelve pairs of ribs, all mating posteriorly with the thoracic vertebrae. The costal cartilages of the first seven pairs of ribs attach directly to the sternum, and the costal cartilages of ribs 8 to 10 attach to the costal cartilages of the immediately superior ribs. The last two rib pairs are known as floating ribs because they do not attach anteriorly to any other structure.

The thoracic cavity is lined with a thin, double-layered membrane called the pleura. The pleural cavity is a narrow space between the pleural membranes that is filled with a layer of pleural fluid secreted by the membranes. The pleural fluid enables the lungs to move against the thoracic wall with minimal friction during breathing.

Bronchial Tree and Lungs

The primary bronchial tubes branch obliquely downward from the trachea at about the level of the seventh thoracic vertebra (**Figure 15-4**). The primary bronchi enter the lungs posterior to the major pulmonary vessels, then

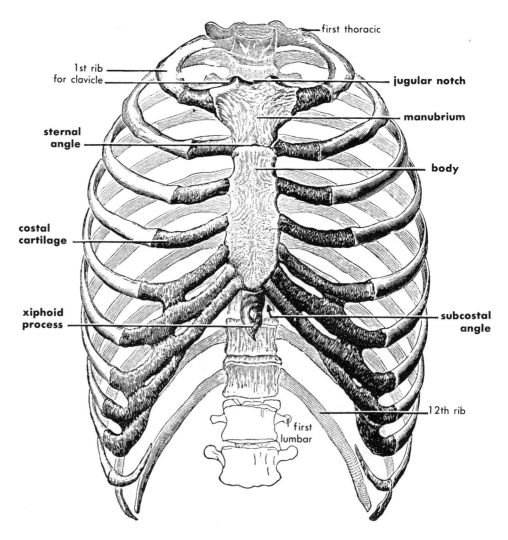

Fig. 15.3: The thoracic cage. Note that only the first seven pairs of ribs articulate anteriorly with the sternum through the costal cartilages.

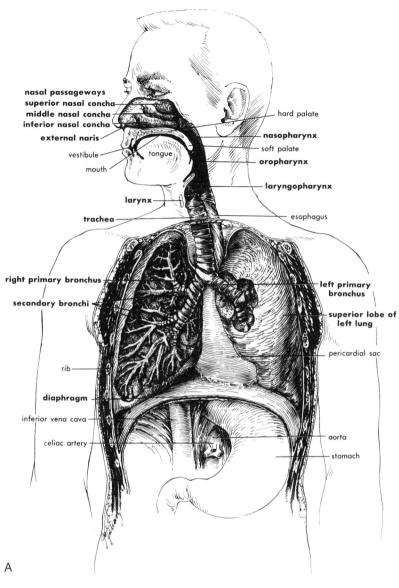

A

nasal passageways
superior nasal concha
middle nasal concha
inferior nasal concha
external naris
vestibule
mouth
tongue
larynx
trachea
right primary bronchus
secondary bronchi
rib
diaphragm
inferior vena cava
celiac artery

hard palate
nasopharynx
soft palate
oropharynx
laryngopharynx
esophagus
left primary bronchus
superior lobe of left lung
pericardial sac
aorta
stomach

Fig. 15.4: The respiratory system. (A) The anterior walls of the lungs have been removed to show the bronchi and bronchioles. (B) The terminal ends of the bronchial tree are alveolar sacs where oxygen and carbon dioxide are exchanged.

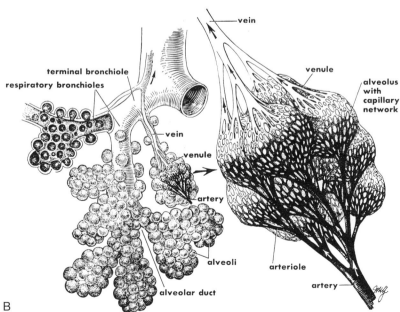

B

terminal bronchiole
respiratory bronchioles
vein
venule
alveoli
alveolar duct

vein
venule
arteriole
artery

alveolus with capillary network

Alveoli
Air sacs at the terminal ends of the bronchial tree where oxygen and carbon dioxide are exchanged between the lungs and surrounding capillaries

Pulmonary circuit
Blood vessels that transport unoxygenated blood to the lungs from the right heart ventricle and oxygenated blood from the lungs to the left heart atrium

Systemic circuit
Blood vessels that transport unoxygenated blood to the right heart atrium and oxygenated blood from the left heart ventricle

Atria
Two superior chambers of the heart that pump blood into the ventricles

Ventricles
Two inferior chambers of the heart that pump blood from the heart; one to the pulmonary circuit and one to the systemic circuit

branch into secondary bronchi, which branch into tertiary bronchi, and so forth, with approximately 23 levels of subsequent branching occurring. Terminal bronchioles are smaller than 0.5 mm in diameter. Tiny air sacs called **alveoli** serve as diffusion chambers where oxygen from the lungs enter adjacent capillaries, and carbon dioxide from the blood is returned to the lungs.

Healthy lungs consist of an elastic network of air passageways and spaces bound together by connective tissue. Although the lungs occupy the majority of the thoracic cavity, each lung weighs only approximately 0.6 kg (1.25 lb). The left lung is smaller than the right lung, containing a concavity known as the cardiac notch in which the heart is nestled.

Heart

The heart and lungs have an intimate relationship both physically and functionally. The right side of the heart pumps blood to the lungs, where it is oxygenated and carbon dioxide is given off. The left side of the heart receives the freshly oxygenated blood from the lungs and pumps it out to the systemic circulation. The vessels interconnecting the heart and lungs are known as the **pulmonary circuit**, whereas the vessels that supply the body are known as the **systemic circuit (Figure 15-5)**.

The heart is positioned obliquely to the left of the midline of the body. It is divided into four chambers—the right and left **atria** superiorly, and the right and left **ventricles** inferiorly (**Figure 15-6**). The heartbeat consists of

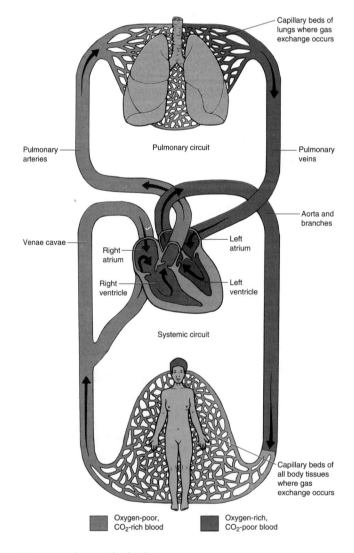

Fig. 15.5: The pulmonary and systemic circuits.

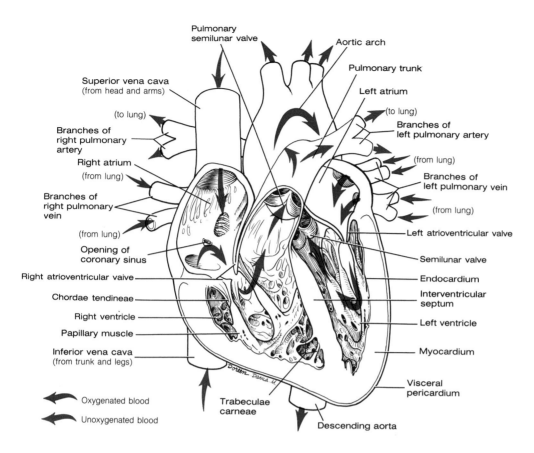

Fig. 15.6: The heart. Note that the direction of blood flow through the chambers of the heart is indicated by arrows.

a simultaneous contraction of the two atria followed immediately by a simultaneous contraction of the two ventricles. The contraction phase is known as systole. The phase in which the chambers are relaxing and filling with blood is known as diastole.

Two pairs of valves within the heart ensure that the flow of blood within the heart is unidirectional. The **atrioventricular valves** seal off the atria during contraction of the ventricles to prevent the backflow of blood. The aortic and pulmonary **semilunar valves** prevent flow of blood from the aorta and pulmonary artery back into the ventricles.

Muscles of the Thorax

The locations, primary functions, and innervations of the muscles of the thoracic region are summarized in **Table 15-1 (Figures 15-7, 15-8)**. Included are the major muscles of respiration.

The major respiratory muscle is the diaphragm, a powerful sheet of muscle that completely separates the thoracic and abdominal cavities. During relaxation the diaphragm is

dome-shaped. During contraction it flattens, thereby increasing the size of the thoracic cavity. This increase in cavity volume causes a decrease in intrathoracic pressure, resulting in inhalation of air into the lungs.

The heart and lungs lie in the thoracic cavity where they are protected by the pleural lining of the cavity and, external to the cavity, by the rib cage and sternum.

ANATOMY REVIEW OF THE VISCERAL REGION

An individual is complaining of pain and cramping in the lower right abdominal quadrant. What possible structures might account for this pain?

The visceral region includes all organs and structures between the diaphragm and pelvic floor. The solid organs include the spleen, liver, pancreas, kidneys, and adrenal glands. The hollow organs include the stomach, small and large intestines, bladder, and ureters. The pelvic girdle protects the lower abdominal organs. The major organs are discussed in detail.

Blood pressure is read as pressure during systole over pressure during diastole (e.g., 120/80)

Atrioventricular valves
Heart valves that prevent the backflow of blood from the ventricles to the atria

Semilunar valves
Heart valves that prevent the backflow of blood from the pulmonary artery and aorta to the ventricles

Table 15–1. Muscles of the Thorax.

Muscle	Proximal Attachment	Distal Attachment	Primary Action(s)	Nerve Innervation
Pectoralis minor	Coracoid process of the scapula	Anterior surfaces of ribs 3–5	With ribs fixed pulls scapula forward and downward; with scapula fixed pulls ribs upward	Medial pectoral (C_7, C_8, T_1)
Serratus anterior	Vertebral border of scapula	Ribs 1–8 or 9	Protraction and rotation of the scapula	Long thoracic (C_5-C_7)
Subclavius	Groove on inferior surface of clavicle	Costal cartilage of rib 1	Assists with stabilization and depression of shoulder girdle	Nerve to subclavius (C_5, C_6)
Levator scapulae	Transverse process of the first four cervical vertebrae	Vertebral border of the scapula	Lateral flexion of the neck	C_3-C_4 nerve roots Dorsal scapular (C_5)
Trapezius	Occipital bone, ligamentum nuchae, C7 and T1-12	Acromion and spine of scapula and lateral clavicle	Stabilizes, elevates, retracts, and rotates scapula, lateral extension of neck	Accessory (Cranial nerve XI)
Rhomboids	C7, T1-T5	Medial border of scapula	Retracts, rotates, and stabilizes scapula	Dorsal scapular (C_4, C_5)
External inter-costals (11 pairs between ribs)	Inferior border of rib above	Superior border of rib below	Elevation of rib cage; assists the diaphragm with inspiration	Intercostal nerves (T_1-T_{11})
Internal inter-costals (11 pairs between ribs)	Inferior border of rib above	Superior border of rib below	Depress rib cage; assists with expiration	Intercostal nerves (T_1-T_{11})
Diaphragm	Inferior border of rib cage and sternum; costal cartilages of ribs 6–12; lumbar vertebrae	Central tendon	Inspiration	Phrenic nerve (C_3-C_5)

Pelvic Girdle and Abdominal Cavity

The pelvic girdle, hip girdle, or pelvis, consists of the sacrum, ilium, ischium, and pubis (**Figure 15-9**). The joints between these bones are fused in adults, with no movement allowed. The pelvis forms a protective basin around the internal organs of the abdomen and transfers loads between the spine and the lower extremity through the hip joint. The pelvis also provides a mechanical link between the upper and lower extremities. Its primary role is to stabilize the lower trunk while motion occurs in the extremities.

Visceral Organs

The stomach is a J-shaped bag positioned between the esophagus and small intestine (**Figure 15-10**). Food is stored in the stomach

The pelvis forms a protective basin around the internal organs of the lower abdomen and transfers weight between the spine and lower extremity through the hip joint

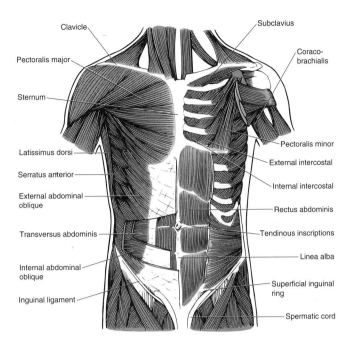

Fig. 15.7: Anterior muscles of the trunk.

for approximately four hours during which time it is broken down by hydrochloric acid secreted in the stomach into a paste-like substance known as **chyme**. Only a few substances, including water, electrolytes, aspirin, and alcohol are absorbed into the blood stream across the stomach lining without full digestion. The chyme then moves into the small intestine where it is progressively absorbed.

The small intestine is a loosely convoluted tube of about 2 m (6 ft) in length that connects the stomach to the large intestine. Using digestive enzymes secreted by the pancreas, the small intestine carries out most of the digestion and absorption of food. Food is propelled through the small intestine in approximately three to six hours by a process called **peristalsis**.

Chyme
Paste-like substance into which food is churned in the stomach

Peristalsis
Periodic waves of smooth muscle contraction that propel food through the digestive system

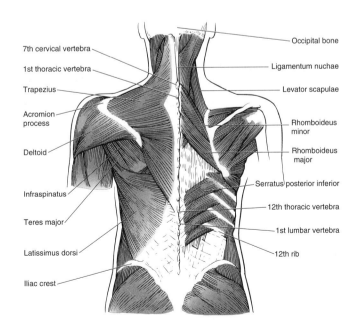

Fig. 15.8: Posterior muscles of the trunk.

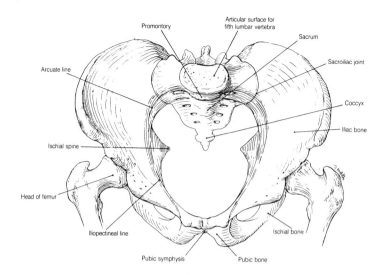

Fig. 15.9: The pelvic girdle.

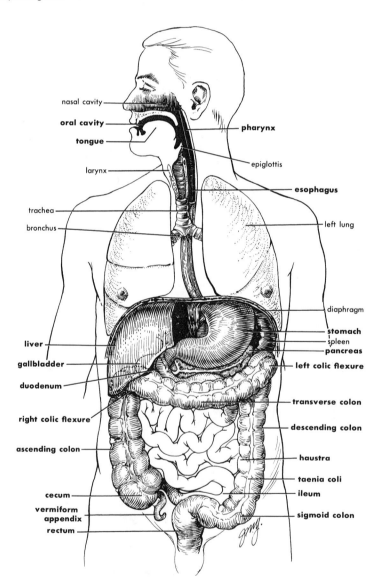

Fig. 15.10: Anterior view of the visceral organs.

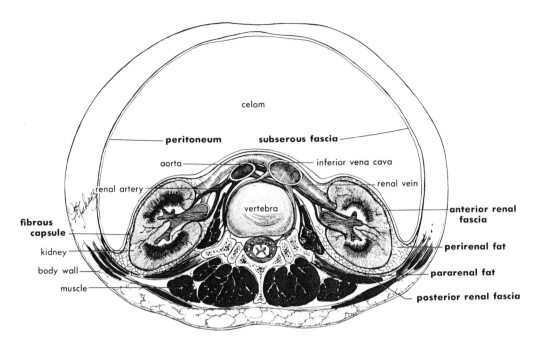

Fig. 15.11: Mid-transverse section of the body showing the kidneys and renal fascia.

The large intestine, or colon, stretches to approximately 1.5 m (4 ft), almost completely encircling the coils of the small intestine, and connecting the intestine to the anus. The different sections of the colon are named according to the direction in which they travel. Thus, there are the ascending, transverse, and descending sections of the colon, and finally the S-shaped sigmoid colon joins to the anus. In the colon, water and electrolytes are further absorbed during the next 12 to 24 hours from the stored material. Mass peristaltic movements pass through the intestines several times per day to move the feces to the rectum.

The vermiform appendix is a twisted, coiled tube of approximately 8 cm in length that protrudes from the large intestine in the right lower quadrant of the abdomen. Since the appendix is twisted, it presents a protected environment for the accumulation of bacteria. Inflammation of the appendix is known as appendicitis.

The liver is a large, versatile organ that lies in the upper right quadrant under the diaphragm where it is largely protected by the rib cage. As part of the digestive system, the liver produces bile, a greenish liquid that helps break down fat in the small intestine. The liver also absorbs excess glucose from the blood stream and stores it in the form of glycogen for later use. Among its other functions are processing fats and amino acids,

manufacturing blood proteins, and detoxifying certain poisons and drugs. These functions can be severely impaired with alcohol abuse, which can result in **cirrhosis** of the liver. **Hepatitis** is inflammation of the liver caused by a viral infection that can also reduce the liver's efficiency.

The gallbladder is a small, muscular sac located in an indentation on the inferior side of the liver. It functions as an accessory to the liver to store concentrated bile on its way to the small intestine.

The spleen, the largest of the lymphoid organs, is located on the posterior wall of the abdomen behind the stomach. It performs four vital functions: (1) cleansing the blood of foreign matter, bacteria, viruses, and toxins; (2) storing excess red blood cells for later reuse and releasing others into the blood for processing by the liver; (3) producing red blood cells in the fetus; and (4) storing blood platelets.

The pancreas is an abdominal gland with two primary functions. One is to secrete most of the digestive enzymes that break down food in the small intestine. The other is to secrete the hormones insulin and glucagon, which respectively lower and elevate blood sugar levels.

The kidneys are not abdominal or pelvic organs, but rather lie posterior to the abdominal cavity (**Figure 15-11**). The kidneys filter and cleanse the blood. They are vital for fil-

Cirrhosis
Progressive inflammation of the liver usually caused by alcoholism

Hepatitis
Inflammation of the liver

The pancreas secretes digestive enzymes into the small intestine where most of the digestion and absorption of nutrients occur

tering out toxins, metabolic wastes, drugs, and excess ions that leave the body via urine, while returning needed substances, such as water and electrolytes to the blood. The kidneys are positioned posterolaterally between the eleventh and twelfth ribs and third lumbar vertebra and are somewhat protected by a surrounding perirenal fat pad.

The urinary bladder is an expandable sac that sits on the floor of the pelvic cavity poste-rior to the pubic symphysis. The muscled walls of the bladder enable it to expel, as well as store urine.

Blood Vessels of the Trunk

The aorta serves as the trunk of the arterial tree in the systemic circuit (**Figure 15-12**). Ascending upward from the left ventricle of the heart, the aorta arches to the left, then

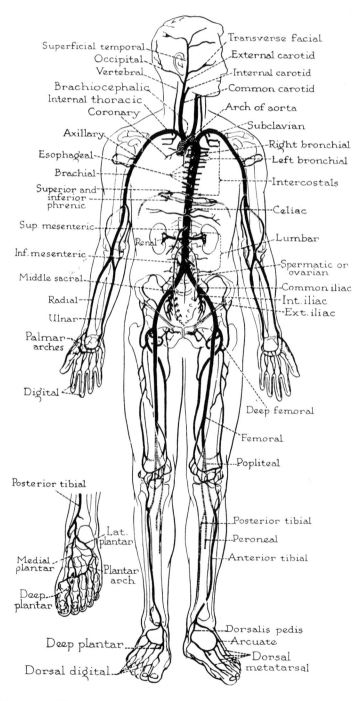

Fig. 15.12: Arterial system of the trunk.

travels downward through the thorax and abdomen.

A number of arteries branch from the ascending aorta and aortic arch. The left and right coronary arteries branch from the ascending aorta to supply the heart muscle. The first arterial branch from the aortic arch is the brachiocephalic artery, which splits into the right common carotid artery and right subclavian artery. The second and third branches from the aortic arch are the left common carotid artery and left subclavian artery, respectively.

More major arteries branch from the lower regions of the aorta. From the thoracic aorta come 10 pairs of intercostal arteries to supply the muscles of the thorax, the bronchial arteries to the lungs, the esophageal artery to the esophagus, and the phrenic arteries to the diaphragm. The first branch of the abdominal aorta is the celiac trunk. It branches to form the left gastric artery to the stomach, the splenic artery to the spleen, and the common hepatic artery to the liver. Other branches of the abdominal aorta include the superior and inferior mesenteric arteries to the small intestine and the first half of the large intestine, the renal arteries to the kidneys, the ovarian arteries (in females) and the testicular arteries (in males). Also branching from the abdominal aorta are several pairs of lumbar arteries to the abdominal and lumbar muscles, and the common iliac arteries, which divide into an internal iliac artery to the organs of the pelvis, and an external iliac artery, which enters the thigh to become the femoral artery.

Muscles of the Pelvic Girdle

As is the case throughout the neck and trunk, muscles in the pelvic region are named in pairs, with one located on the left and the other on the right side of the body. These muscles cause lateral flexion or rotation when they contract unilaterally, but contribute to spinal flexion or extension when bilateral contractions occur. The locations, primary functions, and innervations of the major muscles of the pelvic girdle are summarized in **Table 15-2**.

Table 15–2. Muscles of the Pelvic Girdle.

Muscle	Proximal Attachment	Distal Attachment	Primary Action(s)	Nerve Innervation
Rectus abdominis	Costal cartilage of ribs 5–7	Pubic crest	Flexion, lateral flexion	Intercostal nerves (T_6-T_{12})
External oblique	External surface of lower eight ribs	Linea alba and anterior iliac crest	Flexion, lateral flexion, rotation to opposite side	Intercostal nerves (T_7-T_{12})
Internal oblique	Linea alba and the lower four ribs	Inguinal ligament, iliac crest, and the lumbodorsal fascia	Flexion, lateral flexion, rotation to same side	Intercostal nerves (T_7-T_{12}, L_1)
Transverse abdominis	Inguinal ligament, lumbodorsal fascia, cartilages of ribs 6–12, iliac crest	Linea alba and pubic crest	Compression of the abdomen	Intercostal nerves (T_7-T_{12}, L_1)
Quadratus lumborum	Last rib, transverse processes of the first four lumbar vertebrae	Iliolumbar ligament, adjacent iliac crest	Lateral flexion	Spinal nerves (T_{12}, L_1-L_4)

💡 *Pain from the lower right abdominal region may emanate from the appendix or lower intestinal tract. If appendicitis is suspected, the individual should be referred immediately to a physician.*

PREVENTION OF INJURIES TO THE THROAT, THORAX, AND VISCERA

❓ *The throat, thorax, and viscera are vulnerable to direct impact injuries. Because this is such a critical area where injury can lead to a life-threatening situation, what measures can be taken to prevent injuries to this region?*

Injuries to the throat, thorax, and abdomen occur in nearly every sport, yet few sports require protective equipment for all players. In sports where high velocity projectiles are present, throat and chest protectors are required for only specific players' positions, i.e., a catcher or goalie. As with other body regions, protective equipment, together with a well-rounded physical conditioning program, can reduce the risk of injury. Although proper skill technique can prevent some injuries, this is not a major factor in this body region.

Protective Equipment

Face masks with throat protectors are required for only fencing, baseball/softball catchers, and for goalies in field hockey, ice hockey, and lacrosse. However, nearly all lacrosse and ice hockey players wear an optional extended pad attached to the mask to protect the throat region. Many sport participants in collision and contact sports also wear full chest and abdominal protection, such as in fencing, ice hockey, baseball/softball catchers, and goalies in field hockey and lacrosse. Shoulder pads can protect the upper thoracic region from direct trauma, and rib protectors can protect the rib and upper abdominal region. For women, sport bras provide added support to reduce excessive vertical and horizontal breast motion during exercise. Abdominal binders may also be used to reduce the discomfort from hernias. Much of this protective equipment was discussed in detail and illustrated in Chapter 6.

Physical Conditioning

Flexibility and strengthening of the torso muscles should not be an isolated program, but should include a well-rounded conditioning program for the back, shoulder, abdomen and hip regions. Range of motion and strengthening exercises should include both open and closed kinetic chain activities. Exercises for the thorax and abdominal region were included in the chapters on the hip, shoulder and spine, and will not be repeated here. As such, the reader should review the appropriate Field Strategies in those chapters to develop a conditioning program for the torso.

💡 *Injuries to the throat, thorax, and viscera can be prevented by wearing appropriate protective equipment. Physical conditioning should include a well-rounded flexibility and strengthening program for the shoulder, back, abdominal, and hip region.*

THROAT INJURIES

❓ *An ice hockey player was checked into the sideboard. The opponent's elbow inadvertently struck the player's anterior neck. The player is now on the ice coughing, and having difficulty swallowing and speaking. How will you control the situation and manage the injury?*

Blunt trauma or lacerations to the anterior neck region can have devastating effects on the larynx and trachea, causing serious airway compromise. Injuries of this nature are commonly seen in hockey, but have been reported in football, softball, wrestling, field hockey, soccer, lacrosse, and gymnastics (1,2). Several sports, such as baseball, softball, field hockey, fencing, lacrosse, and ice hockey now require a neck-protecting extension on masks to protect this vital area (See Chapter 6).

Although uncommon, lacerations to the neck caused by a skate blade can occur. Bleeding is profuse and if sufficiently deep, can damage the jugular vein or carotid artery as they pass deep on the lateral side of the neck. Immediate control of hemorrhage is imperative. In addition to blood loss, air may be sucked into the vein and carried to the heart as an air embolism, which may be fatal. Management involves providing firm, direct pressure over the wound followed by an airway assessment. Once pressure has been applied, it should not be released. If the wound is severe, continuous manual pressure should be applied while the individual is in rapid transit to the nearest medical facility (3).

Contusions and fractures to the trachea, larynx, and hyoid bone frequently occur during hyperextension of the neck when the thyroid cartilage (Adam's apple) becomes prominent and vulnerable to direct impact forces. A

With a major laceration to the anterior neck an air embolism can travel to the heart causing death hockey cross-check or slash, a clothesline tackle in football, or a hit or blow to the neck can injure the cartilage. Immediate symptoms include hoarseness, dyspnea (difficulty breathing), coughing, difficulty swallowing, and pain.

Significant trauma to the region may result in severe pain, **laryngospasm**, and acute respiratory distress. Laryngospasm occurs when the adductor muscles of the vocal cords pull together in a shutter-like fashion, and the upper surface of the vocal cords close over the top, causing complete obstruction. A dangerous factor of this injury can occur after the individual leaves care. The individual may recover on site, leave the area to return home, only to have increasing respiratory problems in route. As the internal hemorrhage and swelling increases, the occlusion becomes more complete, and breathing becomes more difficult. Panic and anxiety increase respiration, thereby compounding the problem. Swelling is usually maximal within six hours, but may occur as late as 24 to 48 hours after injury (3). Cyanosis and loss of consciousness may occur with complete occlusion. Blows to the anterior throat should be reported to another individual, such as a parent or roommate, so observation continues should delayed respiratory problems occur.

Sudden inability to breathe produces immediate panic and anxiety in any individual. Often the person becomes agitated and avoids any assistance, therefore, reassuring the individual and maintaining an open airway is a priority. In cases involving severe anterior neck trauma or spasm, it is important to consider an associated injury to the cervical spine (4). Carefully place and maintain the individual's neck in a neutral position, and apply a cervical collar. Slide the chin forward with strong pressure behind the angle of the jaw (jaw-thrust maneuver; see Chapter 3). This action pulls the hyoid bone and surrounding ligaments away from the vocal cords and opens the airway. As the spasm relaxes, usually in a minute, a loud inspiratory crowing sound is often heard (2). The individual should be immediately transported to a medical facility. **Field Strategy 15-1** summarizes signs, symptoms, and management of tracheal and laryngeal injuries.

> Contusions or fractures to the anterior neck produce immediate signs and symptoms, such as a change in voice, dyspnea, coughing, difficulty swallowing, and pain

> **Laryngospasm**
> Spasmodic closure of the glottic aperture leading to shortness of breath, coughing, cyanosis and even loss of consciousness

> As the laryngospasm relaxes, usually in a minute, a loud, inspiratory, crowing sound is heard

 Field Strategy 15–1. Management of Tracheal and Laryngeal Injuries.

Signs and Symptoms
- Mild bruising and redness
- Shortness of breath
- Hoarseness or loss of voice
- Pain and point tenderness
- Subcutaneous crepitation
- Difficulty when swallowing or coughing
- Spasmodic coughing
- Presence of hemorrhage with blood-tinged sputum
- Loss of contour of the Adam's apple (thyroid cartilage)
- Cyanosis

Management
- Talk calmly to the individual. Loosen any restrictive clothing or equipment
- Reassure the individual to reduce panic and anxiety. Tell the individual you are there to help them
- If a laceration is present, control hemorrhage with firm, manual pressure and maintain it while the individual is transported to the nearest medical facility
- Ensure an open airway
- If obvious deformity in the pharynx is present, manually straighten the airway
- Place the individual in a chin-up position and apply ice if appropriate to control swelling. Use the jaw-thrust maneuver if necessary
- If severe anterior throat trauma occurred, assume the presence of a possible cervical spinal injury and treat accordingly until ruled out
- Summon EMS and transport the individual to the nearest medical facility

To care for the injured hockey player, did you reassure the individual and attempt to place the chin in a forward position to straighten the airway? If breathing does not return to normal within a few minutes summon EMS.

THORACIC INJURIES

During a collision in a bike race, a rider fell forward onto the handlebars and is now complaining of pain on the lower right side of the rib cage, aggravated with deep breathing and coughing. What possible injuries might be involved in this accident?

Thoracic injuries are frequently caused by sudden deceleration and impact, leading to compression and subsequent deformation of the rib cage. High-speed collisions in football, skiing, cycling, hockey, skateboarding, car racing, and falls in equestrian events are activities where these injuries may occur. The extent of damage is dependent on the direction and magnitude of force, and point of impact. For example, a glancing blow may contuse the chest wall. A baseball that directly impacts the ribs may fracture a rib, driving bony fragments internally and causing subsequent lung or cardiac damage. Recognizing the potential for serious underlying problems is vital to provide emergency care to an injured individual.

Stitch in the Side

A "**stitch in the side**" refers to a sharp pain or spasm in the chest wall, usually on the lower right side, during exertion. It is thought to be caused by spasm or localized ischemia in the diaphragm and lower intercostal muscles. This condition is seen in untrained individuals, in an individual returning to activity after a long lay-off, or in someone who has recently eaten a large meal. Most individuals can run through the sharp pain by (a) forcibly exhaling through pursed lips; (b) breathing deeply and regularly; (c) leaning away from the affected side; or (d) stretching the arm on the affected side over the head as high as possible. The frequency of a stitch usually diminishes as the individual becomes more fit.

Breast Injuries

The breast includes the mammary glands and surrounding tissues, the overlying skin, and underlying musculature, in essence, the anterior chest wall (**Figure 15-13**). The supporting ligaments, particularly Cooper's ligaments, hold and support the breast on the chest wall. These ligaments are strands of connective tissue that separate the lobules of the breast and are not strong. During the running motion, there is a tendency for vertical and horizontal displacement (5,6). Excessive

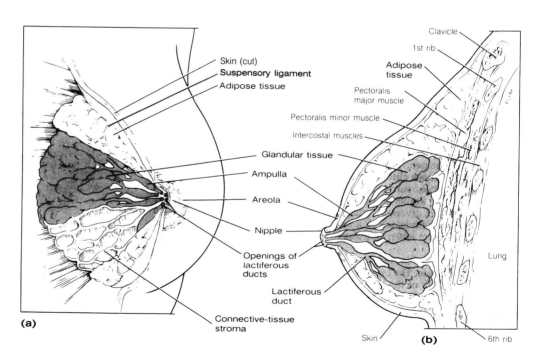

Fig. 15.13: The breast. (A) Anterior view. (B) Sagittal view.

breast motion can lead to soreness and contusions. Additional injuries may be caused by direct impact, friction, and cold. Although breast injuries are associated with females, men may also have them. For information on sport bras, see Chapter 6.

Contusions

Contusions to the breast are managed with ice and support. Although there is no relationship between a blow to the breast and breast cancer, traumatic fat necrosis secondary to a direct blow can result in a suspicious image on a mammogram. This may cause some concern to a physician trying to differentiate a firm mass from a tumor. Blows to the breast should be recorded in medical records to avoid any erroneous conclusions.

Nipple Irritation

Nipple irritation is commonly seen in distance runners when the shirt rubs over the nipples. The resulting friction can lead to abrasions, blisters, or bleeding (**runner's nipples**). This condition can be prevented by applying petroleum jelly, band-aids, or tape over the nipples to reduce irritation (3,7). Initial treatment involves thorough cleansing of the wound, application of a medicated ointment, and covering the wound with a nonadhering sterile gauze pad. Infection, secondary to the injury, may involve the entire nipple region and may necessitate referral to a physician. **Cyclist's nipples** is a condition not caused by friction, but rather from the combined effects of perspiration and windchill that produce cold, painful nipples that may last for several days. Wearing a windproof jacket and rewarming the nipples after completion of the event can prevent the irritation.

Gynecomastia

Gynecomastia involves an excessive development of the mammary glands, particularly in the adolescent male, and is usually bilateral. The nipple is sore and tender to pressure, and more prone to irritation through friction from a shirt. Often it is physiologic and will resolve spontaneously in 6 to 12 months. Gynecomastia is increasingly being seen in weight lifters and football players known to be taking anabolic steroids (8). Other causes include testicular, pituitary, and adrenal pathology. Occasionally resection of

extra breast tissue may be indicated for psychologic reasons, or a biopsy may be performed to rule out malignancy.

Rupture of the Pectoralis Major Muscle

The pectoralis major muscle can rupture on the chest wall from a direct blow, or at the distal humeral attachment when the muscle is at full tension and an additional overload is added. Total ruptures may occur in power lifting, particularly while bench pressing, in water skiing, wrestling, basketball, or in sudden violent deceleration maneuvers, such as when punching in boxing or blocking with an extended arm in football (9). A higher incidence of this injury is seen with anabolic steroid abuse. This may result from muscle hypertrophy and an increase in power secondary to rapid strength gain not accompanied by a concomitant increase in tendon size (3).

Pain is a frequent complaint and is often described as an aching or fatigue-like pain, rather than a sharp pain. Weakness and a popping or snapping sensation at the time of rupture is the most frequently reported symptom (9,10). With a rupture of the proximal attachment, the muscle will retract toward the axillary fold causing it to appear enlarged. Swelling and ecchymosis will be limited to the anterior chest wall. If the distal attachment is ruptured, the muscle will bulge medially into the chest region causing the axillary fold to appear thin (**Figure 15-14**). Swelling and ecchymosis will occur on the anterior chest wall and upper arm. Shoulder motion will be limited by pain. Horizontal adduction and internal rotation of the shoulder will be weak and accentuate the deformity (10,11).

Treatment is dependent on the extent of damage and follows standard protocol for other muscle strains. Mild and moderate strains (Grades I and II) begin with control of inflammation, protected range of motion exercises, and gradual strengthening. Once range of motion has been achieved, strength, endurance, and power are restored. Third degree ruptures of the muscle are treated surgically (10).

Costochondral Injury

Costochondral sprains commonly occur in contact sports. A blow to the anterolateral aspect of the chest may occur during a colli-

A direct blow to the breast can lead to traumatic fat necrosis that can appear as a suspicious image on mammography

Runner's nipples
Nipple irritation due to friction as the shirt rubs over the nipples

Cyclist's nipples
Nipple irritation due to the combined effects of perspiration and windchill producing cold, painful nipples

Gynecomastia
Excessive development of the male mammary glands

Weakness and a popping or snapping sensation are common symptoms after a rupture to the pectoralis major muscle

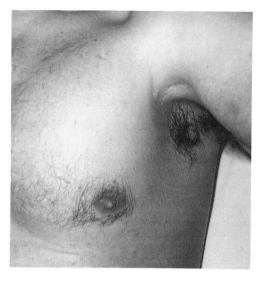

Fig. 15.14: Rupture of the distal attachment of the pectoralis major can lead to swelling and ecchymosis over the muscle belly.

sion with the boards in hockey, a pile-on in football, or a severe twisting motion in wrestling or rugby. This action can sprain or separate the costal cartilage where it attaches to the rib or sternum **(Figure 15-15)**. The individual may report hearing or feeling a pop. If a separation has occurred, the localized sharp pain may be followed by intermittent stabbing pain as the displaced cartilage overrides the bone. A deformity may be visible and localized pain can be palpated at the involved joint. The discomfort usually

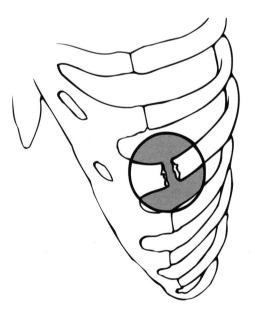

Fig. 15.15: Undisplaced costochondral separation.

resolves itself with three or four weeks of rest and anti-inflammatory medication. However, in sports that require a great deal of twisting, the discomfort may persist for more than six weeks. Occasionally a physician may choose to inject the site with steroid medication to relieve chronic pain.

Sternal Fractures

The sternum is rarely fractured in sports. More frequently, fractures occur as a result of rapid deceleration and high-impact into an object, such as when an individual impacts the steering column (12). Uncomplicated transverse fractures involve a superior and inferior segment. Localized pain directly over the sternum is aggravated with deep inspiration. Treatment is conservative. Because of the anatomical location, any fracture should be assessed for underlying cardiac injury, such as a cardiac contusion. If the individual shows signs of shock, is pale, or has a rapid weak pulse, immediate transportation to the nearest medical facility is warranted.

Rib Fractures

Direct blows or compression of the chest can lead to rib fractures, and rarely involve more than one or two ribs. Stress fractures may be caused by an indirect force, such as a violent muscle contraction in a golf swing or baseball pitch. Most rib fractures are minor and undisplaced. In massive injuries to the chest, however, multiple fractures can penetrate the lungs or intra-abdominal viscera leading to serious complications. A **flail chest** involves three or more consecutive ribs on the same side of the chest wall that are fractured in at least two separate locations **(Figure 15-16)**. The upper four ribs are rarely fractured, since they are well protected by the scapula and clavicle. The fifth through ninth ribs are the most commonly fractured **(Figure 15-17)**. The lower two ribs have greater movement, being attached to only the thoracic vertebrae, and are difficult to injure (13).

A rib fracture will result in intense local pain aggravated with deep inspiration. Shallow breathing may be present. Often the individual will sit very still leaning toward the fracture site, stabilizing the area with a hand to prevent excessive movement of the chest to ease the pain. A visible contusion and palpable crepitus may be present at the impact site. Trunk rotation and lateral flexion of the trunk

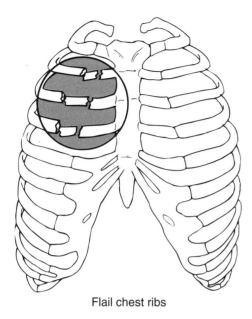

Flail chest ribs

Fig. 15.16: Flail chest involving the ribs.

away from the fracture site will place tension on the involved rib, increasing pain. Manual compression of the rib cage in an anteropos-

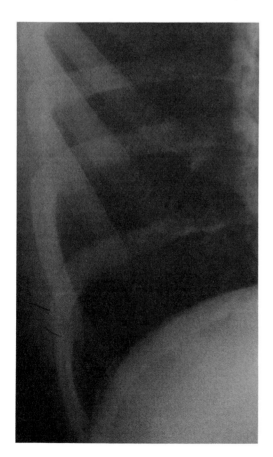

Fig. 15.17: Undisplaced fractured rib.

terior direction, and lateral compression will produce pain over the fracture site (See **Figure 15-26**). If pain is intense or multiple fractures are suspected, a sling and swathe can be applied to immobilize the chest. An individual with a suspected rib fracture should be referred to a physician, as a bone scan may be necessary to show the fracture site. **Field Strategy 15-2** summarizes the signs, symptoms, and management of fractures to the rib cage.

If intense pain or multiple fractures are present, a sling and swathe can be used to immobile the chest

🔲 **Field Strategy 15–2. Management of Rib Fractures.**

Signs and Symptoms
- History of direct blow, compression of the chest, or violent muscle contraction
- Individual may lean toward the fractured side, stabilizing the area with a hand to prevent movement of the chest
- Localized discoloration or swelling over the fracture site
- Slight step deformity may be visible
- Palpable pain and crepitus at fracture site
- Increased pain on deep inspiration
- Increased pain on trunk rotation and lateral flexion away from the fracture site
- Increased pain on manual compression of the rib cage in an anteroposterior direction or with lateral compression
- Shallow breathing and cyanosis may be present
- Rapid, weak pulse and low blood pressure will be present with multiple fractures, in a fracture that has damaged intercostal vessels and nerves, or if the lung or pleura sac has been penetrated

Management
- Rule out underlying internal complications
  —Look for any coughing up of blood, especially bright red or frothy blood
  —Listen to air exchange in lungs for abnormal, or absent sounds
  —Record rate and depth of respirations
  —Record strength and pulse rate
  —Note pupillary response to light
- Apply sling and swathe
- If there is a chance that three or more ribs are fractured, summon EMS
- Treat for shock
- Transport individual to the nearest medical facility

Treatment involves ice and prescribed non-steroidal anti-inflammatory drugs (NSAIDs). Depending on the sport, fracture site, the presence of a displaced or nondisplaced fracture, and the number of ribs involved, this individual may be excluded from sport participation during the full healing process. Strapping or taping to reduce chest movement is not recommended since it may aggravate the condition. In a simple fracture, as discomfort subsides, a flak jacket or canvas rib vest can be worn to protect the area from reinjury **(Figure 6-15)**.

The bicyclist has ecchymosis on the anterolateral aspect of the rib cage at the level of the ninth rib. Palpation causes increased pain and crepitus. Deep breathing and lateral flexion away from the site also increase pain. Did you determine that a possible rib fracture is present? If so, you are correct.

INTERNAL COMPLICATIONS

The second baseman fielded a line drive and threw the ball to first base. By accident, the ball struck a runner going to second base directly on the sternum. The runner immediately collapsed on the base path. You arrived at the scene to find the player in obvious pain and gasping for air. How will you manage this situation? What underlying serious problems can occur as a result of direct impact to the sternum or ribs?

Several conditions can alter breathing and cardiac function. Hyperventilation is associated with an inability to catch one's breath, and in most instances, is not a serious problem. Direct trauma to the thorax, however, can lead to serious underlying problems, although in sport participation, these conditions are rare. Among the more serious complications are pulmonary contusion, pneumothorax, tension pneumothorax, hemothorax, and heart contusions. Sudden death as a result of cardiac malfunction is another serious condition that has been highlighted in the media during recent years. Each condition has specific signs and symptoms indicating that immediate action is necessary.

Hyperventilation

Hyperventilation is a respiratory condition often linked to pain, stress, or trauma in sport participation (14). During activity large amounts of energy are expended, increasing the respiratory rate. Rapid, deep inhalations draw more oxygen into the lungs. Conversely, decreasing levels of carbon dioxide in the blood result from long exhalations. This sets the stage for a chemical imbalance when too much carbon dioxide is exhaled.

Signs and symptoms of hyperventilation include an inability to catch one's breath, numbness in the lips and hands, spasm of the hands, chest pain, dry mouth, dizziness, and even loss of consciousness (15). An immediate concern is to calm the individual down, as panic and anxiety only complicate the condition. Although breathing into a paper bag has proven to be quite successful in restoring the oxygen-carbon dioxide balance, many individuals find it embarrassing. An alternative treatment involves concentrating on slow inhalations through the nose and exhaling through the mouth until symptoms have ceased. The use of breathing into a paper bag is not needed except in severe cases.

Pulmonary Contusion

Pulmonary contusion is the most common intrathoracic injury in nonpenetrating chest trauma, although like other serious internal complications, it rarely occurs as the result of sport participation. The condition occurs during forceful contact with another individual or a hard surface, such as landing on a football or a body slam onto the hard ground. Most injuries are not serious and go undetected except when an individual coughs up blood or has other underlying problems, such as pneumothorax, rib fractures, or **subcutaneous emphysema** (16). Individuals who cough up blood after a chest injury should always be referred to a physician. Confirmation of the condition can only be made through radiographs or CT scans. Mild contusions or lacerations heal within days with the individual returning to full participation in as few as 10 days (16). In more severe cases, the individual is usually hospitalized and monitored with ventilatory support.

Pneumothorax

Pneumothorax is a condition whereby air is trapped in the pleural space causing a portion of a lung to collapse. It seldom occurs bilaterally. Although fractured ribs from direct trauma is the leading cause, pneumothorax may occur as a spontaneous rupture of lung tissue. In a traumatic injury when lung tissue is lacerated, air escapes into the pleural cavity with each inhalation. The pressure builds around the lung, preventing it from fully expanding (**Figure 15-18**). Shortness of breath and severe chest pain on the affected side are the most common symptoms. Spontaneous pneumothorax occasionally follows strenuous physical activity. The pain can stop abruptly after onset, leading to delay in treatment. Shortness of breath and chest discomfort will gradually increase until the individual finally seeks medical care. On the other hand, the symptoms may flair up suddenly, producing acute pain and difficulty in breathing. Pain may be referred to the shoulder tip. Other symptoms may include asymmetric chest expansion, confusion, fatigue, anxiety, or restlessness. If not recognized and treated promptly, the condition can develop into tension pneumothorax.

Tension Pneumothorax

Tension pneumothorax occurs when the mediastinum of the pleural sac is displaced to the opposite side, compressing the uninjured lung and thoracic aorta. Signs and symptoms may include tracheal deviation away from the tension pneumothorax, severe difficulty in breathing, absence of breath sounds, distention of neck veins, and circulatory complications leading to cyanosis and possible death. This is a true emergency with immediate

referral to the nearest medical facility necessary to prevent total collapse of the lung.

Traumatic Asphyxia

Traumatic asphyxia results from direct massive trauma to the thorax. Classic symptoms include a bluish tinge over the neck and facial regions, subconjuctival hemorrhage, ecchymosis, and minute hemorrhagic spots on the face (**Figure 15-19**). Immediate impairment or loss of vision has also been reported as a result of retinal edema, but vision may promptly improve within hours or days (17). Again, immediate recognition and referral to the nearest medical facility is necessary for prompt care.

Hemothorax

Hemothorax involves the loss of blood into the pleural cavity rather than air. Fractured ribs may tear lung tissue and blood vessels in the chest or chest cavity. Signs and symptoms are similar to pneumothorax, including severe pain during breathing, difficulty breathing, cyanosis, coughing up frothy blood, and shock. This condition is a true medical emergency. Treat for shock and immediately transport this individual to the nearest medical facility. **Table 15-3** lists several signs and symptoms indicating blunt injury to the thorax.

Tension pneumothorax
Condition in which air continuously leaks into the pleural space causing the mediastinum to displace to the opposite side compressing the uninjured lung and thoracic aorta

Traumatic asphyxia
Condition involving extravasation of blood into the skin and conjunctivae due to a sudden increase in venous pressure

Hemothorax
Condition involving the loss of blood into the pleural cavity, but outside the lung

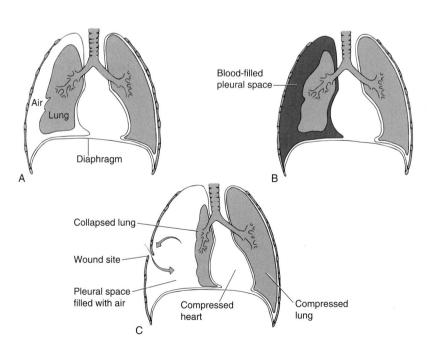

Fig. 15.18: Internal complication to the lungs. (A) Pneumothorax. (B) Hemothorax. (C) Tension pneumothorax. Each condition can become life-threatening if the lung collapses.

Arrhythmia
Disturbance in the heart beat rhythm

Cardiac tamponade
Acute compression of the heart due to effusion of fluid or blood into the pericardium from rupture of the heart or penetrating trauma

In nearly all cases, the individual collapses within seconds and goes into respiratory arrest

Sudden death
Nontraumatic, unexpected death occurring instantaneously or within minutes of an abrupt change in an individual's previous clinical state

Hypertrophic cardiomyopathy
Excessive hypertrophy of the heart, often of obscure or unknown origin

Causes of sudden death for individuals under 30 include:
  hypertrophic cardiomyopathy
  coronary arteries abnormalities
  aortic rupture associated with Marfan's syndrome
  mitral valve prolapse
  cardiac conduction system disorders

Marfan's syndrome
Inherited connective tissue disorder affecting many organs, but commonly resulting in the dilation and weakening of the thoracic aorta

Auscultation
Listening for sounds, often with a stethoscope to denote the condition of the lungs, heart, pleura, abdomen and other organs

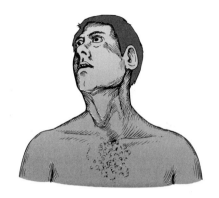

Fig. 15–19. With traumatic asphyxia, the individual will have distended neck veins and bloodshot, bulging eyes. The pale skin will quickly turn dark blue or purple in the head, neck, and shoulders when cyanosis sets in.

Table 15–3. Indications of Severe Blunt Trauma to the Chest.

- Shortness of breath or difficulty in breathing
- Deviated trachea
- Anxiety, fear, confusion, or restlessness
- Distended neck veins
- Eyes may be bulging or bloodshot
- Individual may cough up bright red or frothy blood
- Severe chest pain aggravated with deep inspiration
- Abnormal or absent breath sounds
- Rapid, weak pulse
- Low blood pressure
- Cyanosis

Heart Injuries

Direct blows to the chest due to deceleration can compress the heart between the sternum and spine leading to myocardial contusion. The right ventricle is often injured because it lies directly posterior to the sternum. The blow causes leaking of red blood cells and fluid into the surrounding tissues, thereby decreasing local circulation to the heart muscle. This can result in localized cellular damage and necrosis of the heart tissue (18). Decreased cardiac output secondary to **arrhythmias** are of major concern.

Blunt trauma can also lead to **cardiac tamponade**, the leading cause of traumatic death in youth baseball (19,20). This condition has also occurred from projectiles in other sports, such as softball, hockey, and lacrosse (21–23). Internal damage can lead to rupture of the ventricles, interventricular septum, chordae tendineae, or the cardiac valves **(Figure 15-6)** (24). In nearly all cases, the individual collapses within seconds and goes into respiratory arrest. In many cases, resuscitation is unsuccessful even though it is given immediately after injury. This may be due to gross structural cardiac disruption due to the trauma (25). Treatment is the same for any other chest trauma: maintain an open airway, initiate breathing and chest compressions if necessary, and immediately transport the individual to the nearest medical facility.

Sudden Death in Athletes

Another condition of grave concern in sports participation is sudden death in athletes. **Sudden death** is usually defined as an event that is nontraumatic, unexpected, and occurs instantaneously or within minutes of an abrupt change in an individual's previous clinical state (26). Causes in individuals under 30 years of age stem from **hypertrophic cardiomyopathy**, abnormalities in the coronary arteries, aortic rupture associated with Marfan's syndrome, mitral valve prolapse, and cardiac conduction system disorders (26–28).

Marfan's syndrome is an inherited connective tissue disorder that may affect several organs, but more commonly results in the dilation and weakening of the thoracic aorta. Individuals with Marfan's syndrome commonly have excessively long tubular bones. Because of the long tubular bones, the individual will be tall with an arm span greater than height. In cases of sudden death from Marfan's syndrome in individuals over 30 years of age, severe atherosclerotic coronary artery disease is almost always present.

It is difficult to identify individuals at risk for sudden death. During preparticipation exams, an extensive history should include information on: (1) past history of rheumatic fever, hypertension, cardiac problems, or chronic diseases such as diabetes mellitus; (2) symptoms of syncope (fainting), near syncope, palpitations, low exercise tolerance, chest discomfort on exertion, or dyspnea; and (3) family history of syncope, hypertension, premature coronary disease (prior to age 50), or sudden death (26,29). The physical exam should include measurement of blood pressure and pulse; **auscultation** of the heart for cardiac rhythm, murmurs, and abnormal heart sounds; and palpation of peripheral pulses. Additional symptoms, such as chest pains, sudden onset of fatigue, heartburn or indigestion, and excessive breathlessness during exercise should signal the need for immediate referral to a physician for further investigation. **Table 15-4** lists several cardiovascular conditions that are considered contraindications to vigorous exercise because of the risk for exercise-related sudden death (26).

Athletic Heart Syndrome

Athletic heart syndrome is a benign condition associated with physiologic alterations in the heart (30). Changes in the heart muscle may be brought on by intensive repetitive physical training. These changes may produce abnormalities on electrocardiograms (ECG) but do not in themselves represent a contraindication to exercise. Individuals with athletic heart syndrome must be fully evaluated by a physician to rule out serious underlying cardiovascular disorders that may place them at risk.

The baseball runner is in obvious respiratory distress. The impact of the ball may have caused hyperventilation or more serious internal complications. Initiate a primary survey, talk to the individual to calm them down, and assess breathing and circulation. If respirations do not return to normal

---

Table 15–4. Cardiovascular Conditions that Prohibit Vigorous Exercise.

- Hypertrophic cardiomyopathy
- Idiopathic concentric left ventricular hypertrophy
- Marfan's syndrome
- Coronary heart disease
- Congestive heart failure
- Congenital anomalies of the coronary arteries that may reproduce myocardial ischemia and/or serious arrhythmias
- High-grade ventricular arrhythmias or long QT syndrome
- Constriction of the aorta
- Acute inflammation of the muscular walls of the heart
- Cyanotic congenital heart disease
- Pulmonary hypertension

---

within minutes, or if respiratory or cardiac irregularities are present, summon EMS.

ABDOMINAL WALL INJURIES

A gymnast did a sudden back hyperextension movement after landing on a vault, and felt a sharp pain in the abdominal region. There is marked tenderness and muscle guarding slightly below and to the right of the umbilicus. No swelling or discoloration is visible, however, it hurts to do a modified sit-up. What condition may be present? How will you manage it?

The muscles of the abdominal wall are strong and powerful, yet flexible enough to absorb impact. Consequently, injuries to the abdominal wall are usually limited to minor skin abrasions, contusions, and muscle strains. There are, however, other conditions, such as a contusion to the solar plexus and hernias that can affect sport participation.

Skin Wounds and Contusions

Skin abrasions may occur during contact with the ground, as in sliding or in a fall. Abrasions are best handled with thorough cleansing to prevent contamination, covering the wound with a sterile nonstick dressing, and securing the dressing around the wound to prevent friction directly over the abrasion. Lacerations that penetrate the abdominal wall muscles or deeper should be referred immediately to the nearest medical facility. Because further examination is necessary to rule out intra-abdominal injuries, ointments or creams should not be placed on the wound. Instead, irrigate the wound with sterile water and cover the area with an absorbent pad to control hemorrhage.

Contusions to the abdominal wall may lead to hemorrhage into the subcutaneous fat and connective tissue. The closed wound often appears more traumatic than it really is. Early application of ice and compression will usually limit the amount of hemorrhage. A pressure dressing can be applied if a large hematoma forms.

Muscle Strains

Muscular strains are caused by direct contusion, sudden twisting, or overstretching, but are often overlooked because the signs and symptoms mimic an intra-abdominal injury. The rectus abdominis is the most commonly

Symptoms such as chest pains, sudden onset of fatigue, heartburn or indigestion, and excessive breathlessness during exercise should signal the need for immediate referral to a physician for further investigation

Athletic heart syndrome
Benign condition associated with physiologic alterations in the heart

Lacerations that penetrate the abdominal wall muscles or deeper should be referred immediately to the nearest medical facility

Marked tenderness and muscle guarding along with abdominal pain on straight leg raising or hyperextension of the back indicates an abdominal muscle strain

Solar plexus punch
A blow to the abdomen that results in an immediate inability to breath freely

Celiac plexus
Nerve plexus that innervates the abdominal region

Loosen any restrictive equipment and clothing around the abdomen, and have the individual flex the knees toward the chest

Hernia
Protrusion of abdominal viscera through a weakened portion of the abdominal wall

Hernias can be aggravated by a direct blow, strain, or abnormal intra-abdominal pressure, such as that exerted during weight lifting or shot-putting

injured muscle. Avulsion injuries to the external obliques (hip pointers) were discussed in Chapter 9.

Complications arise in a rectus abdominis strain when the epigastric artery or intramuscular vessels are damaged, leading to hematoma formation. Nearly 80% of the hematomas occur below the umbilicus. The individual will complain of severe abdominal pain with or without swelling. Nausea, vomiting, and fever may also be present. After ruling out possible rib fracture, examination will reveal marked tenderness and muscle guarding in the region. Abdominal pain on straight leg raising or hyperextension of the back will be present. A palpable mass may or may not be present. If a mass is present, it will become fixed with contraction of the muscle (31). Treatment consists of ice, rest, and early use of NSAIDs for the first 36 to 48 hours. Hydrocollator packs and whirlpools can be used with activity modification until the hematoma and soreness ends. Activities, such as twisting, turning, or sudden stretching should be avoided until painful symptoms subside.

Solar Plexus Contusion ("Wind Knocked Out")

A blow to the abdomen with the muscles relaxed is referred to as a "**solar plexus punch**," and results in an immediate inability to breath freely (dyspnea). Fear and anxiety complicate the condition. Although the true cause of the breathing difficulty is unknown, it is thought to be caused by diaphragmatic spasm and transient contusion to the sympathetic **celiac plexus** (3). Assessment should include a thorough airway analysis. Remove any mouthguard or partial plates. Loosen any restrictive equipment and clothing around the abdomen and have the individual flex the knees toward the chest. Normal breathing usually returns rapidly.

A concern with this type of injury is that a severe blow has occurred to an unprotected abdomen. As such, there may be some degree of an intra-abdominal injury. Observe the individual throughout the practice session. At the conclusion of the session another full assessment should be completed to rule out any rib or visceral injury that may have been overlooked.

Hernias

A **hernia** is a protrusion of abdominal viscera through a weakened portion of the abdominal

wall, and can be congenital or acquired. Congenital hernias are present at birth and may be related to family history. Acquired hernias occur after birth and may be aggravated by a direct blow, strain, or abnormal intra-abdominal pressure, such as that exerted during heavy weight lifting or shot-putting. The three most common hernias are the indirect and direct inguinal hernias, and the femoral hernia.

Indirect inguinal hernias account for 50 to 75% of all hernias and typically occur in men under the age of 30 (32). A weakness in the peritoneum around the deep inguinal ring allows a sac to protrude through the ring into the inguinal canal, and occasionally extends into the scrotum (**Figure 15-20A**). This weakness in the peritoneum is usually absent in women, thus decreasing their risk of acquiring this type of hernia. Large indirect hernias may reduce spontaneously because they cannot extend easily into the inguinal canal.

Direct hernias result from a weakness in an area of fascia, bounded by the rectus abdominis muscle, the inguinal ligament, and the epigastric vessels (**Figure 15-20B**). Direct hernias commonly occur in men over 40.

Femoral hernias are rare and more commonly seen in women. It is hypothesized that the femoral rings may be enlarged due to a narrow insertion of the posterior inguinal wall onto the lacunar ligament, establishing a congenitally weak area for herniation (33). Abdominal viscera (often the small intestine), protrudes through the femoral ring into the femoral canal compressing the lymph vessels, connective tissue, and fat. The herniation is similar to a direct hernia, however, the protrusion extends posterior to the inguinal ligament, and can be palpated just inferior to the inguinal ligament. Initially the herniation is small, but can enlarge and pass inferior through the saphenous opening into the loose connective tissue of the proximal thigh. The herniation presents as a mass inferolateral to the pubic tubercle and medial to the femoral artery and vein (**Figure 15-21**).

Symptoms vary, but for most hernias the first sign is a visible tender swelling. Others may complain of an aching feeling in the groin. Many hernias are asymptomatic until the preparticipation exam when the physician palpates the protrusion by invaginating the scrotum with a finger (**Figure 15-22**). Protrusion of the hernia increases with coughing. The danger of a hernia in an active sport par-

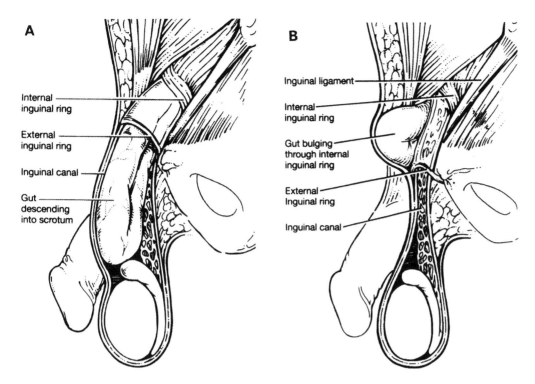

Fig. 15–20: Hernia. (A) Indirect hernia with a portion of the small intestine extending into the scrotum. (B) Direct hernia with a portion of the small intestine extending through a weakening in the internal inguinal ring.

ticipant lies in continued trauma to the weakened area during falls, blows, or increased intra-abdominal pressure exerted during activity. The hernia can twist on itself and produce a strangulated hernia, which can become gangrenous.

Large hernias are surgically repaired and often demand a long healing period. Individuals with an indirect hernia repair can begin walking, mild upper extremity exercises, and bicycling within six weeks of surgery. Return to noncontact sport participation can occur in seven weeks and contact sports within 8 to 10 weeks (34). Repair of direct inguinal and femoral hernias are more extensive. All strenuous activities are prohibited for three weeks postsurgery. Return to noncontact sports can occur after 8 weeks and contact sports in 12 weeks. Activities that stretch or pull the abdominal muscles should be avoided follow-

A hernia can twist on itself, closing off circulation, thus leading to possible gangrene

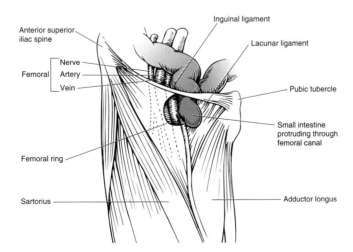

Fig. 15.21: Similar to a direct hernia, a femoral hernia protrudes posterior to the inguinal ligament medial to the femoral artery.

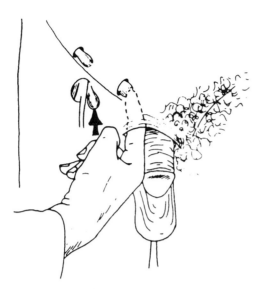

Fig. 15.22: Inguinal hernias in men can be palpated by invaginating the scrotum and feeling the mass, or pressure of the lesion, particularly during coughing.

Peritonitis
Inflammation of the peritoneum that lines the abdomen

ing surgical repair. Recommended activities include swimming, biking, and weight training for the upper extremity (34). Individuals with an unrepaired hernia can participate in noncontact sports, however, surgical repair is recommended to prevent recurrent irreducible hernias that can lead to small bowel obstruction.

The individual experienced sharp abdominal pain after sudden hyperextension of the back. No swelling or discoloration is present, however, pain increases with active contraction of the abdominal muscles. If you determined a possible strain of the rectus abdominus you are correct. Application of ice, compression, and rest will reduce the acute hemorrhage and inflammation.

INTRA-ABDOMINAL INJURIES

A twenty-two-year-old football player was struck in the abdomen with a helmet and experienced a sudden onset of abdominal pain in the upper left quadrant that seemed to radiate into the upper chest and left shoulder. Weakness and light-headedness are also present. Blood pressure is 96/72, and pulse is weak at 96 beats per minute. With what possible injury might you be dealing?

Trauma to the abdomen can lead to severe internal hemorrhage if organs or major blood vessels are lacerated or ruptured. Injuries can be open or closed, with closed injuries typically due to blunt trauma. The solid organs

are more commonly injured in sport participation. Hollow viscera, if damaged, can leak the contents into the abdominal cavity causing severe hemorrhage, **peritonitis**, and shock.

Although specific injuries will be discussed in detail, many signs and symptoms indicating an intra-abdominal injury are similar in nature regardless of the organ involved. Variations arise in the area of palpable pain and site of referred pain. Knowing which organs are located in each quadrant can help identify the injured organ (**Figure 15-23**). Signs and symptoms indicating a general intra-abdominal injury include the absence of normal abdominal movement during the respiratory motion, localized tenderness and abdominal rigidity on palpation, rebound tenderness with release of deep pressure, absence of normal bowel sounds, referred pain into the shoulder, back, or groin, decreased blood pressure, and a rapid, weak pulse. **Table 15-5** summarizes the signs and symptoms of intra-abdominal injury.

Acute management of suspected intra-abdominal injuries is also very similar, regardless of the injured organ. Initially, keep the

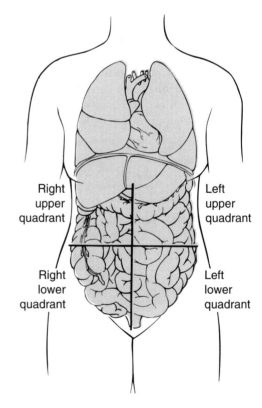

Fig. 15.23: Four quadrants of the abdominal wall and abdominopelvic cavity.

Table 15–5. Signs and Symptoms Indicating an Intra-abdominal Injury.

- Abdominal pain, often starting as mild then rapidly increasing in severity
- Referred pain to the shoulder tip, back, or groin
- Nausea
- Weakness
- Thirst
- Individual may lean forward and bring the knees to the chest to reduce tension in the abdominal muscles
- Shallow breathing. Abdominal respiratory motion may be absent
- Coughing up or vomiting blood that looks like used coffee grounds
- Diffuse hemorrhage or distention of the abdomen
- Palpable local tenderness or rigidity over the injured organ
- Cramps or muscle guarding (splinting)
- Rebound pain on deep palpation
- Absence of bowel sounds
- Rapid, weak pulse
- Low blood pressure
- Cyanosis

 Field Strategy 15–3. Management of Suspected Intra-abdominal Injuries.

- Assess vital signs
  - —Record the rate and depth of respiration. Rapid shallow breathing indicates shock
  - —Record strength and pulse rate. Rapid, weak pulse indicates shock
  - —Record blood pressure. A marked drop in both systolic and diastolic indicates shock
  - —Note pupillary response to light. Lackluster, dilated pupils indicate shock
- Control any external hemorrhage with a sterile dressing
- Lay the individual supine with the knees flexed to relax the abdominal muscles. *Do not* extend the legs or elevate the feet
- Be alert for vomiting. If the individual vomits, roll the person on their side to allow for excretion, making certain the airway remains open
- Treat for shock
- Give nothing by mouth
- Transport immediately to the nearest medical facility

---

individual relaxed while a primary survey is completed. Then summon EMS. Place the individual supine and flex the knees. This position relaxes the low back and abdominal muscles. Monitor vital signs regularly and treat for shock. If external bleeding is present, control bleeding and apply an absorbant sterile dressing. **Field Strategy 15-3** summarizes acute management of intra-abdominal injuries.

Splenic Rupture

The normal spleen is rarely injured in sport participation even when significant direct impact occurs. However, after certain systemic disorders it may become enlarged and vulnerable to injury. A collision with another individual or stationary object that impacts the left upper abdominal quadrant or lower left chest can rupture an enlarged spleen. It remains the most frequent cause of death due to abdominal blunt trauma in sport. The most common condition that leaves the spleen enlarged and weakened is **infectious mononucleosis** caused by the Epstein-Barr virus (EBV). The danger with a ruptured

spleen lies in the ability to splint itself and stop hemorrhage, only to produce delayed hemorrhage days, weeks, or months later after a seemingly minor jarring motion, such as a cough. Because of this delayed action, information should be provided to a parent or other individual to inform them of signs indicating a possible splenic rupture so immediate care can be sought.

Indications of a splenic rupture include a history of blunt trauma to the left upper quadrant. After the initial sharp pain subsides, a dull pain in the left side persists. In some instances as the blood continues to hemorrhage, the individual may develop pain in the left shoulder, referred to as **Kehr's sign**. This referred pain is due to irritation of the diaphragm innervated by the phrenic nerves, which arise from the ventral rami of segments C_3 to C_5. The free blood can also irritate the right side of the diaphragm, in which case, pain will be referred to the dermatome patterns in the right shoulder (35). The individual is often cold, clammy, and will show signs of shock at the time of injury. Nausea and vomiting may also be present.

Infectious mononucleosis
Viral condition caused by the Epstein-Barr virus that attacks the respiratory system and leaves the spleen enlarged and weak

A ruptured spleen can splint itself and then produce delayed hemorrhage days, weeks, or months later

Kehr's sign
Referred pain into the left shoulder due to a ruptured spleen

Internal hemorrhage will produce signs and symptoms of shock including rapid, weak pulse shallow breathing pale, cold, clammy skin dilated pupils and lackluster eyes

Conservative, nonoperative
treatment includes intra-
venous therapy, strict bed
rest, and intensive monitoring of vital signs

Appendicitis
Inflammation of the appendix

McBurney's point
A site one third the distance
between the ASIS and
umbilicus that with deep palpation produces rebound tenderness indicating appen-
dicitis

Blood in the urine is not
always indicative of the
magnitude of injury

Hematuria
Blood or red blood cells in
the urine

Proteinuria
Abnormal concentrations of
protein in the urine

With a bladder contusion,
the individual will be able to
void, however, with a bladder rupture, the individual is
usually unable to void

Running with an empty
bladder can increase the
chances of gross hematuria
since no fluid cushion
exists between the poste-
rior wall and base of the
bladder

Today, even significant trauma-induced bleeding rarely necessitates splenectomy. The treatment of choice is conservative nonoperative treatment with intravenous therapy, strict bed rest, and intensive monitoring of vital signs (36). Following a week of hospitalization the individual should restrict activities for at least three weeks. Return to vigorous physical activity is not recommended until two to three months after injury. If surgical repair is indicated, a three month period is needed for the abdominal musculature to heal and regain adequate strength before return to vigorous activity. Most physicians recommend a six month interval after a splenectomy before return to contact sports (3).

Liver Contusion and Rupture

Damage to the liver ranks second in intra-abdominal injuries as a result of blunt trauma. A direct blow to the upper right quadrant can cause subscapular hemorrhage that produces significant palpable pain, point tenderness, and hypotension. Pain may be referred to the inferior angle of the right scapula (see Chapter 4). Shock is also commonly seen. As with the spleen, systemic diseases such as hepatitis can enlarge the liver, making it more susceptible to injury. Lacerations of the liver are rare in contact sports and typically require surgical repair.

Appendicitis

The vermiform appendix is a pouch extending from the cecum (**Figure 15-10**). If it becomes obstructed (for example, with hardened fecal material), venous circulation may be interfered with. This interference leads to a reduction in oxygen supply and permits bacteria to flourish. The resulting inflamed appendix becomes filled with pus, called **appendicitis,** and can lead to ischemia and gangrene. If the appendix ruptures, feces containing bacteria are sprayed over the abdominal contents causing peritonitis. Signs and symptoms include acute abdominal pain in the lower right quadrant that can be referred to the low back region. Loss of appetite, nausea and vomiting, and a low-grade fever may be present. Rebound pain can be elicited at **McBurney's point**, which is one third the distance between the anterior superior iliac spine (ASIS) and the umbilicus.

Kidney Contusion

Serious injury to the kidneys most likely occurs when the body is extended and the abdominal muscles are relaxed, such as when a receiver leaps to catch a pass. Suspicion should be high if impact is to the midback region, especially if persistent back or flank pain is present. Pain can be referred posteriorly to the low back region, sides of the buttocks, and anteriorly to the lower abdomen. Individuals may complain of blood in the urine (hematuria), although this is not always indicative of the magnitude of injury (37). After acute care to manage shock and associated injuries, the individual should be referred to the nearest medical facility. Treatment for most individuals involves a radiograph or CT scan to determine the extent of injury. Most injuries are managed conservatively with rest and fluid management. Spontaneous healing and return of good renal function can be expected.

Bladder Injuries

Direct damage to the bladder is rare and often associated only with massive pelvic trauma. However, other conditions, such as hematuria and proteinuria can occur. **Hematuria** is characterized by blood or red blood cells in the urine. **Proteinuria** involves abnormal concentrations of protein in the urine.

Massive external trauma associated with pelvic fractures can damage the bladder, leading to lower abdominal pain and tenderness. Bruising in the lower abdominal region may be visible. Palpation may reveal abdominal tenderness, muscle guarding, or rigidity (38). With a bladder contusion, the individual will be able to void and hematuria is present, either gross or microscopically. With a bladder rupture, the individual is usually unable to void, and a specimen obtained by catheter reveals hematuria in the pelvic cavity.

Hematuria may also occur when the flaccid posterior wall of the bladder impacts against the base of the organ. This condition is commonly seen in long distance runners and has earned the name "runner's bladder" (39,40). Most sport participants void prior to running and competition. Running with an empty bladder increases the risk of gross hematuria, since no fluid cushion exists between the posterior wall and base of the bladder.

Occasionally blood in the urine is visible to the naked eye, however, it is often identified only with microscopic examination of urinary sediment. A heavy concentration of visible blood in the urine signifies a significant problem. The individual should be referred to a physician to rule out more serious causes. Hematuria due to running rapidly resolves within 24 to 48 hours of rest.

🔆 *The football player had a history of direct trauma to the abdomen, pain in the upper left quadrant, referred pain to the left shoulder, and showed signs of shock. This indicates a possible splenic rupture. Summon EMS.*

ASSESSMENT OF THROAT, THORAX, AND VISCERAL INJURIES

❓ *A twenty-one-year-old female gymnast finished practice an hour ago but is now complaining of vague chest discomfort and shortness of breath. She is also experiencing pain on the top of the right shoulder. How will you progress through this assessment to determine the extent and seriousness of injury?*

Injury assessment for thoracic and visceral injuries is the same as all sport injuries. However, with thoracic and visceral injuries it is particularly important to focus on the primary survey, vital signs, and history of the injury. Chest or abdominal trauma, although initially appearing superficial and minor, can mask underlying complications that can seriously compromise function of the vital organs. Internal hemorrhage and swelling can slowly deteriorate the individual's condition leading to alterations in breathing or circulation. General observations and palpations can confirm the possibility of a serious underlying condition. However, a good understanding of the history of the injury and constant monitoring of vital signs will be a stronger assessment tool. Therefore, always be aware of internal complications and alert to the signs and symptoms indicating their presence.

While approaching the individual, assess consciousness, respirations, and circulation. If the individual is having difficulty breathing, anxiety and panic may make the task more difficult. After ruling out possible spinal injury, place the individual in a comfortable position that facilitates breathing. This position is typically supine with the knees flexed. Make sure the airway is open and clear of any blood or vomitus. The trachea should be in the middle of the throat and should not move during respirations. Speak in a slow, calm, confident manner. If the difficulty in breathing does not improve significantly in a minute or two, assume that a serious internal injury exists. It is important at this time to take vital

signs so a baseline of information is established. Blood pressure, pulse, respirations, and pupillary response to light should be documented with comparisons made later in the assessment. While progressing through the evaluation, do not hesitate to summon EMS if internal injuries are suspected. It is better to have EMS in route as the assessment is completed than to wait and see if the condition gets any better. Several conditions intensify in severity with time, thereby seriously compromising the health of the injured party.

🔆 *It is important to remember not to give any water or food to an individual with an acute abdominal injury. Not only can the condition be aggravated, but if surgery is needed, any food or fluid in the gastrointestinal tract will make the surgery more dangerous. When the assessment is completed, continue to monitor vital signs and treat for shock until the ambulance arrives.*

HISTORY

❓ *You have completed the primary survey on the gymnast. She is obviously conscious but does have some shortness of breath. Her pulse is somewhat elevated but you are not sure if that is due to anxiety or an injury. What questions are you going to ask to determine the cause of this condition?*

The history of a chest or abdominal injury is extremely important to provide vital information about the injury. Since few special tests are available for the region, assess the condition based on information provided in the history. Gather information on the cause or mechanism of injury, the extent of pain or disability due to the injury, previous injuries to the area, and family history which may have some bearing on this specific condition. Remember that some conditions, such as a ruptured spleen, can delay hemorrhage for hours, days, or weeks after the initial trauma. Other injuries with an acute onset may have signs and symptoms which subside only to recur later. In addition to the general questions discussed in Chapter 4, specific questions that can be asked for chest and abdominal injuries can be seen in **Field Strategy 15-4**.

🔆 *The gymnast has vague mild chest discomfort on the right side that began about a half hour after practice. Since then the discomfort has intensified and now she feels pain on the top of the right shoulder. She*

Chest or abdominal trauma, although initially appearing superficial and minor, can mask underlying complications that can seriously compromise function of the vital organs

Blood pressure, pulse, respirations and pupillary response to light should be documented after the primary survey so comparisons can be made as you continue to monitor the vital signs

Never give water or food to an individual with an acute abdominal injury

Field Strategy 15–4. Developing a History of the Injury.

Determine (a) primary complaint including location, onset, and current nature of the problem; (b) mechanism of injury; (c) characteristics of the symptoms including the nature, location, severity, frequency, and duration of pain or disability; (d) functional deficits relative to ADLs (Activity of Daily Living), occupation, and recreational/athletic pursuits; and (e) related medical history. ASK:

- Why are you here? What is the problem? Where is the pain located? On a scale of one to ten with ten being very severe, how would you rate your pain? Can you describe the pain (dull ache, sharp, nagging, radiating, or burning)? Does it hurt to take a deep breath?
- How did the injury occur? Do you remember what position you were in? What direction was the force (glancing, direct, or violent muscle contraction)?
- Did the pain/dyspnea come on suddenly or gradually? Was the pain/dyspnea severe at first? Did the pain disappear only to gradually increase (spontaneous pneumothorax, ruptured spleen)? How long has the pain/dyspnea been present? Are you nauseous, lightheaded, or weak?
- Did you hear any sounds during the incident? Any snaps, pops, or cracks (rib fracture, costochondral separation, cutaneous emphysema)? Did you notice any swelling or discoloration at the time of the injury? How soon did it occur? What did you do for the swelling? Have you had any muscle spasms or cramps with the injury?
- What motions aggravate the symptoms? In what position are you most comfortable in? Are there certain activities you are unable to perform because of the pain? Which ones? How old are you?
- Have you noticed blood in the urine? Does it occur after long distance running? Is it painful when you urinate? Have you had any recent problems with diarrhea or constipation (bowel obstruction)?
- Have you ever injured this area before? Who evaluated the injury? What did you do for it? Have you seen a physician about this condition? What was the diagnosis? What occurred during that visit? Has there been any improvement in your condition?
- Do you have a history of diabetes mellitis, rheumatic fever, Marfan's syndrome, low or high blood pressure, or high cholesterol?
- Do you have a history of cardiovascular disease, congenital coronary artery anomalies, heart murmurs, heart palpitations, chest pains, or shortness of breath? Have you ever fainted before? Have any of these previous conditions occurred after strenuous exercise? Has anyone in your family had a history of any of these conditions?
- Have you had any medical problems recently? (Look for problems that may refer pain to the area from visceral organs, heart, and lungs. Remember that some injuries, such as a ruptured spleen can splint itself and produce delayed hemorrhage). Do you have any allergies? Are you on any medication?

reports being short of breath and unable to take a deep inhalation without pain. She does not recall any previous chest trauma or injury that might have accounted for her present state, nor does she recall any member of her family having a similar problem.

OBSERVATION AND INSPECTION

You suspect a pulmonary complication because of the pain on deep inspiration. However, you are not sure if it is superficial or internal. What factors can you observe that might provide clues to help determine if there is an injury to the chest wall or an internal complication?

Observation of body position can give an indication of the site, nature, and severity of injury. For example, in an acute thoracic injury, the individual may lean toward the injured side using an arm or hand to stabilize the region. In an acute abdominal injury, the individual will lie on the injured side and bring the knees toward the chest to relax the abdominal muscles (**Figure 15-24**). Facial expressions can confirm the individual's hesitation to perform any movement due to

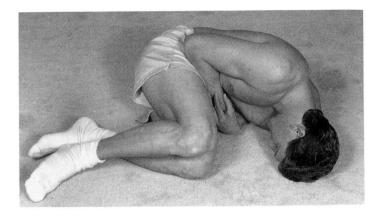

Fig. 15.24: Typical position seen with severe abdominal trauma.

severe pain. Chest expansion can reveal the rate and depth of respirations.

The individual should be sufficiently undressed to observe the injury site. Inspect the neck, back, chest, abdomen, and groin. Look for deformity, edema, bruising, ecchymosis, and skin color. Deformity may indicate a sternal or rib fracture, costochondral separation, or muscle rupture. An abrasion or localized bruising on the chest wall could suggest a possible rib fracture or internal complication. Diffuse bruising in the axilla and chest wall may indicate a ruptured pectoralis major. A bruise or ecchymosis in the umbilical area indicates intraperitoneal bleeding. Distention in the abdomen may indicate internal hemorrhage. Pale, cold and clammy skin is associated with shock. Cyanosis, or a bluish tinge, indicates a lack of oxygen due to internal pulmonary or cardiac problems. Coughing up bright red or frothy blood indicates a severe lung injury. Vomitus that contains blood that looks like used coffee grounds indicates that blood has been swallowed and partially digested.

Observe the rate and depth of respirations; note any difficulty in catching the breath. If the condition is only transitory, that is, the wind has been knocked out, breathing and color should return to normal quickly. If breathing does not return to normal quickly, or if the individual's condition rapidly deteriorates, the injury is significant and EMS should be summoned. Note the symmetrical rise and fall of the chest. **Field Strategy 15-5** provides specific observations that can help determine the extent and severity of thoracic or abdominal injuries.

🔦 *The gymnast is thin but otherwise healthy with no sign of trauma on the chest wall or shoulder region. While sitting, she leans to the right side using her right arm to stabilize the chest. Breathing is rapid and shallow. Skin color is pale and some anxiety is evident in the facial expression.*

PALPATIONS

❓ *You suspect a thoracic injury to the right side of the chest, but can not totally rule out a visceral injury because of the possibility of referred pain. What anatomical structures in the region can be palpated?*

Palpations of the chest and abdominal region can help narrow suspicions to confirm information gathered in the history and observation phase of the assessment. It is important to begin away from the painful area so pain cannot be carried over into other areas. Begin with gentle circular motions and feel for deformity, crepitus, swelling, rigidity, muscle guarding, or tenderness. Place the individual in a supine position with the knees flexed for more comfort.

Palpate the trachea during breathing to ensure that it does not move, as movement may indicate tension pneumothorax. Both hands should be used to palpate the symmetry and depth of respirations. Place the tips of the thumbs on the xiphoid process, resting the hands over the lower rib cage (**Figure 15-25**). Note the rise and fall of the rib cage. It should be symmetrical. If not, internal pulmonary complications may be present.

Palpate the clavicle, ribs, costochondral cartilage, and sternum for deformity and crepitus. Possible fractures and costochondral separations are assessed with gentle pressure applied to the sternum and vertebrae in an anteroposterior direction (**Figure 15-26A**). This action causes the rib cage to

If breathing does not return to normal quickly or the individual's condition rapidly deteriorates, the injury is significant and EMS should be summoned

Lateral movement of the trachea during breathing may indicate tension pneumothorax

Field Strategy 15–5. Observation and Inspection of the Thorax and Viscera.

- In what position is the individual (standing, leaning to one side, knees drawn to the chest, hands stabilizing an area to prevent excessive movement)? Do the facial expressions indicate pain, anxiety, or panic? Is cyanosis present?
- Is the trachea centered or deviated to one side (tension pneumothorax)? Does the trachea move during breathing? Are the neck veins distended (traumatic asphyxia)?
- Both shoulders should have a well-rounded musculature with no prominent bony structures. The pectoralis major, anterior axillary fold, and abdominal muscles should look symmetrical
- Note any bruising, ecchymosis, deformity, or muscular atrophy that may be present in the chest and abdomen
- Does the rib cage look symmetrical with no bony protrusions or deformities? Does the rib cage move symmetrically with each breath? Does the abdomen move with each breath? Is breathing normal or is shallow breathing present? Is the individual coughing up a bright red or frothy blood?
- Are abrasions, blisters, or bleeding present at the nipples? Are the nipples and breasts bilaterally the same size (gynecomastia)?
- Is the space between the arms and body the same on both sides? Are both hands held in the same position?
- Are the folds of the waist at the same height? Does the pelvis appear to be level? Is there any bruising or ecchymosis present in the abdomen (bruising in the umbilical area indicates intraperitoneal bleeding)? Is the discoloration localized or diffuse? Are there any soft tissue protrusions in the lower abdomen or groin (hernia)?
- Is the individual grasping an area with the hand? This may indicate where the pain is or where it is referred. Is the individual pale, cold, clammy, lethargic (shock)?

> Compression in an antero-posterior direction can detect possible rib fractures; lateral compression can detect possible costochondral separations

bow out laterally. Lateral compression on the sides of the rib cage causes strain on the costochondral junctions (**Figure 15-26B**). Begin compression superiorly and move down in an inferior direction until the entire area is covered. Pain at a specific site indicates a positive sign.

Palpate the abdomen with the hips flexed to relax the abdominal muscles. Use the flat

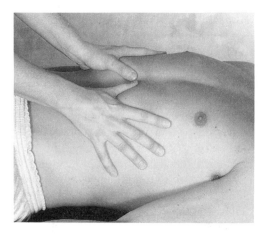

Fig. 15.25: Assessing rib symmetry during breathing.

part of several fingers with both hands moving in small circular motions (**Figure 15-27**). Do not poke or make sudden moves as this may cause the individual to jerk and tighten the muscles. Always begin away from the injured site and move across the abdomen in a straight line. Note any muscle guarding or rigidity. Muscle guarding that can not be voluntarily relaxed may indicate internal peritoneal hemorrhage. Palpate for tenderness, muscle resistance, and superficial masses or deficits in the continuity of the abdominal wall. Deeper palpation can detect rigidity, swelling, or masses. Rebound tenderness at McBurney's point is indicative of appendicitis. The rebounding pain is caused when the inflamed appendix is impacted by the viscera returning to their normal position. However, this phenomenon can also occur with peritonitis.

❓ *You completed palpations and found no irregularities or pain in the abdominal region. In the thorax, pain could not be elicited with palpation but you did notice that the right side of the rib cage is not expanding at the same level as the left side. The gymnast is beginning to have more difficulty breathing and pain is increasing.*

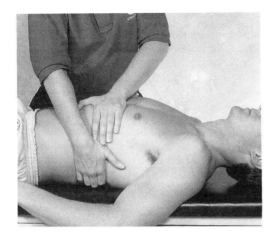
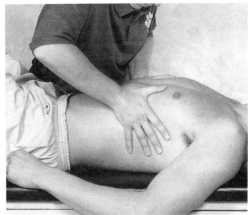

Fig. 15.26: Compression of the rib cage in a supine position. (A) Anteroposterior compression for rib fracture. (B) Lateral compression for costochondral separation.

SPECIAL TESTS

💡 *The condition of the gymnast is slowly deteriorating. Although she remains conscious and fully able to speak, you still have not determined the cause of the problem. What is your next course of action?*

There are very few special tests for the thorax and visceral area. Most of the information must be gathered during the primary survey, history, observation, and palpation phase of the assessment. If the condition is not serious and a muscular strain is suspected, active, passive, and resisted muscle testing can be performed. Neck and trunk motion was described in Chapter 14 and included flexion, extension, lateral flexion, and rotation. Note the individual's willingness to perform the motion, ease of motion, and bilateral comparison of motions where applicable.

Auscultation and Percussion

Auscultation utilizes a stethoscope to listen very carefully for the presence or absence of sounds in the body. In the thorax, the flow of air should be heard throughout the various regions of each lung **(Figure 15-28).** Abnormal sounds include gurgling, popping, snoring, or a high-pitched whistling sound.

Auscultation utilizes a stethoscope to listen very carefully for the presence or absence of sounds

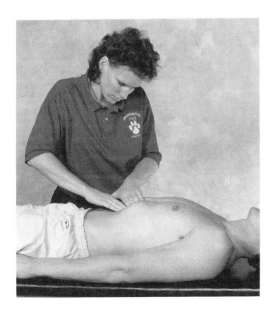

Fig. 15.27: Palpation of the abdomen.

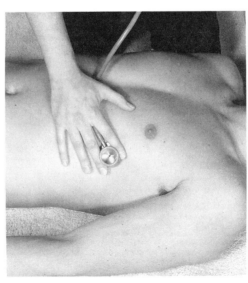

Fig. 15.28: Auscultation is done with a stethoscope to listen for air exchange in the lobes of the lungs.

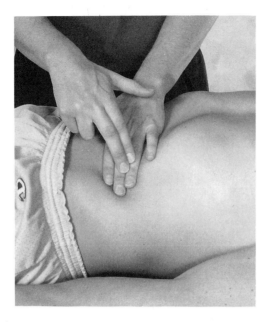

Fig. 15–29. Percussion is used in the abdominal region to indicate internal complications, and should be performed prior to palpation.

Absence of air flow indicates pneumothorax, tension pneumothorax, hemothorax, or traumatic asphyxia. Normal bowel sounds in the abdomen make a gurgling sound. Absence could indicate an obstruction or internal hemorrhage. Any abnormal sounds or absence of sounds indicates a serious underlying problem. Immediate referral to the nearest medical facility is warranted.

Percussion is typically used over a bony structure to determine a possible fracture, however, it can be used in the abdominal region to indicate internal complications. The nondominant hand is placed on the individual's abdomen over the various internal organs. The second and third finger of the dominant hand taps on the distal interphalangeal (DIP) joint of the middle finger with a quick rapid motion (**Figure 15-29**). The tone indicates if the organ is hollow (tympanic) or solid (full). The four quadrants are tested with facial expressions noted to indicate any discomfort in that region.

If auscultation or percussion is used in the assessment, both should be completed *prior* to palpation. Since the visceral organs are interconnected by connective tissue, any palpation in the abdomen will move the internal organs, thus giving inaccurate or false sounds.

Neurological Testing

Neurological testing in the thorax and abdomen is somewhat limited. Dermatomes vary and often overlap. Although the dermatomes tend to follow the ribs, the absence of only one dermatome may lead to no loss in sensation. **Figure 15-30** demonstrates dermatomes in the thoracic and visceral region. Sites for referred pain can indicate the origin of injury and are illustrated in **Figure 15-31**.

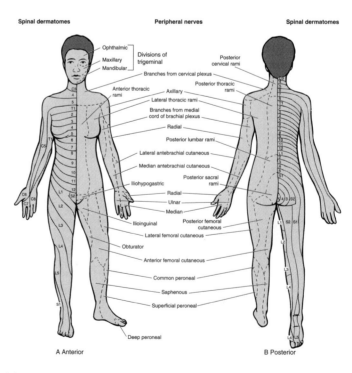

Fig. 15–30. Spinal dermatomes.

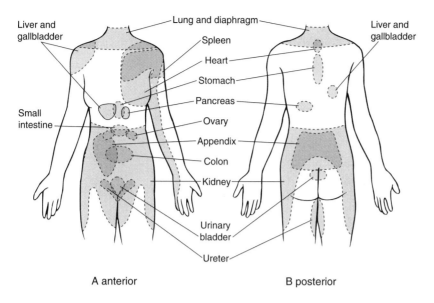

Liver and gallbladder — Lung and diaphragm — Liver and gallbladder

Spleen

Heart

Stomach

Pancreas

Small intestine — Ovary

Appendix

Colon

Kidney

Urinary bladder

Ureter

A anterior   B posterior

Fig. 15.31: Sites of referred pain.

Table 15–6. Common Sites of Referred Pain.

Organ/Condition	Localization of Pain
Appendicitis	Lower right quadrant; umbilicus
Bladder	Lower pelvic region over pubic bone; posterior buttocks
Heart	Left shoulder; down medial left arm; can extend into neck and jaw
Kidneys	Posterior lumbar region radiating to flanks and groin
Liver and gallbladder	Upper right quadrant; right shoulder; inferior angle of scapula
Lung and diaphragm	Upper shoulders and neck
Pancreatitis	Below xiphoid process; posterior lateral mid-back
Small intestines	Umbilicus
Spleen	Left shoulder; proximal 1/3 of left arm
Stomach	Below xiphoid process; posterior back over T4-T10 vertebrae
Ureters	Groin and medial thighs

Table 15-6 summarizes the most common sites of referred pain for injury to the internal organs of the torso. Myotome testing includes finger abduction and adduction (T_1), and hip flexion (L_1-L_2). No other myotome testing exists for the axial region. In addition, there are no deep tendon reflexes for the region, however, it is always wise to test the deep tendon lumbar and sacral reflexes (patellar reflex and Achilles reflex). **Field Strategy 15-6** lists the steps in an injury assessment of the thorax and visceral region.

You determined that muscle testing was not necessary in this assessment, since a more serious internal pulmonary problem exists. During auscultation, decreased air flow sounds were heard in the lower right lung. The gymnast may be experiencing spon-taneous pneumothorax. This individual needs to be transported to the nearest medical facility for further examination.

SUMMARY

Severe blunt trauma to the anterior neck region, thorax and viscera can have devastating effects leading to serious ventilatory and circulatory compromise. Certain injuries may not develop until hours, days, or weeks later. As such, the presumption of possible intrathoracic or intra-abdominal injuries with any blunt trauma necessitates a more complete and thorough assessment. Always assume a serious internal injury is present until it is ruled out by a physician.

Pre-existing conditions, such as hypertrophic cardiomyopathy, abnormalities in the

Field Strategy 15–6. Assessment of the Thorax and Visceral Region.

PRIMARY SURVEY
- Assess the ABCs and maintain an open airway
- Take vital signs including blood pressure, pulse, respirations, and pupillary response to light

HISTORY
- Primary complaint including:
  - Description and mechanism of current injury
  - Onset of symptoms
- Pain perception and discomfort
- Disability and functional impairments from the injury
- Past musculoskeletal injuries, congenital abnormalities, childhood diseases, allergies, or cardiac, respiratory, vascular, or neurological problems
- Family history

OBSERVATION AND INSPECTION
- Observe the general body for:
  - Body position that indicates injury site
  - Difficulty in breathing, shortness of breath, or diminished chest movement
  - Facial expressions that indicate severity of pain
  - Signs of shock

- Inspect the injured area for:
  - Muscle symmetry   Hypertrophy or muscle atrophy
  - Swelling   Visible congenital deformity
  - Discoloration   Surgical incisions or scars

PALPATION
- Bony structures to rule out fracture with:
  - Compression in an anteroposterior direction for rib fracture, and lateral compression for costochondral separation
- Soft tissue structures to determine temperature, point tenderness, rigidity, and muscle spasm or guarding. Note any swelling or loss of continuity in muscle, rebound tenderness on deep palpation, and superficial protrusion or palpable mass

SPECIAL TESTS
- Active and resistive movements for muscular strains (if appropriate)
- Auscultation and percussion for abnormal or absent sounds. Complete this step *prior* to palpation
- Neurological testing for dermatome patterns and referred or radiating pain

coronary arteries, Marfan's syndrome, mitral valve prolapse, cardiac conduction system disorders, and atherosclerotic coronary artery disease can place the sport participant at risk for sudden death. Although it is difficult to identify these individuals, anyone who experiences chest pains, sudden onset of fatigue, heartburn or indigestion, excessive breathlessness during exercise, or has a history of cardiovascular disease should be referred to a physician for further investigation.

Injury assessment for the thorax and visceral region should focus on the primary survey, vital signs, and history of the injury. Observation, palpation, and sites of referred pain can confirm suspicions of an existing internal injury. If at anytime signs and symptoms indicate an intrathoracic or intra-abdominal injury, EMS should be summoned immediately. Constant monitoring of the vital signs can indicate if the individual is improving or deteriorating. If the individual recovers on site, however, they should be informed of signs and symptoms that might develop, indicating the condition is getting worse, and then seek immediate medical care. Conditions that warrant immediate action are listed in **Table 15-7**.

Table 15–7. Conditions that Warrant Immediate Action.

General body signs and symptoms including:
- Uncontrolled anxiety, fear, confusion, or restlessness
- Eyes that are bulging or bloodshot
- Distended neck veins
- Deviated trachea or trachea that moves during breathing
- Individual who coughs up bright red or frothy blood, or vomits blood that looks like used coffee grounds
- Signs of shock
- Sudden fatigue, weakness, palpations, or chest pain during exercise
- Cyanosis in the face or neck region
- Radiating or referred pain to the shoulder tip, back, or groin

Throat signs and symptoms including:
- Hoarseness or loss of voice
- Difficulty swallowing
- Laryngospasm
- Presence of hemorrhage with blood-tinged sputum
- Loss of contour of the Adam's apple

Thoracic conditions including:
- Shortness of breath or difficulty in breathing
- Suspected rib or sternal fracture
- Severe chest pain aggravated with deep inspiration
- Abnormal chest movement on affected side
- Abnormal or absent breath sounds

Abdominal conditions including:
- Severe abdominal pain
- Nausea
- Vomiting
- Diffuse hemorrhage or distention of the abdomen
- Tenderness, rigidity, or muscle spasm
- Rebound pain on deep palpation
- Absence of bowel sounds
- Blood in the urine or stool

REFERENCES

1. Storey, MD, Schatz, CF, and Brown, KW. 1989. Anterior neck trauma. Phys Sportsmed, 17(9): 85–96.
2. McCutcheon, ML, and Anderson, JL. 1985. How I manage sports injuries to the larynx. Phys Sportsmed, 13(4):100–112.
3. Reid, DC. *Sport injury assessment and rehabilitation.* New York: Churchill Livingstone, 1992.
4. Fabian, RL. 1989. Sports injury to the larynx and trachea. Phys Sportsmed, 17(2):111–118.
5. Lorentzen, D, and Lawson, L. 1987. Selected sports bras: A biomechanical analysis of breast motion while jogging. Phys Sportsmed, 15(5):128–139.
6. Gehlsen, G, and Albohm, M. 1980. Evaluation of sports bras. Phys Sportsmed, 8(10):89–96.
7. Haycock, CE. 1987. How I manage breast problems in athletes. Phys Sportsmed, 15(3):89–95.
8. Cowart, V. 1987. Steroids in sports: After four decades, time to return these genies to bottle? JAMA, 257(4):421–427.
9. Kretzler, HH, and Richardson, AB. 1989. Rupture of the pectoralis major muscle. Am J of Spts Med, 17(4):453–458.
10. Reut, RC, Bach, BR, and Johnson, C. 1991. Pectoralis major rupture: Diagnosing and treating a weight-training injury. Phys Sportsmed, 19(3):89–96.
11. McEntire, JE, Hess, WE, and Coleman, SS. 1972. Rupture of the pectoralis major muscle: A report of eleven injuries and a review of fifty-six. J Bone Joint Surg, 54A(Jul):1040–1046.
12. Jones, HK, McBride, GG, and Mumby, RC. 1989. Sternal fractures associated with spinal injury. J of Trauma, 29(3):360–364.
13. Miles, JW, and Barrett, GR. 1991. Rib fractures in athletes. Sports Med, 12(1):66–69.
14. Karofsky, PS. 1987. Hyperventilation syndrome in adolescent athletes. Phys Sportsmed, 15(2):133–138.
15. Joorabchi, B. 1977. Expressions of the hyperventilation syndrome in childhood: Studies in management, including an evaluation of the effectiveness of propranolol. Clin Pediatr, 16(12):1110–1115.
16. Wagner, RB, Sidhu, GS, and Radcliffe, WB. 1992. Pulmonary contusion in contact sports. Phys Sportsmed, 20(2):126–136.
17. Lee, MC, Wong, SS, Chu, JJ, Chang, JP, Lin, PJ, Shieh, MJ, and Chang, CH. 1991. Traumatic asphyxia. Ann Thorac Surg, 51(1):86–88.
18. Hammond, SG. 1990. Chest injuries in the trauma patient. Nurs Clin of N Am, 25(1):35–43.
19. Rutherford, GW, Kennedy, J, and McGee, L. *Hazard analysis: Baseball and softball related injuries to children 5–14 years of age.* US Consumer Product Safety Commission, 1984.
20. King, AI, and Viano, DC. *Baseball related chest impact: Final report to the consumer product safety commission.* US Consumer Product Safety Commission, 1986.
21. Green, ED, Simson, LR, Kellerman, HH, Horowitz, RN, and Sturner, WQ. 1980. Cardiac concussion following softball blow to the chest. Ann Emerg Med, 9(3):155–157.

22. Karofsky, PS. 1990. Death of a high school hockey player. Phys Sportsmed, 18(2):99–103.
23. Edlich, RF, Jr, Mayer, NE, Fariss, BL, Phillips, VA, Smith JF, Chang, DE, and Edlich, RF. 1987. Commotio cordis in a lacrosse goalie. J Emerg Med, 5(0):181–184.
24. Abrunzo, TJ. 1991. Commotio Cordis: The single, most common cause of traumatic death in youth baseball. Am J Dis of Children, 145(1):1279–1282.
25. Liedtke, AJ, Allen RP, and Nellis, SH. 1980. Effects of blunt cardiac trauma on coronary vasomotion, perfusion, myocardial mechanics, and metabolism. J Trauma, 20(9):777–785.
26. Van Camp, SP. "Sudden death." In *Clinics in sports medicine*, edited by JC Puffer, vol. 11, no. 2. Philadelphia: WB Saunders, 1992.
27. Maron, BJ. 1993. Hypertrophic cardiomyopathy in athletes: Catching a Killer. Phys Sportsmed, 21(9):83–91.
28. Allison, TG. 1992. Counseling athletes at risk for sudden death. Phys Sportsmed, 20(6):140–149.
29. Braden, DS, and Strong, WB. 1988. Preparticipation screening for sudden cardiac death in high school and college athletes. Phys Sportsmed, 16(10):128–143.
30. Alpert, JS, Pape, LA, Ward, A, and Rippe, JM. 1989. Athletic heart syndrome. Phys Sportsmed, 17(7):103–107.
31. deShazo, WF. 1984. Hematoma of the rectus abdominis in football. Phys Sportsmed, 12(9):73–75.
32. McCarthy, P. 1990. Hernias in athletes: What you need to know. Phys Sportsmed, 18(5):115–122.
33. McVay, CB, and Savage, LE. 1961. Etiology of femoral hernia. Ann Surg, 154(Supl):25-32.
34. Haycock, CE. 1983. How I manage hernias in the athlete. Phys Sportsmed, 11(8):77–79.
35. Danneker, DA, Mandetta, DF, and Rockower, R. 1979. Case report: Intra-abdominal injury in a gymnast. Phys Sportsmed, 7(6):119–000.
36. Morden, RS, Berman, BM, Nagle, CE, and Jafri, SZH. 1992. Spleen injury in sports, Part II: Avoiding splenectomy. Phys Sportsmed, 20(4): 126–139.
37. Klein, S, Hons, S, Fujitani, R, and State, D. 1988. Hematuria following blunt abdominal trauma: The utility of intravenous pyelography. Arch Surg, 123(9):1173–1177.
38. Cass, AS. 1989. Diagnostic studies in bladder rupture: Indications and techniques. Urol Clin North Am, 16(2):267–273.
39. York, JP. 1990. Sports and the male genitourinary system: Kidneys and bladder. Phys Sportsmed, 18(9):116–129.
40. Blacklock, HJ. 1980. Bladder trauma from jogging. Am Heart J, 99(6):813–814.

Special Conditions Related to Sports

Special Conditions Related to Sports

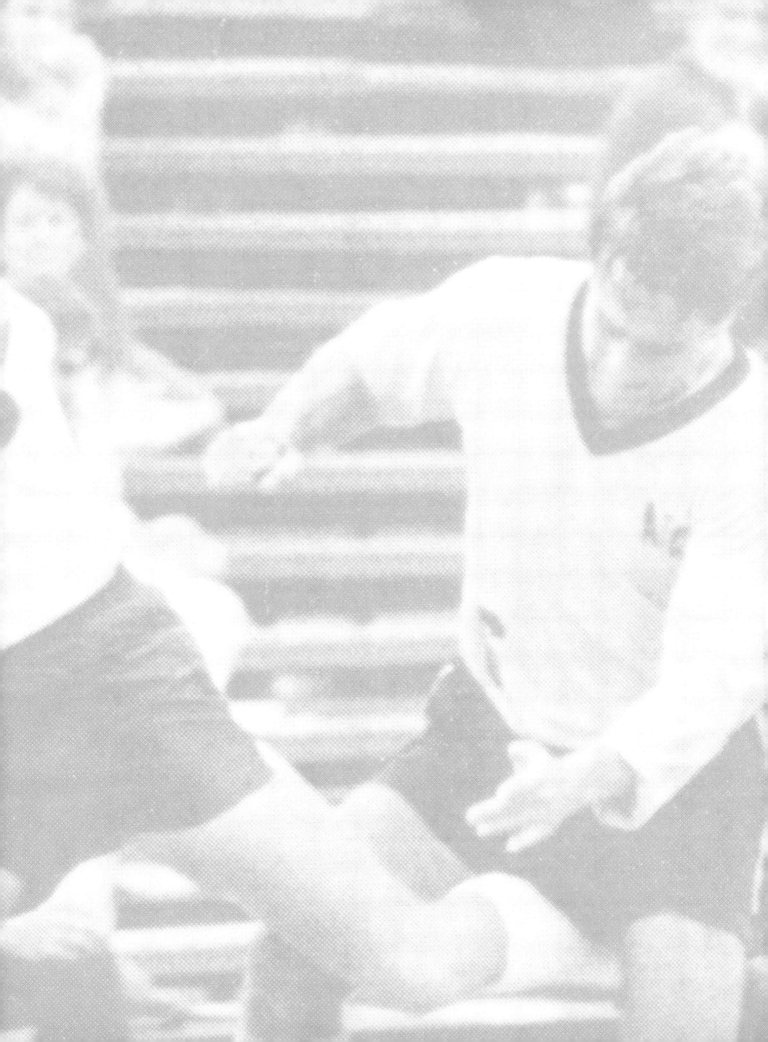

Marsha Grant, M.Ed., A.T.,C.

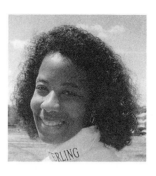

Marsha Grant was the first African-American woman certified by the NATA. As a noted educator, she has served as an athletic trainer at the Division I, II, and III levels. She is currently the Head Athletic Trainer at Sterling High School in Somerdale, New Jersey.

While playing field hockey at East Stroudsburg University, I got hurt twice within a two-week period. As I visited the training room daily, I got to see the trainer, Lois Wagner, in action. What she did really sparked an interest in me. After talking with her about the field, I switched from wanting to be a health and physical education instructor to an athletic trainer. After completing my master's degree in education at the University of Virginia, I got my first taste of training and teaching at Western Illinois State University.

Although I've worked at all three competitive levels of intercollegiate sports, I really enjoy my new job at the high school level. I work full-time with a tremendous staff of administrators and coaches. Typically, I start my day at 1 o'clock in the afternoon and go until all the practices are over. I travel with football unless there is a home game, in which case I stay home to provide coverage there. It's a heavy workload in the fall, but because of the limited daylight I don't go quite as late. I make up for it in the winter season, however. We have a large variety of sports, and each sport may suit up three different levels of teams, so the number of athletes I service daily is immense.

One great thing about this position is that we have a superb staff. Our school nurse always comes to the games, and takes an active interest in the athletes. She also communicates with me daily about any player who may see her during the day. The athletic director also visits practice often to see how things are going, and holds the coaches and athletes responsible for their actions. The athletes are aware of this sincere interest in their welfare, and are grateful for what I do for them. It is really fun to see these athletes enjoy participating in sports for the love of it. They have a good time, and I like being a part of that.

Although working on the college level was exciting because I got to travel all over the United States and interact with some outstanding colleagues, it just doesn't compare to working with this level. On the college level, I put in very long hours, seven days a week for three seasons. Most people don't understand that you need a life outside of the training room and classroom. I honestly don't recall any coach ever asking me what time would be good for me to schedule a weekend practice. I could never make plans to do anything because I was expected to be present at every practice. There is also a significant financial parity in training on the college level. Some coaches with whom I worked were making $80,000 and up, and there I was, responsible for the entire health care of the scholarship athletes, making less than half of their salary.

It's different on the high school level. Salaries are more equitable, and there seems to be more respect from the coaches and administrators about the value you bring to their program. Parents, however, still do not necessarily see the importance of your daily presence. There are budget and equipment limitations, and it is sometimes difficult to convince parents to purchase needed protective braces for their daughters or sons. It may take two to three weeks to convince them to purchase the brace, whereas on the college level, I could walk into the storeroom and pull one out and fit the athlete right there.

Each level of competition has its pros and cons. As a woman in athletic training, you still have to fight the subtle notion that women aren't supposed to be trainers for men's intercollegiate teams. Had I not had the academic preparation and support at a school with an approved curriculum, I think my transition into the marketplace would have been more difficult. To succeed, you need to apply yourself in the classroom and in the clinical rotations. Utilize your resources and ask questions. Do clinical rotations at a variety of settings including summer sports camps to find out where you feel most comfortable. And most importantly, respect your skills and your profession. You are qualified to work with athletes, regardless of gender. Don't let anyone tell you that you can't. If you apply yourself, you will succeed and have fun doing it. It's a great profession.

Conditions Related to the Reproductive System

After you have completed this chapter, you should be able to:

- List the primary and accessory organs in the female and male reproductive systems

- Explain how hormones affect the human body

- Identify the signs and symptoms of common injuries to the female and male genitalia, and explain their management

- Describe the mode of transmission, signs, and symptoms of hepatitis and acquired immunodeficiency syndrome (AIDS), and indicate specific steps to prevent the spread of these diseases

- Identify the various menstrual irregularities and what implications they may have on sport participation

- Describe how sport performance may be affected by the use of oral contraceptives and IUDs

- Specify indications and contraindications for sport participation during pregnancy

Injuries to the reproductive organs in sport participation are rare, particularly in the female. In the male, direct blows to the groin region can injure external genitalia, however, protective equipment is available to reduce this risk. Sexually transmitted diseases, such as hepatitis and AIDS, may also be transmitted via blood or blood products and remain a major concern for all health care providers. Coaches, athletic trainers, and sport supervisors should observe strict adherence to universal safety precautions to prevent the spread of many of these diseases.

This chapter begins with an anatomical review of the female and male reproductive systems and discusses the role of hormones in the overall development of the body. Common injuries or conditions associated with the various structures are then discussed. Next, the mode of transmission, signs and symptoms, and current management of common sexually transmitted diseases are summarized. Detailed information on hepatitis and AIDS is then presented, including risk factors and implications for the work environment. Finally, information on sport participation during menstruation, ingestion of oral contraceptives, and pregnancy is presented.

ANATOMY OF THE GENITALIA

? *Can the pelvic girdle totally protect the male and female reproductive systems from injury? Which structures may not be protected?*

The reproductive organs of the female and male include the primary and accessory sex organs. The **primary sex organs**, the ovaries and testes, produce gametes or germ cells, specifically ovum and sperm, that when joined together develop into a fetus. Important sex hormones influence sexual differentiation, development of secondary sex characteristics, and in the female, regulate the reproductive cycle. All sex hormones are predominantly produced by the primary sex organs and belong to the general family known as **steroids**. In the female, estrogen and progesterone are produced by the ovaries. In the male, the adrenal cortex and testes produce hormones collectively known as androgens, the most active being testosterone. The **accessory sex organs** transport, protect, and nourish the gametes after they leave the ovaries and testes. In females the accessory sex organs include the fallopian tubes, uterus, vagina, and vulva (**Figure 16-1**). In males, the accessory

Primary sex organs
Reproductive organs responsible for producing gametes (ovum and sperm)

Steroids
A large family of chemical substances including endocrine secretions and hormones

Accessory sex organs
Organs that transport, protect, and nourish gametes

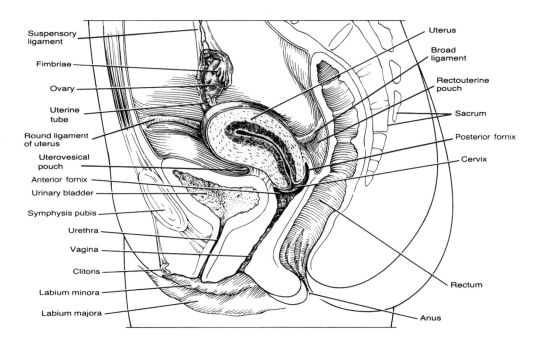

Fig. 16.1: Median section of the female pelvis.

sex organs include the epididymis, ductus deferens, seminal vesicles, prostate gland, bulbourethral glands, scrotum, and penis **(Figure 16-2)**.

Female Reproductive System

The female reproductive system includes: the ovaries, that produce ova (female eggs); the fallopian tubes, that transport, protect, and

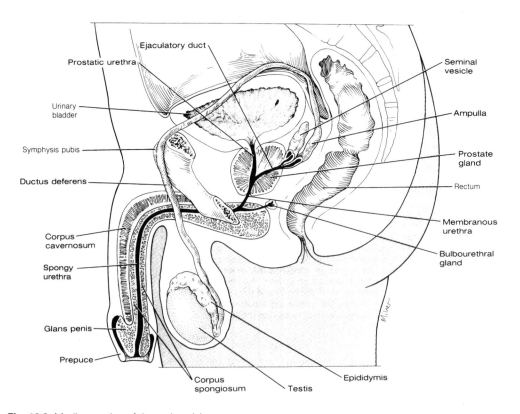

Fig. 16.2: Median section of the male pelvis.

nourish the ova; the uterus, that provides an environment for the development of the fertilized embryo; and the vagina, that serves as the receptacle for the sperm (**Figure 16-1**). These structures are protected by the pelvic girdle and are seldom injured during sport participation.

The ovarian cycle begins at puberty with a release of an ovum, or egg, from the ovary. The ovum, released at ovulation, travels through a fallopian tube to the uterus where it embeds itself in the uterine wall. The menstrual cycle, lasting anywhere from 28 to 40 days, involves a repeated series of changes within the lining of the uterus, and is controlled by the ovarian cycle. **Menses**, or the menstrual flow, is a phase in the menstrual cycle lasting three to six days when the thickened vascular walls of the uterus, the unfertilized ovum, and blood from the damaged vessels of the endometrium are lost.

The hormones estrogen and progesterone are produced by the ovaries. **Estrogens** help regulate the menstrual cycle and influence the development of female physical sex characteristics, such as the appearance of breasts, pubic and axillary hair, increased subcutaneous fat—especially in the hips and breasts—and widening and lightening of the pelvis. Estrogens are also responsible for the rapid growth spurt seen in girls between the ages of 12 and 13 years. However, this growth is short-lived, as increased levels of estrogen cause earlier closure of the epiphyses of long bones, leading to females reaching their full height between the ages of 15 to 17 years. In contrast, males may continue to grow until the age of 19 to 21 years. **Progesterones** are responsible for regulating the menstrual cycle and stimulating the development of the uterine lining in preparation for pregnancy.

The external genital organs of the female are known as the vulva, or pudendum. The outer rounded folds, the labia majora, protect the vestibule into which the vagina and urethra open.

Male Reproductive System

The male reproductive system includes: the testes, that produce spermatozoa, a number of ducts that store, transport, and nourish the spermatozoa, several accessory glands that contribute to the formation of semen, and the penis, through which urine and semen pass (**Figure 16-2**). The primary hormones pro-

duced by the testes are collectively called **androgens**, the most important being testosterone. Testosterone stimulates the growth and maturation of the internal and external genitalia at puberty, and is responsible for sexual motivation. Secondary sex characteristics that are testosterone-dependent include the appearance of pubic, axillary, and facial hair, enhanced hair growth on the chest or back, and a deepening of the voice as the larynx enlarges. Androgens also increase bone growth, bone density, and skeletal muscle size and mass.

💡 *The pelvic girdle does provide strong protection for internal structures of the reproductive systems. However, pelvic fractures can seriously damage these structures. In addition, the external male genitalia are virtually unprotected from direct blows and can be injured with direct trauma.*

INJURIES AND CONDITIONS OF THE GENITALIA

❓ *A soccer player was struck in the groin by an opponent's foot. He was not wearing a protective cup at the time. He immediately fell to the ground and drew the knees to the chest while grasping the genital region. What possible conditions can occur as a result of direct trauma to the genitalia? How should this injury be managed? What signs and symptoms would indicate that immediate referral to a physician is warranted?*

The male genitalia is more susceptible to injury than female genitalia, since several structures in the male reproductive system are external to the body, thus exposed to direct trauma. Protective cups can protect the penis and scrotum from injury, and are required for baseball catchers and hockey goalies (see **Figure 6-21**). Direct trauma can damage the penis, urethra, and scrotum that holds the testes. In addition, congenital variations in testicular suspension make certain individuals susceptible to torsion of the testicle.

Male Genital Injuries

Direct trauma to the groin from a knee, implement, or straddle-like injury, such as falling on a bar, can cause severe pain and dysfunction to the testes and penis (**Figure 16-3**). Lacerations to the penis are rare, however, swelling and hemorrhage inside the scrotal sac is seen more often. To assist in

Menses
Phase in the menstrual cycle when the thickened vascular walls of the uterus, the unfertilized ova, and blood from damaged vessels are lost during the menstrual flow

Estrogens
A class of hormones that produce female secondary sex characteristics and affect the menstrual cycle

Estrogens are responsible for the rapid growth spurt in girls between the ages of 12 and 13 years

Progesterone
Hormone responsible for thickening the uterine lining in preparation for the fertilized ovum

Androgens
A class of hormones that promote development of male genitals and secondary sex characteristics, and influence sexual motivation

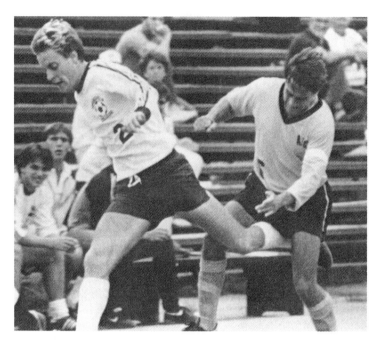

Fig. 16.3: Direct trauma to the groin region can injure the penis or lead to swelling and hemorrhage in the scrotal sac.

assessment and follow-up management of an injury to the male genital organs, the injured individual should be instructed to do periodic self assessment for pain and swelling, and should be given guidelines on seeking further medical care if necessary.

Penis Injuries

Superficial wounds to the penis may involve a contusion, abrasion, laceration, avulsion, or penetrating wound. In addition, the urethra can be damaged. In most cases, however, injuries resolve without specific treatment. Superficial bleeding is controlled with a sterile dressing. Cold compresses with mild compression will control swelling. Referral to a physician is only necessary if hemorrhage persists or swelling impairs function of the urethra.

Bikers may develop transient paresthesia of the penis as a result of pressure on the pudendal nerve. Adjusting the saddle height, tilt, and number of cycling bouts usually resolves the condition. Raising up on the pedals occasionally will also relieve pressure temporarily.

Scrotal Injuries

Blunt scrotal trauma can cause a contusion, hematoma, torsion, dislocation, or rupture of the testicle. If the tunica vaginalis ruptures, the vascular and tubercle components of the testes can be seriously damaged (**Figure 16-**

4). Commonly a knee, foot, or elbow to the groin compresses the testicle against the pelvis, leading to a nauseating, painful condition. Immediate internal hemorrhage, effusion, and muscle spasm occur. Testicular spasm can be relieved by placing the individual on his back and flexing the knees toward the chest to relax the muscle spasm (**Figure 16-5**). After pain has diminished, cold compresses should be placed on the scrotum to reduce swelling and hemorrhage.

Occasionally blunt trauma leads to swelling in the tunica vaginalis, resulting in a traumatic **hydrocele (Figure 16-6A)**. In 9 to 19% of men, the plexus of veins on the posterior testicle can become engorged constituting a **varicocele**. These lesions may be described as "a bag of worms" adjacent to the testicle and cord (**Figure 16-6B**). If the plexus ruptures, due to blunt trauma, a rapid accumulation of blood occurs in the scrotum, leading to a **hematocele**. In nearly 50% of patients with traumatic hematocele, testicular rupture is also present (1).

Pain is not a good indicator of which structure is damaged. Swelling and hemorrhage inside the scrotal sac can enlarge the sac to the size of a tennis ball or grapefruit. Each condition can lead to irreparable testicular damage if evaluation and treatment by a physician is delayed (2,3). Treatment for swelling inside the scrotal sac involves aspira-

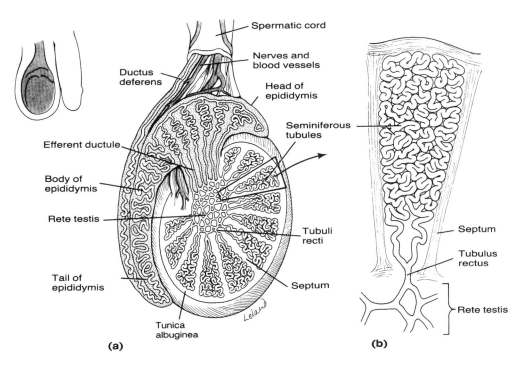

Fig. 16.4: (A) Sagittal section of the testicle. (B) Seminiferous tubules within a single compartment of the testicle. If the tunica vaginalis ruptures, the vascular and tubercle components of the testes can be seriously damaged.

tion of fluid and injection of a solution to toughen the involved tissues. Symptoms disappear in 85 to 90% of the cases with this treatment (4,5).

Torsion of the testicle may or may not have a history of trauma (6). Congenital variations in the testicular suspension can cause rotational twisting of the vascular pedicle and

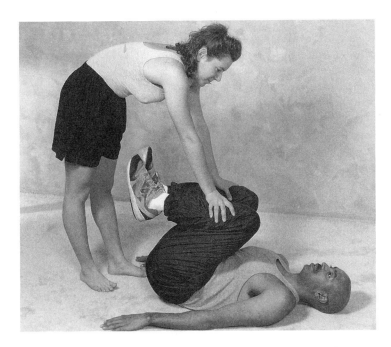

Fig. 16.5: To relieve testicular spasm, place the individual on his back and flex the knees toward the chest. After pain has diminished, apply ice to control swelling and hemorrhage.

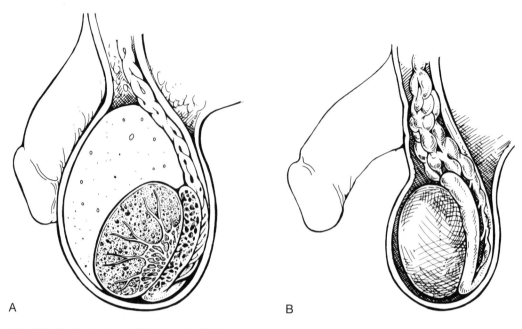

Fig. 16.6: Testicular injury. (A) Hydrocele. (B) Varicocele.

spermatic cord, producing varying degrees of circulatory compromise **(Figure 16-7)**. It is typically seen at or around puberty, manifesting itself after physical activity (7). Groin pain may develop gradually or rapidly, sometimes with associated nausea and vomiting. Immediate referral to a physician is necessary if correction of the condition is to be successful. High-resolution ultrasound can determine the extent and severity of injury. If corrected within six to eight hours, recovery is nearly 100 percent.

A scrotal mass may also be indicative of testicular cancer, the most common malignancy in 16-to-35-year-old males (7). Men who have an undescended or partially descended testicle are at a higher risk of developing testicular cancer than others. The first sign is a slightly enlarged testicle and a change in its consistency. The mass is separate from the cord and epididymis **(Figure 16-8)**. Pain may be absent, but often a dull ache or sensation of dragging and heaviness is present in the lower abdomen or groin. Diagnosis is made with transillumination with a bright light or ultrasound. Early detection and surgical treatment yields an excellent survival rate.

Female Genital Injuries

Injuries to the vulva usually involve straddling or penetration trauma, or by falls resulting in tears from forced perineal stretching during sudden leg abduction. These injuries have occurred in gymnastics, water-skiing, snow-mobiling, motorcycling, bicycling, sledding, cross-country skiing, and while riding horses (8). Nearly all injuries are easily treated by ice application, mild compression, and bed rest. Occasionally high-speed water-skiing injuries result in water being forced under high pressure into the vulva and vagina, leading to rupture of the vaginal walls. The water may also be forced through the fallopian tubes, leading to localized pelvic peritonitis. These injuries

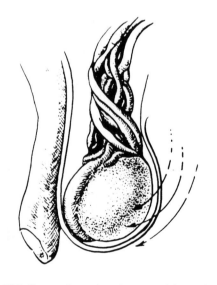

Fig. 16.7: Spermatic cord torsion around the tunica vaginalis.

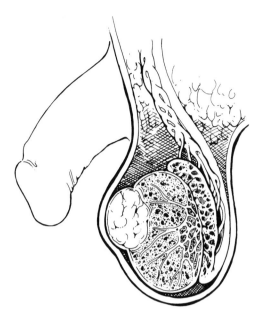

Fig. 16.8: A mass separate from the cord and epididymis demands immediate referral to a physician to rule out possible testicular cancer.

are easily preventable by wearing a neoprene wetsuit or nylon-reinforced suit.

Dermatological Conditions

Conditions affecting the skin of the genital region include tinea cruris, or "jock itch," pediculosis pubis, more commonly known as pubic lice, and chafing of the skin ("chub rub"). These conditions, if recognized early, are easily treated.

Tinea Cruris (Jock Itch)

Tinea cruris or "jock itch" is a common fungal infection involving the genitalia, seen more commonly in men than women. A dark, warm, moist environment is optimal for fungal growth. Perspiration can accumulate between the scrotum and skin of the thigh. This, augmented with wearing constrictive clothing, such as an athletic supporter, tight shorts, or spandex, encourages fungal growth. In addition, tight garments cause chafing and irritation.

The crual or perineal folds between the scrotum and inner thighs are usually the first areas to exhibit small patches of erythema and scaling. The scrotum and penis are seldom involved. Infection can spread to the thighs, perineal area, buttocks, and abdomen. Diffuse thickening and darkening is present over the inflamed region, and weeping vesi-

cles or pustules may be present at the margins of inflammation. Severe itching is also common. When scrotal redness or scaling occurs, it typically results from an allergic reaction to skin medications used prior to seeing the physician, or a chronic skin inflammation caused by scratching or long-term irritation (9).

Treatment involves antifungal medication and changing the warm, moist environment. Over-the-counter medications may include miconazole (Micatin), clotrimazole (Lotrimin, Mycelex), and tolnaftate (Tinactin). These are typically applied twice daily for at least one month. A two to five week regimen of prescribed medication may include Naftifine (Naftin), ciclopirox (Loprox), fluconazole (Diflucan), or an imidazole compound. There is a reported 95% cure rate (9,10). During treatment the groin area should be kept clean and dry. Loose, absorbent clothing should be worn. **Field Strategy 16-1** summarizes the signs, symptoms, and management of tinea cruris.

Pediculosis Pubis (Crabs)

Pubic lice are parasitic insects, called biting lice, found in the pubic hair and skin. The condition is commonly transmitted during sexual contact when pubic areas are brought together, but can be transmitted via the fingers to the armpits, scalp, or eyelashes. The insects (louse) are yellowish-gray in appearance and visible to the naked eye. An adult louse grips a pubic hair and embeds its head into the skin where it feeds on capillary blood. Crabs, as they are commonly called because of their resemblance to a crab, can live away from the body for as long as one day. They may drop off the host onto undergarments, bed sheets, and other apparel. Even after being successfully treated, the host can become reinfected by being exposed to the lice on their own unwashed undergarments or linens. **Pruritus**, or intense itching, is usually the only complaint.

Treatment involves an over-the-counter preparation known as A-200 pyrinate. Kwell and Lindaine 1% are also available but must be prescribed. The solution is applied to all areas of body hair and left on for eight hours, then washed off. A second treatment is repeated seven days later (eggs take seven days to hatch), and may need to be repeated a third time. All clothes and sheets used 48 hours prior to the treatment must be thoroughly dry-cleaned or washed in hot water and

Tinea cruris grows optimally in a dark, warm, moist environment

Diffuse thickening and darkening is present over the inflamed region, and weeping vesicles may be present at the margins

Crabs may drop off the host onto undergarments, bed sheets, and other apparel

Pruritus
Intense itching

All clothes and sheets used 48 hours prior to the treatment must be thoroughly dry-cleaned or washed in hot water and bleach

Field Strategy 16–1. Management of Tinea Cruris.

Signs and Symptoms
- Erythema and scaling on the crual or perineal folds between the scrotum and inner thighs
- Infection can spread to the thighs, entire perineal area, buttocks, and abdomen and may appear thickened and dark
- Weeping vesicles or pustules may appear at the margins of the inflammation
- Severe itching

Management
- Keep genital region clean by washing the region daily and after physical exertion, being careful to thoroughly rinse all soap residue from the region and completely dry the area. Apply powder liberally
- Frequently change and wash the athletic supporter and undergarments. Wear loose, non-restrictive clothing
- Apply ointments twice daily for at least a month. Begin by using over-the-counter medications, such as miconazole (Micatin), clotrimazole (Lotrimin, Mycelex), or tolnaftate (Tinactin)
- If the condition does not clear up, seek medical assistance to rule out candidiasis, dermatitis, psoriasis, or other skin disorders. A two to five week regimen of prescribed medication may include Naftifine (Naftin), ciclopirox (Loprox), fluconazole (Diflucan), or an imidazole compound

bleach. Household members and close contacts also need to be checked for infestation.

Chafing of the Skin

Chafing of the skin (intertrigo) is a superficial dermatitis caused by moisture, warmth, friction, sweat retention, or infectious agents. The condition may occur between the creases of the neck, in the axillary region, or beneath large breasts, but is primarily seen in the groin region in individuals with muscular thighs or in obese individuals. It is sometimes referred to as "chub rub." The condition is characterized by erythema, maceration, burning, itching, and sometimes erosion, fissures, and exudations. The condition can be prevented by wearing loose, soft, cotton underwear to keep the skin dry, clean, and friction-free. The area should be cleansed daily with mild soap and water, followed by an application of hydrocortisone cream.

The position of the player will relieve testicular spasm. After the spasm has eased, remove the player from the field, apply cold compresses to reduce swelling and hemorrhage, and encourage the individual to do periodic self assessment. If swelling of the testicle occurs, the individual should seek immediate medical attention.

SEXUALLY TRANSMITTED DISEASES

A basketball player is complaining of painful urination and open sores on the penis, and is very concerned he may have a sexually transmitted disease. How will you address these concerns and help this individual seek medical care? What can be done in the work environment to prevent the spread of these diseases?

Infections of the genital tract are common health complaints. These complaints, called sexually transmitted diseases (STDs), strike both genders, all socioeconomic classes, and all ages, however, transmission is twice as high in teenagers aged 15 to 19 years old (11). It is not the intent of this book to discuss in detail the various sexually transmitted diseases. A summary of the mode of transmission, incubation period, signs, symptoms, and treatment of the more common STDs can be seen in **Table 16-1**. Notwithstanding, viral hepatitis and AIDS can be transmitted via blood and blood products. Therefore, these two conditions will be discussed in more detail.

Hepatitis

Hepatitis is classified into five major types, each caused by a different virus (**Table 16-2**). Hepatitis A (HAV) is primarily spread via the fecal-oral route with an incubation period ranging between 5 and 50 days. Epidemics are known to have occurred because food handlers failed to wash their hands properly after using the bathroom. An outbreak of hepatitis A has also been associated with swimming in a public pool (12). Hepatitis B

Table 16–1. Common Sexually Transmitted Diseases (STDs).

STD	Transmission	Incubation	Symptoms	Treatment
+Bacterial vaginosis	Caused by *Gardnerella vaginalis* bacterium, it is primarily spread through coitus	1–3 weeks	Women: a pungent, fishy or musty smelling thin gray vaginal discharge resembling flour paste Men: often asymptomatic; inflammation of the foreskin and glans of the penis, urethritis and cystitis may be present	Oral metronidazole (Flagyl), clindamycin, amoxicillin, or imipenem
+Candidiasis (yeast infection)	The *Candida albicans* fungus may accelerate growth when the vaginal chemical balance is disturbed; it may also be transmitted through coitus	2 weeks to 1 month	Women: may range from thin, clear watery discharge to a white, "cheesy" discharge. Intense itching, swelling, irritation, and burning of the vaginal and vulval tissues may lead to a dry rash that makes coitus painful	Vaginal suppositories or creams, such as miconazole, nystatin, terconazole, clotrimazole and fluconazole. Over-the-counter medication includes Monistat and Gyne-lotrimin
+Trichomoniasis	Caused by the parasite *Trichomonas vaginalis;* it is passed through sexual contact, or less frequently by towels, toilet seats, or bathtubs used by an infected person	24 hours in men; 2–3 days in women	Women: a white or yellow vaginal discharge with an unpleasant odor; vulva is sore and irritated Men: often asymptomatic with only mild itching and burning during urination and a white discharge from the penis	Oral metronidazole (Flagyl) for all cases except pregnant women
+Chlamydia	Caused by *Chlamydia trachomatis,* it is passed through sexual contact, or less frequently by fingers from one body site to another	7–28 days	Women: asymptomatic until condition invades upper reproductive tract leading to PID (see below). Complications: ectopic pregnancies, postpartum endometritis, spontaneous abortion, premature labor, blindness or death in a newborn Men: a watery discharge, burning during urination, rectal pain, groin pain, fever, chills, and/or a sense of heaviness in the affected testicle(s), inflammation of scrotal skin, and a small hard, painful swelling at the bottom of the testicle	Tetracycline, doxycycline in men and nonpregnant women; erythromycin for pregnant women and others who cannot use tetracycline
+Gonorrhea ("clap")	Caused by *Neisseria gonorrhea,* it spreads through sexual contact	1–5 days in men; 2 weeks in women	Women: asymptomatic until PID develops; a green or yellowish discharge may be present. Complications include sterility and ectopic pregnancy Men: a pungent, thick, milky yellow or greenish discharge, and a burning sensation during urination. Complications include unilateral scrotal pain, malaise, headache	Ceftriaxone, spectinomycin, and penicillin drugs amoxicillin or ampicillin

(continued)

Table 16–1. Common Sexually Transmitted Diseases (STDs). *(continued)*

STD	Transmission	Incubation	Symptoms	Treatment
+Pelvic inflammatory disease (PID)	Caused by multiple infections including chlamydia and gonorrhea. Risk factors include less than 25 years of age, multiple partners, excessive douching and use of feminine hygiene sprays, and lower tract infections	Results from complications of other infections	Chronic lower abdominal pain that increases sharply with exercise, vaginal discharge, menstrual dysfunction, fever, headache, nausea, vomiting. Complications include ectopic pregnancy and sterility	Must treat the initial cause; may include injections of ceftriaxone or cefoxitin, followed by 10 days of oral doxycycline
+Nongonococcal urethritis (NGU)	Most commonly caused by *Chlamydia trachomatis* and *Urea-plasma urealyticum,* but may also result from other sources. Passed through coitus	7–28 days, but may disappear after 2–3 months	Women: asymptomatic; may have mild itching, burning on urination and a slight vaginal discharge of pus Men: a penile discharge and burning during urination	Tetracycline, doxycycline, temafloxacin, or erythromycin
+Syphilis	Caused by the spiral-shaped bacterium *Treponema pallidum,* it is spread from open lesions through penile-vaginal, oral-genital, or genital-anal contact	10–90 days with infected individuals contagious during the early stages of the disease and during the first year of the latent stage	*Primary stage:* a painless ulcer or chancre is visible at the site of entry. In men, usually on the glans of penis, penile shaft, or scrotum. In women, on the inner vaginal walls, cervix, or labia *Secondary stage* (6 weeks to 6 months): the chancre disappears and a low-grade fever, sore throat, swollen glands, and a skin rash may develop over the entire body or on the palm of the hands and soles of the feet *Latent stage* (several months to a lifetime): there may be no observable symptoms *Tertiary stage* (3–40 years): heart failure, blindness, mental disturbance, among others, and eventual death	In the first year, a single intramuscular injection of benzathine penicillin, doxycycline, tetracycline, or erythromycin. After 1 year, 3 successive weekly intramuscular injections are used
*Herpes	Oral herpes virus (HSV-1) is spread primarily by nongenital contact including orogenital sexual habits. Genital herpes virus (HSV-2) is transmitted primarily by vaginal, anal, or oral-genital intercourse, but can be transmitted through auto-inoculation (touching the lesion, then scratching or rubbing elsewhere)	3–5 days; occasionally less than 24 hours	Small, painful red bumps (papules) appear on the genitals (genital herpes) or mouth (oral herpes). Papules become painful blisters that eventually rupture to form wet, open sores that form a yellow crust and heal within the next 10 days. Other symptoms include vaginal discharge, fever, muscle aches, swollen lymph nodes in the groin, and headache	No known cure; oral or intravenous acyclovir (Zovirax) may reduce symptoms, promote healing, and suppress recurrent outbreaks

Table 16–1. Common Sexually Transmitted Diseases (STDs). *(continued)*

STD	Transmission	Incubation	Symptoms	Treatment
*Genital warts	Caused by the *human papilloma virus,* it spreads primarily through vaginal, anal, or orogenital sexual interaction	3 weeks to 18 months (3 months average)	On dry skin, warts appear hard and yellow-gray. In moist regions, warts appear soft pinkish-red with a cauliflower-like appearance	Topical agents of podophyllin, trichloroacetic acid, and a 5-fluorouracil cream, or cauterization, freezing, surgical removal, or vaporization by carbon dioxide laser
*Viral hepatitis (See Table 16-2)				
*Acquired immuno-deficiency syndrome (AIDS)	HIV has only been found to be transmitted in blood, semen, and vaginal secretions through sexual contact or needle sharing among IV drug users or steroid users	Unknown	Varies depending on the degree to which the immune system is impaired. Symptoms include fever, night sweats, fatigue, weight loss, white spots in the mouth, persistent dry cough, swollen lymph nodes, diarrhea and/or bloody stools, atypical bruising or bleeding, blotches or bumps on or under the skin, and severe headache	At present, there is no effective cure or vaccine. Therapy focuses on controlling the symptoms, azidothymidine (AZT) being the most common

+   Can be successfully treated if recognized early
*   Symptoms may be treated, but no effective cure is available

Table 16–2. Major Viruses Known to Cause Hepatitis in Humans.

	Hepatitis A	Hepatitis B	Hepatitis C	Hepatitis D	Hepatitis E
Virus group	Picornavirus	Hepadnavirus	Pesti/Flavivirus	Plant virus-like	Calcivirus-like
Genetic material	RNA	DNA	RNA	RNA	RNA
Transmitted	Fecal-oral	Blood-borne Vertical Sexual	Blood-borne Vertical Sexual?	Blood-borne	Fecal-oral
Incubation Period	2–6 weeks	2–6 months	4–20 weeks	3–12 weeks	3–7 weeks
Chronicity	No	Yes	Yes	Yes	Yes
Special features	Ig-prophylaxis effective	Pre- and post - exposure prophylaxis available. Associated with hepatocellular carcinoma	Asymptomatic in many; main cause of post-transfusion hepatitis	Co-infection with hepatitis B or infection super-imposed on chronic hepatitis B	High mortality in pregnant women. Large epidemics associated with contaminated water supplies

Hepatitis B (HBV) is the most common form of viral hepatitis and is transmitted via blood or blood products, semen, vaginal secretions, and saliva

A noticeable sign is a yellowing of the whites of the eyes, and a yellowish, or jaundiced, skin appearance in light-complexioned individuals

Currently there is no specific drug therapy to cure hepatitis, although there is a vaccine for immunization against the virus

Retroviruses
Any virus of the family Retroviridae known to reverse the usual order of reproduction within the cells they infect

The greatest number of AIDS cases is related to the HIV-1 virus

(HBV) is the most common form of viral hepatitis and has an incubation period of 45 to 160 days. HBV is transmitted via blood or blood products (post-transfusion hepatitis), semen, vaginal secretions, and saliva. Manual, oral, or penile stimulation of the anus are practices strongly associated with the spread of this virus. Hepatitis C (HCV) is transmitted primarily via blood or blood products, and less frequently through sexual intercourse and saliva. HCV has a similar incubation period to HBV, and is largely responsible for post-transfusion hepatitis (PTH) and development of primary liver cancer (13,14).

Hepatitis primarily attacks the liver, severely impairing function. Early symptoms include mild flu-like symptoms, such as poor appetite, nausea, dizziness, diarrhea, general muscle and joint pain, fatigue, and headaches. As the condition progresses, high fever, vomiting, severe abdominal pain, and dark urine will be present. Among the most notable signs is a yellowing of the whites of the eyes, and a yellowish, or jaundiced, skin appearance in light-complected individuals. Hepatitis may increase the risk for developing cancer of the liver and, in rare cases, is fatal.

Currently there is no specific drug therapy for the various types of viral hepatitis A and B. Bed-rest and adequate fluid intake can prevent dehydration, but the disease must run its course. Chronic hepatitis C does respond to therapy with interferon alfa-2b (15). The vaccine immune globulin (IG) can provide protection before and after exposure to HAV. Immune globulin B (IGB) can prevent hepatitis B, and should be administered to individuals who may be at risk for coming in contact with the virus. These risk groups include: (1) health care workers who are exposed to blood, including athletic trainers, nurses, and physicians; (2) staff and residents of institutions for the developmentally disabled; (3) staff and patients in kidney dialysis

units; (4) gay men; (5) sexually-active heterosexuals with multiple partners; and (6) recipients of blood products on a regular basis (**Table 16-3**). Although not specifically mentioned, coaches, referees, officials, and recreational sport supervisors should also be vaccinated, since they are often first on the scene of an acute injury involving hemorrhage. In 1992 this vaccine became a standard childhood immunization.

Acquired Immunodeficiency Syndrome (AIDS)

AIDS results from the viral infection *human immunodeficiency virus* (HIV). HIV falls within a special category of viruses called **retroviruses**, that is, they reverse the usual order of reproduction within cells they infect. The first virus identified and diagnosed in 1981, and the one responsible for the greatest number of AIDS cases, is HIV-1. HIV-2, diagnosed in 1987, causes AIDS in some but not all people it infects. There have been case studies where individuals have developed AIDS-like symptoms but did not test positive for either HIV-1 or HIV-2, leading some experts to speculate on a possible new HIV strain.

In 1992, most cases (50.8%) were attributed to transmission of the human immunodeficiency virus among homosexual/bisexual men; the number of cases attributed to injecting-drug-use (IDU) accounted for nearly one fourth of reported cases (16). These figures represent a decline in the number of reported cases in homosexual/bisexual men, and an increase (17.1%) in heterosexual contact (16). In the United States, high risk groups include intravenous drug users, gay men, people with blood disorders who require frequent blood transfusions or use of blood products, female and male prostitutes, and anyone who has resided in Haiti or central Africa (**Table 16-4**). A sexual partner of anyone in these groups

---

Table 16–3. Individuals at Risk for Exposure to the Hepatitis Virus.

- Health care workers who are exposed to blood, including athletic trainers, student athletic trainers, nurses, and physicians
- Staff and residents of institutions for the developmentally disabled
- Staff and patients in kidney dialysis units
- Gay men
- Sexually active heterosexuals with multiple partners
- Recipients of blood products on a regular basis

Table 16–4. Individuals at Risk for Exposure to the HIV Virus.

- Intravenous drug users
- Gay men
- People with blood disorders who require frequent blood transfusions or the use of blood products
- Female and male prostitutes
- Anyone who has resided in Haiti or central Africa
- Heterosexual women and men who:
  have anal intercourse
  have multiple sexual partners
  have multiple contacts with an infected partner
  use oral contraceptives

is also viewed as a high risk individual. In addition, risk factors for heterosexual transmission of HIV to women include anal intercourse, multiple sexual partners, multiple contacts with an infected partner, and the use of oral contraceptives (17).

HIV virus has been isolated in saliva, semen, cervical and vaginal secretions, tears, breast milk, amniotic fluid, brain tissue, cerebrospinal fluid, alveolar fluid, urine, serum, and blood (18). Currently, HIV has only been found to be transmitted in blood, semen, and vaginal secretions. Transmission through blood or blood products can occur with transfusions or through blood-contaminated needles shared by intravenous drug users or steroid users. Since 1985 all donated blood is screened and heat-treated to inactivate the virus (19). Currently, HIV infection accounts for less than 1% of the risk of death from infected blood transfusions, while hepatitis B and non-A and non-B hepatitis account for 97 to 98% of the risk of death from infected blood transfusions (19).

The HIV virus attacks and destroys several cells in the body's immune system, particularly the lymphocyte known as the helper T-cell. In a healthy individual, these cells stimulate the immune system to fight disease. In an infected individual, a gradual deterioration of the immune system leaves the body vulnerable to a variety of infections and cancers, such as herpes, oral candidiasis, pneumonia, encephalitis, cytomegalovirus, tuberculosis, meningitis, retinitis, and dementia. In 1993 the CDC broadened its definition of AIDS to include HIV-infected individuals who have 200 or fewer CD4 or T-cells per cubic millimeter of blood. (Normal levels are about 1000 per cubic millimeter).

In sports, the risk of AIDS is rare, although AIDS was recently reported in a body builder who injected anabolic-androgenic steroids into his body with a contaminated needle (20). In boxing, football, or wrestling, where participants may have a bloody nose or open cuts, close contact with the competitor may also pose a health risk. Repeatedly using blood-stained towels after injury clearly establish an environment for transmission of the HIV virus and many other highly contagious infections, such as hepatitis B, hepatitis C, herpes, and cytomegalovirus (CVM), a condition where cells or organs become enlarged (21). **Field Strategy 16-2** is a position statement by the American Academy of Pediatrics concerning HIV and AIDS in an athletic setting.

The term "HIV disease" describes all manifestations of the infections prior to the development of AIDS, whereas AIDS is the final, fatal stage of HIV infection. Signs and symptoms vary, depending on the degree to which the immune system is impaired. Common symptoms include persistent fever or night sweats, extreme fatigue not explained by physical activity or mental depression, unexplained weight loss, white spots or unusual blemishes in the mouth, persistent, dry cough unrelated to smoking, persistent, unexplained diarrhea, easy bruising or atypical bleeding from any body opening, blotches or bumps on or under the skin, and persistent severe headaches (18). Some researchers have suggested that HIV disease is more severe in women than in men and runs a swifter course (12). **Table 16-5** lists these and other common symptoms that may indicate the presence of the HIV virus.

To date there is no effective cure or vaccine for AIDS. Few drugs have been

HIV has only been proven to be transmitted in blood, semen, and vaginal secretions

HIV infection accounts for less than 1% of the risk of death from infected blood transfusions, while hepatitis B and non-A and non-B hepatitis account for 97 to 98%

Sharing water bottles and using blood-stained towels from an injury can transmit the HIV virus and other infections, such as hepatitis B, hepatitis C, herpes, and cytomegalovirus

Field Strategy 16–2. American Academy of Pediatrics. Human Immunodeficiency Virus [Acquired Immunodeficiency Syndrome (AIDS) Virus] in the Athletic Setting

1. Athletes infected with HIV should be allowed to participate in all competitive sports. This advice must be reconsidered if transmission of HIV is found to occur in the sports setting
2. A physician counseling a known HIV-infected athlete in a sport involving blood exposure, such as wrestling or football, should inform him of the theoretical risk of contagion to others and strongly encourage him to consider another sport
3. The physician should respect an HIV-infected athlete's right to confidentiality. This includes not disclosing the patient's status of infection to the participants or the staff of athletic programs
4. All athletes should be made aware that the athletic program is operating under the policies in Recommendations 1 and 3
5. Routine testing of athletes for HIV infection is not indicated
6. The following precautions should be adopted:
   a. Skin exposed to blood or other body fluids visibly contaminated with blood should be cleaned as promptly as is practical, preferably with soap and warm water. Skin antiseptics (e.g., alcohol) or moist towelettes may be used if soap and water are not available
   b. Even though good hand-washing is an adequate precaution, water-impervious gloves (latex, vinyl, etc.) should be available for staff to use if desired when handling blood or other body fluids visibly contaminated with blood. Gloves should be worn by individuals with nonintact skin. Hands should be washed after glove removal
   c. If blood or other body fluids visibly contaminated with blood are present on the surface, the bleach solution made for immediate use is as follows: 1 part bleach in 10 parts of water, or 1 tablespoon bleach to 1 pint water (hereafter called "fresh bleach solution"). For example, athletic equipment (e.g., wrestling mats) visibly contaminated with blood should be wiped clean with fresh bleach solution and allowed to dry before using
   d. Emergency care should not be delayed because gloves or other protective equipment are not available
   e. If the care-giver wishes to wear gloves and none are readily available, a bulky towel may be used to cover the wound until an off-the-field location is reached where gloves can be used during more definitive treatment
   f. Each coach and athletic trainer should receive training in first aid and emergency care and be provided with the necessary supplies to treat open wounds
   g. For those sports with direct body contact and other sports where bleeding may be expected to occur:
      1. If a skin lesion is observed, it should be cleansed immediately with a suitable antiseptic and covered securely
      2. If a bleeding wound occurs, the individual's participation should be interrupted until the bleeding has been stopped and the wound is both cleansed with antiseptic and covered securely or occluded
   h. Saliva does not transmit HIV. However, because of potential fear on the part of those providing cardiopulmonary resuscitation, breathing (Ambu) bags and oral airways for use during cardiopulmonary resuscitation should be available in athletic settings for those who prefer not to give mouth-to-mouth resuscitation
   i. Coaches and athletic trainers should receive training in prevention of HIV transmission in the athletic setting; they should then help implement the recommendations suggested above

Committee on Sports Medicine and Fitness, 1990 to 1991

approved by the Federal Drug Administration (FDA) for use in controlling the symptoms, azidothymidine (AZT) being the most commonly prescribed. Oral fluconazole is used to treat AIDS-related meningitis (22).

The best defense against the virus is education and prevention through behavioral changes. Mandatory testing of individuals for the HIV virus is not a viable alternative to educational programs. Behavioral changes

Table 16–5. Common Signs and Symptoms Indicating the HIV Virus.

- Persistent fever or night sweats
- Unexplained weight loss and loss of appetite
- Extreme fatigue not explained by physical activity or mental depression
- White spots or unusual blemishes in the mouth, or a whitish coating on the tongue
- A persistent dry cough unrelated to smoking
- Persistent unexplained diarrhea or bloody stools
- Easy bruising or atypical bleeding from any body opening
- Blotches or bumps on or under the skin
- Persistent severe headaches

should include maintaining a monogamous relationship, practicing safer sex through regular use of dental dams and condoms with Nonoxynol 9 spermicide, using sterile needles, and practicing universal precautions in dealing with blood and blood products.

In the athletic training room or clinic setting, specific steps should be taken to prevent contact with the virus and were outlined in **Table 3-1**. Latex gloves should be worn when touching any blood, bodily fluids, skin that is not intact, such as abrasions, and in handling materials that are soiled with blood or bodily fluids. Gloves should be worn for routine procedures such as caring for bleeding wounds, blisters, pustules or boils, and changing dressings. If a wound could potentially generate droplets of fluid, protective masks and eyewear should be worn to prevent aerosolization of fluids into the mouth, nose and eyes of the health care provider. Immediately after accidental exposure, any contaminated areas should be thoroughly cleansed with a 1:10 bleach solution. Hands should be washed thoroughly after gloves are removed. Needles, scalpels, and other "sharp" sticks, gloves, and soiled bandages should be disposed of in a marked biohazard container.

Health care workers with open lesions should refrain from direct contact with individuals until the lesion is healed. Saliva, although not presently implicated in HIV transmission, necessitates the use of oral airways should mouth-to-mouth rescue breathing be needed. Any soiled linen or towels should be bagged separately and washed in detergent and bleach. Soiled bandages or dressings should be disposed of in a biohazard receptacle. At athletic events, universal precautions should be implemented when dealing with any situation where bodily fluids or blood may be encountered.

For further information and publications on AIDS, contact:
National AIDS Hotline (CDC)
1-800-342-AIDS
1-800-344-7432 (Spanish)
1-800-243-7889 (Deaf Access, TTY)
National AIDS Information Clearing House (for AIDS publications/educational material) 1-800-458-5231

The basketball player complained of painful urination and open sores on the penis. This individual should be referred to a physician and tested for possible STDs. Furthermore, he should be counseled to avoid any sexual activity with another individual until seen by the physician.

MENSTRUAL IRREGULARITIES

A lean sixteen-year-old distance runner has reported she has not had a menstrual period in three months and is concerned she may be pregnant. What other menstrual irregularities could account for this absence of menses?

There continues to be a high participation rate of girls and women at all levels of sport. Many of these participants will, at one time or another, be affected by menstrual irregularities. Research is just beginning to explore the effects of conditioning and training on gynecological function, yet much needs to be done. Menstrual irregularities may include dysmenorrhea, luteal phase deficiency, anovulation, and exercise-associated amenorrhea.

Dysmenorrhea

Dysmenorrhea, or menstrual cramps, is usually caused by the overproduction of prostaglandins, a group of chemicals produced in the body. Uterine prostaglandins

Latex gloves should be worn when touching any blood, bodily fluids, skin that is not intact, and in handling materials that are soiled with blood or bodily fluids

Surfaces that are contaminated with bodily fluids or blood should be cleansed with a 1:10 bleach solution

Health care workers with open lesions should refrain from direct contact with individuals until the lesion is healed

Dysmenorrhea
Difficult or painful menstruation; menstrual cramps

Oligomenorrhea
Infrequent menstrual cycles

Amenorrhea
Absence or abnormal cessation of menstruation

Osteopenia
Decreased calcification or density of bone

cause the muscles of the uterus to contract. Under most conditions the contractions are minor and go unnoticed. With more severe contractions, abdominal aching or pain results. The condition usually begins with the onset of menses and continues during the first days of a woman's period. Other symptoms include bloating, nausea, vomiting, diarrhea, headache, breast tenderness, fatigue, irritability, or nervousness (23). The condition is very common in adolescent girls and is responsible for a high degree of absenteeism in school (23).

Relief for mild to moderate discomfort can be gained through a variety of methods. Regular exercise and a diet high in fluids and fiber and low in salt can alleviate bloating and swelling caused by water retention. Over-the-counter medications, such as Midol, Advil, Ibuprofen, aspirin, or Tylenol can relieve pain and cramping. Severe or persistent discomfort may necessitate physician referral to rule out pelvic inflammatory disease (PID), benign uterine tumors, obstruction of the cervical opening and endometriosis, a condition whereby endometrial cells from the uterine lining implant themselves in the abdominal cavity.

Luteal Phase Deficiency

The luteal phase of menses extends from ovulation until the onset of the next menstrual period, normally about 14 days. The hormone progesterone is produced only after ovulation. During this period both estrogen and progesterone levels are high. Luteal deficiency is characterized by a shortened luteal phase length and insufficient progesterone production (24). The menstrual cycle is usually normal, however, the cycle occurs more frequently. Research on the condition is lacking. Some researchers postulate this condition is the first stage in the development of amenorrhea (25). Others have found it to be normal for active women (26). Adverse conditions related to luteal phase deficiency include infertility, recurrent spontaneous abortions, lower bone density, and endometrial hyperplasia (overgrowth of the endometrium) and adrenocarcinoma (24).

Anovulation

Anovulation is associated with chronic, unopposed estrogen production that leads to continuous endometrial stimulation and lower levels of progesterone. Several different patterns of irregular bleeding range from very

short (less than 21 days) to long cycles with 35 to 150 days between bleeding (27). The latter pattern is referred to as **oligomenorrhea**. Bleeding is unpredictable and can be very heavy (menorrhagia), leading to iron depletion and anemia, both of which affect athletic performance. Monthly progestin therapy will mature the endometrium, cause regular bleeding, and protect against endometrial hyperplasia (24). Oral contraceptives may also control the menstrual cycle.

Exercise-Associated Amenorrhea

Amenorrhea is the absence of menstruation and is more prevalent among athletes, particularly runners, than the general population. Amenorrhea is a symptom, not a disease, and has been linked to prepubertal exercise, premature ovarian failure, central nervous system tumors, infections, pituitary or hypothalamic hormonal imbalances, chronic diseases, and malnutrition (28). Delayed menarche results in prolonging the hypoestrogenic state of menses, which can lead to **osteopenia** (bone mineral loss) at an age when bone density should be increasing (29). Scoliosis and increased risk of stress fractures may also result (26,28).

There are two types of amenorrhea, primary and secondary. Primary amenorrhea is the failure to begin menstruation at puberty or by age 16. Secondary amenorrhea involves the disruption of an established menstrual cycle resulting in the absence of menstruation for 3 to 12 consecutive menstrual periods. This can result from pregnancy or dysfunction in the ovaries, endometrium, pituitary gland, or hypothalamus. A recent study reported that smoking one or more packs of cigarettes per day, multiple binge-eating behaviors combined with laxative use or self-induced vomiting, and weight fluctuation due to weight control in an adolescent population contributed to secondary amenorrhea (30).

Exercise associated amenorrhea is a form of hypothalamic amenorrhea, and has been reported in women participating in virtually every sport. Amenorrhea has been shown to affect up to 50% of competitive runners, 44% of ballet dancers, 25% of noncompetitive runners, and 12% of cyclists and swimmers (30). Drinkwater defines the amenorrheic athlete under the following criteria (32):

1. Individual has had three or less periods in the past year (none in the last six months)

2. Regular menses began within 18 months of menarche
3. Training began before the onset of amenorrhea
4. No birth control pills were taken in the six months prior to the onset of amenorrhea
5. No signs of pregnancy, ovarian failure, pituitary tumor, hyperandrogenism, or hyperprolactinemia are present

It is commonly accepted that amenorrhea and decreased estrogen predispose women to reduced bone density, leading to increased stress fractures, particularly in the lumbar vertebrae and lower extremity, and increased musculoskeletal injuries (25,28,33). Within the first three months of amenorrhea, a woman should be fully evaluated to rule out pregnancy, counseled on the risks of bone density loss, and encouraged to alter training regimens. Currently, decreasing training, increasing food intake, or hormonal therapy has been used to manage menstrual dysfunctions.

Research suggests that menses returns in some amenorrheic women after gaining weight or decreasing exercise, or both (33). This is accomplished by reducing the number of training days, mileage, or intensity. Diet should be evaluated to ensure adequate caloric intake matches high energy output. Hormone therapy including oral contraceptives and cyclic estrogen/progesterone therapy does not increase bone mass, but prevents further bone loss, vaginal and breast atrophy, and osteopenia. However, individuals may choose not to take oral contraceptives because of adverse side effects, such as increased incidence of vaginitis, weight gain, acne, breast tenderness, or mood alterations. Women who remain amenorrheic should be examined annually.

Secondary amenorrhea is common in adolescent distance runners. However, the woman should be referred to a physician to rule out pregnancy and then counseled accordingly.

BIRTH CONTROL AND SPORT PARTICIPATION

Many women use oral contraceptives for birth control. Think for a minute about what implications this may have on athletic performance. What adverse effects might occur?

IUDs (intrauterine devices) and oral contraceptives are two birth control methods used by women who participate in sport. IUDs are small plastic objects inserted into the uterus through the vaginal canal and cervix (**Figure 16-9**). Once inserted, the device prevents implantation of the fertilized ovum in the uterine lining. Discomfort, cramping, bleeding, or pain may occur during insertion, but these symptoms usually clear up within a few days. In addition, 5 to 20% of women who use IUDs expel the device within the first year, typically during menstruation (35).

The most serious complication with an IUD is an increased risk for PID if bacteria is introduced into the upper genital tract during insertion. This normally occurs within the first four months of use. The attached string may also serve as a pathway for bacteria (35). Other conditions linked to IUDs include: history of ectopic pregnancies, active PID, chlamydia, or gonorrhea, current or suspected pregnancy, or conditions such as endometriosis, anemia, heavy menstrual flow or cramping, a small or malformed uterus, uterine fibroids, and heart disease.

Intrauterine devices have been associated with increased prevalence of heavy menstrual bleeding and dysmenorrhea, each of which can affect sport performance (37). For those women who choose IUDs in place of oral contraceptives or other birth control methods, however, this highly effective contraceptive protection may outweigh the discomfort.

Oral contraceptives (OCs) are used by fewer women athletes than the general population. Much of this is due to early studies that reported decreased maximal oxygen uptake, decreased isometric strength and endurance time, and reduction in mitochondrial citrate (an oxidative enzyme) with OC use (38). However, recent studies have reported that certain adverse effects are counteracted by exercise (39,40). The pills essentially prohibit ovulation, reduce menstrual cramps, and decrease the amount and duration of the menstrual flow. Medications, such as antibiotics, analgesics, antihistamines, and drugs used to treat tuberculosis, epilepsy, and depression may interfere with the effectiveness of the pill (40).

Regular exercise is known to increase protective high-density lipoprotein cholesterol, reduce deleterious low-density lipoprotein cholesterol, lower total triglyceride levels, and activate the fibrinolytic system responsible for converting fibrin to soluble products.

Amenorrhea and decreased estrogen predispose women to reduced bone density, leading to increased stress fractures and musculoskeletal injuries

Decreasing training, increasing food intake, or hormonal therapy can successfully manage many menstrual dysfunctions

Hormone therapy does not increase bone mass but prevents further bone loss, vaginal and breast atrophy, and osteopenia

A major complication with an IUD is an increased risk for pelvic inflammatory disease if bacteria is introduced into the upper genital tract

IUDs have been associated with increased prevalence of heavy menstrual bleeding and dysmenorrhea, each of which can affect athletic performance

Oral contraceptives prohibit ovulation, reduce menstrual cramps, and decrease the amount and duration of the menstrual flow

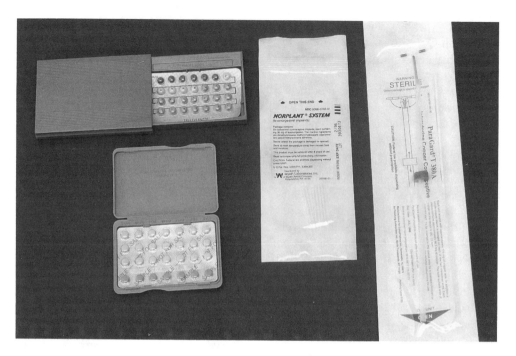

Fig. 16.9: Intrauterine devices (IUDs) and oral contraceptives are two common methods of birth control used by sexually-active women. The Norplant, recently approved in the United States, has flexible capsules that are implanted under the skin of a woman's upper arm. These capsules release the synthetic progestin gradually into the blood stream over a five-year period to prevent contraception.

In addition, most trained women have lower arterial blood pressures, lower body fat, and higher lean body weight and do not smoke, all factors that put sedentary women at risk for complications (38). As such, for healthy active young women, benefits of oral contraceptives outweigh the risks.

💡 *Oral contraceptives can increase risk for certain conditions, however, low-dose oral contraceptives and regular exercise can offset many of the risks, providing a safe, effective birth control method for the active woman.*

PREGNANCY AND SPORT PARTICIPATION

❓ *A recreational tennis player is three months pregnant. She plays at least three times a week. Is there a possibility that her body's physiological needs during exercise may harm the fetus? What actions can avoid complications?*

The impact of exercise on an active pregnant woman and her developing fetus is an area of concern, particularly when chemicals and nutrients pass freely in placental blood flow. Certainly any factors that compromise this fetal blood supply would be of major con-cern in counseling a pregnant woman regarding exercise during pregnancy. Few controlled studies on the effects of physical exercise on uterine circulation and fetal development have been completed for obvious ethical reasons. Much of what is known is based on animal studies.

In early pregnancy blood volume and cardiac output is increased, and arterial blood pressure is slightly decreased until week 22 of gestation. After that, blood pressure slowly increases to prepregnancy levels (34). As pregnancy progresses, the uterus expands in the abdominal cavity, elevating the diaphragm. The thoracic cage compensates by increasing its dimensions so that more air can be inspired. The respiratory rate does not change, however, tidal volume gradually increases. Maximum oxygen uptake increases only slightly due to enhanced maternal costs of renal, cardiac, and respiratory work (34).

Gains in body weight and fat accumulation are an obvious adaptation to pregnancy and can have some effect on weight-bearing exercise. The hormones progesterone and relaxin increase joint laxity, making articulations widen and become more mobile during the later stages of pregnancy (34). Ballistic movements (bouncing) must be avoided during daily activities and exercise.

Blood volume and cardiac output is increased during pregnancy, and arterial blood pressure is slightly decreased until week 22 of gestation

Gains in body weight and fat accumulation during pregnancy can affect weight-bearing exercise

Postural adaptations to compensate for the weight of the uterus lead to increased lordosis and upper spine extension. The woman's center of gravity shifts upward and forward, often leading to lower back pain. Exercises to strengthen the abdominal and hip extensors (hamstrings, gluteus maximus) as well as relaxing and/or stretching the erector spinae and hip flexors (iliopsoas, rectus femoris) can relieve some of this pain. Proper lifting techniques to relieve stress on the low back area should be incorporated in daily activities.

Studies have shown that oxygen uptake by the uteroplacental tissues and fetus during exercise is maintained by a facilitated unloading of oxygen from the available maternal blood supply. For a previously active, healthy woman during an uncomplicated pregnancy, moderate aerobic exercise does not produce circulatory alterations that compromise fetal oxygen supply. In looking at fetal development, fetoplacental growth, prematurity, fetal stress/distress, and condition during labor and at birth, it was found that women who exercise regularly do not experience an increase in abortion, congenital abnormalities, abnormal placentation, premature rupture of the membranes, or preterm labor (41). Although increases were found in fetal heart rate after exercise, no adverse effects were seen.

Pregnant women should be aware of the potential for fetal hypoglycemia during exercise. Under prolonged exercise, the maternal blood sugar may decrease. The pregnant woman needs to consume extra calories to meet the demands of pregnancy and if she exercises, additional calories are needed. In addition, after the fifth month of pregnancy maternal hypotension can exist if she exercises in the supine position. In this position the uterus compresses the vena cava, slowing venous return and causing a decrease in fetal circulation as well as maternal hypotension. Some physicians believe that women in good physical condition do not have an increased risk and can exercise briefly without adverse results. Medical conditions where exercise is contraindicated include cardiovascular disease, respiratory disease, thyrotoxicosis, infection, anemia, prior poor pregnancy results such as miscarriage, hypertension, uterine bleeding, premature rupture of membranes, and anticoagulant therapy.

The American College of Obstetricians and Gynecologists has established guidelines for exercise during pregnancy. These can be seen in **Field Strategy 16-3**. Many physicians, however, believe the guidelines do not take into account the woman's prepregnancy fitness level. Exercise programs for the pregnant woman need to be individualized. All women should consult their physician about their exercise program. It is not recommended that a vigorous exercise program such as jogging be instituted during pregnancy.

Aerobic classes may be modified to decrease the amount of ballistic movements and time spent in exercising in the supine position. A 5 to 10 minute warm-up, low or no impact aerobics, and careful monitoring of heart rate followed by a cool-down and stretching period is recommended. Weight training with light weights and higher repetitions can be continued during pregnancy when the goal is strength maintenance, not gain. Proper lifting and breathing technique, such as exhaling during exertion, must be maintained. Free-weight exercises that place the joints in traction, thereby stressing the ligaments, should be avoided. Weight-loading activities, such as volleyball, basketball, or horseback riding should be avoided. In running programs, distance and intensity of the workout will need to be decreased as the pregnancy progresses. **Table 16-6** summarizes some running problems of pregnant women and suggested recommendations (42).

The recreational tennis player should consult her physician about exercise during pregnancy. The physician will be able to identify any factors or health conditions that may compromise fetal blood supply during exercise as the pregnancy progresses.

SUMMARY

Injuries to the reproductive organs in sport participation are rare, particularly in the female. In the male, direct blows to the groin can injure external genitalia, leading to a hydrocele, varicocele, or hematocele. Sexually transmitted diseases, such as hepatitis and AIDS, may also be transmitted via blood or blood products and remain a major concern for all health care providers. Any individual who experiences a vaginal or penile discharge, itching or burning during urination, or has open lesions in the genital or oral region should seek medical treatment imme-

Postural adaptations to compensate for the weight of the uterus lead to increased lordosis and upper spine extension

Pregnant women should be aware of the potential for fetal hypoglycemia during exercise

Exercise programs for the pregnant woman need to be individualized

Field Strategy 16–3. Guidelines for Exercise During Pregnancy and Postpartum.

1. During pregnancy, women can continue to exercise and derive health benefits even from mild-to-moderate exercise routines. Regular exercise (at least three times per week) is preferable to intermittent activity

2. Women should avoid exercise in the supine position after the first trimester. Such a position is associated with decreased cardiac output in most pregnant women; because the remaining cardiac output will be preferentially distributed away from splanchnic beds (including the uterus) during vigorous exercise, such regimens are best avoided during pregnancy. Prolonged periods of motionless standing should also be avoided

3. Women should be aware of the decreased oxygen available for aerobic exercise during pregnancy. They should be encouraged to modify the intensity of their exercise according to maternal symptoms. Pregnant women should stop exercising when fatigued, and not exercise to exhaustion. Weight-bearing exercises may, under some circumstances, be continued at intensities similar to those prior to pregnancy throughout pregnancy. Nonweight-bearing exercises, such as cycling or swimming, will minimize the risk of injury and facilitate the continuation of exercise during pregnancy

4. Morphologic changes in pregnancy should serve as a relative contraindication to types of exercise in which loss of balance could be detrimental to maternal or fetal well-being, especially in the third trimester. Further, any type of exercise involving the potential for even mild abdominal trauma should be avoided

5. Pregnancy requires an additional 300 kcal/d in order to maintain metabolic homeostasis. Thus, women who exercise during pregnancy should be particularly careful to ensure an adequate diet

6. Pregnant women who exercise in the first trimester should augment heat dissipation by ensuring adequate hydration, appropriate clothing, and optimal environmental surroundings during exercise

7. Many of the physiologic and morphologic changes of pregnancy persist 4–6 weeks postpartum. Thus, prepregnancy exercise routines should be resumed gradually based on a woman's physical capability

Contraindications to exercise include:
- Pregnancy-induced hypertension
- Preterm rupture of membranes
- Preterm labor during the prior or current pregnancy or both
- Incomplete cervix/cerclage
- Persistent second- or third-trimester bleeding
- Intrauterine growth retardation
- In addition, women with certain other medical or obstetric conditions, including chronic hypertension or active thyroid, cardiac, vascular, or pulmonary disease, should be evaluated carefully in order to determine whether an exercise program is appropriate

diately. Many STDs can be cured if early treatment is sought; however, those associated with viruses cannot be cured. Health care providers should be immunized against hepatitis and use universal safety precautions in the clinic and training room to prevent the spread of contagious diseases.

Menstrual disorders, such as dysmenorrhea and amenorrhea, can affect the sport participant. Amenorrhea in particular has been associated with reduced bone-mineral density, leading to an increased incidence of stress fractures and postural deviations. Evidence points to the fact that sport participation is not adversely affected by the use of oral contraceptives and can be beneficial to the pregnant woman.

Table 16–6. Running Problems of Pregnant Women.

Problem	Recommendation
Poor balance	Slow down and run cautiously, being alert to changes in terrain. Experiment with posture changes that make you more stable while running.
Overheating and dehydration	Drink plenty of liquids prior to the run. Do not run mid-day in hot weather, but rather early morning or late evening. If you must run mid-day, run shorter distances. If you feel dizzy or nauseated, stop running and cool down.
Leg, hip, or abdominal pain	Always stretch and warm up prior to running regardless of the distance. Wear well-cushioned shoes with a very firm midsole, a straight last, and a high degree of hindfoot stability. Stop running and walk for a short distance if you have specific pain in an area rather than just mild discomfort.
Concern from others about safe exercise during the pregnancy	Educate yourself about the subject. Talk to your physician and identify problems that may arise. Exercise with other women who may have run or remained active during their pregnancy. Be assertive about exercise during pregnancy, but do it in a cautious, reasonable manner. Run with friends when you can, and keep a positive attitude.

REFERENCES

1. Munter, DW, and Faleski, EJ. 1989. Blunt scrotal trauma: Emergency department evaluation and management. Am J Emerg Med, 7(2):227–34.

2. Briner, WW, Howe, WB, and Jain, RK. 1990. Scrotal injury in a high school football player. Phys Sportsmed, 18(11):64–68.

3. Noujaim, SE, and Nagle, CE. 1989. Acute scrotal injuries in athletes: Evaluation by diagnostic imaging. Phys Sportsmed, 17(10):125–132.

4. Lund, L, and Bartolin, J. 1992. Treatment of hydrocele testis with aspiration and injection of polidocanol. J Urol, 147(4):1065–1066.

5. Fuse, H, Niskikawa, Y, Shimazaki, J, and Katayama, T. 1991. Aspiration and tetracycline sclerotherapy of hydrocele. Scand J Urol Nephrol, 25(1):5–7.

6. York, JP. 1990. Sports and the male genitourinary system: Genital injuries and sexually transmitted diseases. Phys Sportsmed, 18(10):92–100.

7. Melekos, MD, Asbach, HW, and Markou, SA. 1988. Etiology of acute scrotum in 100 boys with regard to age distribution. J Urol, 139(5):1023–1025.

8. Gianini, GD, Method, MW, and Christman, JE. 1991. Traumatic vulvar hematomas: Assessing and treating nonobstetric patients. Postgrad Med, 89(4):115–118.

9. Ramsey, ML. 1990. How I manage jock itch. Phys Sportsmed, 18(8):63–72.

10. Montero-Gei, F, and Perera, A. 1992. Therapy with fluconazole for tinea corporis, tinea cruris, and tinea pedis. Clin Infect Dis, 14(Suppl 1):S77–81.

11. Goldsmith, MF. 1993. 'Invisible' epidemic now becoming visible as HIV/AIDS pandemic reaches adolescents. JAMA, 270(1):16–19.

12. Mahoney, FJ, Farley, TA, Kelso, KY, Wilson, SA, Horan, JM, and McFarland, LM. 1992. An outbreak of hepatitis A associated with swimming in a public pool. J Infect Dis, 165(4):613–618.

13. Schvarcz, R. 1991. Chronic posttransfusion non-A, non-B hepatitis and autoimmune chronic active hepatitis—aspects on treatment, prognosis and relation to hepatitis C virus. Scand J Infec, 79(Suppl).

14. Dusheiko, GM. 1990. Hepatocellular carcinoma associated with chronic viral hepatitis. Br Med J, 46(2):492–511.

15. Keating, MR. 1992. Antiviral agents. Mayo Clin Proc, 67(2):160–178.

16. Centers for Disease Control. 1993. Update: Acquired immunodeficinecy syndrome—United States, 1992. JAMA, 270(8):930–933.

17. Williams, AB. 1992. The epidemiology, clinical manifestations and health-maintenance needs of women infected with HIV. Nurse Practit, 17(5):27, 31–37.

18. Seltzer, DG. 1993. Educating athletes on HIV disease and AIDS: The team physician's role. Phys Sportsmed, 21(1):109–115.

19. Carson, JL, Russell, LB, Taragin, MI, Sonnenberg, FA, Duff, AE, and Bauer, S. 1992. The risks of blood transfusion: The relative influence of acquired immunodeficiency syndrome and non-A, non-B hepatitis. Am J Med, 92(1):45–52.

20. Sklarek, HM, Mantovani, RP, Erens, E, Heisler, D, Niederman, MS, and Fein, AM. 1984. AIDS in a bodybuilder using anabolic steroids, letter. N Engl J Med, 311(26):1701.

21. Calabrese, LH, and Kelley, D. 1989. AIDS and athletes. Phys Sportsmed, 17(1):127–132.

22. Fairbanks, KD, and Sharp, V. 1992. AIDS update. Clinic Rev, 2(2):114–125.

23. Wilson, CA, and Keye, WR, Jr. 1989. A survey of adolescent dysmenorrhea and premenstrual symptom frequency: A model program for prevention, detection, and treatment. J Adolesc Health Care, 10(4):317–322.

24. Otis, CL. "Exercise associated amenorrhea." In Clinics in sports medicine, edited by JC Puffer, vol. 11, no. 2. Philadelphia: WB Saunders, 1992.

25. Shangold, MM. "Menstruation." In Women and exercise: Physiology and sports medicine, edited by MM Shangold and G Mirkin. Philadelphia: FA Davis, 1988.

26. Loucks, AB. 1990. Effects of exercise training on the menstrual cycle: Existence and mechanisms. Med Sci Sports Exerc, 22(3):275–280.

27. Prior, JC, Vigna, YM, Schechter, MT, and Burgess, AE. 1990. Spinal bone loss and ovulatory disturbances. N Engl J Med, 323(18):1221–1227.

28. Shangold, M, Rebar, RW, Wentz, AC, and Schiff, I. 1990. Evaluation and management of menstrual dysfunction in athletes. JAMA, 263(12):1665–1669.

29. Ayers, JWT, Gidwani, GP, Schmidt, IMV, and Gross, M. 1984. Osteopenia in hyperestrogenic young women with anorexia nervosa. Fertil Steril, 41(2):224–228.

30. Johnson, J, and Whitaker, AH. 1992. Adolescent smoking, weight changes, and binge-purge behavior: Associations with secondary amenorrhea. Am J Public Health, 82(1):47–54.

31. Worthington, G. 1991. Athletic amenorrhea: Updated review. JNATA, 26(3):270–273.

32. Drinkwater, BL. *Female endurance athletes*. Champaign, IL: Human Kinetics Publishers, 1986.

33. Lloyd, T, Triantafyllou, SJ, Baker, ER, Houts, PS, Whiteside, JA, Kalenak, A, and Stumpf, PG. 1986. Women athletes with menstrual irregularity have increased musculoskeletal injuries. Med Sci Sports Exerc, 18(4):374–379.

34. Drinkwater, BL, Nilson, K, Ott, S, and Chestnut, CH, III. 1986. Bone mineral density after resumption of menses in amenorrheic athletes. JAMA, 256(3):380–382.

35. Treiman, K, and Liskin, L. 1988. IUDs—A new look. Populat Rep, 16:1–31.

36. Woods, NF. 1987. Women's health: The menstrual cycle. Premenstrual symptoms: Another look. Public Health Reports, 102(Suppl):106–112.

37. Shangold, MM. "Gynecologic concerns in exercise and training." In *Women and exercise: Physiology and sports medicine*, edited by MM Shangold and G Mirkin. Philadelphia: FA Davis, 1988.

38. Wells, CL. *Women, sport, & performance: A physiological perspective*. Champaign, IL: Human Kinetics Publishers, 1991.

39. Gray, DP, Harding, E, and Dale E. 1983. Effects of oral contraceptive on serum lipid profiles of women runners. Fertil Steril, 39(4):510–514.

40. Szoka, P, and Edgren, R. 1988. Drug interactions with oral contraceptives: Compilation and analysis of an adverse experience report database. Fertil Steril, 49(Suppl):31–37.

41. Clapp, JF. 1991. Exercise and fetal health. J Dev Physiol, 15(1):9–14.

42. Slavine, JL, Lutter, JM, Cushman, S, and Lee, V. "Pregnancy and exercise." In *Sport Science Perspectives for Women*, edited by JL Puhl, CH Brown, and RO Voy. Champaign, IL: Human Kinetics Books, 1988.

Other Health Conditions Related to Sports

After you have completed this chapter, you should be able to:

■ Identify what impact environmental conditions such as altitude and poor air quality have on sport performance

■ Describe the signs, symptoms, and management of common respiratory tract infections

■ Describe the signs, symptoms, and management of common disorders of the gastrointestinal tract

■ Explain the physiological factors involved in diabetes, and differentiate the management of diabetic coma from insulin shock

■ Identify common contagious viral diseases

■ Describe the signs and management of an individual experiencing an epileptic seizure

■ List common substances abused by sport participants and the impact each will have on the individual's health and sport performance

■ Describe the various eating disorders and explain guidelines for safe weight loss and weight gain

There are several conditions unrelated to trauma that can influence the health of a sport participant. Environmental considerations, such as altitude and air pollution, can interfere with the body's ability to utilize oxygen at the cellular level. Respiratory tract infections can be contagious and infect the entire team. Gastrointestinal tract problems, such as indigestion, diarrhea, or constipation are common in sport participants. In addition, individuals with systemic conditions, such as diabetes mellitus, epilepsy, hypertension, or anemia may need special supervision to develop an exercise program to fit their needs. Despite education and drug testing efforts, substance abuse and eating disorders continue to be a major concern, as abuse is being seen increasingly more often in younger athletes.

This chapter begins with a discussion on environmental conditions, and the impact of altitude and air pollution on athletic performance. Next, prevalent infections or conditions of the respiratory tract and gastrointestinal system are discussed, including their signs,

symptoms, and management. Information on diabetes, epilepsy, hypertension, and anemia is then presented. Finally, an overview of substance abuse and eating disorders are discussed, relative to implications for the individual's health and sport performance.

ENVIRONMENTAL CONSIDERATIONS

The track and field team is competing in three weeks at nationals in Denver, Colorado. Because of the high altitude, what can be done to reduce the impact of altitude on the athletes' performance?

Environmental conditions can affect performance in even the best conditioned athlete. Athletic contests are often held on hot, humid days, or in cold, windy conditions where hyperthermia and hypothermia, respectively, may impact performance. These conditions were discussed in detail in Chapter 3. Other conditions, such as altitude and air quality, may also affect performance, and will be discussed here.

Hypoxia
Reduction of oxygen supply to tissue despite adequate blood flow

Altitude Disorders

The percentage of oxygen in the atmosphere at an altitude of 10,000 ft is exactly the same as that at sea level. However, the density of air decreases progressively as you ascend above sea level. The decreased partial pressure of ambient oxygen, or density of oxygen molecules, makes it more difficult to deliver oxygen to the working muscles of the body, leading to a reduction in work capacity directly proportionate to the altitude. This will have little if any effect on short bursts of energy, but can have a significant impact on sustained aerobic activities. Often the individual's body will compensate for this decrease in maximum oxygen uptake by hyperventilating or experiencing tachycardia (rapid heart beats). Stroke volume may also be reduced and fewer red blood cells will be available to transport the needed oxygen (1).

Altitude sickness is a disorder related to **hypoxia** at high altitudes. Acute mountain sickness is the mildest form of altitude sickness and will usually appear during the first few days at altitudes of about 3048 m or higher (1). There is a time lag of 6 to 36 hours between arrival at the altitude and the onset of symptoms. The symptoms are directly proportional to the rapidity of the ascent, the duration and degree of exertion, and are inversely proportional to acclimatization and physical conditioning (2). Initial symptoms include headache, dizziness, fatigue, nausea, vomiting, difficulty sleeping, dyspnea (labored respirations), and tachycardia on exertion (1,2). Appetite suppression can be severe during the early days of high altitude stay, and can result in an average reduction in energy intake of about 40% and an accompanying loss of body mass (1). Diets high in carbohydrates and low in salt can lessen the effects of altitude. In addition, acclimatization and physical conditioning can enhance altitude tolerance, reduce the severity of mountain sickness, and decrease the physical performance decrements during the early stages of altitude exposure.

For unknown reasons, some individuals at altitudes over 9,000 ft experience a severe aspect of mountain sickness, called high altitude pulmonary edema or HAPE. It may develop on the first exposure, but often develops after descent and re-ascent. The lungs typically accumulate fluid within the alveolar walls and may progress to pulmonary edema. After the symptoms of acute mountain sickness subside, shortness of breath, headache, decreased cognitive flexibility, decreased concentration, increased respirations and an irritating cough with substernal chest pain develop (2). The cough produces bloody, frothy sputum. It is imperative that these individuals return to a lower altitude quickly and be given oxygen when possible. When at a lower altitude, the condition rapidly resolves.

Preventing Altitude Illness

Acclimatization is the single most important factor to prevent the onset of altitude sickness. In general, the length of the acclimatization period depends on the altitude. Individuals who are native to areas with high altitude have a larger chest capacity, more alveoli, more capillaries that transport blood to tissues, and a higher red blood cell level. As a result, these individuals clearly have an advantage in endurance activities at higher altitudes. Although some researchers recommend two to three weeks of adjustment before competition, most now believe that three days prior to competition is time enough to recover from both the journey and any immediate acid/base disturbances in the body, but will not be long enough to induce a major decrease of blood volume or maximum cardiac output (3). The benefits of acclimatization are probably lost within two to three weeks after returning to sea level.

Air Pollution

Air pollution is becoming more of an issue across the United States, not just in metropolitan areas, but also in rural areas. The pollutants of major concern to sport participants are ozone, sulfur dioxide and carbon monoxide.

Ozone (triatomic oxygen) is formed by a complex union of oxygen, nitrogen oxides, hydrocarbons, and sunlight, and is thus designated a photochemical oxidant. Under conditions of minimal exertion, little change is seen in functional capability. When maximal exertion is required, this irritant may lead to coughing, chest tightness, shortness of breath, pain during deep breaths, nausea, eye irritation, fatigue, and a lowered resistance to lung infections (4). Individuals who reside in regions of high ozone levels may become desensitized to the irritating effects of ozone after repeated exposures.

Sulfur dioxide (SO_2) is a colorless gas produced from burning coal or petroleum products. By itself, sulfur dioxide has little effect on lung function in normal individuals, but can be a potent bronchoconstrictor in asthmatics. Exposed to just a trace of this gas during brief periods of heavy exercise (10 minutes), asthmatics show a marked decrease in airway conductance. Asthmatics can prevent problems in breathing with a prior administration of disodium cromoglycate or by breathing through the nose (4).

Carbon monoxide is a colorless, odorless gas that reduces the ability of hemoglobin to transport oxygen and restricts the release of oxygen at the cellular level. In smokers, carbon monoxide reduces both aerobic power and the ability to sustain heavy submaximal exercise. It not only interferes with maximal performance during exercise but can also impair attentiveness, decision-making, psychomotor, behavioral, or attention-related tasks. The major group at risk from carbon monoxide exposure includes individuals with cardiovascular disorders, such as angina pectoris, ischemic cardiovascular disease, or intermittent claudication (4).

The track team should arrive at least three days prior to competition. This allows the body time enough to recover from both the journey and any immediate acid/base disturbances in the body. Team members should get plenty of rest, eat a high-carbohydrate diet, and drink plenty of water.

RESPIRATORY TRACT CONDITIONS

A thirty-seven-year-old male with asthma is seeking advice about how to improve his cardiovascular endurance. What activities might you recommend, and what guidelines should be followed in developing the exercise program?

Conditions of the respiratory tract are common in sport participants. Many factors, such as fatigue, chronic inflammation from a localized infection, environmental factors (allergens, dust, smog), and psychological stress brought on by stressful life events can suppress resistance to these conditions (5). Respiratory tract conditions include the common cold, sinusitis, pharyngitis, influenza, allergic rhinitis (hay fever), bronchitis, bronchial asthma, exercise-induced asthma, and infectious mononucleosis.

Common Cold

The common cold (coryza) is an acute infection that may result from aspirin sensitivity, use of oral contraceptives, topical deconges-

tant abuse, cocaine abuse, presence of nasal polyps or deviated septum, bacterial, viral, or allergic conditions. Symptoms include a rapid onset of a clear nasal discharge (**rhinorrhea**), nasal itching, sneezing, and associated itching and puffiness of the eyes. In the viral condition associated with the common cold, a low grade fever, chills, and **malaise** (feeling lousy or tired) are often present. Although most cold symptoms are benign and confined to the upper respiratory tract, colds can lead to middle ear infections and bacterial sinusitis when air flow is obstructed by swollen nasal membranes. **Field Strategy 17-1** provides suggestions for preventing a cold.

Although there is no treatment or cure for the viral common cold, over-the-counter medications can alleviate or lessen symptoms. Studies do not support decreases in the incidence of colds with vitamin C supplements, however, decreases in the duration of cold episodes and severity of symptoms have been found (6). If environmental factors, allergens, bacterial infections, or stressful life events are the cause, treatment involves reducing contributing factors, rest, and topical therapy delivered through a pump spray, rather than systemic therapy. Pump sprays offer dosage control and provide less irritation to the interior of the nose, particularly the septum (7). Topical medications may include anti-inflammatory agents (cromolyn sodium), antihistamines (levocabastine), corticosteroids (beclomethasone, flunisolide), and anticholinergics (nasal ipratropium, atropine in saline) (7). Observe caution when any of the preceding medications is used with competitive athletes, as any agent may be on the list of banned drugs, particularly at high competitive levels.

Sinusitis

Sinusitis is an inflammation of the paranasal sinuses (**Figure 17-1**). Sinusitis can be acute, lasting less than 30 days; subacute, lasting 3 weeks to 2 months; or chronic, lasting longer than 2 months (8). The condition is often triggered by an obstruction of the passageway between the sinuses (ostium) due to local mucosal swelling, local insult, or mechanical obstruction. Local mucosal swelling may be secondary to an upper respiratory tract infection, allergy, or direct trauma. Obstruction may be due to a deviated septum, concha bullosa (vesicle of serum or blood located on the concha inside the nose), or nasal masses from polyps or tumors (9,10).

Carbon monoxide reduces the ability of hemoglobin to transport oxygen and restricts the release of oxygen at the cellular level

The common cold is an acute infection that may result from aspirin sensitivity, use of oral contraceptives, topical decongestant abuse, cocaine abuse, presence of nasal polyps or deviated septum, bacterial, viral, or allergic conditions

Rhinorrhea
Clear nasal discharge

Malaise
General discomfort; feeling out-of-sorts

Vitamin C supplements do not decrease the incidence of colds, but can reduce the duration of cold episodes and severity of symptoms

Sinusitis
Inflammation of the paranasal sinuses

Sinusitis is often triggered by an obstruction to the passageway between the sinuses, due to mucosal swelling, local insult, or mechanical obstruction

- Avoid contact with individuals who have upper respiratory tract infections, particularly children, as they tend to have more frequent respiratory infections
- In the presence of individuals who have upper respiratory infections, avoid touching objects or sharing objects that they have touched
- Wash your hands frequently during the cold season and avoid touching your eyes and nose with your fingers. This will prevent many viruses from reaching the mucosal membranes
- If exercising in cold weather dress appropriately, however, colds are not caused by exposure to the cold. Rather, body chills may be an early symptom of a cold
- Drink plenty of fluids
- Although vitamin C supplements will not decrease the incidence of colds, they have been found to decrease the duration and severity of symptoms
- Reduce environmental factors (dust, smog, allergens) that may preclude you to rhinitis
- Reduce stress
- If using topical decongestant therapy, follow the instructions carefully and do not prolong its use, as rebound rhinitis may occur. Use decongestants during the day and antihistamines at night because of their sedative effect
- If cold symptoms are mild, exercise is safe. If, however, symptoms include headache, fever, muscular aches, hacking productive cough, or loss of appetite, exercise should cease. Rest is best

Chronic sinusitis is characterized by chronic nasal congestion, rhinorrhea or postnasal discharge, accompanied by perinasal pressure, and headache not associated with a migraine or muscle tension

Signs and symptoms of acute sinusitis include nasal congestion, facial pain or pressure over the involved sinus, pain in the upper teeth, or retro-orbital pain and pressure. Other symptoms may include purulent nasal discharge (anterior or posterior), palpable pain over the involved sinus, night-time and daytime coughing, and in severe cases perinasal and eyelid swelling, fever, and chills (10). Chronic sinusitis is characterized by chronic nasal congestion, rhinorrhea or postnasal discharge accompanied by perinasal pressure, and headache not associated with a migraine or muscle tension. The individual will often pinch the bridge of the nose to demonstrate the area of discomfort or will report discomfort aggravated by eyeglasses.

Treatment involves controlling the infection, reducing mucosal edema, and allowing for nasal drainage. Oral antibiotics include

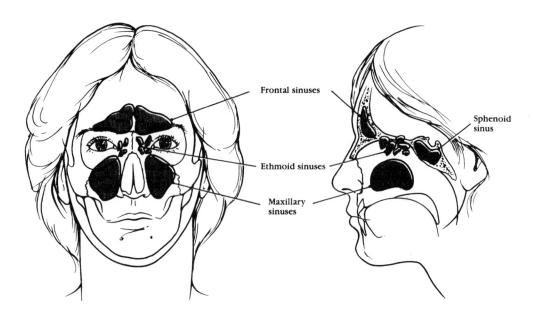

Fig. 17.1: The frontal and ethmoid sinuses are most commonly involved in sinusitis.

amoxicillin (Amoxil, Wymox), cefaclor (Ceclor), cefuroxime (Ceftin), and for those allergic to penicillin, either trimethoprim-sulfamethoxazole (Bactrim) or erythromycin. Topical agents, such as phenylephrine hydrochloride (Neo-Synephrine) or oxymetazoline hydrochloride (Afrin) can be used during the first three to four days of treatment to facilitate drainage, but their value has been unproven (10,11). Longer use of decongestants lead to a rebound effect whereby excessive mucus production and edema are increased. In severe cases surgical intervention may be necessary to drain the sinuses.

Pharyngitis (Sore Throat)

Pharyngitis results from a viral, bacterial, or fungal infection of the pharynx, leading to a sore throat. The condition may result from a common cold, influenza, streptococcus infection, diphtheria, Herpes simplex 1 and 2, Epstein-Barr virus, gonococcal bacteria, chlamydia, or candidiasis. Complications arise when pharyngitis is caused by *Streptococcus pyogenes*. Streptococcal pharyngitis, if inadequately treated, can lead to peritonsillar abscess, scarlet fever, rheumatic fever, or rheumatic heart disease.

Pain is aggravated by swallowing and may radiate along the distribution of the glossopharyngeal nerve (cranial nerve IX) to the ears (12). The throat typically appears dark red and inflamed with the tonsils red and swollen. A pussy discharge may be visible. Other symptoms include rhinorrhea, swollen lymph glands, hoarseness, headache, cough, a low grade fever, and malaise.

Throat swab cultures are used to identify about 90% of individuals with *Streptococcus pyogenes* in the pharynx. Of those, less than 50% are actually infectious. The others are incidental or chronic carriers who are not at risk themselves nor likely to infect others. Treatment for streptococcal pharyngitis includes a 10 day administration of oral penicillin or erythromycin, or a single injection of benzathine penicillin (12). In cases not involving streptococcal pharyngitis, treatment involves bed rest, plenty of fluids, warm saline gargles, throat lozenges, and mild analgesics (aspirin, Advil, Ibuprofen).

Influenza

Influenza, or "flu," is a specific viral bronchitis caused by *Haemophilus influenzae* type A, B, or C. It often occurs in epidemic proportions, particularly in school age children. Immunization for the influenzae type A and B virus is available to individuals at high risk, including pregnant women, individuals with chronic illness such as diabetes mellitus and disorders of the pulmonary or cardiovascular system, children, and individuals with immunocompromised systems. Individuals with a fever should not be immunized until the fever has passed.

Signs and symptoms of influenza include a fever of 39 to 39.5°C (102 to 103°F), chills, malaise, headache, general muscle aches, a hacking cough, and inflamed mucosal membranes. Rapid onset of symptoms can occur within 24 to 48 hours after exposure to the virus. Sore throat, watery eyes, sensitivity to light (photophobia), and a nonproductive cough may linger up to five days. The cough may progress into bronchitis. Treatment consists of rest, plenty of fluids, saltwater gargles, cough medication, and analgesics (aspirin, Advil, Ibuprofen) to control fever, aches, and pains. Amantadine is useful in a therapeutic and prophylactic role in the management of influenza A virus (13).

Allergic Rhinitis (Hay Fever)

Allergic **rhinitis** is a common upper respiratory tract condition affecting nearly 20% of all children and adults in the United States. Although not absolute classifications, it is often divided into seasonal allergic rhinitis, or "hay fever," and perennial allergic rhinitis.

Hay fever usually involves a specific period of symptoms in successive years caused by airborne pollens and/or fungus spores associated with that season. Normally mild in most individuals, it can produce serious bouts of continual sneezing, profuse rhinorrhea, and unremitting itching and watery eyes.

In contrast, perennial allergic rhinitis occurs year-round if continually exposed to allergens. Unremitting nasal obstruction and rhinorrhea may be caused by food allergens (e.g. shellfish, bread mold), dust, and animal emanations (e.g. cat hair, feathers). Postnasal drainage leads to a chronic sore throat and bronchial infection. Furthermore, the pharyngeal openings of the eustachian tubes can become blocked by swollen mucosa or enlarged lymphoid tissue, or exudate. Without normal air flow, increasing negative pres-

Treatment for sinusitis involves controlling the infection with penicillin or erythromyocin, reducing mucosal edema, and maintaining an open ostium to allow for drainage

Pharyngitis
Viral, bacterial, or fungal infection of the pharynx, leading to a sore throat

Pharyngitis, if inadequately treated, can lead to peritonsillar abscess, scarlet fever, rheumatic fever, or rheumatic heart disease

Influenza
Acute infectious respiratory tract condition characterized by malaise, headache, dry cough, and general muscle aches

Influenza immunization should be administered to pregnant women, individuals with chronic illness, children, and individuals with immunocompromised systems

In influenza, a sore throat, watery eyes, photophobia, and a nonproductive cough may linger up to 5 days with the cough progressing into bronchitis

Rhinitis
Inflammation of the nasal membranes with excessive mucus production resulting in nasal congestion and postnasal drip

Hay fever
Seasonal allergic rhinitis caused by airborne pollens and/or fungus spores

Unremitting nasal obstruction and rhinorrhea may be caused by food allergens, dust, and animal emanations

Bronchitis
Inflammation of the mucosal lining of the tracheobronchial tree characterized by bronchial swelling, mucus secretions, and dysfunction of the cilia

With bronchitis, coughing, wheezing, and large amounts of purulent mucus are present

Infectious mononucleosis
Acute viral disease caused by the Epstein-Barr virus manifested by malaise and fatigue

Infectious rates are highest in individuals between 15–25 years of age, with 25–50% of these developing classic symptoms

Advanced signs and symptoms include severe sore throat, fever, swollen eyelids, abnormal liver chemistries, and enlarged lymph nodes, tonsils, and spleen

Easy training may resume 3 weeks after onset of the illness provided the spleen is not enlarged or painful, and liver function is normal

sure in the middle ear results in fluid accumulation and chronic serous otitis, leading to a partial hearing loss and recurrent middle ear infections (14).

Management involves reducing exposure to the allergen or irritant, suppressive medication to alleviate symptom severity, and specific hypersensitization to reduce responsiveness to unavoidable allergens. For example, if dust is an allergen, having bare floors, pillows and mattresses encased in plastic covers, minimizing cloth curtains, and avoiding cluttered table tops can reduce the amount of dust in a home. Antihistaminic drugs have been effective agents in reducing symptoms of allergic rhinitis. However, in competitive sport participants, drowsiness, lethargy, mucous membrane dryness, and occasional nausea and light-headedness may be unwanted side effects. Medications including ephedrine (Fedrine, Ephedd II, Efedron nasal jelly), isoephedrine, and phenylpropanolamine acting as mucosal decongestants can offset sedative effects of antihistamine agents. Cromolyn sodium can reduce the symptoms of allergic rhinitis and conjunctivitis.

Bronchitis

Bronchitis results from infection and inhalants leading to inflammation of the mucosal lining of the tracheobronchial tree, and may be acute or chronic. Acute bronchitis, commonly seen in sport participants, involves bronchial swelling, mucus secretion, and dysfunction of the cilia, leading to increased resistance to expiration. With a significant airway obstruction, coughing, wheezing, and large amounts of purulent mucus will be present (15). Once the stimulus is removed, the swelling decreases and airways return to normal.

Chronic bronchitis is characterized by individuals who have a productive daily cough for at least three consecutive months in two successive years. Irritation may result from cigarette smoke, air pollution, or infections (16). This condition can progress to increased airway obstruction, heart failure, and cellular changes in the respiratory epithelial cells that may become malignant. Signs and symptoms include marked cyanosis, edema, large production of sputum, and abnormally high levels of carbon dioxide and low levels of oxygen in the blood. The condition is often seen simultaneously with emphysema.

Infectious Mononucleosis

The Epstein-Barr virus (EBV) in the Herpes family is the organism known to cause **infectious mononucleosis**, an acute viral disease manifested by a general feeling of malaise and fatigue. The condition is often transmitted in saliva, and as such, is commonly called the "kissing disease," although many cases develop with no known point of contact. Infectious rates are found highest in individuals between 15 to 25 years of age, with 25 to 50% of these developing classic symptoms. After age 35, infectious mononucleosis is rare (17). The association of EBV with "chronic fatigue syndrome" is still debatable.

The incubation period is 30 to 50 days. Within three to five days of developing mononucleosis, headache, fatigue, loss of appetite, malaise, and muscular aches and pains begin to develop. Within 5 to 15 days, additional symptoms, including a moderate to severe sore throat, tonsil enlargement, tonsillar exudate, fever with or without cold sweats, enlarged lymph nodes, swollen eyelids, spots on the palate, and in 90% of patients, inflammation of the liver lead to atypically-shaped white blood cells (18). By the second week, an enlarged spleen can be palpated. In 10 to 15% of infections, jaundice and a rubella-like rash are present (19). Complications arise if enlarged tonsils and adenoids obstruct the airway, or if neurological and cardiac changes occur. Individuals with mononucleosis should not participate in contact or collision sports where trauma could rupture the enlarged and vulnerable spleen.

The overwhelming majority of individuals with mononucleosis will recover uneventfully. Anti-inflammatory medication may be used to control headaches, fever, and general muscle aches and pain. Lozenges, saltwater gargles and viscous lidocaine (Xylocaine) can ease throat pain. Corticosteroid therapy (prednisone) is used only on individuals with specific indications, such as imminent airway obstruction, severe mono-hepatitis, or in the presence of neurological, hematological, or cardiac complications (18). The decision to return to sport participation will rest with the supervising physician. If the spleen is not markedly enlarged or painful, and liver function is normal, easy training may be resumed three weeks after onset of the illness. Strenuous exercise and return to contact sports can occur four to five weeks after onset of the illness provided the spleen is not enlarged or painful, and liver function is normal (19). A flak jacket can be worn to protect the spleen from injury.

Bronchial Asthma

Asthma is a disease caused by hyper-responsiveness of the trachea and bronchi to various stimuli, resulting in recurrent episodes of reversible airway narrowing, separated by periods of relatively normal ventilations. The obstruction may be due to **bronchospasm**, or the presence of inflammation due to increased mucosal edema and mucous secretions. The condition is classified as intermittent, seasonal, or chronic asthma. Intermittent asthma is characterized by symptoms of relatively short duration, usually occurring less than five days per month with extended symptom-free periods. Symptoms of seasonal asthma occur for prolonged periods only in response to exposure to seasonal inhalant allergens. Chronic asthma may occur daily or near daily with absence of extended symptom-free periods (20).

During an asthma attack there is a constriction of bronchial smooth muscles, increased bronchial secretions, and mucosa swelling, all leading to an inadequate airflow during respiration (especially expiration) **(Figure 17-2)**. Since many narrowed airways cannot fill or empty adequately, there is an uneven lung aeration and a loss of matching ventilations and pulmonary blood flow. The pressure of trapped air tends to flatten the diaphragm, interfering with the ability of the diaphragm and lower chest to function. Thus, the accessory muscles must work harder to enlarge the chest during inspiration. The increased workload to maintain breathing leads to a rapid onset of fatigue when the individual tires and can no longer hyperventilate enough to meet the increased oxygen need. Acute attacks may occur spontaneously but are often provoked by a viral infection.

Wheezing is a common sign and results from air squeezing past the narrowed airways. A large amount of thick, yellow or green sputum is produced by the bronchial mucosa. As dyspnea (difficult breathing) continues, anxiety, panic, loud wheezing, sweating, rapid heart rate, and laboring to breathe is apparent. In severe cases, respiratory failure may be indicated by cyanosis, decreased wheezing, and decreased levels of consciousness (15).

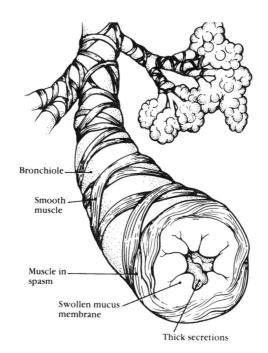

Fig. 17.2: Bronchospasm occurs during an asthma attack when the bronchiole is obstructed on expiration by muscle spasm, increased bronchial secretions, and mucosa swelling.

Individuals diagnosed with asthma typically carry medication delivered by a compressor-driven nebulizer or inhaler to alleviate the attack. However, the value of bronchodilators in children and young adults has been debated. Medications typically involve selective beta$_2$-agonists (albuterol, pirbuterol, terbutaline, and bitolterol), aerosol corticosteroids (budesonide, beclomethasone), or cromolyn sodium, an antiasthmatic drug that prevents the release of chemical mediators that cause bronchospasm and mucous membrane inflammatory changes (20–22). Once the attack has subsided the lungs usually return to normal. There is, however, a significant relationship between asthma and development of chronic obstructive lung disease later in life.

Exercise-Induced Asthma

Exercise-induced asthma (EIA) affects up to 80% of asthmatics, developing shortly after six to eight minutes of strenuous exercise between 65 and 85% of maximum workload (23). Despite its prevalence, the precise mechanisms responsible for EIA are still unknown. Theories include hyperventilation, resulting in airway heat and water loss, carbon dioxide loss with hyperventilation, and release of mast cell mediators causing bron-

Asthma
Disease of the lungs characterized by constriction of the bronchial muscles, increased bronchial secretions, and mucosa swelling, all leading to airway narrowing and inadequate airflow during respiration

Bronchospasm
Contraction of the smooth muscles of the bronchial tubes, causing narrowing of the airway

During an asthma attack the diaphragm and lower chest cannot function effectively, thus the accessory muscles must work harder to enlarge the chest during inspiration, leading to a rapid onset of fatigue

Wheezing results from air squeezing past the narrowed airways

EIA develops shortly after 6 to 8 minutes of strenuous exercise between 65 and 85% of maximum workload

Signs and symptoms of EIA include chest tightness or a burning sensation, wheezing, coughing, and shortness of breath shortly after or during exercise

Vigorous activities are well-tolerated provided exercise includes adequate warm-up and cool-down, and repetitive bouts of exercise (less than 5 minutes) are performed no less than 40 minutes apart

chospasm. These theories, however, have not been substantiated (24). It is thought that breathing dry, cold air through the mouth stimulates bronchospasm. Breathing through the nose can warm and humidify air, and lessen the onset of symptoms. Swimming in an indoor pool where the air is typically warm and humid may also prevent the onset of symptoms.

Signs and symptoms of EIA include chest tightness or a burning sensation, wheezing, coughing, and shortness of breath shortly after or during exercise. Individuals suffering from allergies, sinus disease, or hyperventilation may be at increased risk for EIA. In addition, bronchitis, bronchopulmonary disease, and emphysema can exacerbate symptoms. Medications routinely used for asthma and allergy may be banned by the International Olympic Committee (IOC) or National Collegiate Athletic Association (NCAA), so it is advised to check the lists prior to using medication (See **Table 17-8**). Medications include those used in regular asthma treat-

ment including beta$_2$-agonists, cromolyn sodium, and theophylline.

Children and young adults who have asthma and are physically fit and free of significant airway obstruction respond to exercise similar to nonasthmatic individuals. Activities such as tennis, running, and football are well-tolerated, provided exercise includes pre-exercise warm-up and postexercise warm-down, and repetitive bouts of exercise (less than 5 minutes) are performed no less than 40 minutes apart (23). Use of a bronchodilator 15 minutes prior to activity can delay symptoms for two to four hours. **Field Strategy 17-2** summarizes exercise strategies for individuals with asthma.

 The asthmatic individual should be seen by a physician before starting an exercise program. In general, the program can include a 5 to 10 minute warm-up of moderate stretching, 10 to 15 minutes of low intensity exercise, keeping the pulse below 140 beats/minute. This can be followed by repetitive intensive exercise for less than 5 minutes

---

Field Strategy 17–2. Exercise Strategies for Exercise-Induced Asthma.

- Before beginning an exercise program, consult a physician
- Take medications for asthma (e.g., inhaled bronchodilators and corticosteroids, oral antihistamines) as prescribed by the physician to achieve good overall control of asthmatic symptoms, including those caused by exercise and airborne allergens (pollens, dust, etc)
- Use a bronchodilator containing a beta-agonist and/or cromolyn sodium 15 minutes prior to exercise
- Perform a 5 to 10 minute warm-up of moderate stretching before vigorous exercise
- Work out slowly for the first 10 to 15 minutes, keeping the pulse rate below 140 beats per minute. If symptoms occur during exercise, try to "run through" them and/or use the bronchodilator
- The goal of aerobic training is to do continuous and rhythmic exercise for 20 to 30 minutes at least three times a week at 70 to 80% of maximum heart rate
- Increase the time and intensity of the workout as tolerated, especially if the activity is new
- Breathe slowly through the nose to warm and humidify the air. Exercise in a warm, humid environment, such as a heated swimming pool is also beneficial
- In cold, dry environments, breathe through a mask or scarf. Alternatively, consider different forms or locations of exercise during cold winter months, such as swimming, running, or cycling indoors
- Avoid exposure to air pollutants and allergens whenever possible. For example, try to exercise indoors when air quality is poor, or exercise in residential areas to avoid emissions from automobile traffic. Avoid exercise in the early morning hours when the concentration of ragweed pollen is highest
- Do a graduated 10 to 30 minute warm-down (or cool-down) after a vigorous workout to avoid rapid thermal changes in the airways. This can be achieved by slowing to a less intense pace while jogging, cycling, stretching, or possibly weight lifting

---

performed 40 minutes apart with a 10 to 30 minute cool-down. Use of a bronchodilator 15 minutes prior to exercise can also be used to delay symptoms for 2 to 4 hours.

THE GASTROINTESTINAL TRACT

(?) *A male distance runner has reported the consistent need to stop and have a bowel movement while training. Is this normal for runners? What can be done about it?*

The gastrointestinal tract extends from the mouth to the anus. Often nervous tension produces indigestion, diarrhea, or constipation that can adversely affect sport participation. Many seemingly minor disorders can be the first sign of more serious underlying conditions. If symptoms persist with any disorder, referral to a physician is warranted. In this section, gastroenteritis (stomach flu), diarrhea, constipation, and hemorrhoids are discussed.

Gastroenteritis

Gastroenteritis is an inflammation of the mucous membrane of the stomach or small intestine. The condition may be caused by viruses, bacteria, allergic reactions, medications, ingested contaminated food (food poisoning), or emotional stress. In mild cases, increased secretion of hydrochloric acid in the stomach may lead to indigestion (dyspepsia), characterized by nausea, flatulence (gas) and a sour stomach. In moderate to severe cases, abdominal cramping, diarrhea, fever, and vomiting can lead to fluid and electrolyte imbalance. The condition usually clears up in two to three days. Treatment is symptomatic and includes eliminating irritating foods from the diet, avoiding factors that bring on anxiety and stress, and avoiding dehydration by drinking clear fluids or electrolyte-containing fluids (i.e., Gatorade, Phipps).

Diarrhea

Diarrhea is a common and troublesome disorder characterized by abnormally loose, watery stools. This is due to food residue rushing through the large intestine before that organ has had sufficient time to absorb the remaining water. Prolonged diarrhea can lead to dehydration and depletion of electrolytes, particularly sodium, bicarbonate, and potassium.

Diarrhea is common among runners, although its cause is unknown. In one study, five patterns of bowel dysfunction were found in runners **(Table 17-1)**, and include:

1. Nervous diarrhea prior to competition
2. The need to stop and have a bowel movement while training
3. The need to stop and have a bowel movement while competing
4. Cramps and diarrhea without blood in the stool after hard running
5. Cramps and diarrhea with blood in the stool after hard running

Diarrhea may respond to Pepto-Bismol, loperamide (Imodium), or diphenoxylate with atropine (Lomotil), however, these should not be used on a regular basis. Eliminating foods

Gastroenteritis
Inflammation of the mucous membrane of the stomach or small intestine

Gastroenteritis may be caused by viruses, bacteria, allergic reactions, medications, food poisoning, or emotional stress

Diarrhea
Loose or watery stools resulting when food residue rushes through the large intestine before there is sufficient time to absorb the remaining water

---

Table 17–1. Patterns of Bowel Dysfunction Found in Runners.

1. Nervous diarrhea prior to competition.
   Found to be slightly more common in women, more likely to occur if the runner had irregular bowel function when not running, and a history of lactose intolerance
2. The need to stop and have a bowel movement while training.
   Found to be more common in men occurring in the first few miles of a run, in runners with irregular bowel function, in those that ate prior to running, or did their runs in the morning before breakfast
3. The need to stop and have a bowel movement while competing.
   Found to be infrequent and its occurrence unclear
4. Cramps and diarrhea without blood in the stool after hard running.
   Found to be common, and frequently associated with severe lower abdominal cramps, nausea, and vomiting
5. Cramps and diarrhea with blood in the stool after hard running.
   Found to be associated with diarrhea, severe lower abdominal cramps, and rectal bleeding. Gastrointestinal bleeding may be the result of intestinal mucosal ischemia

Constipation
Infrequent or incomplete bowel movements

Constipation may be caused by lack of fiber in the diet, improper bowel habits, lack of exercise, emotional distress, diabetes mellitus, pregnancy, laxative abuse, or drug-induced

An increase in daily aerobic exercise, a high fiber diet, and plenty of fluids can alleviate symptoms

Hemorrhoids
Dilations of the venous plexus surrounding the rectal and anal area that can become exposed if they protrude internally or externally

Pain, itching, and the passage of bright red blood on defecation, separate from the feces, are common signs and symptoms of hemorrhoids

that trigger bowel irritation, including lactose intolerance, and improving hydration before and during exercise may increase plasma volume to decrease intestinal mucosal ischemia. Eating a low fiber diet 24 to 36 hours prior to competition may also help. An attempt should be made to defecate at a regular daily time, taking advantage of the morning gastrocolic reflex. Peristalsis and defecation can be stimulated by drinking coffee or tea, or performing a light morning warm-up run or workout.

Constipation

Constipation is described as infrequent or incomplete bowel movements, and is not a disease but rather a description of symptoms that may indicate more serious underlying conditions. Identifiable causes range from lack of fiber in the diet, improper bowel habits, lack of exercise, emotional distress, diabetes mellitus, pregnancy, laxative abuse, or drug-induced (diuretics, bile acid binders, drugs that lower serum cholesterol, and analgesics that slow bowel transit) (25).

Management of constipation is dependent on the origin. In most cases, eating high fiber foods such as cereals, grains, and vegetables, increasing daily exercise, particularly aerobic exercise, and adequate fluid intake can alleviate symptoms. Laxatives or suppositories are useful but should be used sparingly. In chronic constipation, surgical intervention may be necessary.

Hemorrhoids

Hemorrhoids are dilations of the venous plexus surrounding the rectal and anal area. The dilated sacs become exposed if they protrude internally (prolapse) into the rectal and

anal canals, or externally around the anal opening. Several factors may increase the incidence of hemorrhoids including constipation, diarrhea, straining during physical exertion, pelvic congestion, enlargement of the prostate, uterine fibroids, rectal tumors, varicose veins, and pregnancy (26). Pain, itching, and the passage of small amounts of bright red blood on defecation, separate from the feces, are the most common signs and symptoms. The condition will normally heal within two to three weeks. Pain or swelling can be relieved by following suggestions listed in **Field Strategy 17-3**. If these suggestions are not successful, physician referral is indicated and surgery may be necessary.

Athletes involved in contact or collision sports (i.e., boxing, hockey, and football) may normally experience small amounts of blood on defecation. In many endurance runners, blood in fecal material is due to gastrointestinal bleeding and is quite common. This bleeding can lead to iron-deficiency anemia and will be discussed later in the chapter. However, if a moderate amount of blood is mixed with feces, a full evaluation by a physician should be carried out.

The runner's condition is not unusual. Find out if he has a history of irregular bowel function, eating prior to running, or running before breakfast. A high fiber diet, an increase in daily exercise and fluid intake, and over-the-counter medication may be recommended. If the condition continues, he should see a physician to rule out other conditions.

THE DIABETIC ATHLETE

A diabetic basketball player is halfway through a practice session when suddenly the player begins to feel weak and faint.

 Field Strategy 17–3. Reducing the Inflammation of Hemorrhoids.

- Take sitz baths in warm water for 15 minutes several times a day, especially after bowel movements
- Use stool softeners to prevent constipation, and products to ease friction (i.e., petroleum jelly)
- Eat a diet high in fiber by adding unprocessed bran to breakfast cereals and eating high-roughage food
- Drink plenty of water and other fluids
- Do not ignore the urge for bowel movements, as delay builds up pressure in the rectum and increases the chance of constipation and development of hemorrhoids
- Exercise to promote good muscle tone
- Avoid pushing too hard or too long during bowel movements

---

658 Section 6 Special Conditions Related to Sports

The skin appears pale and moist, and respirations are shallow. What condition has occurred? How will you manage this athlete?

Diabetes mellitus is a chronic systemic disorder characterized by near or absolute lack of the hormone insulin, or insulin resistance, or both. Insulin, secreted by the pancreas, is needed to transfer glucose from the blood after carbohydrate ingestion, into skeletal and cardiac muscles, and promotes glucose storage in muscles and the liver in the form of glycogen. **Figure 17-3** illustrates the action of normal and deficient insulin in an individual.

Diabetes mellitus ordinarily is divided into two classes: Type I or insulin-dependent diabetes (formerly called juvenile-onset diabetes), and Type II or non-insulin-dependent diabetes (formerly called adult-onset diabetes) **(Table 17-2)**. Type I has an onset prior to age 30 in people who are not typically obese. It is associated with an absolute deficiency of insulin. Individuals generally have a more severe abnormality of glucose homeostasis, the effects of exercise on the metabolic state are more pronouced, and the management of exercise-related problems are more difficult (1). Only 10% of these individuals have a family history of diabetes. Type II has an onset after age 30 with nearly 70 to 80% of affected people obese (27). This type is associated with significant resistance to insulin's actions, an abnormal but relatively well-maintained insulin secretion, and normal to elevated plasma insulin levels (1). Oral gliclazide used alone or in combination with insulin has had positive results in treating Type II diabetes (28). Several factors increase the frequency and severity of diabetes including heredity, increasing age, obesity, being female, stress, infection, and a diet high in carbohydrates and fat.

Diabetes
Metabolic disorder characterized by near or absolute lack of the hormone insulin, or insulin-resistance, or both

Insulin is needed to transfer glucose from the blood after carbohydrate ingestion into skeletal and cardiac muscles, and promotes glucose storage in muscles and the liver in the form of glycogen

Type I has an onset prior to age 30 in people who are not typically obese. Type II has an onset after age 30 with nearly 70 to 80% of affected people obese

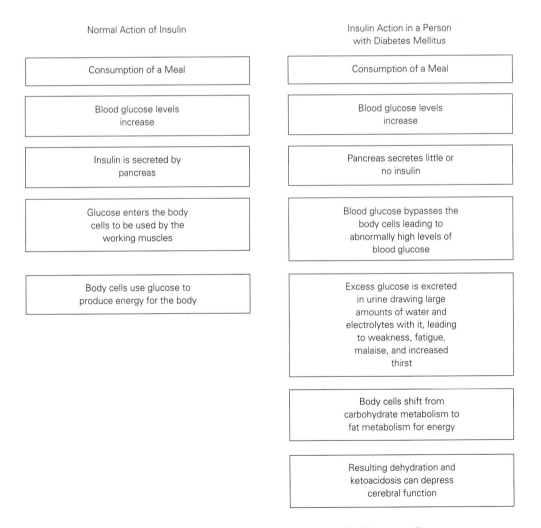

Fig. 17.3: The normal action of insulin and insulin action in a person with diabetes mellitus.

Table 17–2. A Comparison of Type I and Type II Diabetes.

	Type I	Type II
Previous names	Juvenile-onset	Adult-onset
Age of onset	Usually before 30	Usually after 30
Type of onset	Abrupt (days to weeks)	Usually gradual (weeks to months)
Nutritional status	Almost always lean	Usually obese
Insulin production	Negligible to absent	Present, but may be in excess and ineffective due to obesity
Insulin	Needed for all patients	Necessary in only 20–30% of patients
Diet	Mandatory along with insulin for control of blood glucose	Diet alone is frequently sufficient to control blood glucose
Family history	Minor	Common link

Hyperglycemia
Abnormally high levels of glucose in the circulating blood that can lead to diabetic coma

Acetone, formed as a by-product of fat metabolism, is volatile and blown off during expiration, giving the breath a sweet or fruity odor

If in doubt, give sugar to the individual. The additional glucose will not worsen the condition, provided they are transported immediately

Hypoglycemia
Abnormally low levels of glucose in the circulating blood that can lead to insulin shock

Signs and symptoms of insulin shock have a rapid onset and include dizziness, aggressive behavior, intense hunger, fainting, pale, cold and clammy skin, profuse perspiration, salivation, and drooling

In diabetes, lack of insulin or insulin resistance leads to **hyperglycemia**. In essence, adequate amounts of glucose levels in the blood fail to enter the cells, causing blood glucose levels to increase to abnormally high levels. Increased osmotic blood pressure drives fluid from the cells into the vascular system, leading to cell dehydration. The excess glucose is passed into the kidneys and excreted in urine, drawing large amounts of water and electrolytes (polyuria). An electrolyte imbalance leads to weakness, fatigue, malaise, and increased thirst (polydypsia). In response, the body shifts from carbohydrate metabolism to fat metabolism for energy. This produces an excess of ketoacids and results in acidosis. Acetone, formed as a by-product of fat metabolism, is volatile and blown off during expiration, giving the breath a sweet or fruity odor. If the condition is not rectified with insulin injection, further dehydration and ketoacidosis can depress cerebral function. The individual becomes confused, drowsy, and may lapse into a diabetic coma and die.

Controlled diabetes rests on a balance of glucose levels, insulin production, diet, and exercise. Alterations in this equilibrium can lead to two separate conditions: diabetic coma and insulin shock.

Diabetic Coma

Without insulin, the body is unable to metabolize glucose, leading to hyperglycemia in the blood. As the body shifts from carbohydrate metabolism to fat metabolism, an excess of ketoacids (ketoacidosis) in the blood can lower the blood pH to as low as 7.0 (normal pH is 7.35 to 7.45). The symptoms appear gradually and can occur over several days. The individual may become increasingly rest-less, confused, complain of a dry mouth and intense thirst. Abdominal cramping and vomiting are common. As the individual slips into a coma, signs include dry, warm skin, eyes that appear sunken and deep, sighing respirations, rapid, weak pulse, and a sweet acetone breath, similar to nail polish remover (29).

As the name implies, coma is a serious condition and considered a medical emergency. If unsure of the condition and unable to determine if the individual is in insulin shock or a diabetic coma, give the individual glucose or glucose in orange juice. If recovery is not rapid, a medical emergency exists and EMS should be summoned. The additional glucose will not worsen the condition, provided the individual is transported immediately.

Insulin Shock

Exercise lowers blood sugar, hence, any exercise must be counterbalanced with increased food intake or decreased amounts of insulin. If blood glucose falls below normal levels, **hypoglycemia**, or insulin shock, results. During a prolonged session of moderate exercise, hepatic glucose production may not keep pace with the increased demand of glucose by the exercising muscles. Contrary to the slow onset of a diabetic coma, the signs and symptoms of hypoglycemia have a rapid onset and include dizziness, aggressive behavior, intense hunger, fainting, pale, cold and clammy skin, profuse perspiration, salivation, and drooling.

Since glucose levels in the blood are low compared to high levels of insulin, treatment centers on getting sugar into the system quickly. Use table sugar (sucrose), honey, sugared candy, orange juice or soda (only in a conscious person). Do not use a sugar substitute or diet soda, as artificial sweeteners will not help the individual (29). Place sugar or honey under the tongue in an unconscious person as it will be absorbed through the mucosal membrane. Recovery is usually rapid, however, even when blood glucose has returned to normal, physical performance and judgment may still be impaired (30). **Field Strategy 17-4** compares the two conditions and provides further information on the cause, signs and symptoms, and management of the condition.

Exercise and Diabetes

Strenuous exercise is contraindicated for some people with diabetes. With the advent of blood glucose self-monitoring, however, exercise is encouraged if certain precautions are followed. Emphasis should be placed on aerobic low-resistance activities, such as walking, jogging, or swimming. Sports that require resistance strength training are also permissible. Prior to any exercise program, a physician should be consulted and normal blood glucose (BG) levels documented. This allows both the physician and individual to

 Field Strategy 17–4. Management of Diabetic Emergencies.

Insulin Shock	Diabetic Coma
CAUSES	CAUSES
Too much insulin has been taken or not enough food was eaten to provide adequate sugar intake	Insulin was not taken or too much food was eaten, flooding the blood with glucose
The individual may have overexercised, reducing blood glucose levels, or vomited a meal	
SIGNS AND SYMPTOMS	SIGNS AND SYMPTOMS
Rapid onset of symptoms	Gradual onset of symptoms
Dizziness and headache	Dry mouth and intense thirst
Hostile or aggressive behavior	Abdominal pain and vomiting
Normal blood pressure	Increased restlessness and confusion followed by stupor
Full, bounding pulse	Fever is common
Normal or shallow respirations	Coma with these signs:
Intense hunger	Deep, exaggerated respirations
Pale, cold, clammy skin	Rapid, weak pulse
Profuse perspiration	Dry, red, warm skin
Fainting or convulsions	Eyes that appear sunken
Severe salivation and drooling	Slightly lower blood pressure
	Sweet, fruity acetone breath
MANAGEMENT	MANAGEMENT
Look for a medic alert tag	**Look for a medic alert tag**
In a conscious person:	Administer sugar. If no response summon EMS
Administer sugar, such as granular sugar, honey, a lifesaver or other sugared candy under the tongue, or have them drink orange juice or a soda	Transport immediately to the nearest hospital
In an unconscious person:	
Do not give liquids	
Place sugar under the tongue	
Transport to the nearest hospital	

see how exercise affects BG. Gradual exercise over several weeks should precede any competitive sport participation. This allows better regulation of food intake and insulin dosage. Blood glucose levels should be taken before and after exercise.

For the diabetic athlete, it is best to eat complex carbohydrates one to three hours prior to exercise, and ingest 15 to 30 grams of carbohydrates every 30 minutes of intense exercise. A snack of carbohydrates should also follow the exercise period. When exercise lasts for several hours, insulin requirements are decreased, hence total insulin intake dosage should be decreased 20 to 50% (30). Injection administration is timed so that peak activity does not take place when high insulin levels are present (two to four hours after injection). If this is not possible, due to rain delays in competition or other associated factors, the individual should eat a high carbohy-

drate snack like juice and crackers, or milk and cookies about 30 minutes prior to the resumption of activity. Avoid exercising in the evening when hypoglycemia is more apt to be present. Because exercise leads to increased circulation in the arms and legs, insulin should be given in the abdomen. If this is not possible, avoid exercising for one hour those muscles into which short-acting insulin was injected (1). In addition, all diabetic athletes should avoid alcohol immediately prior to and after exercise. Alcohol increases the risk of hypoglycemia. **Field Strategy 17-5** provides guidelines to prevent hypoglycemia or hyperglycemia with exercise.

The basketball player suddenly felt weak and faint. The skin was pale, moist, and respirations were shallow. If you determined possible insulin shock, you are correct. Get the player to the sideline and provide a source of sugar, such as a candy bar, orange juice, or

 Field Strategy 17–5. Preventing Hypoglycemia or Hyperglycemia with Exercise.

Before Exercise:
- Estimate the time of day, intensity, duration, and energy expenditure for the exercise bout
- Schedule the exercise at the same time in the day
- Eat a meal 1-2 hours prior to exercise
- Avoid exercising in the late evening
- Administer insulin more than 1 hour before exercise
- Decrease the insulin dose with:
  a. Intermediate-acting insulin—decrease the dose by 30 to 35% on the day of exercise
  b. Intermediate- and short-acting insulin—omit the dose if it precedes exercise
  c. Multiple doses of short-acting insulin—reduce the dose prior to exercise by 30% and supplement carbohydrate intake
  d. Continuous subcutaneous insulin infusion—eliminate mealtime bolus or insulin increment that precedes or follows exercise
- Avoid exercising muscles in the region where short-acting insulin was injected for at least 1 hour
- Measure blood glucose before exercise, particularly if exercise is in the morning or 3 to 4 hours after eating
  If blood sugar is low (<100 mg/dL), eat 30 g of carbohydrates (about two slices of bread)
  If blood sugar is high (>250 mg/dL), delay exercise

During Exercise:
- Ingest 15 to 30 g of carbohydrate foods every 30 minutes of strenuous exercise
- Drink plenty of fluids
- Monitor blood glucose during long duration exercise or if exercise is done in the evening

After Exercise:
- Measure blood glucose. If low, eat carbohydrate snacks
- Increase caloric intake for 12-24 hours after activity, based on the intensity and duration of exercise
- Reduce insulin peaking in evening and night, based on intensity and duration of exercise

sugared candy. If this is the first episode, the individual should see a physician.

COMMON CONTAGIOUS VIRAL DISEASES

❓ *An adolescent soccer player has come to the field with a red rash over the body. The glands in the neck are very swollen, and opening the mouth is painful. Is this serious? What should you suggest to this individual and the parents?*

Although it is not the purpose of this book to discuss all contagious viral diseases to which sport participants may be exposed, there are several common diseases that may confront the coach, athletic trainer, or sport supervisor. Several are considered childhood diseases that have immunization standards. However, an alarming increase in the number of cases is being seen in inner city populations where children may not be vaccinated. In addition, older populations may not receive necessary booster shots to prevent the onset of the illness. Chicken pox, mumps, measles (rubeola), and German measles

(rubella) are common viral infections transmitted through the DNA or RNA within a cell. Incubation periods range from 7 to 21 days, and treatment is totally symptomatic. **Table 17-3** summarizes the main features of common viral infections.

💡 *This individual should be removed from the vicinity of the other players. The parents should be immediately notified to take the individual to a physician to determine the possibility of mumps or measles.*

EPILEPSY

❓ *During warm-up, a softball player suddenly gets a glassy stare on the face, begins to smack the lips, and walks aimlessly around the field as if intoxicated. What condition might this individual have? How will you manage the situation?*

Epilepsy is a brain disorder characterized by recurrent episodes of sudden, excessive discharges of electrical activity in the brain. The discharge may trigger altered sensation, perceptions, behavior, mood, level of consciousness, or convulsive movements.

Epilepsy
Disorder of the brain characterized by recurrent episodes of sudden, excessive discharges of electrical activity in the brain

Table 17–3. Common Viral Infections.

Disease	Epidemiology	Incubation Period	Clinical Symptoms	Duration
Chicken pox (varicella)	Respiratory droplet Very contagious	10–21 days	Fever, vesicular eruptions profuse on trunk and on oral mucosa	1–2 weeks
German measles (rubella)	Nasopharyngeal droplets Very contagious	14–21 days	Light rash on face that spreads to trunk and extremities, low-grade fever and enlarged lymph nodes. Can cause congenital heart defects in an infant if acquired by the mother in the first trimester of pregnancy	1–5 days
Measles (rubeola)	Respiratory droplet Very contagious	7–14 days	Rash on face and body, rhinitis, cough, photophobia, fever, and pneumonia may also be present	4–7 days
Mumps	Respiratory tract secretions: very contagious	15–21 days	Enlarged salivary glands, fever, headache, malaise, and males may have swollen and tender testes	10 days

The three types of epileptic seizures include:
Absence attacks
(petit mal)
Complex partial seizures
(psychomotor)
Tonic-clonic seizures
(grand mal)

Clonic state
Movement marked by repetitive muscle contractions and relaxation in rapid succession

Tonic state
Steady rigid muscle contractions with no relaxation

Protect the individual's head at all times, but never place your fingers or any other object in the mouth

Individuals with epilepsy should consult their neurologist prior to participating in contact sports, water sports, and activities where there is a danger of falling

Although nearly 10% of the population will have a seizure sometime in their life, only 2% of the population will develop epilepsy (31). There are three recognizable types of epileptic seizures: absence attacks (petit mal), complex partial seizures (psychomotor), and tonic-clonic seizures (grand mal).

Absence attacks are characterized by blank staring into space for 5 to 10 seconds. Slight twitching of the facial muscles or fluttering of the eyelids may occur. Onset is usually about age five with attacks most prevalent in childhood (31).

Complex partial seizures are characterized by disorientation, loss of contact with reality, uncontrolled motor activity in isolated muscle groups, such as hand clapping or lip smacking, or walking about aimlessly. The average seizure is one to five minutes and may be followed by disorientation (31).

Tonic-clonic seizures are the most severe form of generalized epilepsy. Many individuals experience a sensory phenomenon, such as a particular taste, smell, or aura prior to the seizure. The person loses consciousness and displays intense convulsions, either clonic or tonic. A **clonic state** is movement marked by repetitive muscle contractions and relaxation in rapid succession. A **tonic state** involves steady rigid muscle contractions with no relaxation. A fracture to the neck of the humerus, greater trochanter, clavicle, vertebrae, and ankle, or a shoulder or hip dislocation may occur due to the magnitude of muscular contraction. Loss of bowel and bladder control is common and severe biting of the tongue may occur, although this is relatively uncommon. The average seizure lasts from 50 to 90 seconds, then muscles relax, the person awakens, but may not remember what happened (31).

Management of any seizure is directed toward protecting the individual from self-injury. Nearby objects should be removed so the individual does not strike them during uncontrollable muscle contractions. Protect the individual's head at all times, but do not stop or restrain the person. Although the individual may bite their tongue during the seizure, never place fingers or any other object into the mouth. Wait until the seizure has come to an end and ensure an adequate airway. Do not move the individual as a spinal cord injury may be present. Usually a single seizure is not considered an emergency. However, if seizure activity is continuous or if

another attack occurs in rapid succession, the individual should be transported to the nearest medical facility by ambulance. **Field Strategy 17-6** summarizes management of a seizure.

In nearly all instances, epilepsy can be controlled with proper medication. Participation in sports, particularly those with a danger of falling, contact sports, and water sports, should be carefully evaluated with a neurologist prior to participation. It is highly recommended that children be allowed to participate in physical education and athletics provided that proper medical management, good seizure control, and proper supervision is available at all times (32). Individuals who

Field Strategy 17–6. Management of an Epileptic Seizure.

During the seizure:
- Remove harmful objects from the proximity of the person
- Do not stop or restrain the person. You cannot stop the seizure
- Help the individual into a supine position and place something soft under the head
- Remove glasses and loosen tight clothing
- Do not place your fingers or any other object into the mouth

After the seizure:
- Ensure an adequate airway
- Turn the individual to one side to allow saliva to drain from the mouth
- Protect the person from curious bystanders
- Do not leave the person until the individual is fully awake
- If this is a first-time seizure the individual should be seen by a physician
- If seizure activity is continuous or if another attack occurs in rapid succession, the individual should be transported to the nearest medical facility by ambulance
- If transported:
  A written description of the type of seizure activity should be sent with the individual. Include whether it was generalized or localized, how it started, the length of time from the moment of onset until the individual regained consciousness, and the number of seizures experienced by the individual

experience frequent seizures should choose activities accordingly.

💡 *The softball player is probably having a complex partial seizure. Do not stop or restrain the person, but help them lie down and place something soft under the head. Clear the other ball players away from the area. The person may be confused or disoriented after the seizure. If this is their first seizure, refer the individual to a physician.*

HYPERTENSION

❓ *A football player has just learned during his pre-participation exam that his blood pressure is high. What implications will this have on his participation?*

Hypertension is defined as a sustained elevated blood pressure above the accepted norms of 140 mm Hg systolic or 90 mm Hg diastolic. Nearly 25% of the general population will develop hypertension by age 50. The onset is generally between ages 20 and 50 with the frequency greater in African Americans. Certain prescribed medications, anabolic steroids, amphetamines, oral contraceptives, chronic alcohol use, nasal decongestants containing sympathomimetic amines, and some non-steroidal anti-inflammatory drugs (NSAIDs) may elevate blood pressure (33). The condition is classified as benign or malignant. Benign hypertension progresses slowly, whereas malignant hypertension rapidly accelerates, leading to severe organ damage. Longstanding hypertension often attacks the heart, brain, kidneys, and eyes. Any individual who has mild or moderate hypertension should not participate in competitive sports until cleared by a physician.

Aerobic type exercises have been shown to modestly reduce high blood pressure, but specific mechanisms are still unknown. This decrease may result from decreased body fat, relaxation during exercise, or decreased smoking and alcohol consumption (34). Twenty to thirty minutes of aerobic exercise at 60 to 85% of maximum heart rate, three to four times a week, is recommended. Daily walking at a moderate speed is excellent, however, isometric exercises and heavy resistance training should be avoided. In more serious cases, sodium and alcohol restrictions, weight loss, reduction of other cardiovascular risk factors, calcium channel blockers, and angiotensin-converting enzyme (ACE) inhibitors are used to manage the condition (33,34).

💡 *The football player should see the physician to determine the degree of severity. A supervised exercise program may include sodium restrictions, weight control, and possible medications. The individual should not participate in activity until cleared by the physician.*

ANEMIA

❓ *A middle-aged female endurance runner is complaining of chronic fatigue and malaise, particularly during running. She appears somewhat pale and tired, but otherwise is fine. While taking her history, she reports that she tends to have a heavy menstrual flow. What condition might you suspect?*

A reduction in either the red blood cell volume (hematocrit) or hemoglobin concentration is called **anemia**. Although there are five classifications of anemia, all are caused by either impaired red blood cell (RBC) formation or excessive loss or destruction of RBCs. A family history of anemia, past history of anemia, intermittent jaundice early in life, chronic blood loss through heavy menstruation or gastrointestinal bleeding, certain drugs and toxins, chronic inflammatory disease, malignant diseases, and patients with diminished hepatic, renal, or thyroid function are all at increased risk for developing the disorder (35). In sport participation, anemia reduces maximum aerobic capacity and anaerobic threshold, decreases efficiency at submaximal levels, and decreases exercise time to exhaustion (19). Several specific anemic conditions occur in sport participants.

Iron-Deficiency Anemia

The most common cause of anemia in the world is iron-deficiency characterized by deficient hemoglobin synthesis. In infancy and early childhood, inadequate diet may be an underlying factor; in older children and adults blood loss or impaired absorption of iron should be suspected (36). It is particularly prevalent in women of childbearing age, secondary to menstrual losses and to increased iron demand during pregnancy. Iron-deficiency anemia is also seen in endurance athletes and in those who maintain a lower percent body fat.

Symptoms may include fatigue, tachycardia, blood mixed with feces, and pallor with epithelial abnormalities, such as a sore tongue. Later symptoms include cardiac

Hypertension
Sustained elevated blood pressure above the norms of 140 mm Hg systolic or 90 mm Hg diastolic

Twenty to thirty minutes of aerobic exercise at 60 to 85% maximum heart rate, three to four times a week, has been shown to reduce high blood pressure

Anemia
Abnormal reduction in red blood cell volume or hemoglobin concentration

Individuals at risk for anemia include those that have:
  Family history of anemia
  Past history of anemia and intermittent jaundice early in life
  Chronic blood loss through heavy menstruation or gastrointestinal bleeding
  (On) medication that limits absorption of iron
  Chronic inflammatory disease and malignant diseases
  Diminished hepatic, renal, or thyroid function

Iron-deficiency anemia is commonly seen in women of childbearing age secondary to menstrual losses, pregnant women, endurance athletes, and athletes maintaining a lower percent body fat

Sickle cell anemia
Abnormalities in hemoglobin structure resulting in a characteristic sickle- or crescent-shaped red blood cell that is fragile and unable to transport oxygen

Infarcts
Clumping together of cells that block small blood vessels leading to vascular occlusion, ischemia, and necrosis in organs

Individuals with sickle cell trait should limit running to no more than ½ mile without rest, avoid activity in extremely hot, humid weather, and altitudes greater than 2500 feet

Drugs are divided into three types:
   Therapeutic
   Performance-enhancing
   Recreational

Therapeutic drugs
Prescribed or over-the-counter medications used to treat an injury or illness

murmurs, congestive heart failure, loss of hair, and pearly sclera. Treatment may involve dietary iron supplementation (ferrous sulfate, ferrous gluconate) and ascorbic acid (Vitamin C) to enhance iron absorption. Avoid colas, coffee, or tea, as caffeine hampers iron absorption. Surgery may be needed if active bleeding from polyps, ulcers, malignancies, or hemorrhoids is the cause.

Sickle Cell Anemia

Sickle cell anemia, more commonly seen in African Americans, results from abnormalities in hemoglobin structure that produce a characteristic sickle- or crescent-shaped red blood cell that is fragile and unable to transport oxygen. Because of its rigidity and irregular shape, sickle cells clump together and block small blood vessels, leading to vascular occlusion, or **infarcts** in organs, such as the heart, lungs, kidneys, spleen, and central nervous system. Although an individual with the sickle cell trait may be asymptomatic for their entire life, exercising in excessively high heat, humidity, and/or altitude may lead to dehydration, predisposing an individual to an increase in protein concentration in the circulating blood cells. This high concentration increases blood viscosity and impairs blood flow, which can lead to a stroke, congestive heart failure, acute renal failure, pulmonary embolism, or sudden death (37).

Signs and symptoms may include swollen, painful, and inflamed hands and feet, irregular heart beats, severe fatigue, headache, skin pallor, muscle weakness, or severe pain due to oxygen deprivation. Currently there is no known treatment to reverse the condition. Since dehydration can complicate the condition, individuals should hydrate maximally before, during, and after exertion. Liquids with caffeine, such as colas, coffee, and tea should be avoided because of their potential diuretic effect. Individuals with sickle cell trait should limit running to no more than ½ mile without rest, and avoid activity in extremely hot, humid weather, and at altitudes greater than 2500 ft (37).

The endurance runner may have iron-deficiency anemia. Her age, distance running, and heavy menstrual flow are all factors that put her at risk for the condition. Refer her to a physician to rule out other underlying conditions.

SUBSTANCE ABUSE

A 16-year-old football player returned from summer vacation thirty pounds heavier and able to bench press 50 additional pounds. He reported he was on an aggressive weight-training program over the summer, but you question how these gains were made in such a short time. What implications might this have on his health and performance?

Drugs are divided into three types: (1) therapeutic—those taken to manage an injury or illness; (2) performance-enhancing—those used to enhance one's athletic performance; and (3) recreational—those taken to alter one's mood (for entertainment or to escape reality). These are not exclusive categories, as some therapeutic and performance-enhancing drugs may be used recreationally to alter one's mood. Drugs sold over-the-counter, or nonprescription drugs, generally have a dosage of less than 200 mg of medication, and are designed to relieve pain and inflammation. Prescription drugs may range from 200 to 700 mg of medication and are designed to relieve symptoms and cure a disease or condition. In most cases, you will only be concerned with nonprescription drugs. Extreme caution must be exercised with all medication, however.

Therapeutic Drugs

Therapeutic drugs are used to treat an injury or illness, and depending on the dosage, may be prescribed or over-the-counter medications. Prescribed medications include nonsteroidal anti-inflammatories (NSAIDs), major pain relievers, diuretics, beta blockers, beta-agonists, local anesthetics, corticosteroids, barbiturates or tranquilizers, amphetamines, and oral contraceptives. Over-the-counter medications include analgesics, decongestants and antihistamines, laxatives and antidiarrheal agents, and weight-loss medications (38). The use and side effects of therapeutic drugs can be seen in **Table 17-4**.

Prescription Drugs

Prescription drugs are used to reduce pain, inflammation, fever, and associated symptoms after an injury, illness, or surgery. Each category of drugs has adverse effects that can alter sport performance or body metabolism. Examples of common medications are listed with each group.

Table 17–4. Therapeutic Drugs

Prescription	Intended Use	Side/Adverse Effects
NSAIDs	Reduce inflammation, pain and fever	Gastrointestinal bleeding, drowsiness, diarrhea, prolonged clotting time, dizziness, tinnitus, headaches, elevated liver enzymes, renal failure
Dimethyl sulfoxide (DMSO)	Anti-inflammatory to promote vasodilation and decrease pain	Rash, dermatitis, headache, nausea, dizziness, cataracts, and can weaken tendons and ligaments
Diuretics	Control hypertension, reduce edema, congestive heart failure, promote fluid and electrolyte balance	Hyperglycemia, hypotension, decreased sport performance, reduced blood volume, dehydration, electrolyte imbalance, muscle cramps
Beta-blockers	Reduce tremors, lower heart rate, control hypertension, angina, stage fright, certain cardiac arrhythmias, anxiety	Hypotension, edema, nausea, impotence, fatigue, diarrhea, constipation, insomnia, nightmares, depression, dyspnea, peripheral vascular disease
Beta-agonists	Respiratory disorders, asthma and bronchospasm	Dizziness, flushing, swelling of the face, lips, or eyelids, headache, tremors, tachycardia
Local anesthetics	Local anesthesia during treatment and examination, local anti-inflammatory effect, arthritis, bursitis, tendinitis	Allergic reactions, localized edema, masks pain, hypotension, may delay healing, local infections, and cardiac arrhythmias
Corticosteroids	Chronic inflammation and pain reduction	Gastrointestinal bleeding, nausea, vomiting, fluid retention, insomnia, hyperglycemia, depression, hallucinations, oral candidiasis
Barbiturates	Seizure disorders, tremors, depression, fatigue, lethargy, anxiety, and insomnia	Decreased performance and attention span, slurred speech, impaired gait, blurred vision, drowsiness, dependence, tolerance, addiction, and in large doses, respiratory depression, coma, and death
Amphetamines	Narcolepsy and short-term appetite suppression	Insomnia, restlessness, hyperactivity, headache, tremors, twitches, palpitations, nausea, vomiting, constipation, and drug dependence
Oral contraceptives	Prevent unwanted pregnancies and osteopenia in amenorrheic athletes	Dizziness, weight gain, fluid retention, migraine headaches, lethargy, depression, hypertension, breast tenderness and enlargement, urinary tract infections, breakthrough bleeding, and dysmenorrhea

(continued)

Table 17–4. Therapeutic Drugs *(continued)*

Prescription	Intended Use	Side/Adverse Effects
Analgesics	Reduce pain, inflammation and fever	Nausea, vomiting, GI bleeding, allergic reactions, prolonged clotting, tinnitus, diarrhea, abdominal pain, renal failure, hepatic coma, convulsions, death
Decongestants and antihistamines	Control upper respiratory tract infections, colds, allergies	Nervousness, dizziness, headaches, tachycardia, confusion, cerebral hemorrhage, stroke, arrhythmias
Laxatives and antidiarrheals	Relieve or control constipation and diarrhea	Gas pains, pain with bowel movement, fluid and electrolyte imbalance, dry mouth, constipation
Weight-loss drugs	Control and lose weight	Hyperactivity, nervousness, tremors, headache, nausea, vomiting, constipation

Antipyretic
Medication used to bring a fever down

NSAIDs are used to reduce pain, inflammation, and fever through vasodilation

Diuretics promote the excretion of water, sodium, and to a lesser extent, other electrolytes by stimulating the kidneys

Beta-blockers reduce tremors, and lower heart rate and blood pressure

Beta-agonists are used to manage respiratory disorders, particularly asthma and bronchospasm

NSAIDs (e.g., Motrin, Indocin, Butazolidin, Feldene, Clinoril) are used to reduce pain, inflammation, and fever (**antipyretic**) through vasodilation of blood vessels. This promotes heat loss from the vessels to the skin surface. NSAIDs are used in acute injuries in conjunction with ice, compression, and elevation after the acute phase has ceased. They are commonly used in chronic injuries and certain arthritic conditions. To reduce the risk of gastrointestinal irritation, NSAIDs should always be taken with food or fluid.

Dimethyl sulfoxide (DMSO) is used as an anti-inflammatory to stimulate a histamine response at the cellular level to promote vasodilation, and decrease pain by blocking the C nerve fibers. In sports, it is used to decrease joint swelling, hematomas, ecchymosis, and promote the healing process, but its effectiveness remains highly controversial. In nearly all states, DMSO is not approved for use by humans. DMSO is absorbed rapidly into the skin and spreads systemically within five minutes of application, leaving a characteristic taste or breath smelling of garlic. Because of the rapid absorption, it is sometimes used to assist systemic application of hydrocortisone into the body. Side effects include a localized rash, dermatitis, headache, nausea, dizziness, and in large doses, cataracts. Prolonged treatment can weaken tendons and ligaments.

Diuretics (e.g., Diamox, Hydrodiuril, Osmitrol, Lasix, Diuril) promote the excretion of water, sodium, and to a lesser extent, other electrolytes by stimulating the kidneys to work. They are used to control hyperten-

sion, reduce edema, and assist in the treatment of congestive heart failure. Essentially, they regulate fluid and electrolyte balance when kidney function is compromised, or aid in reducing vascular fluid and edema. Athletes may use them to achieve rapid weight loss, while others may use them to dilute urine to mask the presence of banned substances during drug testing. Using diuretics to "make weight" has been associated with lower plasma and blood volume, depletion of liver glycogen stores, increased electrolyte loss, impairment of body temperature regulation, lower aerobic capacity, and reduction in muscular strength and work performance (39).

Beta-blockers (e.g., Secral, Tenormin, Lopressor, Inderal) are used to reduce tremors and lower heart rate, such as in archery or shooting sports. The medications block the fight-or-flight response of the sympathetic nervous system by decreasing the rate and force of cardiac contractions, thereby reducing blood pressure. Hypertension, angina, stage fright, and certain cardiac arrhythmias are treated with this medication (40).

Beta-agonists (e.g., Proventil, Maxair, Bronkosol, Brethaire) are used to manage respiratory disorders, particularly asthma and bronchospasm, and may have some performance-enhancing effects. As such, many are on the banned substance lists for most sport-governing bodies. Products, such as Bronkaid mist and Primatene mist, are sold over-the-counter, and in the inhaled forms, are acceptable for therapeutic use in athletes (38). The medications relax the smooth muscles of the bronchial walls and can stimulate the heart and central nervous system.

Clenbuterol, a veterinary beta-agonist drug, is used in Europe to build muscle mass and strength in livestock. The drug is being used illegally by some athletes in hopes of achieving the same effects in humans. Like most steroid alternatives, the long-term side effects are not fully understood. In 1990, 135 individuals became seriously ill after eating beef liver that contained traces of clenbuterol residue. Their symptoms included rapid pulse rate, muscle tremors, severe headache, dizziness, nausea, fever, and chills. The symptoms appeared between 30 minutes and 6 hours after consumption of the beef, and lasted for nearly 2 days (41). Some athletes use the drug with anabolic steroids thinking they can derive from 10 to 25% of the effect of anabolic steroids with daily use. However, this practice may lead to serious cardiovascular complications, and should be strongly discouraged.

Local anesthetics (e.g., lidocaine, procaine) are used by physicians and dentists to provide local anesthesia during examination or treatment. The injected drugs produce a loss of sensation by blocking pain conduction, and as such, could cause a serious injury if an individual participates in sport while the area is anesthetized. Fortunately, the abuse rate is low. Topical anesthetics can inhibit peripheral pain receptors through rapid cooling with the use of spray coolants or alcohol, or with counterirritants, such as liniments and analgesic balms that irritate skin receptors, leading to a localized increase in blood circulation, temperature, and erythema.

Corticosteroids (e.g., cortisone, prednisone) increase blood levels of adrenocorticosteroid hormones normally secreted by the adrenal gland. They influence body systems by affecting fluid, electrolyte balance, and metabolic activities in the major systemic systems of the body (42). Their use in acute injuries remains debatable. Some researchers believe they limit pain and swelling, whereas others believe they hinder the healing process, delaying recovery (38). Chronic inflammatory conditions are the main indication for use. Extreme caution must be used, however, to avoid injecting corticosteroids directly into tendons, such as the Achilles or patellar tendons, as eventual rupture of the tendon may occur.

Barbiturates (e.g., phenobarbital, pentobarbital, Mebaral, Amytal), or tranquilizers, are seldom prescribed for sport participants. Barbiturates are used to treat seizure disorders and tremors; tranquilizers are used to treat depression, anxiety, and insomnia. Barbiturates reduce reaction time, visual tracking skills, and ability to concentrate (40).

Amphetamines (e.g., pemoline, methylphenidate, Desoxyn) stimulate the central nervous system, resulting in respiratory stimulation, appetite suppression, increased energy, and increased mental alertness. This medication is used to treat narcolepsy, a condition characterized by uncontrolled disposition toward sleep, and for short-term appetite suppression. Amphetamines can cause insomnia, restlessness, hyperactivity, headache, tremors, twitches, palpitations, nausea, vomiting, constipation, and drug dependence (42).

Oral contraceptives are used by female sport participants to prevent unwanted pregnancies, and prevent osteopenia (diminished bone mineral density) in amenorrheic athletes. There is virtually no potential for abuse.

Over-the-Counter Medications

There are numerous over-the-counter medications available to any individual. Although the abuse rate is low, individuals trying to lose weight have been known to use excessive amounts of laxatives and weight-loss medications to attain their goals.

Analgesics include aspirin, acetaminophen (Anacin-3, Panadol, Tylenol), and ibuprofen (Advil, Medipren, Nuprin, Motrin). Aspirin can reduce pain, fever, inflammation, and prevent the clotting of blood for up to seven days. Because of its anti-clotting factor, aspirin should never be administered during the acute phase of an injury. Fever is reduced by peripheral vasodilation, perspiring, and heat dissipation. Acetaminophen does not have the antiplatelet activity of aspirin, nor does it cause gastrointestinal bleeding. However, acetaminophen has limited anti-inflammatory properties. Ibuprofen, like aspirin, reduces pain, fever, and inflammation. If used in excess, ibuprofen and aspirin can lead to gastrointestinal bleeding, resulting in anemia. As such, analgesic drugs should be taken after a meal or with sufficient fluid to dilute GI irritation.

Decongestants and antihistamines (e.g., ephedrine, Benadryl) are frequently used to control symptoms of upper respiratory tract infections and allergies. Histamine is a protein that, when released in the general circu-

Anesthetics produce a loss of sensation by blocking pain conduction

Corticosteroids are commonly used to treat chronic inflammatory conditions

Barbiturates are used to treat seizure disorders and tremors; tranquilizers are used to treat depression, anxiety, and insomnia

Oral contraceptives are used to prevent unwanted pregnancies and osteopenia in amenorrheic athletes

Aspirin can reduce pain, fever, inflammation, and prevent the clotting of blood for up to 7 days

lation, causes an allergic-like reaction, such as dilated capillaries, flushed skin, and a rise in temperature. Antihistamines block histamine action, however, they are known to decrease reaction time and cause drowsiness, lethargy, mucous membrane dryness, and occasionally nausea and light-headedness. Decongestants do not result in any appreciable side effects. Therefore, decongestants should be used during the day and antihistamines used at night when the side effects of antihistamines will not have as severe an effect. These drugs increase blood pressure, cause moderate tachycardia, increase cardiac output, coronary, cerebral, and muscle blood flow (42). Bronchodilation reduces airway resistance and improves air movement following an episode of bronchospasm. In severe allergic reactions, antihistamines alone may not control the symptoms, and additional epinephrine or dexamethasone is needed to prevent anaphylactic shock. Many of these medica-

tions are on the banned substance lists through the various sport-governing bodies (See **Table 17-8**).

Laxatives and antidiarrheal agents are used to control constipation and diarrhea. These agents should never be used on a regular basis as it places the individual at risk for dehydration and heat illnesses. Individuals with eating disorders and those who want to "make weight" are frequent abusers of these drugs. These individuals should receive intensive therapy and dietary counseling.

Weight-loss medications (e.g., Dexatrim, Acutrim) can also be abused. Wrestlers, boxers, swimmers, and gymnasts are at a high risk for abusing these drugs (38). Individuals in competitive sports should have their weight monitored. If it is necessary to lose weight, specific goals and dietary manipulation should be done under proper supervision. (See **Field Strategy 17-7** for guidelines for supervised weight loss.)

 Field Strategy 17–7. Guidelines for Safe Weight Loss and Weight Gain.

- One pound of body fat contains approximately 3,500 calories
- Caloric needs are dependent on age, gender, basal metabolic rate, physical condition, body weight, composition, and activity level
- Weight loss is best achieved by reducing daily caloric intake by 500 to 1000 calories, thus averaging 1 to 2 pounds of body fat lost per week. Weight reduction should begin in the off-season and should not exceed 3 to 4 pounds per week. Weight loss during the season should not exceed 2 to 3 pounds per week
- Moderate exercise for one half hour three times a week burns over 1050 calories. Consequently, one need only reduce weekly caloric intake by 2450 calories to lose one pound per week. Exercise 5 days a week coupled with reduced caloric intake (1200 to 1500 calories/day) would result in more weight loss
- Aerobic exercise, such as walking, running, rope-skipping, cycling, and swimming are excellent. Weight reduction without exercise causes a significant loss in muscle mass
- Drink plenty of water and avoid caffeine
- A well-balanced diet should include fresh fruits and vegetables, cereal and grains, milk and milk products, and meat and high-protein foods. Avoid fried foods
- In the first 3 days of weight loss, 70% is attributed to water loss. At least 2 months of weight reduction is necessary for any substantial fat loss
- Rapid weight loss to "make weight" is often achieved through water loss, which can be harmful. Dehydration can lead to muscle cramping, fatigue, weakness, and impaired heat regulation
- Laxatives or diuretics should never be used in weight loss, as chronic abuse can lead to serious complications
- Weight gain can be accomplished by consistently eating 3 meals a day and consuming extra servings at mealtime. Eat frequent snacks that are low in fat and primarily carbohydrate, along with some protein, such as granola, GrapeNuts, and bananas. Drink lots of juice and milk, particularly those higher in calories, such as whole milk, cranberry and grape juice, or calorie-containing fluids
- Weight gain should not exceed 1 to 2 pounds per week, and should be combined with continued exercise and weight training
- Maintenance of weight is just as important as weight loss. Yo-yo dieting can be deleterious to your health

Performance-enhancing Drugs

Performance-enhancing drugs include anabolic-androgen steroids (AAS), growth hormone, stimulants including some amphetamines, caffeine, nicotine, and beta-sympathomimetics, erythropoietin (EPO), and beta-blockers (38). Their use and adverse side effects can be seen in **Table 17-5**. There is little to no research proving food supplements such as amino acids, protein or carbohydrate powders, herbs, vitamins, and minerals enhance performance and will not be discussed. Reported side effects of food supplements include stomach pain, nausea, dizziness, vomiting, diarrhea, and cardiovascular problems (43).

Anabolic-androgen steroids (AAS) are synthetic derivatives of the hormone testosterone including Methosarb, Danocrine, Dianabol, Anavar, Drolban, and Maxibolin. These drugs enhance performance by increasing lean body mass and strength. Research has not proven that enhanced recovery from high-intensity workouts, speed, or endurance are affected by their use. Adverse effects include increased acne, changes in liver function, benign and malignant liver tumors, decreased sperm count, sterility or testicular atrophy, gynecomastia, premature epiphyseal closure in prepubescent children, and hypertension. In addition, women may experience masculinization, menstrual irregularities, clitoral hypertrophy, decreased breast tissue, deepened voice, increased growth of facial and body hair, irritability, and aggressiveness. Many of these adverse effects are irreversible and place the individual at risk for atherosclerotic cardiovascular disease (44,45,46).

> Research has not proven that food supplements enhance performance

> Anabolic steroids enhance performance by increasing lean body mass and strength, but can cause severe irreversible damage to the body organs

Table 17–5. Performance Enhancing Drugs.

Drug	Intended Use	Side/Adverse Effects
Anabolic/ Androgen Steroids (AAS)	Increase lean body mass, increase strength	Acne, psychologic changes (increased aggression and libido, mood swings, depression, delusions, hallucinations), decreased high-density lipoproteins, increased low-density lipoproteins, changes in serum cholesterol, hematocrit, and clotting factors, hypertension, risk of cardiovascular disease
Growth hormone	Treat growth hormone deficiency	Excessive linear bone growth, thickened skin, soft tissue swelling, organomegaly, glucose intolerance, cardiomyopathy, hypertension
Amphetamines	Stimulation of CNS to fight narcolepsy, delay onset of fatigue, speed reaction time, increase force of muscle contractions, appetite suppression, decrease body fat	Insomnia, hyperactivity, headache, tremors, twitches, tachycardia, nausea, vomiting, diuresis, drug tolerance, addiction
Erythropoietin (EPO)	Anemia, AIDS, rheumatoid arthritis, patients receiving chemotherapy	Hypertension, chest pain, tachycardia, headache, dehydration, pelvic and limb pain, increased clotting of arteriovenous grafts, death
Beta-blockers	Reduce tremors, lower heart rate, hypertension, angina, stage fright, certain cardiac arrhythmias, anxiety	Hypotension, edema, nausea, impotence, fatigue, diarrhea, constipation, insomnia, nightmares, depression, dyspnea, peripheral vascular disease

Preliminary data also show a psychological dependence on anabolic-androgenic steroids, drug craving, and difficulty stopping despite psychological side effects. Most of these adverse effects are reversible. However, side effects during withdrawal include mood swings, violent behavior, rage, and depression that may lead to thoughts of suicide (47).

Of great concern in the medical community is the practice of cycling and stacking AAS with other drugs. In a recent study involving 14-to-16-year-old students, researchers reported illegal use of AAS in boys (6.5%) and girls (1.9%). Of these, 33% used AAS concurrently with cocaine, injectable drugs, alcohol, marijuana, cigarettes, and smokeless tobacco. Furthermore, 25% of the individuals reported sharing needles to inject the drugs (48). This practice can have serious implications for contributing to the spread of the human immunodeficiency virus (HIV). Anabolic steroids are banned substances and illegal in the United States.

Little research exists on the benefits of the *human growth hormone* (HGH) as a performance enhancer. Its only indication for use is to treat growth hormone deficiency. Although some animal research has shown increased lean body mass and strength, it remains debatable for humans. Adverse effects in individuals with an excess of HGH include gigantism due to accelerated linear bone growth, organomegaly, thickened skin, soft tissue swelling, cardiomyopathy, hypertension, and glucose intolerance (40).

Amphetamines (e.g., Vivarin, caffeine, Dexedrine) stimulate the central nervous system to release stored norepinephrine from nerve terminals, resulting in increased respirations, appetite suppression, increased energy and alertness. These drugs are used to treat attention-deficit disorders, narcolepsy, delay the onset of fatigue, speed reaction time, decrease body fat, and increase the force of contraction (40). Adverse effects include restlessness, tremors, headache, palpitations, paranoia, compulsive behaviors, and drug dependence or tolerance.

Caffeine is found in coffee, tea, chocolate, and many other medications. As little as two cups of coffee can produce adverse effects. Caffeine has been shown to reduce fatigue, and as such, may enhance performance, but its effects are limited. It has been shown to increase blood pressure 5 to 10 mm Hg, dilate bronchial passages in asthmatic patients,

increase gastric secretions, suppress motility in the stomach and small intestine, but relax muscles in the large intestine. As a diuretic, it can increase urination by as much as 30% for up to 3 hours after consumption (49). Combined with exercise, an increase in the release of free fatty acids is seen.

Nicotine from cigarettes or smokeless tobacco (snuff or chewing tobacco) has been shown to significantly increase heart rate, speed the onset of fatigue, decrease endurance performance, but has not been shown to affect reaction time, movement time, or total response time among athletes or nonathletes (50,51). Adverse effects include bad breath, decreased taste perception, periodontal bone loss, tooth loss, nicotine addiction, and various forms of oral infections and cancer.

Adolescent and young adult males continue to use smokeless tobacco at alarming rates. In a recent 1991 study, 45% of professional baseball players were users (52). To address this, professional baseball developed an educational program to help players quit using smokeless tobacco. Several clubs have banned carrying smokeless tobacco while in uniform, and banned tobacco advertising. Sport governing bodies have yet to establish strict policies against its use, however, the NCAA has banned its use on intercollegiate fields.

Beta-sympathomimetics are stimulants found in decongestants used to fight fatigue and enhance explosiveness. Ginseng is an herb that has similar effects and falls into this category. No research has proven any performance enhancing quality (38).

Erythropoietin (EPO) stimulates red blood cell production by causing the tissues of the bone marrow to increase cell division to produce additional red blood cells. It is often linked with blood doping. The drug is currently used to treat anemia, AIDS patients, and patients receiving chemotherapy. Although erythropoietin is a naturally occurring hormone produced by the kidneys, supplementation is thought to help endurance performance, although this has not been proven.

As mentioned earlier, *beta-blockers* are used by competitive athletes to reduce tremors or lower heart rates in archery or shooting sports. The medications block the fight-or-flight response of the sympathetic nervous system by decreasing the rate and force of cardiac contractions, thereby reducing blood pressure. Hypotension, nausea, fatigue, insomnia, and depression are side effects of the drugs.

Recreational Drugs

Recreational drugs are nonprescription drugs used for mood-altering purposes. Alcohol is the major drug abused in the United States and falls within this category. Tobacco, already discussed with nicotine, and illegal drugs, such as marijuana/hashish, heroin, barbiturates, amphetamines, cocaine/crack, hallucinogens (LSD), and PCP (phencyclidine hydrochloride) also fall within this category (38). Their use and adverse side effects can be seen in **Table 17-6**.

Table 17–6. Recreational Drugs.

Drug	Intended Use	Side/Adverse Effects
Alcohol	Powerful CNS depressant; mood-altering to aid in socializing and escape from reality	Decreases alertness, reaction time, hand-eye coordination, accuracy, balance, judgement; chronic use leads to tremors, hallucinations, seizures, delusions, circulatory collapse, death
Tobacco	No role in clinical medicine; thought to improve psychomotor performance through calming effect; appetite suppression	Oral and lung cancer, atherosclerosis, coronary artery cerebrovascular disease, chronic obstructive pulmonary disease; neoplasms in the respiratory and GI systems
Stimulants	Childhood minimal brain dysfunction, attention-deficit disorders, certain CNS diseases to overcome drowsiness	Increases heart, breathing rate, and blood pressure, appetite suppression, blurred vision, insomnia, headache, dry mouth
Sedatives	Seizure disorders and certain psychiatric disorders	Sedation, slurred speech, impaired gait/balance, confusion, impaired memory, dependence, tolerance, respiratory depression, coma
Marijuana	Bronchodilator, decrease intraocular pressure and muscle spasms, reduce some side effects of chemotherapy	Tachycardia, impaired motor coordination, chest pains, increased short-term memory loss, immune system compromised, asthma, bronchitis, emphysema
Opiates (Narcotics)	Moderate to severe pain management, suppresses cough, diarrhea, and dyspnea associated with pulmonary edema	Nausea, vomiting, dizziness, mental clouding, itching, constipation, delirium, addiction, seizures
Psychedelics	No clinical use in medicine	Increased pulse and breath rates, impaired judgment, chills, hallucinations, convulsions, strokes, coma, heart and/or lung failure
Cocaine/crack	Used with epinephrine as topical anesthetic for nasal surgery	Impaired sport performance, ventricular arrhythmias, myocardial infarction, cerebral infarction, addiction, seizures, blindness, delirium, paranoia, liver toxicity, loss of smell, hyperthermia, sudden death

Alcohol has a vasodilation effect on the body and is a powerful central nervous system depressant

Alcohol is a poor source of carbohydrates and should not be consumed prior to or after physical exertion

Neoplasm
Mass of tissue that grows more rapidly than normal, and may be either benign or malignant

When confronting an individual about substance abuse, the individual often denies there is a problem

Alcohol use by intercollegiate athletes is reported to be approximately 89%, however, this percent is no greater than that used by nonathletes on college campuses. Alcohol has a vasodilation effect on the body and acts as a powerful, central nervous system depressant. It has been shown to decrease alertness, reaction time, hand-eye coordination, accuracy, balance, and judgment. Although some sport participants include alcohol consumption in their pre-game meal for carbohydrate loading, alcohol is a poor source of carbohydrates (CHO). One can of regular beer has only 14 gm of CHO (5 gm in light beer), whereas 40 gm of CHO are in 12 oz of juice or 8 oz of a soft drink (53). In addition, alcohol has dehydrating properties that can affect heat tolerance and hinder sport performance. While exercising in the cold, alcohol stimulates blood flow to the skin, leading to a flushed, warm sensation. However, a significant amount of heat loss from the body core can lead to hypothermia. Decreased liver glucose output places the sport participant at greater risk for hypoglycemia (53). Prolonged use of alcohol has been shown to be a precipitator of myocardial infarction in persons with coronary stenosis, and has been identified as a cause of variant angina, arrhythmias, primary myocardial disease, and sudden death (54).

Tobacco products have no clinical use in medicine, although some believe psychomotor skills are enhanced through its calming effects. A reduction in appetite may have some use in weight control, however, the side effects far outweigh the benefits of its use. Smoking and the use of smokeless tobacco are the leading cause of **neoplasms** in the respiratory and gastrointestinal tracts. Other disorders linked to the use of tobacco products include pneumonia, bronchitis, chronic obstructive pulmonary disease, oral and lung cancer, heart disease, growth retardation, and low birth weight in newborns (40).

Illegal drugs, used for mood-altering effects, stimulate neurotransmitters in the body in different combinations. Stimulants (e.g., uppers, speed, ice, meth) increase heart and breathing rates, increase blood pressure, decrease appetite and produce blurred vision, insomnia, profuse sweating, headache, and dry mouth. Sedatives (e.g., downers, ludes, reds, barbs) relax muscles, reduce heart and breathing rates, decrease blood pressure, and produce slurred speech, drowsiness, confusion, and loss of coordination. Marijuana

(e.g., grass, pot, weed) leads to increased pulse rate, impaired motor coordination, chest pains, increased short-term memory loss, impaired functioning of the immune system, and decreased sweating that can impair heat regulation. Continued use can lead to respiratory infections, such as asthma, bronchitis, and emphysema (55).

Opiates (e.g., heroin, morphine, codeine) slow down breathing, increase nausea, and reduce appetite, thirst, and pain perception. In addition, misuse can lead to infections of the heart lining and valves, skin abscesses, and congested lungs. Psychedelic drugs (LSD) increase pulse, breathing rates, blood pressure, temperature, impair judgment, and may cause nausea, chills, hallucinations, convulsions, strokes, coma, heart and/or lung failure. Cocaine and crack increase blood pressure, pulse, breathing rates, temperature, and can lead to ulcers in the mucous membrane of the nose, emphysema, psychological addiction, and malnutrition. Heart arrhythmias, coma, and death can result from even the smallest amounts (55).

Many of these drugs cause additional serious problems to unborn or newborn infants. The risk of AIDS and other infections from sharing needles is a major health concern. Used in combination with alcohol or other drugs, coma and death may result.

Signs of Substance Abuse

The coach, athletic trainer, and sport supervisor must be alert to the signs of possible drug abuse. It is imperative to intervene and get prompt professional help for the individual. Signs that indicate possible drug abuse are included in **Table 17-7**. Be prepared for denial of use by the individual. This barrier, however, must be overcome if the individual is to seek help. It is best to document any suspicions by noting behavioral or physical changes in the individual prior to counseling them. If confronting the individual is uncomfortable, it may be best to discuss the situation first in confidentiality with a professional counselor. The counselor may then intervene to help the suspected user.

Drug Testing

Drug testing began in 1968 at the Olympic Games and was adopted overwhelmingly by the National Collegiate Athletic Association (NCAA) in 1986 at their national convention.

Table 17–7. Signs of Possible Substance Abuse.

1. Abrupt changes in attendance at school, practice, or place of employment
2. Deterioration in work performance
3. Deterioration of physical condition, i.e., less stamina, dressing poorly, unclean or unkept
4. Out of character mood swings, impaired judgment (barbiturates)
5. Overt protection of personal possession, such as equipment, clothing, books, or secretiveness
6. Wearing sunglasses in inappropriate weather or indoors
7. Wearing long-sleeved garments in inappropriate weather
8. Borrowing money often
9. Social withdrawal from usual circle of friends or association with known drug users
10. Stealing items that can be pawned or sold for money to pay for the drug habit
11. Frequent trips to the bathroom, basement, or bedroom
12. Blood-shot eyes, slurred speech, excessive acne, raw red nostrils, hair loss, needle marks on the arms, legs, or between the toes
13. Dilated pupils (alcohol, marijuana, barbiturates). Constricted pupils (heroin and other narcotics)
14. Rapid weight gain, excessive aggression, irritability, nervousness, frequent complaints of "feeling sick"
15. Alcohol odor on breath, excessive bad breath (amphetamines), appears intoxicated, or tends to fall asleep easily

Some of the drugs banned by the NCAA are listed in **Table 17-8**. The major goal of drug testing is to make competition fair and equitable, and safeguard the health and safety of participants. In essence, drug testing involves analyzing a urine sample with thin-layer chromatography (TLC) or gas-liquid chromatography (GLC) for the presence of performance-enhancing and illegal drugs. The athletic trainer should not be involved in the drug-testing process, as it compromises their role as an impartial, unbiased health professional.

Many institutions have adopted their own drug-testing procedures and may include mandatory testing of all athletes—announced or random, or testing only those athletes where reasonable suspicion is present. It is imperative that institutions inform all student athletes of the drug testing protocol. In a 1992 study, over one third of 2,282 student athletes at 11 NCAA institutions were oblivious to the fact that their school did drug testing. Furthermore, 70% of the student athletes were unable to correctly identify their school's drug-testing protocol (56). This has direct implications for informed consent.

Student athletes may be totally unaware of what drugs may be on the banned substance list until they have tested positive for their use. A positive test can result in ineligibility for an extended period of time. Drug-testing

policies should be clearly documented and made available to all student athletes. Further information on drugs and the athlete and drug testing can be obtained from the NCAA, P.O. Box 1906, Mission, Kansas, 66201.

You suspect the football player used anabolic steroids over the summer to increase his size and strength. Did you determine you should talk to him about it? There is no set process. You might want to show your concern about his health, discuss the short- and long-term health consequences of using performance-enhancing drugs, and let him know you are there to help.

EATING DISORDERS

There are rumors that a swimmer was seen eating a large amount of food then disappeared to the restroom to vomit. There is noticeable bilateral soft tissue swelling over the angle of her mandible and calluses over the metacarpophalangeal joint of the middle finger. Her weight appears normal. Do these rumors need to be addressed? Why or why not?

Eating disorders are becoming more prevalent in both competitive and recreational sport participants. Although the disorders are often linked to sports that stress leanness, such as gymnastics, distance run-

Table 17–8. NCAA Banned Drug Classes.

(This is an abbreviated list of some of the medications banned by the NCAA and should be used only to demonstrate the variety of banned substances. Generic names are listed in the left hand column; examples are in the right hand column)

Psychomotor and central nervous system stimulants:

amiphenazole	Dapri, Daptizole	meclofenoxate	Lucidril, Brenal
amphetamine	Benzedrine, Dexedrine	methamphetamine	Desoxyn, Met-Ampi
bemigride	Megimide	methylphenidate	Ritalin
benzphetamine	Didrex	nikethamide	Coramine
caffeine	12 mcg/ml	pemoline	Cylert, Deltamin, Stimul
chlorphentermine	Pre-Sate, Lucofen	pentetrazol	Leptazol
cocaine	Surfacaine	Phendimetrazine	Phenzine, Bontril, Plegine
diethylpropion	Tenuate, Tepanil	phenmetrazine	Preludin
dimetamfetamine	Amphetamine	picrotoxine	Cocculin
ethamivan	Emivan, Vandid	pipradol	Meratran
fencamfamine	Envitrol, Altimine	prolintane	Villescon, Promotil, Katovit

Sympathomimetic Amines:

clorprenaline	Vortel, Asthone	Isoetharine	Bronkosol, Numotac, Dilabron
ephedrine	Bronkaid, Primatene	methoxyphenamine	Ritalin, Orthoxicol cough syrup
etafedrine	Mercodal, Decapryn	methylephedrine	Tzbrine, Methep
phenylpropanolamine	ARM, Allerest, Alka-Seltzer Plus, Contac, Dexatrim, Formula 44, Daldecon, Arnex, Sine-Aid, Sine-Off, Sinutab, Triaminicin, Sucrets Cold Decongestant		
pseudoephedrine	Actifed, Afrinol, Co-Tylenol, Deconamine, Emprazil, Fedahist, Fedrazil, Histalet, Isoclor, Novafed, Poly-Histine, Pseudo-Bid, Sudafed, Triprolidine, Tussend, Chlorafed, Chlortrimeton-DC, Drixoral, Polaramine Expectorant, Rondec		

Anabolic Steroids:

boldenone	Vebonol	nandrolone	Durabolin, Kabolin
clostebol	Sternanobol	norethandrolone	Nilevar
fluoxymesterone	Android-F, Halotestin	Oxandrolone	Anavar
mesterolone	Androviron, Proviron	Oxymetholone	Anadol, Nilevar, Anapolon 50
metandienone	Danabol, Dianabol	Stanozolol	Winstrol, Stroma
metenolone	Primobolan-Depot	testosterone	Malogen, Malogex, Oreton

Substances banned for specific sports (rifle):

alcohol		pindolol	Visken
atenolol	Tenormin	propranolol	Inderal
metoprolol	Lopressor	timolol	Blocadren
nadolol	Corgard		

Diuretics:

acetazolamide	Diamox, AK-Zol	furosemide	Lasix
benzthiazide	Aquatag, Hydrex	hydrochlorothiazide	Esidrix, Oretic, Thiuretic
bumetanide	Bumex	spironolactone	alatone, aldactone
chlorthalidone	Hygroton, Hylidone	triamterene	Dyrenium, Dyazide
ethacrynic acid	Edecrin		

Street Drugs:

heroin		THC (tetrahydrocannabinol)	
marijuana			

ning, swimming, diving, rowing, ballet, cross-country skiing, and wrestling, no sport is exempt. The incidence of eating disorders is difficult to pinpoint because of the secretive nature of those who have the disorder. Many sport participants engage in weight-control practices to afford optimal performance. However, when eating habits are altered because of a distorted body image, serious problems result. There are four specific eating disorders: atypical eating disorders, bulimia nervosa, anorexia nervosa, and combined disorders of anorexia plus bulimia (57). Eating disorders are typically associated with single, white, college-educated females from middle- to upper-class families, however more recent findings indicate gender, race, and social class are becoming less of a factor (58).

Atypical Eating Disorders

Many athletes show signs of disordered eating habits, but do not meet the criteria established for bulimia nervosa or anorexia nervosa. Studies by the American College of Sports Medicine (ACSM) have shown the prevalence of atypical eating disorders among female athletes ranges from 15 to 62% of sport participants (58). Many of these individuals exhibit certain physical features, and psychological and behavioral symptoms that indicate a possible eating disorder, and are listed in **Table 17-9**.

Bulimia Nervosa

Bulimia is the most common eating disorder, and is often characterized by normal weight

The four eating disorders include: bulimia nervosa, anorexia nervosa, atypical eating disorders, and combined disorders of anorexia plus bulimia

---

Table 17–9. Signs and Symptoms of a Possible Eating Disorder.

Physical features:
- Weight that is too low for athletic performance
- Precipitous weight loss
- Extreme fluctuations in weight
- Bloating or edema
- Swollen salivary glands (puffy cheeks or jaw just in front of the ear)
- Amenorrhea
- Yellowish appearance on palms of hands or soles of feet (carotinemia)
- Sores or callouses on knuckles or back of hand from inducing vomiting
- Hypoglycemia
- Cardiac arrhythmias, bradycardia
- Muscle cramps
- Gastrointestinal complaints
- Headaches, dizziness, weakness due to electrolyte disturbances
- Numbness and tingling in limbs due to electrolyte disturbances
- Renal dysfunction due to electrolyte disturbances
- Proclivity to stress fractures
- Loss or thinning of hair
- Downy hair appearing on face, back, or extremities

Psychological and behavioral symptoms:
- Excessive dieting
- Excessive eating without weight gain
- Excessive exercise that is not part of the training program
- Guilt about eating
- Claiming to feel fat at normal weight despite reassurances from others
- Preoccupation with food
- Avoidance of eating in public, denial of hunger
- Hoarding of food
- Frequent weighing
- Evidence of binge eating
- Evidence of self-induced vomiting
- Use of drugs to attempt to control weight (abuse of laxatives, diet pills, diuretics, emetics)

Bulimia

Personality disorder manifested by episodic bouts of binging large amounts of food followed by purging and feelings of guilt, self-disgust, and depression

Signs of bulimia include: Russell's sign, hypertrophy of the salivary glands, and dental erosion

Anorexia nervosa

Personality disorder manifested by extreme aversion toward food, resulting in extreme weight loss, amenorrhea, and other physical disorders

for age and height. **Bulimia nervosa** is defined as recurrent episodes of binge eating with a minimum average of two binge eating episodes a week for at least three months (57). The bulimic maintains a cyclical pattern of ingesting large quantities of food, 1,000 to 10,000 calories during a few minutes to several hours, then fasting. Purging may or may not occur (59). Purging behaviors may include self-induced vomiting, laxative, and diuretic abuse. Other symptoms include strict dieting, vigorous exercise to prevent weight gain, and persistent overconcern with body shape and weight (58). Individuals often lose their gag reflex and can purge without mechanical stimulation, or Ipecac may be used (60).

Depression and low self-esteem associated with perceptual distortions of body size are commonly seen in bulimics. They tend to feel socially undesirable, distrustful and suspicious of others, have higher levels of anxiety, and tend to come from families with conflict-resolution problems (59). Bulimics strive for thinness. This fear, however, manifests itself in either a restrictive eating pattern or purging behavior. Weight fluctuations are common.

The individual often has significant fluid and electrolyte abnormalities resulting in cardiac arrhythmias, hypotension due to low blood volume, metabolic acidosis due to laxative induced diarrhea, and cardiomyopathy. Gastrointestinal complications include esophagitis, possible esophageal perforation, pancreatitis, and constipation secondary to chronic laxative abuse (60). Irregular menses is common, rather than amenorrhea as seen in anorexics. The three most common physical signs associated with bulimics include:

1. Russell's sign, which is a lesion on the dorsum of the hand caused by repetitive trauma to the area during self-induced vomiting. This elongated ulceration, or hyperpigmented callus or scar, is visible on the metacarpophalangeal joint
2. Hypertrophy of the salivary glands, particularly the parotid glands. The individual often has a "chipmunk"-like face
3. Dental erosion caused by acidic gastric secretions that decalcify the teeth during recurrent vomiting episodes

Anorexia Nervosa

Anorexia nervosa is defined as a refusal to maintain body weight over a minimal normal weight for age and height, with body weight

being 15% below what is expected (57). The disorder is typically seen in females during adolescence, although it has been known to occur after menopause.

Anorexics have a distorted body image and maintain a great fear of gaining weight even though they are underweight. They view themselves as "fat" and equate body appearance with self-worth. An obsessive-compulsive nature for perfection and achievement leads many individuals to develop a highly ritualized exercise program for continuation over an entire day. Other characteristics include an overcontrolling ego, irrational logic, depression, sexual inhibition, and fear of maturation (59).

Amenorrhea often occurs prior to significant weight loss and continues for at least three consecutive months. There is a desire to control the body and eating, and remain in a prepuberty state, resulting in a near-starvation behavior. Many complain of being cold even on hot days. Others suffer from severe constipation because of poor food intake.

Low self-esteem and feelings of ineffectiveness are risk factors in the development of the disorder. Many anorexics sense their parents expect them to excel, yet do not believe they receive the support and affection they need to achieve that excellence (57). Feelings of anxiety and depression often result.

Detection of anorexia is easier than bulimia nervosa because of the deteriorated physical state of the individual. Treatment for both conditions is dependent on the presence of a personality disorder. If present, an extensive rehabilitation program of psychological and pharmacological intervention is necessary. If recognized early enough, behavioral and psychoeducational intervention with individual counseling can help (60). Bulimia nervosa and anorexia nervosa may not be curable, but can be managed with a well-structured and supervised rehabilitation program. **Table 17-10** compares bulimia nervosa with anorexia nervosa and lists medical complications that can result from these eating disorders. In extreme cases of eating disorders, the mortality rate is 10 to 18% (58).

Exercise and Weight Management

Weight management is best achieved with a supervised program of exercise and food intake. Sport performance can be adversely affected by improper weight reduction. Rapid

Table 17–10. Comparison of Bulimia Nervosa and Anorexia Nervosa.

Bulimia nervosa	Anorexia nervosa
Normal weight for age and height	Body weight 15% below what is expected
Afflicts women in their teens and twenties, however, it is also seen in wrestlers	Afflicts women in their teens and twenties
Distorted body image for body shape and weight	Distorted body image, so person feels "fat" even when emaciated
Recurrent binge eating, followed by fasting	Near-starvation is commonly seen
Purging may or may not occur	Purging is not common
Laxatives, diuretics, and self-induced vomiting is used for purging	
Low self-esteem and depression is common; obsessive-compulsive behavior is present	Low self-esteem is common; obsessive-compulsive behavior for perfection
Weight fluctuations are common	Weight diminishes steadily
Irregular menses is common	Amenorrhea is common

Complications of Eating Disorders	
Related to Purging	**Related to Weight Loss**
Electrolyte disturbances due to decreased blood volume, metabolic alkalosis, and magnesium deficiency	Loss of fat and muscle mass, including heart muscle
Inflammation of the salivary glands and pancreas	Bloating, constipation, abdominal pain, nausea
	Amenorrhea
Erosion of the esophagus and stomach which can lead to severe GI bleeding	Osteopenia, osteonecrosis, and femoral head collapse
	Peripheral neuropathy
Erosion and decay of dental enamel and discoloration due to gastric juices	Loss of scalp and pubic hair, or increased growth of pigmented baby-like hair over body

weight loss can affect body composition, renal function, electrolyte balance, thermal regulation, testosterone levels, and strength (61). To lose weight, one must increase activity or decrease food intake. The average American consumes 3300 calories a day, much more than is necessary for normal activity.

Weight loss should not exceed three pounds per week. Eating foods low in fat can significantly decrease caloric intake. In addition, fresh fruits, vegetables, water, and foods high in complex carbohydrates (potatoes, rice, and pasta) should provide the bulk of food intake. Competitive athletes should start weight reduction prior to the beginning of the competitive season so as not to affect sport performance.

Individuals who want to gain weight may think that high fat foods are the best choice. Although additional fat may be needed,

intake should not be excessive. Instead, individuals should consume extra servings at mealtime and eat frequent snacks that are low in fat and primarily carbohydrate with some protein. Good food choices include bagels, muffins, English muffins, pretzels, a turkey or lean beef sandwich, fresh fruit, chopped vegetables, soup (tomato, bean, or vegetable), yogurt, low fat crackers, and popcorn (with little or no butter) (58). Weight gain of lean body mass may only increase one to two pounds per week. In addition to increasing dietary intake, the sport participant should continue to exercise and weight train. **Table 17-11** lists activities and caloric expenditures. **Field Strategy 17-7** lists guidelines for safe weight-loss reduction and weight gain.

There was noticeable bilateral soft tissue swelling on the cheeks of the swimmer, and a callus over the MCP joint of the middle

Table 17–11. Calories expended during activity.

Activities	Calories Burned/Hr based on Weight		
	130 lbs	150 lbs	176 lbs
Aerobic dancing (intense)	474	552	648
Basketball	486	564	660
Canoeing (leisure)	156	180	210
Cycling (leisure at 5.5 mph)	228	264	306
Field hockey	474	546	642
Football	468	540	636
Free weights	300	348	408
Golf	300	348	408
Jumping rope (70 beats/min)	576	660	780
Nautilus weight training	330	378	444
Racquetball	630	726	852
Running, horizontal (7 min mile)	834	936	1074
Running, cross-country	576	666	780
Swimming (crawl, slow)	456	522	612
Swimming (breast stroke)	576	660	750
Tennis	384	444	522
Volleyball	180	204	240

finger. This individual is showing definite physical and behavioral signs of an eating disorder. Intervene and talk with her, letting her know you are there to help. Express concern for her health and recommend professional counseling.

SUMMARY

As a health care provider you will be confronted with numerous daily health problems unrelated to trauma. Sport performance can be adversely affected at altitudes or in poor quality air. Upper respiratory tract infections can be contagious and affect other team members. Gastrointestinal tract problems can lead to indigestion, diarrhea, or constipation. Sport participants may also have systemic conditions, such as diabetes mellitus, epilepsy, hypertension, or anemia that may require special adaptations to their exercise program or require immediate care, should their health status rapidly deteriorate.

There is no place in sport for substance abuse. Being under the influence of drugs can lead to self-injury or injury to other players through unintentional actions. In addition, current drug testing can lead to expulsion from sport participation. You should know the common signs that indicate possible drug use, intervene on behalf of the individual, and make sure that individual seeks professional counseling.

Eating disorders are becoming more prevalent and can affect any sport participant. Obsession with losing weight and a distorted body image can lead to atypical eating disorders, bulimia nervosa, or anorexia nervosa. Severe psychological and physical complications can result. Professional counseling and medical care are needed to help the individual overcome their depression and low self-esteem.

REFERENCES

1. McArdle, WD, Katch, FI, and Katch, VL. *Exercise physiology: Energy, nutrition, and human performance.* Philadelphia: Lea & Febiger, 1991.
2. American Academy of Orthopaedic Surgeons. *Athletic training and sports medicine.* Park Ridge, IL: American Academy of Orthopaedic Surgeons, 1991.
3. Shephard, RJ. "Adjustment to high altitude." In *Current therapy in sports medicine 1985–1986,* edited by RP Welsh and RF Shephard. St. Louis: CV Mosby College Publishing, 1985.
4. Folinsbee, LJ. "Air pollution and exercise." In *Current therapy in sports medicine 1985–1986,* edited by RP Welsh and RF Shephard. St. Louis: CV Mosby College Publishing, 1985.
5. Cohen, S, Tyrrell, DAJ, and Smith, AP. 1991. Psychological stress and susceptibility to the common cold. N Engl J Med, 325(9):606–611.
6. Hemila, H. 1992. Vitamin C and the common cold. Br J Nutr, 67(1):3–16.
7. Marby, RL. 1992. Topical pharmacotherapy for allergic rhinitis: New agents. South Med J, 85(2):149–154.
8. Ott, NL, O'Connell, EJ, Hoffman, AD, Beatty, CW, and Sachs, MI. 1991. Childhood sinusitis. Mayo Clin Proc, 66(12):1238–1247.

9. Wald, ER. 1992. Sinusitis in infants and children. Ann Otol Rhinol Laryngol Suppl, 155:37–41.

10. Oppenheimer, RW. 1991. Sinusitis: How to recognize and treat it. Postgrad Med, 91(5):281–286, 289–292.

11. Herr, RD. 1991. Acute sinusitis: diagnosis and treatment update. Am Fam Physician, 44(6):2055–2062.

12. Lang, SDR, and Singh, K. 1990. The sore throat: When to investigate and when to prescribe. Drugs, 40(6):854–862.

13. Keating, MR. 1992. Antiviral agents. Mayo Clin Proc, 67(2):160–178.

14. Solomon, W. "Familiar allergic disorders: Anaphylaxis and the atopic diseases." In *Pathophysiology: Clinical concepts of disease processes*, edited by SA Price and LM Wilson. St. Louis: Mosby-Year Book, 1992.

15. Renfroe, DH. "Obstructive alterations in pulmonary function." In *Pathophysiology: Adaptations and alterations in function*, edited by BL Bullock and PP Rosendahl. Philadelphia: JB Lippincott, 1992.

16. Kuhn, C, and Askin, FB. "Lung and mediastinum." In *Anderson's Pathology*, edited by JM Kissane. St. Louis: Mosby-Year Book, 1990.

17. Peterslund, NA. 1991. Herpes virus infection: An overview of the clinical manifestations. Scan J Infect, 80(Suppl):15–20.

18. Chetham, MM, Roberts, KB. 1991. Infectious mononucleosis in adolescents. Pediatr Ann, 20(4):206–213.

19. Sitorius, MA, and Mellion, MB. "General medical problems in athletes" In *The team physician's handbook*, edited by MB Mellion, WM Walsh, and GL Shelton. Philadelphia: Hanley & Belfus, 1992.

20. Weinberger, M. 1991. Day-to-day management of asthma. Pediatr, 18(4):301–311.

21. Murphy, S, and Kelly, HW. 1991. Management of acute asthma. Pediatr, 18(4):287–300.

22. Reisman, JJ, Canny, GJ, and Levison, H. 1991. Management of asthma in early life. Pediatr, 18(4):280–286.

23. Gong, H, Jr. 1992. Breathing easy: Exercise despite asthma. Phys Sportsmed, 20(3):159–167.

24. Jarjour, NN, and Calhoun, WJ. 1992. Exercise-induced asthma is not associated with mast cell activation or airway inflammation. J Allergy Clin Immunol, 89(1 Pt 1):60–68.

25. Tremaine, WJ. 1990. Chronic constipation: Causes and management. Hosp Prac Off Ed, 25(4A):89–100.

26. Birkett, DH. 1988. Hemorrhoids—diagnostic and treatment options. Hosp Prac Off Ed, 23(1A):99–108.

27. Heaman, D. "Normal and altered functions of the pancreas." In *Pathophysiology: Adaptations and alterations in function*, edited by BL Bullock and PP Rosendahl. Philadelphia: JB Lippincott, 1992.

28. Rifkin, H. 1991. Current status of non-insulin-dependent diabetes mellitus (type II): Management with gliclazide. Am J Med, 90(Suppl 6A):3–7.

29. Grant, HD, Murray, RH, Jr, and Bergeron, JD. Brady's Emergency Care. Englewood Cliffs, NJ: Prentice Hall, 1990.

30. Robbins, DC, and Carleton, S. 1989. Managing the diabetic athlete. Phys Sportsmed, 17(12):45–54.

31. Gates, JR. 1991. Epilepsy and sports participation. Phys Sportsmed, 19(3):98–104.

32. American Academy of Pediatrics Committee on Children with Handicaps and The Committee on Sports Medicine. 1983. Sports and the child with epilepsy. Pediatr, 72:884.

33. Daniels, SR, and Loggie, JMH. 1992. Hypertension in children and adolescents: Part II: Pharmacologic control—what works and why. Phys Sportsmed, 20(4):97–110.

34. Massie, BM. 1992. To combat hypertension, increase activity. Phys Sportsmed, 20(5):89–111.

35. Brown, RG. 1991. Determining the cause of anemia: General approach, with emphasis on microcytic hypochromic anemias. Postgrad Med, 89(6):161–170.

36. Baldy, CM. "Red blood cells." In *Pathophysiology: Clinical Concepts of Disease Process*, edited by SA Price and LM Wilson. St. Louis: Mosby-Year Book, 1992.

37. Browne, RJ, and Gillespie, CA. 1993. Sickle cell trait: A risk factor for life-threatening rhabdomyolysis? Phys Sportsmed, 21(6):80–88.

38. Jones, AP, Sickles T, and Lombardo, JA. "Substance Abuse." In *Clinics in sports medicine*, edited by JC Puffer, vol. 11, no. 2. Philadelphia: WB Saunders, 1992.

39. American College of Sports Medicine. *Position stand: Weight loss in wrestlers*. Indianapolis, 1976.

40. Wadler, GI, and Hainline, B. *Drugs and the athlete*. Philadelphia: FA Davis, 1989.

41. Ropp, KL. 1992. No-win situation for athletes. FDA Consumer, 26(10):8–12.

42. Alfaro-LeFevre, R, Blicharz, ME, Flynn, NM, Boyer, MJ. *Drug handbook*. Redwood City, CA: Addison-Wesley Nursing, 1992.

43. Cowart, VS. 1992. Dietary supplements: Alternative to anabolic steroids? Phys Sportsmed, 20(3):189–198.

44. Uzych, L. 1992. Anabolic-androgenic steroids and psychiatric-related effects: A review. Can J Psych, 37(1):23–28.

45. Cheever, K, and House, MA. 1992. Cardiovascular implications of anabolic steroid abuse. J Cardiovasc Nurs, 6(2):19–30.

46. Catlin, D, Wright, J, Pope, H, and Liggett, M. 1993. Assessing the threat of anabolic steroids. Phys Sportsmed, 21(8):37–44.

47. Rogol, AD, and Yesalis, CE. III. 1992. Clinical review 31: Anabolic-androgenic steroids and athletes: what are the issues? J Clin Endocrinol Metab, 74(3):465–469.

48. DuRant, RH, Rickert, VI, Ashworth, CS, Newman, C, and Slaven, G. 1993. Use of multiple drugs among adolescents who use anabolic steroids. N Eng J Med, 328(13):922–926.

49. Work, JA. 1991. Are java junkies poor sports? Phys Sportsmed, 19(1):83–88.

50. Edwards, WW, Glover, ED, and Schroeder, KL. 1987. The effects of smokeless tobacco on heart rate and neuromuscular reactivity in athletes and nonathletes. Phys Sportsmed, 15(7):141–147.

51. Van Duser, BL, and Raven PB. 1992. The effects of oral smokeless tobacco on the cardiorespiratory response to exercise. Med Sci Sports Exerc, 24(3):389–95.

52. Siegel, D, Benowitz, N, Ernster, VL, Grady, DG, and Hauck, WW. 1992. Smokeless tobacco, cardiovascular risk factors, and nicotine levels in professional baseball players. Am J Public Health, 82(3):417–421.

53. Clark, N. 1989. Social drinking and athletes. Phys Sportsmed, 17(10):95–100.

54. Sheehy, TW. 1992. Alcohol and the heart: How it helps, how it harms. Post Grad Med, 91(5):271–277.

55. National Collegiate Athletic Association. *Drugs and the athlete...A losing combination*. Mission, KS, 1988.

56. Albrecht, RR, Anderson, WA, McGrew, CA, McKeag, DB, and Hough, DO. 1992. NCAA institutionally based drug testing: Do our athletes know the rules of this game? Med Sci Sports Exerc, 24(2):242–245.

57. American Psychiatric Association. *Diagnostic and statistical manual of mental disorders*. Washington D.C., 1987.

58. Wichmann, S, and Martin, DR. 1993. Eating disorder in athletes: Weighting the risks. Phys Sportsmed, 21(5):126–135.

59. Kerr, JK, Skok, RL, and McLaughlin, TF. 1991. Characteristics common to females who exhibit anorexic or bulimic behavior: A review of current literature. J Clin Psychol, 47(6):846–853.

60. Yen, JL. 1992. General overview and treatment considerations of anorexia and bulimia. Comp Ther, 18(1):26–29.

61. Steen, SN, Oppliger, RA, Brownell, KD. 1988. Metabolic effects of repeated weight loss and regain in adolescent wrestlers. JAMA, 260(1):47–50.

Credits

Chapter 1. Courtesy of Lee's Photo Service, Muncie, IN, Fig. 1-3; From American Academy of Pediatrics Committee on Sports Medicine, Pediatrics, 81:737–739, 1988, Table 1–7; From D.L. Herbert, Legal Aspects of Sports Medicine, Canton, Ohio, Professional Reports Corporation, 1990, Field Strategy 1-1; From American Academy of Pediatrics, Sports Medicine: Health Care for Young Athletes. Elk Grove Village, Illinois, 1991, Field Strategies 1-2, 1-4, and 1-5; From M.D. Johnson, Tailoring the preparticipation exam to female athletes, Phys. Sportsmed., 20(7):61–72, 1992, Field Strategy 1-3.

Chapter 2. From M. Nordin and V.H. Frankel, Biomechanics of the Musculoskeletal System, Philadelphia: Lea & Febiger, 1989, Figs. 2-1, 2-7, 2-9; From S. Hall, Basic Biomechanics, St. Louis, Mosby-Yearbook, Inc., 1991, Figs. 2-2, 2-3, 2-4, 2-6; From E.C.B. Hall-Craggs, Anatomy as a Basis for Clinical Medicine, Baltimore: Williams & Wilkins, 1990, Fig. 2-8; From W.D. McArdle, F.I. Katch, and V.L. Katch, Exercise Physiology: Energy, Nutrition, and Human Performance, Philadelphia: Lea & Febiger, 1991, Fig. 2-10; From S.L. Michlovitz, Thermal Agents in Rehabilitation, Philadelphia: F.A. Davis Company, 1990, Fig. 2-11; From A.P. Spence, Basic Human Anatomy, Redwood City: The Benjamin/Cummings Publishing Company, 1990, Figs. 2-13(A), 2-16; Adapted from R.B. Salter, Textbook of Disorders and Injuries of the Musculoskeletal System, Baltimore: Williams & Wilkins, 1983, Fig. 2-15; Courtesy of S.J. Hall, Fig. 2-13(B & C).

Chapter 3. Courtesy of Mueller Sports Medicine, Inc., Prairie du Sac, WI, Fig. 3-4(C); From M.D. McArdle, F.I. Katch, and V.L. Katch, Exercise Physiology: Energy, Nutrition, and Human Performance, Philadelphia: Lea & Febiger, 1991, Fig. 3-6, Table 3-3, Table 3-5, modified; From R.L. Fritz and D.H. Perrin, "Cold exposure injuries: Prevention and treatment," in Clinics in Sports Medicine, edited by R.L. Ray, Vol. 8, No. 1, Philadelphia: W.B. Saunders Company, 1989, Table 3-6 and Field Strategy 3-6 (adapted); From H.D. Grant, R.H. Murray, and J.D. Bergeron, Brady Emergency Care, Englewood Cliffs, NJ: Prentice-Hall, Inc., 1990, Table 3-8 (adapted).

Chapter 4. Courtesy of Springfield College Sports Medicine Department, Springfield, MA, Figs. 4-1 and 4-9; Courtesy of Dr. R. Ortwein, Racine Sports Medicine Clinic, Racine, WI, Fig. 4-17; From H.M. Clarkson and G.B. Gillewich, Musculoskeletal Assessment: Joint Range of Motion and Manual Muscle Strength, Baltimore, Williams & Wilkins, 1989, Tables 4-4 and 4-5 (adapted).

Chapter 5. Courtesy of Dr. R. Ortwein, Racine Sports Medicine Clinic, Racine, WI, Fig. 5-2, 5-6, 5-16, 5-17, 5-18, 5-22, and 5-24; Courtesy of Biodex Medical Systems, Shirley, NY, Fig. 5-7; Courtesy of Lee's Photo Service, Muncie, IN, Fig. 5-8(C); Courtesy of Breg, Inc., Vista, CA, Fig. 5-9(A); Courtesy of Contemporary Design Co., Glacier, WA, Fig. 5-9(C); Courtesy of Aircast, Inc., Summit, NJ, Fig. 5-12; From K.L. Knight, "Guidelines for rehabilitation of sports injuries," in Clinics in Sports Medicine, edited by J.S. Harvey, Vol. 4, No. 3, 1985, Table 5-3 (adapted); From K.L. Knight, Cryotherapy: Theory, Technique and Physiology, Chattanooga, TN: Chattanooga Corporation, 1985, Field Strategy 5-11 (adapted).

Chapter 6. Courtesy of Lee's Photo Service, Muncie, IN, Fig. 6-5; Courtesy of J. P. Polonchek, Bridgewater, MA, Figs. 6-8 and 6-15(A); Courtesy of Brace International, Scottsdale, AZ, Figs. 6-10 and 6-18(B); Courtesy of Mueller Sports Medicine, Inc., Prairie du Sac, WI, Figs. 6-11, 6-12(A), 6-21(A) and 6-25(A); Courtesy of Body Armor, Durham, NC, Figs. 6-12(B) and Fig. 6-19; Courtesy of Pro Orthopedic Devices, Inc., Tucson, AZ, Figs. 6-13(A & B), 6-17(B), 6-20, 6-23(A), and 6-25(B); Courtesy of Jbi, Williston, VT, Fig. 6-16; Courtesy of Adams, U.S.A., Cookeville, TN, Fig. 6-18(A & C); Courtesy of Townsend Design, Bakersfield, CA, Fig. 6-21(B); Courtesy of Innovation Sports, Irvine, CA, Fig. 6-21(C); Courtesy of Aircast, Inc., Summit, NJ, Fig. 6-25(C); Courtesy of Foot Management, Pittsville, MD, Figs. 6-26 and 6-27(A); From S. Wichman and D.R. Martin, "Athletic shoes: Finding the right fit," Phys. Sportsmed., 21(3):204, 1993, Field Strategy 6-4 (adapted).

Chapter 7. From K. Luttgens, H. Deutsch, and N. Hamilton, Kinesiology: Scientific Basis of Human Motion, Dubuque: Brown Communication, Inc., 1992, Fig. 7-2; From A. Agur, Grant's Atlas of Anatomy, Baltimore: Williams & Wilkins, 1991, Figs. 7-3, 7-8, 7-9, and 7-10; From D. Magee, Orthopedic Assessment, Philadelphia: W.B. Saunders, 1992, Fig. 7-5; Courtesy of Charles City Community Schools, Charles City, IA, Fig. 7-25; From H. Kelikian and A.S. Kelikian, Disorders of the Ankle, Philadelphia: W.B. Saunders, 1985, Fig. 7-29; Courtesy of Dr. D. Adelberg, Hawthorn Physical Therapy and Sports Medicine, N. Dartmouth, MA, Fig. 7-33.

Chapter 8. From D.H. O'Donoghue, Treatment of Injuries to Athletes, Philadelphia: W.B. Saunders, 1984, Figs. 8-1(A), 8-2, and 8-5; From J.E. Crouch, Functional Human Anatomy, Philadelphia: Lea & Febiger, 1985, Fig. 8-1(B, C, D); Courtesy of Lee's Photo Service, Muncie, IN, Figs. 8-7 and 8-10; Courtesy of Charles City Community Schools, Charles City, IA, Fig. 8-8; Courtesy of Bridgewater State College Athletic Department, Bridgewater, MA, Fig. 8-9; Courtesy of Dr. D. Adelberg, Hawthorn Physical Therapy and Sports Medicine, N. Dartmouth, MA, Fig. 8-21; Courtesy of Dr. B. Saperia, Morton Hospital and Medical Center, Taunton, MA, Fig. 8-22; From C.C. Norkin and P.K. Levangie, Joint Structure and Function: A Comprehensive Analysis, Philadelphia: F.A. Davis Company, 1992, Table 8-1 (adapted); From American Academy of Orthopaedic Surgeons, Athletic Training and Sports Medicine, Philadelphia: American Academy of Orthopaedic Surgeons, 1991, Table 8-3.

Chapter 9. From A. Agur, Grant's Atlas of Anatomy, Baltimore, Williams & Wilkins, 1991, Fig. 9-1; From J.E. Crouch, Functional Human Anatomy, Philadelphia: Lea & Febiger, 1985, Fig. 9-3; From E.C.B. Hall-Craggs, Anatomy as a Basis for Clinical Medicine, Baltimore: Williams & Wilkins, 1990, Fig. 9-7; Courtesy of Dr. D. Adelberg, Hawthorn Physical Therapy and Sports Medicine, N. Dartmouth, MA, Figs. 9-9 and 9-13; Courtesy of Dr. M. Ehrlich, Rhode Island Hospital, Providence, RI, Fig. 9-15.

Chapter 10. Courtesy of W. Hinshaw, Salisbury Evening Post, Salisbury, NC, Fig. 10-12(A); Courtesy of T.F. Maguire,Jr., Attleboro, MA, Fig. 10-12(B); Courtesy of Lee's Photo Service, Muncie, IN, Fig. 10-12(C & D); Courtesy of Bridgewater State College Athletic Department, Bridgewater, MA, Fig. 10-12(E); From J.A. Nicholas and E.B. Hershman, The Upper Extremity in Sports Medicine, St. Louis: The C.V. Mosby Company, 1990, Fig. 10-14; From D.H. O'Donoghue, Treatment of Injuries to Athletes, Philadelphia: W.B. Saunders, 1984, Figs. 10-16 and 10-19; Courtesy of Dr. D. Adelberg, Hawthorn Physical Therapy and Sports Medicine, N. Dartmouth, MA, Figs. 10-17, 10-22, 10-25, and 10-26; From D.C. Reid, Sports Injury Assessment and Rehabilitation, New York: Churchill Livingstone, Inc., 1992, Fig. 10-20; From A.M. Papas, R.M. Zawacki, and C.F. McCarthy, Rehabilitation of the pitching shoulder, Am. J. Sports Med., 13(4):223–235, 1985, Field Strategy 10-10 (adapted).

Chapter 11. From J.E. Crouch, Functional Human Anatomy, Philadelphia: Lea & Febiger, 1985, Fig. 11-1; Courtesy of T.F. Maguire, Jr., Attleboro, MA, Fig. 11-10; Courtesy of Dr. B. Saperia, Morton Hospital and Medical Center, Taunton, MA, Fig 11-12; Courtesy of Lee's Photo Service, Muncie, IN, Fig. 11-13; From D. Magee, Orthopedic Assessment, Philadelphia: W.B. Saunders, 1992, Fig. 11-15.

Chapter 12. Courtesy of T.F. Maguire, Jr., Attleboro, MA, Fig. 12-1; From D.H. O'Donoghue, Treatment of Injuries to Athletes, Philadelphia: W.B. Saunders, 1984, Figs. 12-13 and 12-22; Courtesy of T. Robichaud, Bridgewater, MA, Figs. 12-14 and 12-30; From R. Cailliet, Hand Pain and Impairment, Philadelphia: F.A. Davis Company, 1984, Figs. 12-18, 12-21, 12-29, and Field Strategy 12-1(A); From J.E. Crouch, Functional Human Anatomy, Philadelphia: Lea & Febiger, 1985, Fig. 12-23; From J.A. Nicholas and E.B. Hershman, The Upper Extremity in Sports Medicine, St. Louis: The C.V. Mosby Company, 1990, Fig. 12-24; Courtesy of Dr. D. Adelberg, Hawthorn Physical Therapy and Sports Medicine, N. Dartmouth, MA, Figs. 12-26 and 12-28; Courtesy of Boston University Sports Medicine Department, Boston, MA, Fig. 13-21(A); From D. Magee, Orthopedic Assessment, Philadelphia: W.B. Saunders, 1992, Fig. 12-31.

Chapter 13. From J.E. Crouch, Functional Human Anatomy, Philadelphia: Lea & Febiger, 1985, Figs. 13-1, 13-4, and 13-7; From E.C.B. Hall-Craggs, Anatomy as a Basis for Clinical Medicine, Baltimore: Williams & Wilkins, 1990, Fig. 13-6; From J.M. Booher and G.A. Thibodeau, Athletic Injury Assessment, St. Louis: Mosby-Year Book, Inc., 1994, Fig. 13-9; From C.C. Alling III and D.B. Osbon, Maxillofacial Trauma, Philadelphia: Lea & Febiger, 1988, Figs. 13-11(A & B), 13-17, 13-19, and Fig. 13-20; Courtesy of Dr. D. Titelbaum, Shields Health Care, Brockton, MA, Fig. 13-12(A & B); From J.S. Torg, Athletic Injuries to the Head, Neck, and Face, St. Louis: Mosby-Year Book, Inc., 1991, Figs. 13-26 and 13-27; From R.C. Cantu, "Criteria for return to competition after a closed head injury," in Athletic Injuries to the Head, Neck, and Face, edited by J.S. Torg, 1991, Table 13-6. St. Louis: Mosby-Year Book, Inc., 1991.

Chapter 14. From J.E. Crouch, Functional Human Anatomy, Philadelphia: Lea & Febiger, 1985, Figs. 14-2, 14-3, and 14-5; From M. Nordin and V.H. Frankel, Basic Biomechanics of the Musculoskeletal System, Philadelphia: Lea & Febiger, 1989, Figs. 14-4, 14-9, and 14-10; From A. Nachemson, "Towards a better understanding of back pain: A review of the mechanics of the lumbar disc," Rheumatol. Rehabil. 14(3):129, 1975, Fig. 14-10 (adapted); From E.C.B. Hall-Craggs, Anatomy as a Basis for Clinical Medicine, Baltimore: Williams & Wilkins, 1990, Figs. 14-6, 14-13, and 14-21; From K. Luttgens, H. Deutsch, and N. Hamilton, Kinesiology: Scientific Basis of Human Motion, Dubuque: Brown Communications, Inc., 1992, Fig. 14-8; Courtesy of Thomas F. Maguire, Jr., Attleboro, MA, Figs. 14-11(A) and Fig. 14-16(A); From J.S. Torg, J.J. Begso, M.J. O'Neill, and B. Sennett, "The epidemiologic, pathologic, biomechanical, and cinematographic analysis of football-induced cervical spine trauma," The American Journal of Sports Medicine, 18(1):52-53, 1990, Figs. 14-11(B) and 14-12; Courtesy of Dr. D. Adelberg, Hawthorn Physical Therapy and Sports Medicine, N. Dartmouth, MA, Fig. 14-15; Courtesy of Dr. B. Saperia, Morton Hospital and Medical Center, Taunton, MA, Fig. 14-18(A); Courtesy of Dr. M. Ehrlich, Rhode Island Hospital, Providence, RI, Fig. 14-18(B); From I. Macnab and J.A. McCullock, Backache, Baltimore: Williams & Wilkins, 1989, Figs. 14-19 and 14-20; From D. Magee, Orthopedic Assessment, Philadelphia: W.B. Saunders, 1992, Fig. 14-31; From A.B. Schultz, "Mechanics of the human spine," Applied Mechanics Review, 27:1487, 1974, and A.A. White and M.M. Panjabi, Clinical Biomechanics of the Spine, Philadelphia: J.B. Lippincott, 1978, Table 14-2.

Chapter 15. From J.E. Crouch, Functional Human Anatomy, Philadelphia: Lea & Febiger, 1985, Figs. 15-1, 15-2, 15-3, 15-4, 15-10, 15-11, and 15-12; From A.P. Spence, Basic Human Anatomy, Redwood City: The Benjamin/Cummings Publishing Company, Inc., 1990, Figs. 15-6 and 15-13; From E.C.B. Hall-Craggs, Anatomy as a Basis for Clinical Medicine, Baltimore: Williams & Wilkins, 1990, Fig. 15-9; From H.H. Gretzer and A.B. Richardson, "Rupture of the Pectoralis Major Muscles," The American Journal of Sports Medicine, 17(4):455, 1989, Fig. 15-14; Courtesy of Dr. D. Adelberg, Hawthorn Physical Therapy and Sports Medicine, N. Dartmouth, MA, Fig. 15-17; From D.C. Reid, Sports Injury Assessment and Rehabilitation, New York: Churchill Livingstone, Inc., 1992, Figs. 15-20 and 15-22; From S.P. van Camp, "Sudden death," in Clinics in Sportsmedicine, edited by J.C. Puffer, Vol. 11, No. 2, Philadelphia: W.B. Saunders Company, 1992, Table 15-4 (adapted); From D.C. Reid, Sports Injury Assessment and Rehabilitation, New York: Churchill Livingstone, Inc., 1992, Field Strategy 15-1 (adapted).

Chapter 16. Courtesy of Springfield College Sports Medicine Department, Springfield, MA, Fig. 16-3; From D.C. Reid, Sports Injury Assessment and Rehabilitation, New York: Churchill Livingstone, Inc., 1992, Fig. 16-7; From R. Schvarcz, "Chronic posttransfusion non-A, non-B hepatitis and autoimmune chronic active hepatitis: Aspects of treatment, prognosis and relation to hepatitis C virus," J. Infect. Dis. 79:(Suppl), p. 7, 1991, Table 16-2 (adapted); From J.L. Slavin, J.M. Lutter, S. Cushman, and V. Lee, "Pregnancy and exercise," in Sport Science Perpectives for Women, Champaign, IL: Human Kinetic Books, 1988, Table 16-6 (adapted); From American Academy of Pediatrics, Field Strategy 16-2; From the American College of Obstetricians and Gynecologists, "Exercise During Pregnancy and the Postpartum Period," ACOG Technical Bulletin #190, February, 1994, Field Strategy 16-3.

Chapter 17. From B.L. Bullock and P.P. Rosendahl, Pathophysiology: Adaptation and Alterations in Function, Philadelphia: J.B. Lippincott Company, 1988, Figs. 17-1 and 17-2; From S.N. Sullivan and C. Wong, "Runner's diarrhea: Different patterns and associated factors." J. Clin. Gastroenterol., 14(2):101, 1992, Table 17-1 (adapted); From R. Alfaro-Levre, M.E. Blicharz, N.M. Flynn, and M.J. Boyer, Drug Handbook: A Nursing Process Approach, Redwood City, CA: Addison-Wesley Nursing, 1992, Tables 17-4 and 17-5 (adapted); From G. Wadler and B. Hainline, Drugs and the Athlete, Philadelphia: F.A. Davis Company, 1989, Table 17-6 (adapted); From National Collegiate Athletic Association, Drugs and the Athlete . . . A Losing Combination, Mission, KS, 1988, Table 17-7 (adapted); From D.M. Garner and L.W. Rosen, "Eating disorders among athletes: Research and recommendations," J. Appl. Sport Sci. Res., 5(2):100, 1991, Table 17-9; From W.D. McArdle, F.I. Katch, and V.L. Katch, Energy, Nutrition, and Human Performance, Philadelphia: Lea & Febiger, 1991, Table 17-11 and Field Strategy 17-5 (adapted); From J. Gong: "Breathing easy: Exercise despite asthma," Phys. Sportsmed., 20(3):159, 1992, Field Strategy 17-2 (adapted).

Glossary

Abduction
Movement of a body segment away from the midline of the body

Abrasion
Skin wound where the external layers have been rubbed or scraped off

Abscess
Localized accumulation of pus and necrotic tissue

Acceleration
An increased velocity

Accessory movements
Movements within a joint that cannot be voluntarily performed by the individual

Accessory sex organs
Organs that transport, protect, and nourish gametes

Acclimatization
Physiological adaptations of an individual to a variation in environment, especially one of climate or altitude

Acidosis
Condition caused by excess accumulation of acid or loss of base in the body; characteristic of diabetes mellitus

Active inhibition
Technique whereby an individual consciously relaxes a muscle prior to stretching it

Active movement
Joint motion performed voluntarily by the individual through muscular contraction

Acute injury
Injury with rapid onset due to traumatic episode, but with short duration

Adduction
Movement of a body segment toward the midline of the body

Adhesions
Tissues that bind the healing tissue to adjacent structures, such as other ligaments or bone

Ad libitum
At pleasure or at will

Afferent nerves
Nerves carrying sensory input from receptors in the skin, muscles, tendons, and ligaments to the central nervous system

Agonist muscles
Muscles that perform the desired movement; primary movers

AIDS
Acquired immunodeficiency syndrome caused by the human immunodeficiency virus (HIV), characterized by severe weight loss, swollen lymph nodes, night sweats, and secondary infections

Airway obstruction
Choking

Alveoli
Air sacs at the terminal ends of the bronchial tree where oxygen and carbon dioxide are exchanged between the lungs and surrounding capillaries

Ambient
Environmental air temperature

Ambulation
Moving or walking about

Ambulatory aid
Assistance used to help an injured individual walk

Amenorrhea
Absence or abnormal cessation of menstruation

Anabolic steroid
Testosterone, or a steroid hormone resembling testosterone, that stimulates anabolism in the body

Analgesia
Conscious state in which normal pain is not perceived, such as a numbing or sedative effect

Analgesic
Agent that produces analgesia

Anaphylactic shock
Shock caused by an allergic reaction that can become life-threatening

Anatomical position
Standardized position with the body erect, facing forward, with the arms at the sides, palms facing forward

Anatomical snuff box
Region directly over the scaphoid bone bounded by the extensor pollicis brevis medially and the extensor pollicis longus laterally

Androgen
A class of hormones that promotes development of male genitals, secondary sex characteristics, and influences sexual motivation

Anemia
Abnormal reduction in red blood cell volume or hemoglobin concentration

Anesthesia
Partial or total loss of sensation

Anesthetic
Agent that produces anesthesia

Aneurysm
Weakened, bulging area of a blood vessel

Anisotropic
Having different strengths in response to loads from different directions

Anode
Positively charged electrode in a direct current system

Anomaly
Deviation from the average or normal state

Anorexia nervosa
Personality disorder manifested by extreme aversion toward food resulting in extensive weight loss, amenorrhea, and other physical disorders

Anoxia
Deficiency or absence of oxygen

Antagonist muscles
Muscles that oppose or reverse a particular movement

Antalgic gait
Walking with a limp to avoid pain

Anterior pelvic tilt
Anterior sagittal plane tilt of the anterior superior iliac spine (ASIS) with respect to the pubic symphysis

Anteversion
Forward displacement or turning forward of a body segment without bending

Antihistamine
Medication used to counteract the effects of histamine; one that relieves the symptoms of an allergic reaction

Antipyretic
Medication used to relieve or reduce a fever

Apnea
Temporary cessation of breathing

Aponeurosis
A fibrous sheet or tendinous expansion connecting a muscle to the part it moves

Apophysis
An outgrowth or projection on a bone where muscles attach

Apophysitis
Inflammation of an apophysis

Appendicitis
Inflammation of the appendix

Appendicular segment
Relates to the extremities of the body, including the arms and legs

Arrhythmia
Disturbance in the rhythm of the heart beat

Arthralgia
Severe joint pain

Arthrogram
Diagnostic tool whereby a radiopaque material is injected into a joint to facilitate taking a radiograph

Arthroscopy
Diagnostic tool whereby the inside of a joint is viewed through a small camera lens (arthroscope) to facilitate surgical repair of the joint and/or joint structures

Aseptic necrosis
The death or decay of tissue due to a poor blood supply in the area

Aspiration
Removing a fluid or gas by suction from a body area, such as a joint cavity. Inspiratory sucking into the airways of fluid or foreign matter, such as vomitus

Assumption of risk
When a sport participant assumes a certain level of risk for injury during an activity, and therefore has no action for negligence

Asthma
Disease of the lungs characterized by constriction of the bronchial muscles, increased bronchial secretions, and mucosal swelling, all leading to airway narrowing and inadequate airflow during respiration

Athletic heart syndrome
Benign condition associated with physiological alterations in the heart

Atrophy
A wasting away or deterioration of tissue due to disease, disuse, or malnutrition

Aura
A peculiar sensation that precedes an epileptic attack

Auscultation
Listening for sounds, often with a stethoscope to denote the condition of the lungs, heart, pleura, abdomen and other organs

Autoinoculation
Spreading of an infection from one body part to another by touching the lesion, then scratching or rubbing somewhere else

Avascular
Devoid of blood vessels

Avascular necrosis
Death of tissues due to insufficient blood supply

Avulsion
A tearing away or forceful separation of a body part or structure

Axial loading
Loading directed along the long axis of a body

Axial segment
Central part of the body including the head and trunk

Ballistic stretching
Increasing flexibility by utilizing repetitive bouncing motions at the end of the available range of motion

Bandage
Material used to cover a wound

Bankart's lesion
Avulsion or damage to the anterior lip of the glenoid as the humerus slides forward in an anterior dislocation

Battery
Unpermitted or intentional contact with another individual without their consent

Battle's sign
Delayed discoloration behind the ear due to basilar skull fracture

Bending
Loading that produces tension on one side of an object and compression on the other side

Bennett's fracture
Fracture-dislocation to the proximal end of the first metacarpal at the carpal-metacarpal joint

Bilateral
Pertaining to both sides

Bimalleolar fracture
Fractures of both medial and lateral malleoli

Bipartite
Having two parts

Blister
Fluid accumulation under the skin caused by friction of the skin over a hard or rough surface causing the epidermis to separate from the dermis

Boutonnière deformity
Rupture of the central slip of the extensor tendon at the middle phalanx resulting in no active extensor mechanism at the proximal interphalangeal joint

Bowler's thumb
Compression of the digital nerve on the medial aspect of the thumb leading to paresthesia in the thumb

Boxer's fracture
Fracture of the 5th metacarpal resulting in a flexion deformity due to rotation of the head of the metacarpal over the neck

Brachial plexus
A complex web of spinal nerves (C_5–T_1) that innervates the upper extremity

Bronchitis
Inflammation of the mucosal lining of the tracheobronchial tree characterized by bronchial swelling, mucus secretions, and dysfunction of the cilia

Bronchospasm
Contraction of the smooth muscles of the bronchial tubes causing narrowing of the airway

Bucket-handle tear
Longitudinal meniscal tear of the central segment that can displace into the joint leading to locking of the knee

Bulimia
Personality disorder manifested by episodic bouts of binging of large amounts of food followed by purging and feelings of guilt, self-disgust, and depression

Bunion
Swelling and prominence of the 1st metatarsal head associated with lateral shift of the great toe (hallus valgus)

Burner
Burning or stinging sensation characteristic of a brachial plexus injury

Bursa
A fibrous sac membrane containing synovial fluid typically found between tendons and bones; acts to decrease friction during motion

Bursitis
Inflammation of a bursa

Calcific tendinitis
Accumulation of mineral deposits in a tendon

Callus
Localized thickening of skin epidermis due to physical trauma. Fibrous tissue containing immature bone tissue that forms at fracture sites during repair and regeneration

Cancellous
Bone tissue of relatively low density

Cardiac tamponade
Acute compression of the heart due to effusion of fluid or blood into the pericardium from rupture of the heart or penetrating trauma

Cardiovascular endurance
The body's ability to sustain submaximal exercise over an extended period of time

Carpal tunnel syndrome
Compression of the median nerve as it passes through the carpal tunnel leading to pain and tingling in the hand

Carrying angle
The angle between the humerus and ulna when the arm is in the anatomical position

Cathode
Negatively charged electrode in a direct current system

CAT scan
Computed tomography scan. A computer assisted x-ray tomogram that provides detailed images of tissue based on their density

Cauda equina
Lower spinal nerves that course through the lumbar spinal canal that resemble a horse's tail

Cauliflower ear
Hematoma between the perichondrium and cartilage of the outer ear; auricular hematoma

Cavitation
Gas bubble formation due to non-thermal effects of ultrasound

Celiac plexus
Nerve plexus that innervates the abdominal region

Center of gravity
Center of mass, or the point at which the mass and weight of a body is balanced in all directions

Cervicitis
Inflammation of the mucous membrane frequently involving the deeper structures of the uterine cervix

Chancre
A raised, red painless sore associated with the primary phase of syphilis

Chemosensitive
Sensitive to chemical stimulation

Chondral fracture
Fracture involving the articular cartilage at a joint

Chrondromalacia patellae
Degenerative condition in the articular cartilage of the patella caused by abnormal compression or shearing forces

Chronic exertional compartment syndrome
Intermittent excessive pressure that reduces blood flow through a muscular compartment causing pain and possible paresthesia

Chronic injury
An injury with long onset and duration

Circumduction
Circular motion of a body segment resulting from sequential flexion, abduction, extension, and adduction or vice versa

Cirrhosis
Progressive inflammation of the liver usually caused by alcoholism

Claw toes
Toe deformity characterized by hyperextension of the metatarsopha-

langeal (MP) joint and hyperflexion of the interphalangeal (IP) joints

Clonic state
Movement marked by repetitive muscle contractions and relaxations in rapid succession

Close packed position
Joint position in which contact between the articulation structures is maximal

Coach's finger
Fixed flexion deformity of the finger resulting from dislocation at the proximal interphalangeal joint

Coccygodynia
Prolonged or chronic pain in the coccygeal region due to irritation of the coccygeal nerve plexus

Coitus
Technical name for penile-vaginal intercourse

Cold allergies
Hypersensitivity to cold leading to superficial vascular reaction manifested by transient itching, erythema, hives or whitish swellings (wheals)

Cold diuresis
Excretion of urine in cold weather due to blood being shunted away from the skin to the core to maintain vascular volume

Cold urticaria
Condition characterized by redness, itching, and large blister-like wheals on skin that is exposed to cold

Collagen
Major protein of the white fibers in connective tissue, cartilage, and bone

Collateral ligaments
Major ligaments that cross the medial and lateral aspects of a hinge joint to provide stability from valgus and varus forces

Colles's fracture
Fracture involving a dorsally angulated and displaced, and a radially angulated and displaced fracture within one and a half inches of the wrist

Collision sport
Activity in which participants use their bodies to deter or block opponents

Compartment syndrome
Condition where increased intramuscular pressure brought on by activity impedes blood flow and function of tissues within that compartment

Compression
A pressure or squeezing force directed through a body in such a way as to increase density

Concussion
Violent shaking or jarring action of the brain resulting in immediate or transient impairment of neurologic function

Conjunctivitis
Bacterial infection leading to itching, burning, watering, and inflamed eye; pinkeye

Constipation
Infrequent or incomplete bowel movements

Contracture
Permanent muscular contraction due to tonic spasm, fibrosis, loss of muscular equilibrium, or paralysis

Contraindication
A condition adversely affected if a particular action is taken

Contralateral
Pertaining to the opposite side

Contrecoup injuries
Injuries away from the actual injury site due to rotational components during acceleration

Contusion
Compression injury involving accumulation of blood and lymph within a muscle; a bruise

Convulsion
Involuntary spasm or series of jerking motions

Coordination
The body's ability to execute smooth, fluid, accurate, and controlled movements

Core temperature
Internal body temperature regulated by the hypothalamus

Cortical
Compact bone tissue of relatively high density

Corticosteroid
Any of the steroid hormones secreted by the adrenal cortex

Counterirritant
A substance causing irritation of superficial sensory nerves so as to reduce pain transmission from another underlying irritation

Cramp
Painful involuntary muscle contraction, either clonic or tonic

Crepitation
Crackling sound or sensation characteristic of a fracture when the bone ends are moved

Cruciate ligaments
Major ligaments that crisscross the knee in the anteroposterior direction providing stability in that plane

Cryokinetics
Use of cold treatments prior to an exercise session

Cryotherapy
Cold application

Current
The actual movement of ions

Curvature
An overdeveloped spinal curve that inhibits proper mechanical functioning

Cyanosis
A dark blue or purple skin color due to deficient oxygen in the blood

Cyclist's nipples
Nipple irritation due to the combined effects of perspiration and windchill producing cold, painful nipples

Cyclist's palsy
Seen when bikers lean on the handlebars for an extended period resulting in paresthesia in the ulnar nerve distribution

Cystitis
An inflammation of the urethra or bladder, characterized by discomfort during urination

Dead arm syndrome
Common sensation felt with a recurrent anterior shoulder dislocation

Débridement
Removal of foreign matter and dead tissue from a wound

Decerebrate rigidity
Extension of all four extremities

Decompression
Surgical release of pressure caused by fluid or blood accumulation

Decorticate rigidity
Extension of the legs with flexion of the elbows, wrists, and fingers

Deformation
Change in the original shape of a structure due to mechanical strain

de Quervain's tenosynovitis
An inflammatory stenosing tenosynovitis of the abductor pollicis longus and extensor pollicis brevis tendons

Dermatome
Region of skin supplied by cutaneous branches of a single spinal nerve

Detached retina
Neurosensory retina is separated from the retinal epithelium by swelling

Diabetes
Metabolic disorder characterized by near or absolute lack of the hormone insulin, or insulin resistance, or both

Diagnosis
Definitive determination of the nature of the injury or illness made only by physicians

Diarrhea
Loose or watery stools

Diastole
Residual pressure in aorta between heart beats

Diathermy
Local elevation of temperaure in the tissues produced by therapeutic

application of high frequency electric current, ultrasound, or microwave radiation

Diffuse injuries
Injury over a large body area, usually due to low velocity-high mass forces

Diplopia
Double vision

Dislocation
Separation of a joint so that the bone ends are no longer in contact; third degree sprain

Distal
Farthest from a point of reference, e.g., the wrist is distal to the elbow

Distention
The act or state of being stretched or inflated

Diuretics
Chemicals that promote the excretion of urine

Dorsum
Relating to the back or posterior surface of a body part

Dorsiflexion
Movement of the forefoot toward the shin

Dressing
Covering over a wound used to hold a bandage in place

Drug
A therapeutic agent used in the prevention, diagnosis, cure, treatment, or rehabilitation of a disease, condition, or injury

Dural sinuses
Formed by tubular separations in the inner and outer layers of the dura mater, these sinuses function as small veins for the brain

Dynamic flexibility
Active range of motion exercises used to improve flexibility

Dysmenorrhea
Difficult or painful menstruation; menstrual cramps

Dyspnea
Labored or difficult breathing

Dysuria
Difficulty, pain, or burning sensation during urination

Ecchymosis
Superficial tissue discoloration

Ectopic bone
Proliferation of bone ossification in an abnormal place

Edema
Swelling resulting from a collection of exuded lymph fluid in interstitial tissues

Efferent nerves
Nerves carrying motor impulses from the central nervous system to the muscles

Effleurage
Stroking technique used in massage

Effusion
The escape of fluid from the blood vessels into the surrounding tissues or joint cavity

Emergency plan
A process that activates emergency health care services of the facility and community

End feel
The sensation felt in the joint as it reaches the end of the available range of motion

Epicondylitis
Inflammation and microrupture of the soft tissues on the epicondyles of the distal humerus

Epididymitis
Inflammation of the epididymis, which is on the back of each testicle where sperm mature

Epilepsy
Disorder of the brain characterized by recurrent episodes of sudden, excessive discharges of electrical activity

Epiphyseal fracture
Injury to the growth plate of a long bone in children and adolescents; may lead to arrested bone growth

Epistaxis
Profuse bleeding from the nose; nosebleed

Estrogens
Hormones that produce female secondary sex characteristics and affect the menstrual cycle

Etiology
The science and study of the causes of disease

Eversion
A turning outward, such as turning the sole of the foot outward

Exostosis
A cartilage capped bony projection arising from any bone that develops from cartilage

Expressed warranty
Written guarantee that states the product is safe for consumer use

Extensor mechanism
Complex interaction of muscles, ligaments, and tendons that stabilize and provide motion at the patellofemoral joint

Extrasynovial
Structures found outside of the synovial cavity and synovial fluid

Extrinsic
Originating outside of the part where it is found or upon which it acts; denoting particularly a muscle

Extruded
Tooth driven in an outwardly direction

Extruded disc
Condition in which the nuclear material bulges into the spinal canal and runs the risk of impinging adjacent nerve roots

Exudate
Material composed of fluid, pus, or cells that has escaped from blood vessels into surrounding tissues following injury or inflammation

Failure
Loss of continuity; rupturing of soft tissue or fracture of bone

Fasciitis
Inflammation of the fascia surrounding portions of a muscle

Felon
Abscess within the fat pad of the fingertip

Fibrositis
Inflammation of fibrous tissue

Flail chest
Three or more consecutive ribs on the same side of the chest wall that are fractured in at least two separate locations

Flexibility
Total range of motion at a joint dependent on normal joint mechanics, mobility of soft tissues, and muscle extensibility

Focal injuries
Injury in a small concentrated area, usually due to high velocity-low mass forces

Force
A push or pull that causes or tends to cause motion, or a change in motion

Forearm splints
Chronic strain to the forearm muscles

Foreseeability of harm
Condition whereby danger is apparent, or should have been apparent, resulting in an unreasonably unsafe condition

Fracture
A disruption in the continuity of a bone

Freiberg's disease
Avascular necrosis that occurs to the second metatarsal head in some adolescents

Galeazzi fracture
Radial fracture with an associated dislocation of the ulna at the distal radial ulnar joint

Gamekeeper's thumb
Rupture of the volar ligament at the metacarpophalangeal joint due to forceful abduction of the thumb while the thumb is extended

Ganglion cyst
Benign tumor mass commonly seen on the dorsal aspect of the wrist

Gastroenteritis
Inflammation of the mucous membrane of the stomach and/or small intestine

Glenoid labrum
Soft tissue lip around the periphery of the glenoid fossa that widens and deepens the socket to add stability to the joint

Goniometer
Protractor used to measure joint position and available joint motion (range of motion)

Gray matter
Brain matter composed of neuron cell bodies, dendrites, and short unmyelinated axons

Gross negligence
By committing or not committing, acting with total disregard for the health and safety of others

Gynecomastia
Excessive development of the male mammary glands

Hallux
The first, or great, toe

Hammer toes
A flexion deformity of the distal interphalangeal (DIP) joint of the toes

Hay fever
Seasonal allergic rhinitis caused by airborne pollens and/or fungus spores

Heat cramps
Painful involuntary muscle spasms caused by excessive water and electrolyte loss

Heel bruise
Contusion to the subcutaneous fat pad located over the inferior aspect of the calcaneus

Hemarthrosis
Collection of blood within a joint or cavity

Hematocele (scrotal)
A rapid accumulation of blood and fluid in the scrotum around the testicle and cord

Hematoma
A localized mass of blood and lymph confined within a space or tissue

Hematuria
Blood or red blood cells in the urine

Hemophilia
Inherited disorder resulting in the inability of blood to clot, which can lead to excessive blood loss

Hemorrhage
Bleeding

Hemorrhoids
Rectal and anal dilations of the venous plexus that can become exposed if they protrude internally or externally

Hemothorax
Condition involving the loss of blood into the pleural cavity, but outside the lung

Hepatitis
Inflammation of the liver

Hernia
Protrusion of abdominal viscera through a weakened portion of the abdominal wall

High-density material
Materials that absorb more energy from higher impact intensity levels through deformation, thus transferring less stress to a body part

Hip pointer
Contusions caused by direct compression to an unprotected iliac crest that crushes soft tissue, and sometimes the bone itself

Homeostasis
The state of a balanced equilibrium in the body's various tissues and systems

Hunting response
Cyclical periods of vasoconstriction and vasodilation after ice application

Hydrocele
Swelling in the tunica vaginalis of the testes

Hyperemia
Presence of increased blood flow into a region or body part once treatment has ended

Hyperesthesia
Excessive tactile sensation

Hyperextension
Extension of a limb or body part beyond the normal limits

Hyperglycemia
Abnormally high levels of glucose in the circulating blood that can lead to diabetic coma

Hypermobility
Increased motion at a joint; joint laxity

Hypertension
Sustained elevated blood pressure above the norms of 140 mm Hg systolic or 90 mm Hg diastolic

Hyperthermia
Elevated body temperature

Hypertrophic cardiomyopathy
Excessive hypertrophy of the heart, often of obscure or unknown origin

Hypertrophy
General increase in bulk or size of an individual tissue not due to tumor formation

Hyperventilation
Respiratory condition where too much carbon dioxide is exhaled leading to an inability to catch one's breath

Hyphema
Hemorrhage into the anterior chamber of the eye

Hypoesthesia
Decreased tactile sensation

Hypoglycemia
Abnormally low levels of glucose in the circulating blood that can lead to insulin shock

Hypomobility
Decreased motion at a joint

Hypothermia
Decreased body temperature

Hypothenar
Mass of intrinsic muscles of the little finger including the abductor digiti minimi, flexor digiti minimi brevis, and opponens digiti minimi

Hypovolemic shock
Shock caused by excessive loss of whole blood or plasma

Hypoxia
Having a reduced concentration of oxygen in air, blood, or tissue, less severe than anoxia

Idiopathic
Denoting a disease or condition of unknown cause

Impingement syndrome
Chronic condition caused by repetitive overhead activity that damages the glenoid labrum, long head of the biceps brachii, and subacromial bursa

Implied warranty
Unwritten guarantee that the product is reasonably safe when used for its intended purpose

Incision
A wound with smooth edges; a surgical wound

Indication
A condition that could benefit from a specific action

Infarcts
Clumping together of cells that block small blood vessels leading to vascular occlusion, ischemia, and necrosis in organs

Infection
Invasion of a host or host tissue by organisms such as bacteria, fungi, viruses, or parasites

Infectious mononucleosis
Acute viral disease caused by the Epstein-Barr virus manifested by malaise and fatigue

Inflammation
Pain, swelling, redness, heat, and loss of function that accompany musculoskeletal injuries

Influenza
Acute infectious respiratory tract condition characterized by malaise, headache, dry cough, and general muscle aches

Informed consent
Consent given by a person of legal age who can understand the nature and extent of any treatment, and available alternative treatments prior to agreeing to receive treatment

Innervation
Nerve supply to a body part

Inspection
Refers to factors seen at the actual injury site, such as redness, swelling, bruising, cuts, or scars

Intracapsular
Structures found within the articular capsule; intra-articular

Intrinsic
Inherent; belonging entirely to a part; muscles with proximal and distal attachments located within the body part

Intruded
Tooth driven deep into the socket in an inward direction

Inversion
Turning the sole of the foot inward

In vivo
Occurring within the living organism or body

Iontophoresis
Technique whereby direct current is used to drive charged molecules from certain medications into damaged tissue

Ipsilateral
Situated on, pertaining to, or affecting the same side, as opposed to contralateral

Ischemia
Local anemia due to decreased blood supply

Jaundice
A yellowish discoloration of the skin, sclera, and deeper tissues often due to liver damage

Jersey finger
Rupture of the flexor digitorum profundus tendon from the distal phalanx due to rapid extension of the finger while actively flexed

Jones's fracture
A transverse stress fracture of the proximal shaft of the 5th metatarsal

Kehr's sign
Referred pain down the left shoulder indicative of a ruptured spleen

Keratolytic agent
An agent that promotes softening and dissolution, or peeling of the horny layer of skin

Kinematic chains
Series of interrelated joints that constitute a complex motor unit so that motion at one joint will produce motion at the other joints in a predictable manner

Kinematics
Study of the spatial and temporal aspects of movement

Kinetics
Study of the forces causing and resulting from motion

Kyphosis
Excessive curve in the thoracic region of the spine

Laceration
Wound that may leave a smooth or jagged edge through the skin, subcutaneous tissues, muscles, and associated nerves and blood vessels

Larsen-Johansson disease
Inflammation or partial avulsion of the apex of the patella due to traction forces

Laryngospasm
Spasmodic closure of the glottic aperture leading to shortness of breath, coughing, cyanosis and even loss of consciousness

Legal duty of care
Recognized standard of care in which an individual is expected to act or behave in providing care

Legg-Calvé-Perthes disease
Avascular necrosis of the proximal femoral epiphysis seen especially in young males ages 3 to 8

Liability
Legal responsibility to act in a reasonable and prudent manner

Ligament
Band of regular fibrous tissue that connects bone to bone

Little leaguer's elbow
Tension stress injury of the medial epicondyle seen in adolescents

Little league shoulder
Fracture of the proximal humeral growth plate in adolescents caused by repetitive rotational stresses during the act of pitching

Load
A force or combination of forces to a structure that is sustained or carried by the matter of the structure

Loose-packed position
Resting position where the joint is under the least amount of strain

Lordosis
Excessive convex curve in the lumbar region of the spine

Low-density material
Materials that absorb energy from low impact intensity levels

Lumbar plexus
Interconnected roots of the first four lumbar spinal nerves

Magnetic resonance imaging (MRI)
Diagnostic technique using magnetism to produce high-quality cross-sectional images of organs or structures within the body without x-rays or other radiation

Malaise
Lethargic feeling of general discomfort; out-of-sorts feeling

Malfeasance
Committing an act that is not your responsibility to perform

Mallet finger
Rupture of the extensor tendon from the distal phalanx due to forceful flexion of the phalanx

Malocclusion
Inability to bring the teeth together in a normal bite

Malpractice
Committing a negligent act while providing care

Marfan's syndrome
Inherited connective tissue disorder affecting many organs, but commonly resulting in the dilation and weakening of the thoracic aorta

McBurney's point
A site one third the distance between the anterior superior iliac spine (ASIS) and umbilicus that with deep palpation produces rebound tenderness indicating appendicitis

Mechanosensitive
Sensitive to mechanical stimulation

Meninges
Three protective membranes that surround the brain and spinal cord

Meningitis
Inflammation of the meninges of the brain and spinal column

Menisci
Fibrocartilagenous discs found within a joint that serve to reduce joint stress

Menses
Phase in the menstrual cycle when the thickened vascular walls of the uterus, the unfertilized ova, and blood from damaged vessels are lost during the menstrual flow

Metatarsalgia
A condition involving general discomfort around the metatarsal's heads

Microtrauma
Injury to a small number of cells due to accumulative effects of repetitive forces

Misfeasance
Committing an act that is your responsibility to perform, but the wrong procedure is followed, or the right procedure is done in an improper manner

Modalities
Therapeutic agents that promote optimal healing while reducing pain and disability

Monteggia's fracture
Ulnar fracture with an associated dislocation of the radial head

Motion segment
Two adjacent vertebrae and the intervening soft tissues; the functional unit of the spine

Muscle spindle
Encapsulated receptor found in muscle tissue sensitive to stretch

Muscular endurance
The ability of muscles to exert tension over an extended period

Muscular power
The ability of muscles to produce force at a given time

Muscular strength
The ability of muscles to produce force during a single maximal contraction

Myopia
Nearsightedness

Myositis
Inflammation of connective tissue within a muscle

Myositis ossificans
Accumulation of mineral deposits within muscle tissue

Myotome
A group of muscles primarily innervated by a single nerve root

Necrosis
Death of a tissue due to deprivation of a blood supply

Negligence
Breach of one's duty of care that causes harm to another individual

Neoplasm
Mass of tissue that grows more rapidly than normal and may be benign or malignant

Nerve entrapment
Condition whereby a nerve is compressed between a bone or soft tissue

Nerve root
The portion of a nerve associated with its origin in the spinal cord, such as C_6 or L_5

Neurapraxia
Injury to a nerve that results in temporary neurological deficits followed by complete recovery of function

Neuritis
Inflammation or irritation of a nerve; commonly found between the 3rd and 4th metatarsal heads

Neuroma
A nerve tumor

Neurotmesis
Complete severance of a nerve

Nightstick fracture
Fracture to the ulna due to a direct blow. Commonly seen in football players

Nociceptors
Specialized nerve endings that transduce pain

Nonfeasance
Failing to perform your legal duty of care

Nongonococcal urethritis
Inflammation of the urethra not caused by gonorrhea

Nonunion fracture
A fracture where healing is delayed or fails to unite at all

NSAID
Nonsteroidal anti-inflammatory drug

Nystagmus
Abnormal jerking or involuntary eye movement

Observation
Visual analysis of overall appearance, symmetry, general motor function, posture, and gait

Oligomenorrhea
Infrequent menstrual cycles or menstruation involving scant blood flow

Orthosis
Devices or appliances used to correct or straighten a deformity

Orthotics
The science concerned with the making and fitting of orthopedic appliances

Osgood-Schlatter disease
Inflammation or partial avulsion of the tibial apophysis due to traction forces

Osteitis pubis
Stress fracture to the pubic symphysis caused by repeated overload of the adductor muscles or repetitive stress activities

Osteochondral fracture
Fracture involving the articular cartilage and underlying bone

Osteochondritis dissecans
Localized area of avascular necrosis resulting in complete or incomplete separation of joint cartilage and subchondral bone

Osteochondrosis
Any condition characterized by degeneration or aseptic necrosis of the articular cartilage due to limited blood supply

Osteomyelitis
Inflammation or infection of the bone and bone marrow

Osteopenia
Condition of reduced bone mineral density that predisposes the individual to fractures

Osteoporosis
Pathological condition of reduced bone mass and strength

Otitis externa
Bacterial infection involving the lining of the auditory canal; swimmer's ear

Otitis media
Localized infection in the middle ear secondary to upper respiratory infections

Overload principle
Physiologic improvements occur only when an individual physically demands more of the muscles than is normally required

Overuse injury
Any injury caused by excessive repetitive movement of the body part

Painful arc
Pain located within a limited number of degrees in the range of motion

Pallor
Skin ashen or pale in color

Palpation
Act of feeling a region with the fingers to detect temperature, swelling, point tenderness, deformity, crepitus, and cutaneous sensation

Papule
Small red elevated painful bump on the skin

Paralysis
Partial or complete loss of the ability to move a body part

Paresis
Partial paralysis of a muscle leading to a weakened contraction

Paresthesia
Abnormal sensations such as tingling, burning, itching, or prickling

Paronychia
A fungal/bacterial infection in the folds of skin surrounding a fingernail or toenail

Parrot-beak tear
Horizontal meniscal tear typically in the middle segment of the lateral meniscus

Partial airway obstruction
Choking where the individual still has some air exchange in the lungs and is able to cough

Passive movement
A limb or body part is moved through the range of motion with no assistance from the individual

Passive stretching
Stretching of muscles, tendons, and ligaments produced by a stretching force other than tension in the antagonist muscles; stretching of body part done by a clinician without the help of the patient

Patella plica
A fold in the synovial lining that may cause medial knee pain without associated trauma

Patellofemoral joint
Gliding joint between the patella and patellar groove of the femur

Patellofemoral stress syndrome
Condition whereby the lateral retinaculum is tight, or the vastus medialis oblique is weak, leading to lateral excursion and pressure on the lateral facet of the patella causing a painful condition

Pathology
The cause of an injury, its development, and functional changes due to the injury process

Percussion
Used to assess abdominal injuries; performed by tapping the nondominant hand with the dominant hand to determine presence and location of hollow versus solid organs, or masses in the abdomen

Periorbital ecchymosis
Swelling and hemorrhage into the surrounding eyelids; black eye.

Periostitis
Inflammation of the periosteum (outer membrane covering the bone)

Peristalsis
Periodic waves of smooth muscle contraction that propel food through the digestive system

Peritonitis
Inflammation of the peritoneum that lines the abdomen

Pes cavus
High arch

Pes planus
Flat feet

Pétrissage
Kneading technique used in massage

Phagocytosis
Process by which white blood cells surround and digest foreign particles, such as bacteria, necrotic tissue, and foreign particles

Pharyngitis
Viral, bacterial, or fungal infection of the pharynx leading to a sore throat

Phlebothrombosis
Thrombosis, or clotting, in a vein without overt inflammatory signs and symptoms

Phonophoresis
The introduction of anti-inflammatory drugs through the skin with the use of ultrasound

Photophobia
Abnormal sensitivity to light

Plantar fascia
Specialized band of fascia that covers the plantar surface of the foot and helps support the longitudinal arch

Plyometric exercise
Type of explosive exercise that maximizes the myotatic on-stretch reflex

Pneumothorax
Condition whereby air is trapped in the pleural space causing a portion of a lung to collapse

Point tenderness
Specific painful area at an injury site that can be palpated

Postconcussion syndrome
Delayed condition characterized by persistent headaches, blurred vision, irritability, and inability to concentrate

Posterior pelvic tilt
Posterior sagittal plane tilt of the anterior superior iliac spine with respect to the pubic symphysis

Post-traumatic memory loss
Forgetting events after an injury

Primary sex organs
Reproductive organs responsible for producing gametes (ova and sperm)

Primary survey
Immediate assessment to determine unresponsiveness and status of the ABCS (Airway, Breathing, Circulation, and Severe bleeding)

Progesterone
Hormone responsible for thickening the uterine lining in preparation for the fertilized ovum

Prognosis
Probable course or progress of an injury or disease

Prolapsed disc
Condition when the eccentric nucleus produces a definite deformity as it works its way through the fibers of the annulus fibrosus

Pronation
Inward rotation of the forearm; palms face posteriorly. At the foot, combined motions of calcaneal eversion, foot abduction, and dorsiflexion

Pronator syndrome
Median nerve is entrapped by the pronator teres leading to pain on activities involving pronation

Prophylactic
To prevent or protect

Proprioceptive Neuromuscular Facilitation (PNF)
Exercises that stimulate proprioceptors in muscles, tendons, and joints to improve flexibility and strength

Proprioceptors
Specialized deep sensory nerve cells in joints, ligaments, muscles, and tendons sensitive to stretch, tension, and pressure that are responsible for position and movement

Proteinuria
Abnormal concentrations of protein in the urine

Proximal
Closest to a reference point, i.e., the elbow is proximal to the wrist

Pruritus
Intense itching

Pulmonary circuit
Blood vessels that transport unoxygenated blood to the lungs from the right heart ventricle and oxygenated blood from the lungs to the left heart atrium

Pulmonary contusion
Contusion to the lungs due to compressive force

Pulmonary embolism
A blood clot that travels through the circulatory system and lodges in the lungs

Pupillary light reflex
Rapid constriction of pupils when exposed to intense light

Purulent
Consisting of, containing, or forming pus

Pus
Fluid product of inflammation composed of white blood cells, debris of dead cells, and a thin fluid

Pyarthrosis
Suppurative pus within a joint cavity

Q-angle
Angle between the line of quadriceps force and the patellar tendon

Raccoon eyes
Delayed discoloration around the eyes from anterior cranial fossa fracture

Raynaud's phenomenon
Condition characterized by intermittent bilateral attacks of ischemia of the fingers or toes, marked by severe pallor, numbness, and pain

Reciprocal inhibition
Technique using an active contraction of the agonist to cause a reflex relaxation in the antagonist allowing it to stretch; a phenomenon resulting from reciprocal innervation

Referred pain
Pain felt in a region of the body other than where the source or actual cause of the pain is located

Reflex
Action involving stimulation of a motor neuron by a sensory neuron in the spinal cord without involvement of the brain

Resilience
The ability to bounce or spring back into shape or position after being stretched, bent, or impacted

Resting position
Slightly flexed position of a joint that allows for maximal volume to accommodate any intra-articular swelling

Retrograde amnesia
Forgetting events that happened before an injury

Retroviruses
Any virus of the family Retroviridae known to reverse the usual order of reproduction within the cells they infect

Rhinitis
Inflammation of the nasal membranes with excessive mucus production resulting in nasal congestion and postnasal drip

Rhinorrhea
Clear nasal discharge

Rotation
Movement around an axis in an angular motion

Rotator cuff
The SITS (supraspinatus, infraspinatus, teres minor, and subscapularis) muscles hold the head of the humerus in the glenoid fossa and produce humeral rotation

Rubor
Reddish skin

Runner's nipples
Nipple irritation due to friction when the shirt rubs over the nipples

Sacral plexus
Interconnected roots of the L_4-S_4 spinal nerves that innervate the lower extremities

Saddle joint
Joint at which one bone surface has a convex saddle-like shape and the articulating bone surface is reciprocally shaped

SAID principle
Specific *a*daptation to *imp*osed *d*emands

Salicylates
Any salt of salicylic acid; used in aspirin

Scapulohumeral rhythm
Coordinated rotational movement of the scapula that accompanies abduction and adduction of the humerus

Scheuermann's disease
Osteochondrosis of the spine due to abnormal epiphyseal plate behavior that allows herniation of the disc into the vertebral body giving a characteristic wedge-shaped appearance

Sciatica
Compression of a spinal nerve due to a herniated disc, annular tear, myogenic or muscle-related disease, spinal stenosis, facet joint arthropathy, or compression from the piriformis muscle

Scoliosis
Lateral rotational spinal curvature

Screwing-home mechanism
Rotation of the tibia on the femur at the end of extension to produce a "locking" of the knee in a closed packed position

Secondary survey
Detailed head-to-toe assessment to detect medical and injury related problems that if unrecognized and untreated could become life-threatening

Seizure
An attack or sudden onset of a disease or condition, such as convulsions

Sequela
Pathological condition that occurs as a consequence of another condition, such as shock as a result of a fracture

Serous otitis
Fluid buildup behind the eardrum associated with otitis media and upper respiratory infections

Sesamoid bones
Short bones embedded in tendons; largest is the patella (knee cap)

Sesamoiditis
Inflammation of the sesamoid bones of the 1st metatarsal

Sever's disease
A traction-type injury, or osteochondrosis, of the calcaneal apophysis seen in young adolescents

Shear
A force directed parallel to a surface

Shin bruise
A contusion to the tibia; sometimes referred to as tibial periostitis

Shock
Collapse of the cardiovascular system when insufficient blood cannot provide circulation for the entire body

Sickle-cell anemia
Abnormalities in hemoglobin structure resulting in a characteristic sickle- or crescent-shaped red blood cell that is fragile and unable to transport oxygen

Sign
Objective measurable physical findings that you can hear, feel, see, or smell during the assessment

Sinusitis
Inflammation of the paranasal sinuses

Smith's fracture
Forearm fracture with volar angulation or displacement; opposite of Colles's fracture

Snapping hip syndrome
A snapping sensation either heard or felt during motion at the hip

Snowball crepitation
Sound similar to that heard when crunching snow into a snowball; indicative of tenosynovitis

Solar plexus punch
A blow to the abdomen that results in an immediate inability to breathe freely

Somatic pain
Pain originating in the skin, ligaments, muscles, bones, or joints

Spasm
Transitory muscle contractions

Spina bifida occulta
Congenital defect in the vertebral canal characterized by absence of the laminae and spinous process

Spinal stenosis
A loss of cerebrospinal fluid around the spinal cord due to deformation of the spinal cord, or a narrowing of the neural canal

Spondylolisthesis
Anterior slippage of a vertebrae resulting from complete bilateral fracture of the pars interarticularis

Spondylolysis
A stress fracture of the pars interarticularis

Sports medicine
Area of health and special services that applies medical and scientific knowledge to prevent, recognize, manage, and rehabilitate injuries related to sport, exercise, or recreational activity

Sprain
Injury to ligamentous tissue

Standard of care
What another minimally competent professional educated and practicing in the same profession would have done in the same or similar circumstances to protect an individual from harm

Stasis
Stagnation of blood or other fluids

Static position
Stationary position in which no motion occurs

Static stretching
Slow and deliberate muscle stretching used to increase range of motion

Stenosing
Narrowing of an opening or stricture of a canal; stenosis

Steroids
A large family of chemical substances including endocrine secretions and hormones

Sticking point
Presence of insufficient strength to move a body segment through a particular angle

Stitch in the side
A sharp pain or spasm in the chest wall, usually on the lower right side, that occurs during exertion

Strain
Amount of deformation with respect to the original dimensions of the structure

Stratum corneum
The outermost layer of the epidermis; horny layer of dead cells

Stress
The distribution of force within a body; quantified as force divided by the area over which the force acts

Stress (fatigue) fracture
Fracture resulting from repeated loading with relatively low magnitude forces

Stretch reflex
The monosynaptic reflex initiated by stretching muscle spindles that results in immediate development of muscle tension

Sty
Infection of the sebaceous gland of an eyelash or eyelash follicle

Subconjunctival hemorrhage
Minor capillary ruptures in the eye globe

Subcutaneous emphysema
Presence of air or gas in subcutaneous tissue, characterized by a crackling sensation on palpation

Subungual hematoma
Hematoma beneath a finger- or toenail

Sudden death
A nontraumatic, unexpected death occurring instantaneously or within a few minutes of an abrupt change in an individual's previous clinical state

Supination
Outward rotation of the forearm; palms facing forward. At the foot, combined motions of calcaneal inversion, foot adduction, and plantar flexion

Symptom
Subjective evidence of an abnormal feeling of pain, weakness, or loss of function perceived by the injured individual

Syncope
Fainting or lightheadedness

Syndesmosis
A joint where the opposing surfaces are joined together by fibrous connective tissue

Syndrome
An accumulation of common signs and symptoms characteristic of a particular injury or disease

Synovitis
Inflammation of a synovial membrane, particularly at a joint

Systemic circuit
Blood vessels that transport unoxygenated blood to the right heart

atrium and oxygenated blood from the left heart ventricle

Systole
Pressure in aorta when left ventricle contracts

Tackler's exostosis
Irritative exostosis on the anterior or lateral humerus

Tapotement
Percussion technique used in massage

Tendinitis
Inflammation of a tendon

Tenosynovitis
Inflammation of a tendon sheath

Tension
A pulling or stretching force directed axially through a body or body part

Tension pneumothorax
Condition in which air continuously leaks into the pleural space causing the mediastinum to displace to the opposite side compressing the uninjured lung and thoracic aorta

Thenar
Mass of intrinsic muscles of the thumb including the flexor pollicis brevis, abductor pollicis brevis, and opponens pollicis

Therapeutic drugs
Prescription or over-the-counter medications used to treat an injury or illness

Thermotherapy
Heat application

Thoracic outlet syndrome
Condition whereby nerves and/or vessels become compressed in the root of the neck or axilla leading to numbness in the arm

Thrombophlebitis
Acute inflammation of a vein

Tibiofemoral joint
Dual condyloid joints between the tibial and femoral condyles that function primarily as a modified hinge joint

Tinea
Ringworm; fungal infection of the hair, skin, or nails characterized by

small vesicles, itching, and scaling; tinea pedis—athlete's foot; tinea cruris—jock itch; tinea capitis—ringworm of the scalp

Tinnitus
Ringing or other noises in the ear due to trauma or disease

Tomogram
Cross-sectional image of an organ or body part at various depths of field produced by an x-ray technique

Tonic state
Steady rigid muscle contractions with no relaxation

Torsion
Twisting around an object's longitudinal axis in response to an applied torque

Tort
A wrong done to an individual whereby the injured party seeks a remedy for damages suffered

Total airway obstruction
Choking where the individual has no air passing through the vocal cords and is unable to speak or cough

Trachoma
Chronic contagious form of conjunctivitis caused by bacterial infection that can lead to blindness

Transitory paralysis
Temporary paralysis

Translation
Refers to anterior gliding of tibial plateau on the femur

Traumatic asphyxia
Condition involving extravasation of blood into the skin and conjunctivae due to a sudden increase in venous pressure

Triage
Assessing all injured individuals to determine the priority of care

Trigger finger
Condition whereby the finger flexors contract but are unable to reextend due to a nodule within the tendon

sheath or the sheath being too constricted to allow free motion

Tunics
Three layers of protected tissues that surround the eye

Unconsciousness
Impairment of brain function whereby the individual lacks conscious awareness and is unable to respond to superficial sensory stimuli

Valgus laxity
An opening on the medial side of a joint caused by the distal segment moving laterally

Valsalva effect
Holding one's breath against a closed glottis resulting in sharp increases in blood pressure

Varicocele
Abnormal dilation of the veins of the spermatic cord leading to engorgement of blood into the spermatic cord veins when standing

Varus laxity
An opening on the lateral side of a joint caused by the distal segment moving medially

Vasoconstriction
Narrowing of blood vessels

Vasodilation
Increased diameter of the blood vessels

Vasospasm
Contraction or spasm of the muscular coats of the blood vessels

Verrucae plantaris
Plantar's warts

Vertigo
Balance disturbance characterized by a whirling sensation of one's self or external objects

Vibration
Rapid shaking technique used in massage

Visceral pain
Pain resulting from injury or disease to an organ in the thoracic or abdominal cavity

Viscoelastic
Responding to loading over time with changing rates of deformation

Vital signs
Objective measurements of the pulse, respirations, blood pressure and skin temperature indicating normal body functions

Volar
Referring to the palm or the sole

Volkmann's contracture
Ischemic necrosis of the forearm muscles and tissues caused by damage to the blood flow

Voltage
The force that causes ions to move

Wedge fracture
A crushing compression fracture that leaves a vertebra narrowed anteriorly

Wheal
A smooth, slightly elevated area on the body that appears red or white and is accompanied by severe itching; commonly seen in allergies to mechanical or chemical irritants

White matter
Brain matter composed of myelinated nerve axons; it is the myelin sheaths that give the tissue its characteristic white coloring

Wrist drop
Weakness and/or paralysis of the wrist and finger extensors due to radial nerve damage

Yield point (elastic limit)
The maximum load that a material can sustain without permanent deformation

Zone of primary injury
Region of injured tissue prior to vasodilation

Zone of secondary injury
Region of damaged tissue following vasodilation

Index

Numbers in italics refer to illustrations; numbers followed by t indicate tables; numbers followed by fs indicate field strategies.

A

AAROM. *See* Range of motion, restoration of, active assisted (AAROM)
ABCs (Airway, Breathing, Circulation)
 emergency assessment, 60
Abdomen
 assessment of, 613–620, *615*, 620fs
  auscultation, *617*, 617–618
  neurological testing, 618
   referred pain, *619*
   reflexes, *618*, 618
  palpation, 616, *617*
  percussion, 617–618, *618*
 binders for
  in weight training, 197–198, *200*
 injury of, 607–612
  hematomas, 608
  hernia, 608–610, *609*, *610*
  intra-abdominal, *610*, 610–612, 611fs, 611t
  muscle strains, 607
  peritonitis, 610
  skin wounds/contusions, 607
  "solar plexus punch," 608
 quadrants of, 105, *106*
Abduction. *See* Valgus
Abrasions, skin, 41
Acanthamoeba
 keratitis infection and, 191
Accidents
 information on, 27t
 report forms for, 20, 23, 28fs
Acclimatization, 71, 75–76
Acetabular labrum, *320–321*, 322
Acetaminophen, 179
Achilles tendon
 apophysitis of calcaneus and, 252
 bursitis of, 240, *241*
 overuse syndrome, 250
 plantar fasciitis and, 249, 249fs
 reflexes, 262, *262*
 rupture, 247–248, *248*
  Thompson's test for, 263, *263*
 strain of, 247–248, *248*
 tendinitis, 250
Acquired immune deficiency syndrome (AIDS), 638–641
 groups at risk, 638–639, 639t
 in athletic setting, 640fs
 signs and symptoms of, 641t
 wound treatment and, 61t
Acromioclavicular (AC) joint, 364, *364*
 sprain of, 380–382, *381*
  management of, 382fs
 test of, 407, *410*
Activities of daily living (ADL)
 injury assessment and, *112*, 113, 115fs
 longterm rehabilitation goals and, 139

Adam's apple, 585, 586
 injury of, 598–599
Adduction. *See* Varus
ADL. *See* Activities of Daily Living (ADL)
Administrators, sports medicine
 responsibilities of, 12
Adrenocorticosteroids, 179
Aerobic training
 American College of Sports Medicine recommendations, 159
 exercises, 160fs
 hypertension and, 665
AIDS. *See* Acquired immune deficiency syndrome (AIDS)
Air pollution
 sports performance and, 650–651
Airway obstruction, 58, *58*
 clearance of, 81–84, *82*, *83*
  foreign object removal, 83, *84*
Alcohol
 abuse of, 11, 666–675
 hypoglycemia and, 662
Allergy(-ies)
 anaphylactic shock and, 64
 Eustachian tube and, 654
 hay fever, 653–654
 to cold, 162
Altitude
 sports performance and, 650
Amenorrhea
 anorexia nervosa and, 678
 bone loss and, 642–643
 defined, 252
 exercise-associated, 642–643
 stress fractures and, 252
Amnesia
 after head injury, 510, 514–515
 retrograde, 510
Analgesic(s), 178–179
 phonophoresis of, 172
Anaphylactic shock, 64
Anatomical position, *104*, 105
Anatomy, human body. *See also* under specific parts of
 abdominal quadrants, 105, *106*
 anatomical position, *104*, 105
 directional terms, 105, 106t–107t
 joint movement terms, 105, *108–109*
 regional terms, 105, *107*
 segments, *104*, 105
Androgens, 627, 629
Anemia, 665–666
 iron-deficiency, 665–666
 menstruation irregularities and, 665
 sickle cell, 666
Anesthetic(s)
 for pain, 172
 phonophoresis of, 172

Ankle joint
 anatomy of, 220–221, *220–222*
  blood vessels, 227, 229, *230*
  nerves, 226–227, 229
 assessment of, 256, 266fs
  anterior drawer test, 263, *264*
  talar tilt, 263, *264*
  Thompson's test, 263, *263*
 injury of, 220–221, 242–267
  fractures
   avulsion, 253
   dislocations, 256
   displaced/undisplaced, 254–256
   malleolar, 246, *246*
   osteochondral, 253–254, *255*
   osteochondritis dissecans, 253–254
   stress, 252–253
  sprains/dislocations, 164fs, 242–246
   lateral, 243–245, *244*, 245fs
   mechanisms of, 243t, 243–244
   medial, *244*, 245–246
  strains, 246–248
   of Achilles tendon, 247–248, *248*
   of peroneal tendon, 247, *247*
   of tibialis posterior tendon, 247
 kinematics of, 230–232, *232*
  gait cycle, 231, *231*
 kinetics of, 232–233
 physical conditioning of, 233, 234–235fs
 protection of, 205, *206*, 223
 rehabilitation of, 264–265, 265fs
Annual reports, 23, 25
Annulus fibrosus, 538
Anorexia nervosa
 amenorrhea and, 678
Anovulation, 642
Anterior drawer test
 of ankle joint, 263, *264*
Anti-inflammatory drugs (NSAIDS), 178–179
Antifungal agent (s)
 for athlete's foot, 238fs
 for jock itch, 633, 634fs
Antipyresis, 178–179
 defined, 178
Aorta, 591, 596, 596–597
Apley's compression test
 of knee meniscus, 311, *311*
Apley's scratch test
 shoulder injury and, 402, *403*
Apnea, 83
Aponeuroses, 40
Apophyseal fracture
 Osgood-Schlatter's disease and, 299–300
Appendicular segment, human body, *104*, 105
Appendix, 595
 inflammation (appendicitis), 612
 McBurney's point, 612, 617